Ways of Living

Self-Care Strategies
for Special Needs

Edited by

Charles Christiansen, EdD, OTR, OT(C), FAOTA

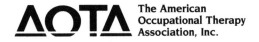

AOTA The American
Occupational Therapy
Association, Inc.

Disclaimers

"This publication is designed to provide accurate and authoritative information in regard to the subject matter covered. It is sold or distributed with the understanding that the publisher is not engaged in rendering legal, accounting, or other professional service. If legal advice or other expert assistance is required, the services of a competent professional person should be sought."

— From the Declaration of Principles jointly adopted by the American Bar Association and a Committee of Publishers and Associations.

It is the objective of the American Occupational Therapy Association to be a forum for free expression and interchange of ideas. The opinions and positions expressed by the contributors to this work are their own and not necessarily those of either the editors or the American Occupational Therapy Association.

It is expected that the procedures and practices described in this book will be used only by qualified practitioners in accordance with professional standards and in compliance with applicable practice statutes. Every effort has been made to assure that the information presented is accurate and consistent with generally accepted practices. However, the authors, editor, and publisher cannot accept responsibility for errors or omissions, or for the consequences of incorrect application of information by individuals or rehabilitation professionals. No warranty, express or implied, is made regarding the contents of this text.

AOTA Director of Nonperiodical Publications: Frances E. McCarrey

Edited by Laura Farr Collins
Designed by Robert Sacheli
Cover illustration by Diana Ong

Printed in the United States of America.

ISBN 1-56900-008-5

Table of Contents

Preface i

Dedication iii

Foreword v
Gail S. Fidler, OTR, FAOTA

Chapter 1: A Social Framework for Understanding
Self-Care Intervention 1
Charles Christiansen, EdD, OTR, OT(C), FAOTA

Chapter 2: The Personal Meaning of Self-Care Occupations 27
Gelya Frank, PhD

Chapter 3: Assessment of Self-Care Skills 51
Catherine Backman, MS, OT(C)

Chapter 4: Principles for Teaching Self-Care Skills 77
Martha E. Snell, PhD

Chapter 5: Self-Care Strategies for Children With
Developmental Deficits 101
Jane Case-Smith, EdD, OTR, FAOTA

Chapter 6: Self-Care Strategies for Persons With Arthritis and
Connective Tissue Diseases 157
Jeanne L. Melvin, MS, OTR, FAOTA

Chapter 7: Self-Care Strategies for Persons With
Spinal Cord Injuries 189
Susan L. Garber, MA, OTR, FAOTA
Theresa L. Gregorio, MA, OTR
Nancy Pumphrey, MOT, OTR
Pam Lathem, OTR

Chapter 8: Self-Care Strategies Following Stroke 227
Kathleen Okkema, MBA, OTR/L

Chapter 9: Self-Care Management for Adults With
Movement Disorders 255

    Margaret McCuaig, MA, OT(C)

Chapter 10: Managing Self-Care in Adults With
Upper Extremity Amputations 277

    Diane J. Atkins, OTR, FISPO

Chapter 11: Self-Care Strategies Following Severe Burns 305

    Cheryl Leman Jordan, MA, OTR/L, FAOTA
    Rebekah Allely, OTR/L
    Joanne Gallagher, MSc, OTR/L

Chapter 12: Self-Care Strategies for Persons With
Cognitive Deficits 333

    Mary Hall, BSc, OT(C)
    Sherida Ryan, BOT(C)
    Estella Tse, BSc, OT(C)

Chapter 13: Self-Care Strategies in Intervention for
Psychosocial Conditions 357

    Carol A. Leonardelli Haertlein, PhD, OTR, FAOTA
    Margaret C. Blodgett, MS, OTR

Chapter 14: Technology for Self-Care 379

    Roger Smith, PhD, OTR, FAOTA
    Margie Benge, OTR
    Marian Hall, MBA, OTR/L

Chapter 15: The Self-Care Environment: Issues of Space
and Furnishing 423

    Pearl Sarah Bates, MA, OTR

Chapter 16: Caregiver Assistance: Using Family Members
and Attendants 453

    Carolyn Baum, PhD, OTR/L, FAOTA
    Patricia LaVesser, MA, OTR/L

Index 483

Preface

This edited volume unfolded over several years. As is so often the case with such projects, neither the destination nor the path traversed were exactly as I envisioned them at the outset. Nevertheless, I hope that the volume contributes to the provision of improved occupational therapy services, which will enable the performance of useful self-care tasks for persons with special needs. That was the intention of the project from the beginning and has been an unwavering goal.

During the volume's journey toward completion, I became dedicated to three beliefs about rehabilitation practice. First, daily life, and thus virtually all we do, is inextricably linked to our shared existence with others as social beings. Thus, self-care tasks, whether related to eating, dressing, or personal hygiene, must be viewed as a foundation for enabling a shared existence with others. Too often, in my view, rehabilitation providers fail to recognize this important relationship.

Second, tasks of living are seldom interpreted as isolated events by their doers, but rather as parts of an unfolding and connected set of events that have powerful meaning for a person's self-identity. Throughout our lives, each of us yearns to understand who we are and to make meaning of our existence. Even self-care tasks, though seemingly mundane, have importance in a person's unfolding story, or self-narrative, through which this identity and meaning take shape. The appreciation of self-narrative as a means for better understanding the patient and the manner in which he or she attributes meaning to various events is, I believe, an important and long overdue development in the rehabilitation professions.

Third, and perhaps most importantly, during the development of this volume I came to believe that the traditional view of independence as performing tasks without assistance is a concept that, while well-intentioned, may be potentially delimiting at best and damaging at worst. In its place, I have promoted a broader and more realistic goal of *interdependence* for self-care intervention. This view recognizes that as participants in a social world, we all must depend on others to meet some of our basic needs. Thus, we are all interdependent. Within this interdependent environment we maintain our sense of self by exercising self-reliance in decision making on matters that affect our daily lives, and ultimately our destinies. The distinction between self-reliance in making decisions that affect our daily lives and *performing* independently is thus an important one. The value of the interdependence perspective will become more apparent as therapists incorporate narrative reasoning into their treatment planning. Through narrative understanding, patients are more likely to be understood by rehabilitation providers as they must be— as protagonists in a story that continues to unfold, and over which they (as patients) must have fundamental control.

Finally, all offerings of scholarship owe a fundamental debt to others whose ideas served as catalysts for reflection and study. Therefore, I acknowledge with appreciation Robert Bing, Florence Clark, Gail Fidler, Maureen Fleming, Gary Kielhofner, Cheryl Mattingly, Anne Mosey, David Nelson, Kenneth Ottenbacher, Joan Rogers, and Wilma

West, whose writings and personal interaction have particularly challenged and stimulated my thinking.

Several other people deserve acknowledgment for their contributions and encouragement as this book took form. I am indebted to my wife, Pamela, an occupational therapist, for her support and professional advice; to Sarah Hertfelder of the Practice Department at the American Occupational Therapy Association (AOTA) for inviting my involvement in the project; to Anne Rosenstein and Laura Farr Collins of the Publications Department at AOTA for their patience and competence; to the many rehabilitation experts in the United States and Canada who agreed to share their wisdom and experience as chapter authors; and to Andrea Crouch of Vancouver, British Columbia, for capable assistance early in the project.

Charles Christiansen

Galveston, Texas

Dedication

I dedicate this book with love and appreciation to my parents, and to Dr. Robert K. Bing, mentor, scholar, humanitarian, and friend, who constantly reminds me and others that the past contains a treasure of very important lessons.

Foreword

Self-care represents a broad sphere of interest and concern within occupational therapy. Viewed as a fundamental component of performance in activities of daily living, it has consistently been a major focus of practice and study, particularly in the treatment and rehabilitation of individuals with a physical disability. Therefore, publication of a volume devoted to strategies of self-care should not be especially noteworthy. However, this work is indeed noteworthy in its exciting challenge for us to revisit the domain of self-care as a humanistic endeavor.

In approaching self-care as "ways of living," the frame of reference that is established emphasizes the care of self as a multidimensional process requiring artful interaction between the self and the self's human and physical world. Emphasis in the Preface and beginning chapters of this volume on key principles over techniques, on individualized reasoning and self-narrative beyond instrumental thinking, offer a refreshing perspective. The context that these create for conceptualizing self-care approaches should provoke in us a timely reminder of the essence of our profession and offer an enlightened dimension to our sometimes perfunctory, marketplace-induced ways of addressing self-care issues.

Many of the fundamental constructs of occupational therapy come alive as one considers the well-developed strategies presented in this work within the context that is established early in the volume. Exploration of the social relevance and meaning of self-care brings sharply into focus the inextricable linkage of self to others. Thus the impact of disability as an insult to self-identity and as a threat to achieving social credibility emerge as critical variables in the design of assessments and interventions. Furthermore, in this context a provocative question is raised regarding our traditional view of independent functioning. Acknowledging that no one is truly independent, that help and support from others is essential to a sense of self in a social world, should our view be one of interdependent rather than independent performance? Distinguishing self-reliance from performing independently, and defining and understanding self-agency are some of the challenging proposals confronted.

Examination of the personal meaning of such tasks as toileting, grooming, or eating, for example, makes it unlikely that self-care could ever again be viewed as a set of rather mundane tasks. Rather, one begins to grasp the reality of self-care as part of an intimate, ego-invested self-portrait, a powerful narrative of one's sense of self and one's relationships with others.

Although the affective component is addressed in a more implicit than explicit manner, its influence is clearly evident. The role of personal interests and motivation, the personal meaning attributed to events, and the importance of a self-narrative that personalizes procedures of daily living are only a few examples of ways in which this volume addresses the affective realm that underlies individual response to disability and to the strategies of occupational therapy. Task performance is subjective; that inner self of affect, ideation, and perception is indeed a weighted variable in the schema of human performance. Throughout this volume, again and again, one is reminded that what an individual can or cannot do is influenced more by how that person views self and defines social credibility than by physical capacity.

Designing interventions congruent with individual needs, interests, values, and goals represents a long-standing standard and value of occupational therapy. "Ways of living" reemphasizes the importance of setting priorities and planning strategies that both protect and reflect the essence of the personal self, as well as sustain and support the integrity of one's relationships with significant others and with one's world.

It should be pointed out that additionally, the nature and relevance of any self-care activity for an individual is shaped and defined from within the context of that person's total way of living. The meaning and dimension of any one domain within a life-style or way of living can only be understood as a part that contributes to the definition of the whole and that is in turn shaped by that whole and its interacting parts. Hopefully this work will give impetus to exploring the ways in which the multidimensional self-care domain relates to, influences, and is shaped by the other significant daily living activities in the process of composing the whole of a life-style. And that furthermore, this work will lead to as thorough and dynamic a study of other domains of concern for occupational therapy.

Understanding self-care as a highly personal, interpersonal, and social activity of daily living precludes ever addressing this component of human performance in a procedural manner, circumscribed by standards of reimbursement. Self-care encompasses an individually poignant narrative that embodies self to self and self to others. When such activity is defined and addressed as one dimension, in concert with other domains that comprise a life-style, a way of living, our practice and study move closer to realizing the full potential of occupational therapy. This work represents a significant move toward that goal.

Gail S. Fidler, OTR, FAOTA
Tamarac, Florida

1

A Social Framework
for Understanding
Self-Care Intervention

Charles Christiansen

*Charles Christiansen, EdD, OTR, OT(C), FAOTA, is Dean of the School of
Allied Health Sciences and Professor in the Department of Occupational Therapy at the
University of Texas Medical Branch at Galveston. During the early stages in the
development of this volume, he was Director of the School of Rehabilitation Sciences and
Professor of Occupational Therapy at The University of British Columbia,
Vancouver, Canada.*

Chapter 1 Outline

Self-Care as a Category of Daily Living Skills

The Significance of Self-Care Tasks in a Social World

The Socioanalytic Perspective of Self-Care

Self-Identity

Disability as an Assault on Self-Identity

Stigma

Decision Making for Self-Care

Considerations in Determining Intervention Strategies

Instrumental Reasoning

Narrative Reasoning

Formulating an Occupational Therapy Diagnosis

Goals of Intervention in Self-Care: Independence or Interdependence?

Planning Self-Care Intervention

Social Considerations in Selecting Adaptive Strategies

General Strategies for Self-Care Intervention

Training

Use of Adaptive Systems and Devices

Environmental Modifications

Use of Family and Personal Care Attendants

Social Skills: Assessment and Intervention

Social Impression Management

Summary

References

Tristram Englehardt (1977) has observed that people define health and illness in terms of the "activities open to them or denied them" (p. 667). Englehardt's statement deserves further elaboration in order to appreciate its meaning fully. An acute illness, such as the flu, creates less of a nuisance because of its pain and discomfort than because of the resulting disruption in our lives. Typically, when people experience such illnesses they impatiently wait for the expected recovery so that they can resume their daily routines and get back to the business of living.

Yet when more catastrophic health problems occur and individuals have much less understanding of what has happened to them, their concerns are much the same. Diagnoses such as "cerebral infarct" or "spinal cord lesion" are not interpretable in the lexicons of everyday interaction. When presented with information involving such medical terminology, patients and families typically want health care professionals to provide a functional translation. "Will I be able to ride my horse again? Or play the piano?" become the defining parameters of the condition. When such questions are raised, it becomes quite evident that what we do (and not how we feel) provides the meaning for our lives. In short, health problems constrain living less from a physiological standpoint than from the standpoint of being.

It is interesting, though not surprising, to note that when they are confronted with a disabling condition that will result in permanent disability, people seldom inquire if they will be able to eat without assistance or go to the toilet. These mundane acts of self-maintenance are taken for granted by able-bodied people to such an extent that their fundamental place in everyday existence is not apparent. It is only when their performance becomes difficult or impossible that the salience of these everyday requirements is evident.

Indeed, people with disabilities who write about their own experiences typically comment about the unexpected challenges presented by their inability to perform routine daily tasks such as dressing and bathing. In the excerpt below, from *The Body Silent*, anthropologist Robert Murphy (1987) provides a personal account of the effects of a spinal tumor that progressively diminished his ability to live independently:

> I was quite self sufficient back in that stage of my disability. I could dress my upper body, though I never did master pants and shoes, and I took care of most of my personal needs. I shaved, brushed my teeth, sponge bathed most of my body, and I used the toilet without assistance. Yolanda would go off to work every day, leaving lunch in the refrigerator, and I would fend for myself. I even managed to reheat coffee. The only time that I required help was in getting dressed in the morning and undressed at night. (p. 62)

The abnormal cells that caused Robert Murphy's tumor created gradual paralysis, which eventually cost him his life. Murphy experienced this sequence of biological events, ranging from cell growth to spinal cord damage and paralysis, as an inability to perform the daily tasks he had previously taken for granted. Moreover, when his inability to walk and his diminished upper extremity strength and coordination compromised his ability to meet the physical and social demands of his home and community, he recognized that his very identity as a college professor, husband and father, and valued and respected member of society had been assaulted.

Robert Murphy was unique in the sense that he had unusual insights into his situation and was able to continue for many years in his role as an academic. In another sense, however, his situation provides a typical illustration of the dynamic consequences of having impaired function that interferes with the requirements of daily living. The ability to participate fully in activities is a quality of life issue that has a profound effect on an individual's satisfaction and well-being. And as we will see, being able to participate in the ordinary routines described earlier in Murphy's excerpt assumes both practical and symbolic significance to those who no longer take such tasks for granted.

Self-Care as a Category of Daily Living Skills

In considering the range of activities that constitute daily living, occupational therapists typically categorize them within three broad domains. Although these domains have been variously labeled, they include daily activities that are productive in a work or educational sense, those that are freely chosen to provide recreation or relaxation, and those that pertain to maintaining the self (see Figure 1). In the latter category, self-maintenance tasks have included a scope of activities ranging from personal care (such as dressing and grooming) to communication, medication management, and socialization. These tasks are collectively referred to in the health care literature under the broad (if somewhat misleading[1]) label of activities of daily living, or ADL.

The specific tasks that have been included under the ADL rubric by different authors have varied. However, this category nearly always includes bowel and bladder functions (toileting), bathing, dressing, eating, and grooming (including oral hygiene). These personal care tasks have come to be known collectively as basic "self-care"[2] (see Figure 2).

In the late 1960s, M. Powell Lawton, a gerontologist, recognized that living independently in the community required a level of competence that enabled the accomplishment of tasks beyond those of basic self-care (which he termed physical self-maintenance). Accordingly, he devised a hierarchy of task performance that included a

Figure 1. Domains of occupational performance.

Self-Maintenance Occupations

Use of time related to performing personal tasks necessary for self-care and social interaction, including communication and mobility.

Work and Productive Occupations

Use of time related to maintaining the living environment, caring for others, engaging in paid employment, education, or volunteerism.

Play or Leisure Occupations

The intrinsically motivated use of time for amusement, relaxation, spontaneous enjoyment, and self-expression.

---

[1]Elsewhere (Christiansen 1992) I have commented on the folk taxonomy that characterizes our view of daily occupations. This taxonomy can be confusing to those outside of health care, because the phrase *activities of daily living* should logically refer to the entire range of daily activities performed during the day, rather than a small subset of them.

[2]In the past decade, within the health sciences, the phrase *self-care* has also taken on the meaning of being able to care for one's health-related needs, rather than simple personal maintenance.

Figure 2. AOTA Recommended terminology for self-maintenance tasks (activities of daily living).

Grooming	Obtainment and use of supplies; removal of body hair (use of razors, tweezers, lotions, etc.); application and removal of cosmetics; washing, drying, combing, styling, and brushing hair; caring for nails (hands and feet); caring for skin, eyes, ears, and eyes; application of deodorant.
Oral hygiene	Obtainment and use of supplies; cleaning mouth; brushing and flossing teeth, or removal, cleaning, and reinsertion of dental orthotics and prosthetics.
Bathing/ showering	Obtainment and use of supplies; soaping, rinsing, and drying of body parts; maintaining bathing position; transferring to and from bathing position.
Toilet hygiene	Obtainment and use of supplies; clothing management; maintaining toileting position; transferring to and from toileting position; cleaning body; caring for menstrual and continence needs (including catheters, colostomies, and suppository management).
Personal device care	Cleaning and maintaining hearing aids, contact lenses, glasses, orthotics, prosthetics, adaptive equipment, and contraceptive and sexual devices.
Dressing	Selection of clothing and accessories appropriate to time of day, weather, and occasion; obtainment of clothing from storage area; dressing and undressing in a sequential fashion; fastening and adjusting clothing and shoes; application and removal of personal devices, protheses, or orthoses.
Feeding and eating	Setting up food; selection and use of appropriate utensils and tableware; bringing food or drink to mouth; cleaning face, hands, and clothing (including management of alternative methods of nourishment). Performance of sucking, masticating, coughing, and swallowing.
Medication routine	Obtainment of medication; opening and closing containers; following prescribed schedules; taking correct quantities; reporting problems and adverse effects.
Socialization	Assessing opportunities and interacting with other people in appropriate contextual and cultural ways to meet emotional and physical needs.
Functional communication	Use of equipment or systems to send and receive information, such as writing equipment, telephones, typewriters, computers, communication boards, call lights, emergency systems, Braille writers, and augmentative communication systems.
Functional mobility	Movement from one position or place to another, such as in bed mobility, wheelchair mobility, transfers (wheelchair, bed, car, tub, toilet, shower, chair, floor); performance of functional ambulation, driving, and transporting objects; obtainment of public or private transportation.
Emergency response	Recognition of sudden, unexpected hazardous situations, and initiation of action to reduce threat to health.
Sexual expression	Recognizing, communicating, and engaging in desired sexual activities.

From *AOTA Uniform Terminology* (3rd ed.), in press, Rockville, MD: AOTA.

second scale of more complex behaviors viewed as representative of the level of competence necessary for living more independently in the community. These more complex tasks were termed instrumental activities of daily living (IADL) and included use of the telephone, food preparation, housekeeping, laundry, shopping, money management, use of transportation, and medication management (Lawton, 1971).

Ultimately, the selection of specific tasks to guide goal-setting in rehabilitation should be arranged in a hierarchy of those competencies viewed as necessary for living in the community with a minimum of assistance, and being able to take responsibility for one's performance needs and desires. This book focuses primarily on personal care tasks and also addresses those processes important to everyday living, such as communication and mobility. The overall cluster of basic self-care tasks and processes is viewed as a foundation for participation in the social world.

Research has shown that self-maintenance activities consume about 10% to 15% of the average able-bodied person's waking day (Szalai, 1972), with a slightly higher proportion of time required for those with disabilities (Lawton, 1990; Yelin, Lubeck, Holman, & Epstein, 1987). These obligatory[3] activities are considered essential for survival and necessary for the satisfactory performance of social roles.

The Significance of Self-Care Tasks in a Social World

To be sure, the essential nature of some self-care tasks cannot be denied, because if we are to continue living we must be able to nourish ourselves. Living in the community requires an ability to acquire and prepare food as necessary, and to eat. Beyond survival, community living requires the ability to conform to societal expectations of hygiene, grooming, and dress, and to communicate effectively.

Although it is seldom emphasized in the occupational therapy literature, all tasks of daily living are embedded within a social framework, and life satisfaction and perceptions of well-being are influenced substantially by participation in and acceptance by social groups (e.g., Cooper & Okamura, 1992; Ishii-Kuntz, 1990). Indeed, social factors have been shown to explain life satisfaction and perceived well-being to a greater extent than functional limitations for persons who must adjust to the consequences of aging (Bowling & Edelmann, 1989), injury (Rintala & Young, 1992), or disease (Affleck & Pfeiffer, 1988).

Thus, being able to gain access to locations where social transactions take place[4] and to "fit in" should also prove to be important elements of a satisfactory life-style, and research has borne this out. Fuhrer and colleagues (Fuhrer, Rintala, Hart, Clearman, & Young, 1992) studied 640 persons with paralysis due to spinal cord injury who were living in the community, to determine the overall level of life satisfaction and those aspects of living that contributed to it. They found that social support, social integration, perceived control, and mobility were all significantly related to life satisfaction in the persons studied. There was no relationship between the extent of a participant's paralysis or neurological status and his or her life satisfaction.

---

[3]In many studies of time use, activity engagement is categorized according to whether it is obligatory (required for living) or discretionary (the individual chooses to engage in the activity).

[4]See Rowles (1991) for an excellent analysis and discussion of the importance of places in maintaining well-being.

To the extent that one or more of the basic and instrumental tasks of living cannot be performed, the ability to meet social role requirements is made more difficult and life satisfaction is compromised (Branholm & Fugl-Meyer, 1992). Thus, a clear and important relationship exists between meeting the essential requirements of daily living and our perceptions of well-being (Yerxa & Baum, 1986). A central theme of this chapter is that by meeting self-care and daily living requirements in a satisfactory manner, social integration is facilitated and greater life satisfaction is enabled (Crisp, 1992).

A Socioanalytic Perspective of Self-Care

Psychologist Robert Hogan (Hogan, 1982; Hogan & Sloan, 1991) provides a basis for understanding the importance of daily self-maintenance activities in his socioanalytic theory of personality. He notes that humans evolved as group-living, culture-bearing, and symbol-using animals, and that groups of people, whether in committees or communities, tend to organize themselves naturally in terms of status hierarchies.

According to Hogan, these characteristics of humans influence daily life in two fundamental ways. First, because we live in groups, it is necessary that we get along with others. Second, because human groups are organized along status lines, much of our well-being requires an ability to compete successfully and to gain status in the group. His theory emphasizes the importance of evolution as an influence on human behavior.

The idea that human behavior may be fundamentally influenced by a need for gaining status within groups is often viewed as a threat to more tranquil, idealistic, and egalitarian views of the world. Nevertheless, the existence of sibling rivalries, the need for second graders to "be first in line," the presence of organizational charts, and the expression "keeping up with the Joneses" all point to the ubiquitous nature of status concerns in society and the extent to which they influence human behavior.

The ability to achieve and maintain status in social groups requires a social identity, and Hogan notes that a good deal of time is spent negotiating, repairing, enhancing, and defending our social identities which, in turn, reflect our claims to status in the group. Identity is achieved principally through our self-presentation, or how we appear to others during interactions. Hogan asserts that the basis for social interaction occurs through roles (such as spouse, parent, friend, or colleague) that are prescribed for us by the group and/ or that we seek to define for ourselves. Since individuals differ in the extent to which they can successfully fulfill their roles, these differences explain variations in status and popularity, which over time take on a more enduring quality, known as reputation. When persons are no longer able to perform their roles competently, both status and reputation can be threatened. Thus, chronic illness and disability can have a profound affect on social identity because they threaten the views others may hold of that person as well as the person's view of self, or self-identity.

Self-Identity

Traditional views of self-identity are based on the belief that a core self-concept evolves based on our interactions with others and through our appraisals of the successes or failures that we accumulate as we mature. Cognitive theorists (e.g., Flavell, 1985; Kagan, 1989) have hypothesized that knowledge of the self and others occurs as a consequence of experiences that reveal individual characteristics. These characteristics serve as a basis for classifying (and differentiating) the self and others. Other theorists (e.g., Cooley, 1902;

Mead, 1934) have proposed that concepts of the self emerge from observing how others respond to us during social encounters.

According to Rogers (1982), if we are to view ourselves as competent individuals who are able to demonstrate mastery of the challenges that confront us, we must have a sense of autonomy. Rogers suggests that autonomy is demonstrated through our ability to make choices and influence the world around us. Psychologists often use the term *human agency* to describe an intrinsic human need to explore and act on the environment. Our sense of self, then, is profoundly influenced by our engagement in the everyday activities of the world in which we live, and our ability to fulfill roles that are appreciated and valued by the social groups in which we claim membership.

Discussions of self-identity are not complete without a consideration of the importance of narrative. Recently it has been suggested that individuals view and understand themselves through narratives or stories. These accounts of events that involve us and are connected over time are described as self-narratives (Gergen & Gergen, 1988). Narrative is pervasive. According to Mancuso and Sarbin (1985), any slice of life, when carefully considered, is interpreted and experienced as part of a story. Indeed, Jerome Bruner (1990) is convinced that the ability to make meaning of life events is so dependent upon narrative structure that he theorizes an innate or biological disposition to interpret events in the world through language.

In speaking of the influence of narrative in self-identity, Polkinghorne (1988) has written that:

> We achieve our personal identities and self-concept through the use of the narrative configuration, and make our existence into a whole by understanding it as an expression of a single unfolding and developing story. We are in the middle of our stories and cannot be sure how they will end; we are constantly having to revise the plot as new events are added to our lives. Self, then, is not a static thing or a substance, but a configuring of personal events into an historical unity which includes not only what one has been but also anticipations of what one will be. (p. 150)

Thus, viewed in the context of narrative, our self-identity is based on our current views of the past and present, and our anticipation of the future. Because we interpret our lives as stories, we also live them as stories with many possible endings. The possible future chapters and endings for our stories involve many anticipated selves. These possible selves influence the choices we make and the behaviors we exhibit on a daily basis. Our behaviors are embedded within our striving to perform our roles in ways that enhance our views of self and the views others have of us.

In life, events happen that make some future chapters and story endings implausible. Thus Robert Murphy, who had imagined himself as an active, highly mobile retiree could no longer entertain that possibility following his spinal surgery. One view of his future self had suddenly become impossible. Moreover, a view he had of himself in the present had been compromised. In short, his self-identify was in transition.

Disability as an Assault on Self-Identity

Mattingly and Fleming (1993) have pointed out that the work of occupational therapists brings them into daily contact with patients whose self-identities are in transition. Many patients will not be able to return to their previous conditions of living and are in the process of trying to make new sense of who they are now and who they will become. They are in a transitional state because their identities are very much dependent on the social roles they occupy, and their performance of valued social roles has now been compromised.

People with traumatic spinal cord injuries offer dramatic examples of how abrupt role transitions are experienced. Spinal cord injury patients are often young, active men in excellent physical condition who were skiing or swimming one instant and suddenly paralyzed for life moments later. During their rehabilitation, these patients encounter considerable anxiety regarding their roles as desirable marital partners, as productive members of the workforce, and as accepted members of their peer groups (Zedjlik, 1992).

However, all persons, whether disabled or not, must confront role transitions during their lives. The process of normal aging leads to a series of role changes at predictable stages in life. A person may move from being a parent responsible for rearing children to a grandparent who may increasingly rely on others for support. Often, as the capacity for self-reliance declines, individuals are placed within living environments where choice and control are limited, and where their sense of self as competent members of society becomes tragically diminished (Rosow, 1985).

In these transitional circumstances, acts that were previously viewed as ordinary or routine assume enhanced significance as symbols of competency. Relearning or retaining the ability to perform tasks of self-maintenance (even with assistance) becomes a means of fostering self-identity. To permit others to perform self-care tasks for us may be interpreted symbolically as occupying a role of one who is dependent—as one who has assumed the sick role. As described by Parsons (1958, 1975), the sick role is a transitional state in which the person is exempted from typical role responsibilities with the expectation that active steps are taken to facilitate recovery.

Unfortunately, as soon as individuals become disabled, they are in danger of being assigned a permanently diminished status by society because they are often viewed as "sick" and thus denied the same status they were accorded as able-bodied persons performing valued social roles. In the words of Goffman (1963) their identity has been "spoiled," and they have become the victims of stigma. The concept of stigma is relevant to an understanding of the importance of self-care to socialization.

Stigma

Stigma describes a social condition where the individual is devalued because he or she cannot meet expected "codes of behavior" in role performance. Goffman (1959) portrayed all interaction as consisting of crediting or discrediting role performances. A discrediting role performance can result from any number of behaviors that vary from those expected within a given situation.

For example, Goffman notes that behaviors such as yawning, stuttering, appearing nervous or self-conscious, problems with balance, losing muscular control, or losing one's temper can each diminish the creditability of a given social encounter. Because persons with physical or emotional disorders may be unable to control some behaviors that would be expected in a given situation, their performances can become discrediting, and they must learn to manage the impressions they convey during social interaction.

Disability may result in a changed body image that alters a person's view of self, as well as the way he or she is viewed. The following excerpt from the book *Able Lives*, written to document the experiences of women with spinal cord injuries, illustrates this reality:

> One of the hardest parts of becoming disabled is acceptance of, and living with, a changed body image. Our body shape and the aids we use (a wheelchair or crutches) are the visible signs of disability. Appearance plays a very important part in interaction with other people. What is more, women face an additional problem in that our

physical attractiveness is generally the way our femininity and sexuality are measured by other people. (Morris, 1988, p. 160)

Thus, as the excerpt reveals, creditable social performance also requires maintaining expected standards of dress and appearance. People are expected to present themselves according to social norms, and the manner of their appearance and dress have been shown to influence perceptions of their status and competence. Thus, being able to manage basic self-care tasks is a fundamental prerequisite for successful social interaction for the able-bodied person, and it is no less important for the person with a disability. Learning to overcome stigma and regaining an acceptable social identity may be the most significant challenge confronting someone with a disability.

The importance of managing stigma and achieving satisfactory social integration is confirmed by recent studies. Fuhrer et al. (1992, 1993) found that depression among persons with spinal cord injury was not related to degree of impairment or disability, but to the extent to which subjects were able to participate in customary social relations and were engaged in work, volunteer activities, self-improvement, or employment. These findings were similar to those reported by Rybarczyk et al. (1992), who found that depression among persons with leg amputations was less likely to occur when subjects reported that they were comfortable with social contacts that involved acknowledgment of their amputation or prosthesis.

Decision Making for Self-Care

The challenge of helping individuals rebuild their self-identities and adjust to their altered circumstances is difficult. Considered from the narrative point of view, it is important for the occupational therapist to recognize that the life story a person has been living must now be rewritten in a manner that is acceptable to the person. The future person he or she has considered being must now be revised. This transition period may take time, and it also requires a period of exploration so that the individual has an opportunity to consider this revised set of possible selves.

In addressing this point, Fidler and Fidler (1978) have observed that the patient acquires a sense of the limitations and potential of self through the exploratory opportunities provided by the therapist. Yerxa (1967) asserted in her 1966 Eleanor Clarke Slagle lecture that therapists meet their responsibilities to clients when they provide opportunities to develop new skills and the ability to substitute for lost capacities. Legitimate therapy forces the client to confront reality by squarely recognizing limitations while simultaneously discovering possibilities. Thus, the role of the therapist is not only to identify and implement intervention strategies for greater autonomy and personal responsibility (if this is desired), but also to provide settings, strategies, and opportunities to enable the person receiving care to explore alternatives and to imagine possible selves. In a narrative sense, the therapist and the person receiving care must determine a course of action that individualizes the goals of therapy and allows untold stories to be enacted (Mattingly, 1991a). By carefully considering the patient in the context of a life story and providing options that are appropriate for a particular person, therapy changes from simply the provision of technical expertise for the acquisition of movements and skills, to a professional intervention that is practical, as well as relevant and meaningful to the individual.

Considerations in Determining Intervention Strategies

In deciding how to proceed in helping their patients manage self-maintenance needs, therapists must determine the nature of the patient's strengths and deficits and many other important technical aspects. However, because of the uniqueness of each person's individual circumstances, making the right choice in deciding a course of action for a patient with a particular kind of deficit requires much more than objective knowledge of strengths and deficits. Rogers (1983) writes that the therapeutic action chosen:

> ...must be the right action for this individual. This implies that it must be as congruent as possible with the patient's concept of the good life. Treatment must be in concert with the patient's needs, goals, life-style and personal and cultural values. A therapeutic program that is right for one patient is not necessarily right for another. (p. 602)

In discussing the right choice, Rogers refers to a decision process that has ethical, as well as technical, implications. In planning intervention, the therapist must continually strive to choose courses of action that are right in an ethical sense and correct in a theoretical or procedural sense. This requires the therapist to base decisions on information from several domains of knowledge.

Instrumental Reasoning

When therapists rely on their knowledge of established frames of reference and their accompanying techniques, they are using procedural or instrumental reasoning (Mattingly, 1991a). Instrumental reasoning is the application of theory to practice and is based on learned knowledge most often gained from textbooks. While instrumental reasoning provides insight into a broad range of general situations, it alone is not sufficient for occupational therapy practice.

Mattingly (1991a) argues that instrumental reasoning does not take into account the unique complexities of a specific person within a specific context. When therapists rely exclusively on instrumental reasoning, they are likely to focus their treatment on components of performance rather than on life tasks. Individualized therapy occurs only when the therapist improvises from the general techniques and procedures of instrumental reasoning and fits the therapy to the unique needs of the particular situation.

In order to fit the therapy to the needs of a specific person, the therapist must have some understanding of what the individual is experiencing. This involves an interpretation of the meaning of the person's condition within that unique set of circumstances that constitutes the person's life. As experienced by the individual receiving care, learning to dress or to transfer from a toilet represents more than the acquisition of a set of self-care skills. Because therapy is embedded within an illness experience, the therapy itself, and the ability to perform these acts, each contribute to an unfolding life story.

Narrative Reasoning

Just as effective occupational therapy depends on the involvement of the person receiving care, good clinical reasoning depends on the ability of the therapist to understand the therapy experience from that person's viewpoint. The commitment of the patient will not be enlisted if a shared understanding between the therapist and the patient is not achieved. Master clinicians know that effective therapy depends on the establishment of an alliance between the therapist and the patient. This occurs only when the therapist has gained a tacit understanding of the individual's viewpoints and values and is thus able to structure the therapy session in a manner that evokes the motivational commitment of the patient.

Mattingly (1991b) calls this process of coming to understand the patient's world *narrative reasoning*, and suggests that therapists use two forms of narrative thinking in their work: story-telling and story-making. In story-telling, disability is portrayed from the patient's point of view, and motivations and commitments come to the forefront as the therapist describes the therapy experience. In story-making, therapy is structured in a narrative way to create dramatic therapeutic events that connect therapy to a patient's life.

In describing the narrative reasoning process, Mattingly (1991b) writes:

> In each new clinical situation then, the therapist must answer the question "What story am I in?" To answer this question, the therapist must make some initial sense of the situation and then act on it. The process of treatment encourages, perhaps even compels, therapists to reason in a narrative mode. They must reason about how to guide their therapy with particular patients by imagining where the patient is now and where this patient might be at some future point after discharge. It is not enough for therapists to know how to do a set of tasks that have an abstract order based on a typical treatment plan; therapists must be able to picture a larger temporal whole, one that captures what they can see in a particular patient in the present and what they can imagine seeing sometime in the future. This picturing process gives them a basis for organizing tasks. (p. 1001)

This narrative reasoning process must contend with the client's frame of mind at any particular point in time. Feelings of guilt, shame, lowered self-esteem, and anger may be expressed as a natural consequence of frustrations experienced during the rehabilitation process. The skillful therapist is able to manage each treatment session with sensitivity and flexibility, which permit almost unnoticeable changes in plans based on the client's mood, physical condition, and unexpected events that occur during the session.

Formulating an Occupational Therapy Diagnosis

While learning the patient's story and having sensitivity toward a patient's possible selves constitute an essential part of clinical reasoning, the therapist also draws on biomedical knowledge and occupational therapy theory and techniques to address self-care problems. The determination of potential intervention strategies for use in addressing self-care limitations occurs as part of the reasoning that accompanies functional assessment.

The focus of functional assessment is the performance of life tasks that support competent role performance and the underlying components that support task performance. As described by Rogers and Holm (1991), functionally oriented clinical reasoning leads to an occupational therapy diagnosis and decisions about intervention. Described simply, the occupational therapy process begins with the identification of a functional problem (diagnosis) and leads to an intervention strategy to resolve the problem. During the diagnostic phase, the therapist calls upon a storehouse of knowledge and often uses data collection protocols to identify cues indicative of dysfunction, to generate hypotheses, and to formulate a diagnosis that serves as the basis for intervention. Specific strategies for formal assessment of self-care capabilities are described in Chapter 3.

The hierarchical views of function and dysfunction from the *International Classification of Impairment Disability and Handicap* (ICIDH) (World Health Organization, 1980) provide a useful means of formulating the diagnostic statement (see Figure 3). This hierarchy permits the therapist to consider the role performance, task performance, and components of task performance in identifying the nature of the performance deficit, the goals of intervention, and possible strategies for meeting those goals (see Figure 4).

Trombly (1993) has emphasized that occupational therapists need to be aware of the specific activities and tasks underlying a patient's roles, and to understand the relationship between components of performance and higher-level function better. She notes

Figure 3. Application of World Health Organization (WHO) terminology to levels of function.

WHO Hierarchy	Pathology ➡	Impairment ➡	Disability ➡	Handicap
OT Functional Assessment Hierarchy	Pathology	Components of task performance	Task performance	Social role performance
Example	Spinal injury at level C-6 (complete)	Loss of sensation and voluntary movement in legs, lower trunk, and hands.	Can perform most self-care tasks without assistance, but may need equipment for bathing, dressing, grooming, and wheelchair transfer.	Transportation and mobility may be restricted, but individual is able to perform most roles with adaptations.

Figure 4. Simplified model of the occupational therapy (OT) process.

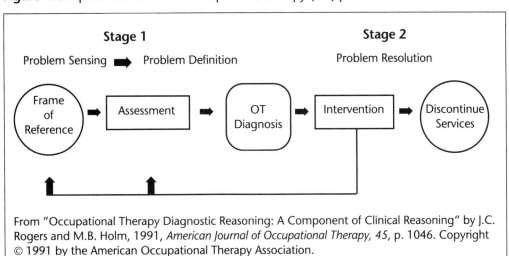

From "Occupational Therapy Diagnostic Reasoning: A Component of Clinical Reasoning" by J.C. Rogers and M.B. Holm, 1991, *American Journal of Occupational Therapy, 45*, p. 1046. Copyright © 1991 by the American Occupational Therapy Association.

that the components of task performance typically assessed by occupational therapists (such as sensorimotor control of the upper extremity) only partially predict the success with which those tasks are accomplished. Nearly 40% of such performance is explained by unidentified factors. The implication is that the therapist must attend to each layer in the performance hierarchy during the assessment process, while ensuring that the assessment begins with a thorough understanding of the unique context that characterizes each patient. When choosing therapeutic options that address performance components, such as balance or sensation, the therapist must explain to the patient the relationship between those abilities and the safe performance of relevant tasks (such as bathing).

Goals of Intervention in Self-Care: Independence or Interdependence?

The occupational therapy diagnosis will lead to a decision about the goals of therapy, which should be decided in collaboration with the patient, the therapist (or treatment team), and (as appropriate) family members or individuals who occupy the living environment within which the patient resides. In this chapter, the social framework for viewing self-care and the rehabilitation process emphasizes the importance of preparing the individual to enact societal roles that contribute to life satisfaction. While this general goal involves complexities of self and environment, little has been said about the *means* by which the goal is achieved.

Traditionally, rehabilitation providers have cited independent living as a valued aim of intervention.[5] However, goals of independence are often inappropriate from a practical standpoint and represent an unreasonable expectation from a social perspective if independence is defined as total self-reliance. It is argued here that the concept of independence may have more to do with determining what is accomplished and setting personal standards for such accomplishment than being involved in the task as the sole performer.

Rogers (1982) argued that when occupational therapists use the term *independence*, they imply autonomy and competence, and the interrelationship between the two concepts within an environmental context. Competencies are based on abilities and skills, while autonomy is based on our freedom to choose courses of action and our ability to appraise and modify our actions according to our own values, needs, and interests. In turn, autonomy and competence occur within an environment that includes physical and social dimensions. Independence requires a degree of mastery over our surroundings. To be able to function independently implies that the demands and obstacles of our physical and social environment have been met and overcome. Note that nothing has been said about how these demands are met.

Thus independence must be defined broadly. One can be considered independent while performing tasks that require the use of adapted devices or environments, or when overseeing others to meet various needs. In truth, few people in the modern world can claim that they are entirely self-reliant. Most of us depend on others extensively as we manage the affairs of our daily lives.

Dever (1989) makes the point that no one is truly independent. We depend on others for practical reasons—on those who transport goods to the market, on those who manufacture and sell goods, and on those who work in service occupations such as policemen, hair stylists, butchers, mechanics, bus drivers, and employees of public utilities.

We also depend on others for emotional support and for providing behavioral models and expectations that guide and influence our behavior. Berger and Luckmann (1967) maintain that our very understanding of the events in our daily lives is derived from shared interpretations of the world around us that have been communicated linguistically. Thus, it can be claimed that we depend on others to provide the very structure that gives us our sense that the reality of daily life has stability and continuity.

---

[5]Therapists are trained (and often required) to document a client's level of independence to establish intervention goals, measure gains, and assist in discharge decisions. Typically, 7-point scales are used (examples of which can be found in Chapter 3), ranging from independent (able to perform the task being rated with or without adaptive equipment), to dependent (defined as unable to do any part of the task). The concept of independence described in this chapter would find the wording on such scales pejorative and limiting. While abilities and skills should be documented, the labels attached to task performance must be reexamined.

Brown and Gillespie (1992) argue that independence as a principal goal in occupational therapy is a misleading and potentially damaging way of viewing recovery or therapy outcome. They contend that adopting a recovery model that recognizes and values interdependence will improve therapy and more accurately reflect the realities of our social existence. Moreover, the view taken in this chapter is that an interdependent view of outcomes in rehabilitation will provide a broader, more socially relevant array of options for the therapist in planning self-care management strategies.

Planning Self-Care Intervention

When planning for intervention, the therapist and patient should ideally examine the range of needs, settings, and resources in a collaborative manner. The overall importance of each task can be measured against the options available, the resources of the patient, and the characteristics of the setting in which the task is likely to be performed.

In considering possible strategies to use in accomplishing self-maintenance tasks, the therapist and patient have several options. The range of options employed falls into two principal categories: (a) restoration of impaired abilities, and/or (b) adaptation to the dysfunction or disability (Trombly, 1993) (see Figure 5).

Restorative approaches may incorporate motor or sensory techniques to fully or partially develop or restore sufficient voluntary control or movement to enable task accomplishment. Techniques derived from theories of neuroscience, biomechanics, and motor control are included among restorative approaches. The objective is to recover sufficient sensation, cognition, and voluntary movement to enable task performance in a safe and effective manner.

When restorative approaches are unlikely to be successful or are too costly in terms of time, energy, or expense, adaptive approaches are necessary (Trombly, 1993). In adaptive approaches, the objective is to identify new ways to accomplish the required task within remaining performance capabilities. Before any strategies are selected it is useful

Figure 5. Occupational therapy diagnosis.

Narrative Reasoning ➡	OT Diagnosis ➡	Intervention Strategies
Learning how patients view occupational dysfunction within their "life stories" and how those stories can be rewritten in terms acceptable to the patient.	The interface between problem sensing and problem resolution	Restorative Approaches • Techniques to regain sensory and motor function
Instrumental Reasoning		Adaptive Approaches • Training • Use of systems and devices • Environmental modifications • Care attendants • Social skills training
Functional assessment of performance that determines abilities and skills for the purpose of applying OT technical knowledge for restoration or adaptation of function.		

for the therapist and patient to examine together and prioritize the array of tasks to be performed. Since the time and energy available for task performance may be limited, learning how to manage and conserve these resources is an important part of adapting to disability. Moreover, by learning how to structure one's daily routine, unnecessary stress and its physical consequences can be avoided. In many cases, while strategies are available to enable completion of certain tasks, the cost in terms of time and energy of doing so without assistance in the face of competing demands makes it necessary and more logical to have others complete them. For many aspects of self-care, what matters most may be the outcome, not the means by which it was achieved. Thousands of hair salons would be out of business if the general public did not hold a similar view.

When personal involvement is desired or necessary, there are many strategies that can be used to adapt a task and the task environment to enable one to meet self-care objectives satisfactorily. First, the individual can be taught to perform a task within his or her capabilities. This is termed *habilitation* or *compensatory training*. Second, the environment can be modified to permit accomplishment of the task despite limitations in ability or skill. Third, systems or devices can be designed or acquired to enable performance, despite limited cognition, strength, or sensory ability. Finally, task requirements can be performed by an agent or caregiver according to the needs of the individual receiving assistance. In this last category, home health personnel, family members, or personal care assistants can help accomplish self-care tasks.

Often, the solutions for a given individual may involve a combination of strategies. For example, persons with a spinal cord injury at level C-6 may learn to use their remaining wrist movement to produce tenodesis action, which extends and flexes the fingers sufficiently to permit grasp with the use of a wrist-driven flexor hinge splint. The movement made possible by the splint allows objects, such as a cup, to be grasped. However, these objects may need special modifications: A cup may have adapted handles or a rim designed to prevent spilling. In other instances, the addition of a flexible straw and lid may improve cup efficiency. When dining in a restaurant, the individual may prefer the assistance of a family member or caregiver and avoid using the splint and adapted cup altogether.

Each possible strategy for assisting with the performance of self-care tasks must be evaluated in terms of its simplicity, cost in time and energy, and perceived benefit to promoting an enhanced quality of life from the standpoint of a particular patient (Weingarden & Martin, 1989). As there are typically many ways to accomplish a given task, several strategies should be identified and used depending on individual preferences and the varied situational contexts in which valued roles must be performed. The context of the rehabilitation setting, including the physical environment, persons involved, and daily routines, varies from that of the patient's home and community. Thus, a self-care strategy appropriate for the clinical setting may not be appropriate for the home or community. Family members or other caregivers are often present in the post-discharge living environment to assist with self-care tasks, and devices may seem awkward, inefficient, or out of place.

It appears that during the first 3 months following discharge, newly established routines and habits determine whether or not a specific device or strategy is going to be used consistently. Studies of the use of devices after discharge confirm that adaptive strategies may change depending on the situation (Bynum & Rogers, 1987; Garber & Gregorio, 1990; Gitlin, Levine, & Geiger, 1993). Moreover, the social acceptability of a given strategy may change depending on the setting, or even depending on the context within the same setting.

Social Considerations in Selecting Adaptive Strategies

Perhaps the most important characteristic of an adaptive strategy from the perspective of the disabled person concerns its social acceptability and the extent to which it permits individuals to present themselves as capable, competent individuals. In a study of adaptive strategies used by a 53-year-old woman with cerebral palsy who lives independently in the community, McCuaig and Frank (1991) found that the choice of strategy used to perform daily tasks, such as eating and communicating, would vary according to the situation.[6] For example, communication occurred by gesture, letter board, typed letter, and Canon Communicator. The method used by the woman depended on whether or not the context involved others (was social) and the extent to which it permitted her to control her activities in a way that influenced perceptions of her as a competent adult. Importantly, the authors emphasized that the woman's need to display herself as mentally able, physically capable, and socially competent influenced her choice of routine and technique more than did functional necessity. This illustrates the use of (and need for) multiple strategies in adapting to the requirements of everyday living. It also underscores the relevance of a social framework in viewing adaptive strategies for self-care (see Figure 6).

General Strategies for Self-Care Intervention

The following sections describe the major adaption strategies for meeting self-care needs. For procedures related to the restoration of sensorimotor control, the reader is referred to the many excellent sources available that provide details on the theory and procedures underlying biomechanical and neurodevelopmental treatment approaches.

Training

Self-care intervention often involves training, and this can take the form of habilitative or compensatory approaches. Habilitation training approaches are used when, as in the case of congenital or developmental disorders, skills are being learned for the first time. Typically, the acquisition of self-care skills takes place over extended periods and involves the careful structuring of tasks, frequent monitoring to correct performance errors, and feedback. Behavior modification techniques, wherein desirable behaviors are rewarded through positive reinforcement and undesirable behaviors are ignored and extinguished, are often useful. Such operant conditioning, often provided through token reward systems, allows successive approximations toward each goal through an incremental process known as shaping. Practice occurs as needed.

Compensatory training is based on the recognition that skills can be successfully accomplished in many ways, and the successful completion of the task is the primary goal. In this approach, alternative techniques may be combined with the use of orthoses, prostheses, or other types of assistive or adaptive devices or systems. For example, the individual with only one functional arm can continue to don and button a shirt, using substitute motions and a device to pull the button through the buttonhole.

Use of Adaptive Systems and Devices

The recent past has been marked by a remarkable increase in the number and types of systems and devices designed to help individuals compensate for lost or diminished functions. Sadly, some studies have shown that because of the difficulty experienced by

---

[6]In Chapter 9, which describes persons with movement disorders, McCuaig details other strategies used by this woman.

Figure 6. Decision making for self-care intervention.

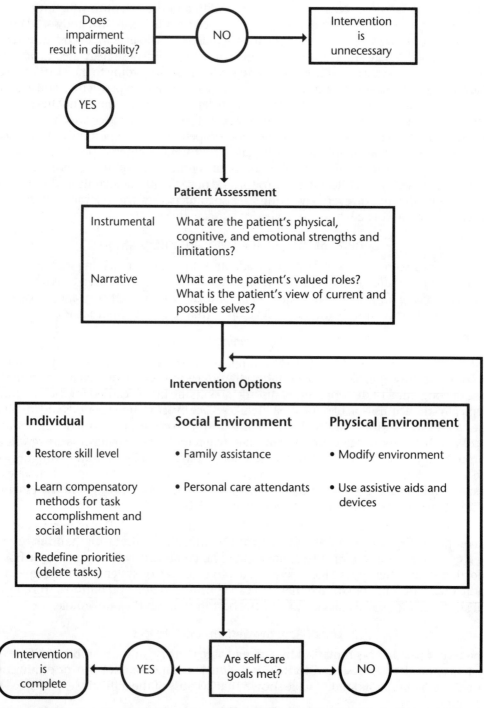

From "Self-Care: Evaluation and Treatment" by C. Christiansen, R. Schwartz, and K. Barnes, in *Rehabilitation Medicine: Principles & Practice* (p. 181) (2nd ed.), by J.A. DeLisa and D.M. Gans (Eds.), 1993, Philadelphia: Lippincott. Copyright © 1993 by Lippincott. Adapted by permission.

the average rehabilitation provider in keeping up with the latest assistive technology, some useful devices and systems are never considered or recommended to individuals who could benefit from them (Newrick & Langton-Hewer, 1984).

Devices range from those described as "low technology," which include such items as special utensils with built-up handles and shoelaces that can be tied with one hand, to high-technology devices, which include electronic remote control devices that activate appliances and speech synthesizers that store and speak words and sentences. Smith (1991) has noted that patients are too often provided with more technology than is necessary, and that therapists should be mindful that the best solution is often the simplest. Often, patients may need equipment at one phase of their rehabilitation but not at another. For example, Haworth (1983) found that patients with a total hip replacement stopped using devices for dressing and toileting once they found they could manage without them.

In other cases, experience after discharge from a rehabilitation setting may result in a change of strategies based on reordering priorities due to time and energy. This was a finding reported by Rogers and Figone (1980) following a study of the use of self-care skills learned during rehabilitation among patients with a cervical spinal cord injury. While the level of self-care attained during rehabilitation was maintained by the majority of patients, both improvement and regression in function was observed.

Cosmetic considerations may also limit the use of prostheses and adaptive devices. Steïn and Walley (1983) reported that 60% of the persons with an upper extremity amputation they studied preferred myoelectric prostheses over conventional devices, even though usage decreased with the myoelectric protheses and they were slower than the conventional devices. Cosmetic considerations were felt to influence this choice.

Clearly, the most important criterion in evaluating an assistive device is whether it meets the needs of the consumer. On what basis, however, do disabled consumers determine whether or not a device meets their needs? Batavia and Hammer (1990) addressed this question through use of the Delphi approach with panels of consumer experts who regularly use an array of mobility and sensory devices. While affordability, durability, effectiveness, and personal acceptability were among the important factors that influenced decisions, the importance of these factors varied according to the type of device evaluated (see Figure 7). Although the authors did not address this point in their study, it is notable that the personal acceptability factor (which pertained to the level of psychological comfort associated with use of the device), was viewed as more important for devices that were more publicly visible and more clearly associated with disability. For example, personal acceptability was a more important factor for a wheelchair than for an environmental control unit. Unfortunately, the authors did not ask the panels to assess self-care devices.

Environmental Modifications

Environmental modifications can range from the rearrangement of furniture to major alterations in the design of rooms or dwellings. Common examples include widening doorways, building ramps, and converting family rooms into bedrooms for facilitating wheelchair access. Within bathrooms, the addition of grab bars, special toilet seats, and other safety equipment can dramatically improve the completion of self-care tasks by persons with limitations.

The Americans with Disabilities Act (ADA) and its related legislation in the United States, as well as efforts by advocacy groups in other countries, have made apparent the

Figure 7. Factors used by disabled consumers to rate assistive devices.

Factor	Ranked Importance of Factor		
	Wheelchair	Robotic Arm	Environmental Control Unit
Effectiveness	1	1	1
Affordability	4	4	6
Operability	2	2	2
Dependability	3	3	3
Durability	8	8	7
Compatibility	13	6	4
Flexibility	7	5	5
Ease of maintenance	6	11	9
Learnability	14	10	11
Personal acceptance	5	7	13
Physical comfort	10	13	14
Supplier repair	9	12	8
Physical security	11	9	10
Consumer repair	12	14	12
Ease of assembly	15	15	15

Note: Securability and portability were also factors identified as being important to consumers.

From "Toward the Development of Consumer-Based Criteria for the Evaluation of Assistive Devices" by A.I. Batavia and G.S. Hammer, 1992, *Journal of Rehabilitation Research, 27,* 425–436.

need to design environments and to make other accommodations so that persons with functional limitations are not deprived of societal access or participation. Unfortunately, individuals with disabilities often encounter bureaucratic obstacles that preclude timely completion of necessary environmental modifications or the acquisition of devices to facilitate adaptation. As societal attitudes reflect improved awareness of environmental barriers, buildings, playgrounds, and access areas will incorporate the curb cuts, ramps, and signage that permit their use by persons with motor and sensory deficits.

Use of Family and Personal Care Attendants

Another strategy available to the patient involves the use of personal care attendants to assist in the performance of various self-maintenance tasks. Relatives or family members may voluntarily provide assistance without compensation. However it may be necessary, or even preferable, to find paid assistance. A study by Nosek (1993) found that inadequate personal care assistance affects the long-term health and well-being of persons who are discharged from rehabilitation facilities, and concluded that a much better system for providing caregivers is needed. Her study found that burnout, fatigue, and other factors typically compromise the quality of care provided by family members. However, because outside attendants are often unavailable or economically infeasible, the study recommended that rehabilitation facilities do a much better job of training family members to provide such services. The study also recommended that rehabilitation facilities ensure that patients are trained to manage personal care attendants adequately.

One of the most important and difficult requirements for the patient will be to define all of the activities for which assistance is required. Some self-care tasks, such as dressing, grooming, and oral hygiene, are performed daily. Others, such as washing the hair, doing the laundry, or changing the bed, are done less frequently. The list of activities must be categorized according to those requiring no assistance, those requiring some assistance, and those that the personal care attendant must perform for the patient. Therapists can assist in the formulation of these lists by helping the patient gain a realistic and thorough understanding of his or her strengths and limitations related to self-care. Chapter 16, by Baum and LeVesser, provides a more in-depth examination of the use of personal care assistants for managing self-care needs.

Social Skills: Assessment and Intervention

Given the social nature of humans and the clear relationship between self-care and socialization, it is surprising that the development of social skills has not been given more attention in the occupational therapy literature. Doble, Bonnell, and Magill-Evans (1991) surveyed therapists to determine the therapists' perceptions of the importance of evaluating social skills and the means by which they attempt to do so. While therapists felt that social skills were relevant to practice, only 29% reported using any formal evaluation of them. The study concluded that a conceptual model was needed to define social skills and to relate social skills to occupational performance more clearly. Moreover, assessment tools must be identified or developed to enable therapists to assess social functioning directly. The study observed that despite the absence of such tools, many therapists do provide intervention directed toward the enhancement of social skills.

Social skills training recognizes that competence in dealing with others involves several dimensions, including social cognition, social skills, and social affect. To be socially competent, individuals must have the ability and skill to understand situations and social expectations, to initiate prosocial behaviors, and to demonstrate those affective characteristics related to self-presentation (see Figure 8) that influence positively how an individual is viewed by others.

Some social skills training has been used effectively as a primary intervention tool in the treatment of persons with mental impairments and emotional problems, as well as in other populations (Brady, 1984, 1985). Typically, these programs use group-oriented approaches that include role-playing, and modeling of behaviors that allows practicing social behaviors under various circumstances. Assertiveness training is often part of such programming. The assumption behind these approaches is that the most problematic aspects of some illnesses are behaviors that are viewed as socially maladaptive and unacceptable. The goal is to improve social behaviors and thereby reduce the alienation and rejection so often experienced by persons with deficits in social competency.

Social Impression Management

Deloach and Greer (1981) have identified a cluster of skills that are designed to help persons with visible disability overcome stigma barriers. They maintain that specific skills can be learned by the individual to reduce the stress of social encounters through influencing or managing the impressions others form during the interaction.

Figure 8. Selected dimensions of social competence.

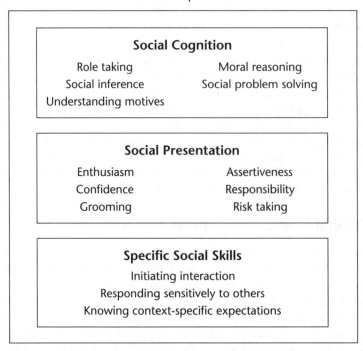

A fundamental goal of social impression management is to be able to present oneself in a creditable manner. This presentation includes appearance, mannerisms, gestures, vocalizations, the management of space and environment, and a host of other considerations. Adequate self-care is a necessary prerequisite to creditable appearance and effective social impression management.

Before impression management strategies can be implemented, individuals must be made aware of those behaviors that may be discrediting or socially troublesome, and provided with practical strategies that can be used to dilute the effects of their discrediting behaviors. For example, it is known that smiles and humor can go a long way toward overshadowing physical imperfections. Other techniques may include those that distract attention away from physical or behavioral characteristics that create discomfort for others.

An important part of impression management is conveying a socially pleasant demeanor. A number of nonverbal behaviors and gestures have been identified which, when used individually or in combination, convey a particular attitude or tone, such as openness, readiness, competence, or courting. Knowing how and when to invoke these gestures to manage social impressions favorably forms the basis of training in impression management.

Although some persons have the abilities and skills to manage impressions favorably (Braithwaite, 1989), others can benefit from social skills training as an important part of their rehabilitation regimen (Halford & Hayes, 1991; Hobart, 1983; Wixted & Morrison, 1988). The use of these strategies seems logically linked to the performance of self-care tasks, such as dressing, grooming, and personal hygiene. Connecting self-care and self-presentation as important tasks of daily living can have beneficial effects on planning and implementing therapy.

While some therapists may prefer to avoid dealing with social issues, which can cause emotional discomfort to providers as well as patients, the importance of these skills in daily living cannot be denied and should not be overlooked. As long as health care and rehabilitation providers themselves demonstrate stigmatized views of persons with disabilities (Gething, 1992; Mercer & Andrews, 1983), some strategies must be provided to help clients overcome the significant barriers to social participation and life satisfaction they are likely to experience.

Summary

In this chapter, self-care tasks have been presented within a social perspective that considers the importance of enabling the patient to maintain valued social roles. Maintaining the self in a manner that permits rewarding social interaction is fundamental to community living and an important factor in life satisfaction.

Because disability imposes an assault on social role performance and self-identity, occupational therapists can perform a valuable service by helping their patients explore and reconstruct alternative views of self that are both acceptable and offer reasonable prospects for personal fulfillment. Adopting a narrative perspective to understand better how the patient is experiencing and interpreting the challenges of disability will assist in this process.

Strategies for managing self-care should be determined in collaboration with the patient from among restorative or adaptive options that include compensatory training, environmental modification, assistive and adaptive devices, and the use of personal care assistants. Social skills assessment and training, including techniques for social impression management, should also be incorporated into the intervention plan for individuals whose personal resources are unlikely to allow them to overcome stigma barriers and to experience meaningful social participation. Ideally, the satisfactory performance of self-care and its relationship to effective social interaction should be communicated to the patient or client. ◆

References

American Occupational Therapy Association (in press). *Uniform terminology for occupational therapy—Third edition*. Rockville, MD: Author.

Affleck, G., & Pfeiffer, C.A. (1988). Social support and psychosocial adjustment to rheumatoid arthritis: Quantitative and qualitative findings. *Arthritis Care and Research, 1*(2), 71–77.

Batavia, A.I., & Hammer, G.S. (1990). Toward the development of consumer-based criteria for the evaluation of assistive devices. *Journal of Rehabilitation Research, 27*, 425–436.

Berger, P.L., & Luckmann, T. (1967). *The social construction of reality*. New York: Doubleday.

Bowling, A.P., & Edelmann, R.J. (1989). Loneliness, mobility, well-being and social support in a sample of over 85 year olds. *Personality and Individual Differences, 10*, 1189–1192.

Brady, J.P. (1984). Social skills training in psychiatric patients: Concepts, methods and clinical results. *Occupational Therapy in Mental Health, 4*(4), 51–68

Brady, J.P. (1985). Social skills training in psychiatric patients: Clinical outcome studies. *Occupational Therapy in Mental Health, 5*(1), 59–74.

Braithwaite, D.O. (1989) An interpretive analysis of the way persons with disabilities make attributions and use impression management strategies in their communication with able bodied persons (Doctoral dissertation, University of Minnesota). *Dissertation Abstracts International, 48*, 5002A.

Branholm, I.B., & Fugl-Meyer, A.R. (1992). Occupational role preferences and life satisfaction. *Occupational Therapy Journal of Research, 12*, 159–171.

Brown, K., & Gillespie, D. (1992). Recovering relationships: A feminist analysis of recovery models. *American Journal of Occupational Therapy, 46*, 1001–1005.

Bruner, J. (1990). *Acts of meaning.* Cambridge, MA: Harvard University Press.

Bynum, H., & Rogers, J.C. (1987). The use and effectiveness of assistive devices possessed by patients seen in home care. *Occupational Therapy Journal of Research, 7*, 181–191.

Christiansen, C. (1992, March). *The study and classification of occupation.* Presented at the AOTF Research Colloquium, Houston, Texas.

Christiansen, C. (1993). Three perspectives on balance in occupation. In F. Clark & R. Zemke (Eds.), *Occupational science: Selections from the symposia.* Philadelphia: F.A. Davis.

Christiansen, C., Schwartz, R., & Barnes, K. (1993). Self-care: Evaluation and treatment. In J.A. DeLisa and D.M. Gans (Eds.), *Rehabilitation medicine: Principles & practice* (2nd ed.) (pp. 178–200). Philadelphia: Lippincott.

Cooley, H.C. (1902). *Human nature and the social order.* New York: Scribner.

Cooper, H., & Okamura, L. (1992). Social activity and subjective well-being. *Personality and Individual Differences, 13*, 573–583.

Crisp, R. (1992). The long term adjustment of 60 persons with spinal cord injury. *Australian Psychologist, 27*(1), 43–47.

Deloach, C., & Greer, B. (1981). *Adjustment to severe physical disability: A metamorphosis.* New York: McGraw-Hill.

Dever, R.B. (1989). A taxonomy of community living skills. *Exceptional Children, 55*, 395–404.

Doble, S., Bonnell, J.E., & Magill-Evans, J. (1991). Evaluation of social skills: A survey of current practice. *Canadian Journal of Occupational Therapy, 58*, 241–249.

Englehardt, H.T. (1977). Defining occupational therapy: The meaning of therapy and the virtues of occupation. *American Journal of Occupational Therapy, 31*, 666–672.

Fidler, G.S., & Fidler, J.W. (1978). Doing and becoming: Purposeful action and self-actualization. *American Journal of Occupational Therapy, 32*, 305–310.

Flavell, J. (1985). *Cognitive development.* Englewood Cliffs, NJ: Prentice Hall.

Fuhrer, M.J., Rintala, D.H., Hart, K.A., Clearman, R., & Young, M.E. (1992). Relationship of life satisfaction to impairment, disability, and handicap among persons with spinal cord injury living in the community. *Archives of Physical Medicine and Rehabilitation, 73*, 552–557.

Fuhrer, M.J., Rintala, D.H., Hart, K.A., Clearman, R., & Young, M.E. (1993). Depressive symptomatology in persons with spinal cord injury who reside in the community. *Archives of Physical Medicine and Rehabilitation, 74*, 255–261.

Garber, S.L., & Gregorio, T.L. (1990). Upper extremity devices: Assessment of use by spinal cord injured patients with quadriplegia. *American Journal of Occupational Therapy, 44*, 126–131.

Gergen, K.J., & Gergen, M.M. (1988). Narrative and the self as relationship. In L. Berkowitz (Ed.), *Advances in experimental and social psychology* (pp. 17–55). New York: Academic Press.

Gething, L. (1992). Judgements by health professionals of personal characteristics of people with a visible physical disability. *Social Science and Medicine, 34*, 809–815.

Gitlin, L.N., Levine, R., & Geiger, C. (1993). Adaptive device use by older adults with mixed disabilities. *Archives of Physical Medicine & Rehabilitation, 74*, 149–152.

Goffman, E. (1959). *The presentation of self in everyday life*. New York: Doubleday.

Goffman, E. (1963). *Stigma: Notes on the management of a spoiled identity*. Englewood Cliffs, NJ: Prentice Hall.

Halford, W.K., & Hayes, R. (1991). Psychological rehabilitation of chronic schizophrenic patients: Recent findings on social skills training and family psychoeducation. *Clinical Psychology Review, 11*(1), 23–44.

Haworth, R.J. (1983). Use of aids during the first three months after total hip replacement. *British Journal of Rheumatology, 22*, 29–35.

Hobart, S.C. (1983) *Improving disability specific social skills: The effects of training and locus of control*. Unpublished doctoral dissertation, University of Alabama.

Hogan, R. (1982). A socioanalytic theory of personality. *Nebraska Symposium on Motivation, 30*, 55–89.

Hogan, R., & Sloan, T. (1991). Socioanalytic foundations for personality psychology. *Perspectives in Personality, 3*(Part B), 1–15.

Ishii-Kuntz, M. (1990). Social interaction and psychological well-being. *International Journal of Aging and Human Development, 30*(1), 15–36.

Kagan, J. (1989). *Unstable ideas: Temperament, cognition and self*. Cambridge, MA: Harvard University Press.

Lawton, M.P. (1971). The functional assessment of elderly people. *Journal of the American Geriatrics Society, 19*, 465–481.

Lawton, M.P. (1990). Age and the performance of home tasks. *Human Factors, 32*, 527–536.

Mancuso, J.C., & Sarbin, T.R. (1985). The self-narrative in the enactment of roles. In T.R. Sarbin & K.E. Scheibe (Eds.), *Studies in social identity* (pp. 233–253). New York: Praeger.

Mattingly, C. (1991a). What is clinical reasoning? *American Journal of Occupational Therapy, 45*, 979–987.

Mattingly, C. (1991b). The narrative nature of clinical reasoning. *American Journal of Occupational Therapy, 45*, 998–1005.

Mattingly, C., & Fleming, M. (1993). *Clinical reasoning: Forms of inquiry in a therapeutic practice*. Philadelphia: F.A. Davis.

McCuaig, M., & Frank, G. (1991). The able self: Adaptive patterns and choices in independent living for a person with cerebral palsy. *American Journal of Occupational Therapy, 45*, 224–234.

Mead, G.H. (1934). *Mind, self, and society*. Chicago: University of Chicago Press.

Mercer, J., & Andrews, H. (1983). The effects of physical attractiveness and disability on client ratings by helping professionals. *Journal of Applied Rehabilitation Counseling, 14*, 41–45.

Morris, J. (Ed.). (1988). *Able lives*. London: The Women's Press.

Murphy, R.F. (1987). *The body silent*. New York: Henry Holt.

Newrick, R., & Langton-Hewer, R. (1984). Motor neuron disease: Can we do better? A study of 42 patients. *British Medical Journal, 289*, 539–542.

Nosek, M.A. (1993). Personal assistance: Its effect on the long term health of a rehabilitation hospital population. *Archives of Physical Medicine and Rehabilitation, 74*, 127–32.

Parsons, T. (1958). Definitions of health and illness in the light of American values and social structure. In E.G. Jaco (Ed.), *Patients, physicians, and illness* (pp. 165–187). New York: Free Press of Glencoe.

Parsons, T. (1975). The sick role and the role of the physician reconsidered. *Health and Society: Milbank Memorial Fund Quarterly, 53*(3), 257–278.

Polkinghorne, D. (1988). *Narrative knowing and the human sciences.* Albany: State University of New York Press.

Rintala, D., & Young, M.E. (1992). Social support and the well being of persons with spinal cord injury living in the community. *Rehabilitation Psychology, 37*, 15–163.

Rogers, J. (1982). The spirit of independence: The evolution of a philosophy. *American Journal of Occupational Therapy, 36*, 709–715.

Rogers, J. (1983). Clinical reasoning: The ethics, science and art. *American Journal of Occupational Therapy, 37*, 601–616.

Rogers, J.C., & Figone, J.J. (1980). Traumatic quadriplegia: Follow-up study of self-care skills. *Archives of Physical Medicine and Rehabilitation, 61*, 316–321.

Rogers, J.C., & Holm, M.B. (1991). Occupational therapy diagnostic reasoning: A component of clinical reasoning. *American Journal of Occupational Therapy, 45*, 1045–1053.

Rosow, I. (1985). Status and role change through the life cycle. In R.H. Shanas & E. Shanas (Eds.), *Handbook of aging and the social sciences* (pp. 62–91). New York: Van Nostrand Reinhold.

Rowles, G.D. (1991). Beyond performance: Being in place as a component of occupational therapy. *American Journal of Occupational Therapy, 45*, 265–271.

Rybarczyk, B.D, Nyenhuis, D.L., Nicholas, J.J., Schulz, R., Alioto, R.J., & Blair, C. (1992). Social discomfort and depression in a sample of adults with leg amputations. *Archives of Physical Medicine and Rehabilitation, 73*, 1169–1173.

Smith, R.O. (1991). Technological approaches to performance enhancement. In C. Christiansen & C. Baum (Eds.). *Occupational therapy: Overcoming human performance deficits* (pp. 747–788.) Thorofare, NJ: Slack.

Stein, R.B., & Walley, M. (1983). Functional comparison of upper extremity amputees using myoelectric and conventional prostheses. *Archives of Physical Medicine and Rehabilitation, 64*, 243–248.

Szalai, A. (Ed.). (1972). *The use of time: Daily activities of urban and suburban populations in twelve countries.* The Hague: Mouton.

Trombly, C.A. (1993). Anticipating the future: Assessment of occupational function. *American Journal of Occupational Therapy, 47*, 253–257.

Weingarden, S.I., & Martin, M.C. (1989). Independent dressing after spinal cord injury: A functional time evaluation. *Archives of Physical Medicine and Rehabilitation, 70*, 518–519.

Wixted, J.T., & Morrison, R.L. (1988). Social skills training in the treatment of negative symptoms. *International Journal of Mental Health, 17*(1), 3–21.

World Health Organization. (1980). *International classification of impairment, disability and handicap.* Geneva, Switzerland: Author.

Yelin, E., Lubeck, D., Holman, H., & Epstein, W. (1987). The impact of rheumatoid arthritis and osteoarthritis: The activities of patients with rheumatoid arthritis and osteoarthritis compared to controls. *The Journal of Rheumatology, 14*, 710–717.

Yerxa, E.J. (1967). Authentic occupational therapy. *American Journal of Occupational Therapy, 21*, 1–9.

Yerxa, E.J., & Baum, S. (1986). Engagement in daily occupations and life satisfaction among people with spinal cord injuries. *Occupational Therapy Journal of Research, 40*, 271–283.

Zedjlik, C. (1992). *Management of spinal cord injury* (2nd ed.). Boston: Jones and Bartlett.

2

The Personal Meaning of Self-Care Occupations

Gelya Frank

Gelya Frank, PhD, *is an Associate Professor in the Departments of Occupational Therapy and Anthropology at the University of Southern California, Los Angeles, CA.*

The writing of this chapter was supported in part by a 3-year grant from the American Occupational Therapy Foundation (AOTF) to the Department of Occupational Therapy at the University of Southern California to establish an AOTF Center for Scholarship and Research (1992–1994) to investigate "The Relationship of Occupation to Adaptation and its Implications for Occupational Therapy." The author's discussion of Arnold Beisser's autobiography closely follows the insightful analysis by Elizabeth J. Yerxa, EdD, LHD, OTR, FAOTA, in her talk, "Searching for an Ethical, Realistic, and Relevant Basis for New Models of Practice for Occupational Therapy," November 15, 1991, at the West Los Angeles V.A. Medical Center, Los Angeles, California. More generally, the author wishes to acknowledge her debt to Dr. Yerxa for directing scholarly attention in the field of occupational therapy to the impact of disability-related experiences upon the identity and dignity of individuals.

Chapter 2 Outline

The Meaning of Symptoms—Illness Narratives

Culture, Ethnicity, and Class

Chronicity and Adaptation Over Time

Defining Symptoms in Occupational Terms

Self-Care Experiences—The Importance of "Self"

"Unspeakable Practices"— Toileting

Architectural Barriers and Special Equipment

Home Care, Family Dynamics, and Rehabilitation Policy

Hospitals and Institutional Care

Feeding, Eating…and Dining

Feeding Oneself—Shame and Pride

Food Choices—Preferences and Limitations

Meals as the Enactment of Social Relationships

Grooming and Dressing as Self-Expression

Stigma and Deviance Disavowal

Cultural Stereotypes of
Beauty and Fashion as Cultural Code

Overcoming Barriers to Self-Expression

Conclusion

References

Nursing home attendant: "Tinkle, tinkle?"

Old woman: "Little star."

Self-care, in the professional language of occupational therapy practice and reimbursement, has come to include the activities of "toileting," "grooming," and "feeding." Something deep in the soul of any occupational therapist worth his or her registration certificate rebels against this language. Even when applied to our primate cousins, the chimpanzees, starkly behaviorist terms such as these are in themselves inadequate. They strip away the rich symbolism that the body and its functions take on in cultural traditions and social interactions.

From the standpoint of the biological sciences, using the bathroom, combing one's hair, putting on clothes, and getting food into one's mouth are relatively objective behaviors that may be described with more or less precision as a set of muscle movements. But when an individual incurs a stroke or spinal cord injury, or becomes the parent of a child with a congenital impairment, he or she quickly discovers worlds of meaning packed into even the mundane activities of self-care.

The Meaning of Symptoms—Illness Narratives

The personal meanings of illness and disability are forged within various kinds of significance accorded to symptoms by culture, family, and the practitioners to whom a patient turns for help. There is very little that is "natural," in a universal biological sense, about the meaning of symptoms. Arthur Kleinman (1988), a psychiatrist and anthropologist, writes that the meaning of illness is manifold: "Illness is polysemic or multivocal. Illness experiences and events usually radiate (or conceal) more than one meaning" (p. 8).

Although certain facial expressions, vocalizations, and gestures can be "read" cross-culturally (Ekman, 1980), they cannot be read very deeply. Human experiences are more complex than the body alone can express. This is due to the capacity of our species to use language, the many languages and dialects spoken in the world, and the idiosyncratic meanings that emerge whenever people interact over time. Historical documents, literary texts, and the stories patients tell are keys, therefore, to the personal meanings of illness and disability.

Culture, Ethnicity, and Class

Medical anthropologists confirm what experienced clinicians in urban areas have long noted: Ethnic groups differ in their responses to suffering—for example, in their expression of pain (Lipton & Marbach, 1984; Wolff & Langley, 1968; Zborowski, 1969). What has been observed more recently is how groups vary in according special local and historical significance to body parts and body functions (Scheper-Hughes & Lock, 1987).

Literary critic Susan Sontag (1978) has shown, for instance, how the equally life-threatening diseases of tuberculosis (TB) and cancer have been very differently conceptualized in Western culture. TB came to be associated with the "upper" region of the body—with the lungs, with breath, and with the spirit. At the same time that TB was romanticized, cancer came to be associated with the lower parts of the body and treated as shameful and disgusting.

Little matter, of course, that TB could be localized in bones and other places, or that cancer could occur in the lungs and everywhere else. Descriptions of the diseases were also tinged with economic concepts: The 19th century description of TB as "consumption" carried with it early capitalist concerns about saving and spending resources; the metaphor of uncontrolled growth dominates descriptions of cancer in the more advanced stages of capitalism in the present century.

Lower class position, membership in stigmatized ethnic or racial groups, and other forms of social marginality associated with patients having a particular disease also influence the disease's socially ascribed or cultural meaning. Moral judgments enter and, typically, the civil rights of sufferers are compromised. During the New York City epidemic of 1832, for example, cholera was assumed to be a disease caused by intemperance, since the first cases appeared in the Four Points District among poor Irish immigrants (Rosenberg, 1988). That these people inhabited a slum, with minimal public services, where raw sewage ran in the streets, seems today a better explanation for the spread of the epidemic than its victims' nationality or consumption of alcohol.

The same phenomenon is demonstrated by the application of harsher public health measures to female prostitutes versus male clients, and to blacks versus whites, to control the spread of syphilis in the early decades of this century (Fee, 1988). Irrational fears about Acquired Immune Deficiency Syndrome (AIDS), its association in North America and Western Europe with stigmatized groups and behaviors, and discrimination against AIDS patients are a current case in point (Bayer, 1989; Brandt, 1988; Treichler, 1988).

Chronic illness and disability offer a free course in culture, complete with a one-way trip to the field, during which individuals may discover social rules they had never before noticed or questioned. Many of the sharpest insights on the cultural shaping of disability have been articulated in recent works by social scientists writing about their own disability experiences.

These authors note a conspiracy of polite silence around disability in American culture. Barbara Webster (1989), a graduate student in anthropology diagnosed with multiple sclerosis at age 37, writes:

> When I was in Egypt, walking with difficulty and using a cane, strangers and passersby asked me directly, "What is wrong with you? Why do you limp? Why are you sitting there? Why are you using a cane?" Walking in a Cairo street, an old woman came up to me, put her arm on mine, pointed to the cane, and patted my hand. I was struck by this; in the United States people don't ask questions of that nature or respond openly to disability. Instead they stare at or ignore me. The open acceptance I experienced in Egypt contrasted starkly with the equally open turning away I have come to expect in this country. (p. 62)

Similar responses were evoked in India by the appearance of sociologist Irving Kenneth Zola (1982), a polio survivor writing in his late forties. When he had visited the country in 1969, Zola used a back support, long leg brace, and cane. Zola's acquaintances, government ministers and bureau heads, did not hesitate to greet him with the question, "What happened to your leg?" They were oblivious to the intrusion upon privacy with which Americans would regard such an inquiry.

Writing at age 62 about his life since developing symptoms of a spinal cord tumor, anthropologist Robert F. Murphy (1987) highlights the lack of interest in his disability evinced in the United States not only by lay persons but also by physicians:

> Nobody has ever asked me what it is like to be a paraplegic—and now a quadriplegic—for this would violate all the rules of middle-class etiquette. A few have asked me what caused my condition, and, after hearing the answer, have looked as though they wished they hadn't. After all, tumors can happen to anybody—even to them. Polite manners may protect us from most such intrusions, but it is remarkable that

physicians seldom ask either. . . . What goes on in the patient's head is another department. . . . (p. 88)

Chronicity and Adaptation Over Time

The timing of symptoms affects their meaning to patients and families. Each person's chronic illness or disability follows its own trajectory—upward, stable, unstable, or downward (Corbin & Strauss, 1988). When symptoms occur during the course of an illness matters. Helen Featherstone (1980), special educator and mother of a multihandicapped child, imagines how happy she would have been if, after a year of increasingly grim diagnoses, her son had been "only" blind or retarded:

> When I learned Jody was blind, I was shocked. I wept for the perfect baby I had lost, for the sunsets he would never see, for the four-year-old who would not be able to play outside unsupervised. But in a few days I learned to live with the idea of blindness, to believe that if he were "only" blind, he could have a rich, rewarding, and independent life. I lived in terror of retardation.
>
> . . .As the months passed, things were both worse and better than I had imagined. Reality was worse: the baby had to cope with cerebral palsy and seizures, as well as with retardation and blindness. He was hydrocephalic. His shunt blocked often; family head colds brought him to the brink of death. He was hospitalized seven times in the first eighteen months of his life. Within the year I would have given worlds for the hope that he would one day walk and talk like the bumbling special-class children of my earlier nightmares. (pp. 26–27)

The meaning of symptoms also changes with the ability to cope and make adaptations. It is important to note that although Featherstone's outer reality was bleaker than her worst fears, her inner reality—feelings about her child and her family's life—had improved. She had faced so many crises and challenges, and had learned to handle them, that her confidence in herself began to overpower her fears about tomorrow. Her child's symptoms were worse, but she felt better.

Defining Symptoms in Occupational Terms

Many social scientists distinguish the terms *illness* and *disease*. *Disease* refers to a disorder as understood through biomedicine. *Illness* refers to the individual's experience of disorder or suffering (Eisenberg, 1977). Kleinman (1988) coins the term "illness problems" to cover the effect of symptoms on the ability to perform one's customary and daily activities. Illness problems are central to the meaning of symptoms.

The functions and meanings of daily activities are the core concern of occupational therapy (Yerxa et al., 1990; Clark et al., 1991). Occupational therapists, whose discipline since 1917 has emphasized the restoration of function in activities of daily living, may greet the good news from medical anthropology with a sense of vindication, if not justifiable impatience:

> Illness problems are the principal difficulties that symptoms and disability create in our lives. For example, we may be unable to walk up our stairs to our bedroom. Or we may experience distracting low back pain while we sit at work. Headaches may make it impossible to focus on homework assignments or housework, leading to failure and frustration. Or there may be impotence that leads to divorce. (Kleinman, 1988, p. 4)

Kleinman (1988) suggests that practitioners have a better chance of providing meaningful care when they have gained an understanding of a patient's illness experience. Chronic illnesses, he notes, are characterized by the oscillation of periods of exacerbation and quiescence of symptoms. Knowledge of the meaning of symptoms for patients can help practitioners to break the vicious cycles that amplify distress. Thus, Kleinman reconceptualizes medical care for chronically sick persons to include, first, "empathic witnessing of the existential experience of suffering," and, second, "practical coping with the major psychosocial crises that constitute the menacing chronicity of that experience" (p. 10). It is a prescription that occupational therapists are ideally qualified to carry out.

Self-Care Experiences—The Importance of "Self"

Narratives by adults and parents of children with a range of chronic illnesses and disabilities reveal the personal meaning of self-care activities. Threats are posed to the individual's sense of self by the body's failure to perform activities that are usually taken for granted (Corbin & Strauss, 1988).

Dancer and choreographer Agnes de Mille (1981) first noticed symptoms of the stroke she suffered in 1975, in her seventies, when her hand didn't work to sign a contract. De Mille registered this performance failure in terms of her lifetime identity: "Please do something fast," she told her doctor, "because I've got to be on the stage in one hour delivering a very difficult lecture and I've never been late for anything in the theater in my life" (pp. 21–22).

Adults who become disabled through disease or injury often report that their bodies or impaired body parts become alien to them, disassociated, and sometimes even seem dead. "Half of me was imprisoned in the other half," writes de Mille (p. 57) about the weeks immediately after her stroke. She describes the residual effect, 6 months after, as if her whole self were split in two:

> My right arm, my right leg, that whole side of my body gone. I was to be two bodies, one of them not my friend, alien. And must I drag this creature about with me, this Siamese horror, forever? Forever not my friend? Very likely. (p. 219)

Poet Audre Lorde (1980), 9 months after a modified radical mastectomy for breast cancer, also expressed longing for a past self who could perform daily activities effortlessly:

> I must be content to see how really little I can do and still do it with an open heart. I can never accept this, like I can't accept that turning my life around is so hard, eating differently, sleeping differently, moving differently, being differently. . . . I want the old me, bad as before. (pp. 11–12)

In moments when the body can become invisible again, taken for granted, the self may flourish. Robert F. Murphy's (1987) personal history was "divided radically into two parts: pre-wheelchair and post-wheelchair." Yet his return to the lecture halls of Columbia University, even in a wheelchair, meant a restoration of self: "Hey, it's the same old me inside this body!" (p. 81)

It is rarely possible to recover the "same old me" without reexamination and reevaluation of the components of one's identity. According to social psychologists in rehabilitation, "adjustment" to disability requires shifting emphasis away from what is missing and placing primary value upon one's assets (Wright, 1983). Taking a sociological approach, some scholars suggest the term, "biographical work," for the efforts evoked by chronic illness and disability to reevaluate and reconstruct personal identity (Corbin & Strauss, 1988).

The narratives of self-care experiences in this chapter represent the biographical work of a variety of individuals. The biographical impact of handicaps in self-care activities is by no means trivial. Agnes de Mille (1981), who finally managed to get to the toilet in the night using a three-pronged cane, without falling or bumping herself, wrote: "My trip to the bathroom in privacy and decency meant more to me than a rave notice in the [New York] Times" (p. 167).

"Unspeakable Practices"—Toileting

With Irving Kenneth Zola's (1982) permission, readers may follow him into the bathroom on the morning of Friday, May 26, 1972. The setting is Het Dorp, a planned independent living community for persons with physical disabilities in the Netherlands, where Zola resided for a week. During his stay, Zola decided to use a wheelchair for the first time in decades, part of a naturalistic experiment that led him to reevaluate and reintegrate his disability into his identity.

Taking the role of participant observer, and as a spokesperson for the Independent Living Movement, Zola approached his morning routine at Het Dorp uniquely. He decided to report how, from his new position in a wheelchair, he handled the "unspeakable practices" of urinating and defecating.

While transferring to and from the wheelchair, and using the toilet from a seated position, Zola realized two things. The bathroom's barrier-free design made this the easiest "toileting" he had ever experienced. Using the grab bar, he was able to raise himself from the toilet despite his weak stomach muscles and legs. He became aware how unnecessary his previous difficulties with toileting had been.

Using the toilet from a seated position was uncomfortable, however, in terms of Zola's sense of himself by gender and age:

> Two difficulties did remain. For lack of a better term I call the first one "cultural" and the second "psychosocial." As a Western man I had been trained to urinate standing with both feet firmly planted on the ground. Thus, to sit and urinate took some getting used to. This did, however, provide a side benefit. Standing I had always needed one hand free to steady myself. Sitting at least made it a more relaxed activity. My second problem was more "psychosocial." Before leaving the bathroom I tried to think if I had "to go" again. Once more I was reduced to the status of a child as I recalled parental admonitions to the effect, "We are starting on a trip so you better use the toilet now." I did the same thing with my own children. What were the toilet facilities like elsewhere in the Village? Would they be as easy to negotiate as the one in my room? (1982, pp. 65–66)

Zola's candid report suggests how individuals' ability and willingness to adapt their behavior—even in the most private situations—can hinge on cultural rules that are deeply embedded with meaning about social identity. Zola's capacity to step back and observe how his reactions were shaped is an asset. Critical abilities can help people make choices, as individuals, about what works for them.

Architectural Barriers and Special Equipment

Robert F. Murphy (1987) shows, too, how accessibility can affect the meaning of symptoms within a trajectory of progressive disablement. Murphy became confined to the first floor of his two-story suburban home after all other options were ruled out. He had considered getting a stairway lift since the bedrooms and his study were upstairs, but the cost was so high that it would have made more sense to buy a new home.

As it turned out, Murphy's disablement soon worsened to the point where he would not have been able to transfer independently to and from the lift and his wheelchairs anyway. All discussion about getting Murphy up to the second floor ended when his son and his son's friend carried him upstairs one day in 1977. Murphy discovered that the bathrooms would have to be torn up to make them accessible. That was the last time he saw the second floor of his house.

Moving permanently to the family room on the 1st floor, to which a half bathroom was added, marked Murphy's change in status within the family. His choice of activities and quality of life were dictated increasingly by his self-care needs in relation to the built environment. Lamenting the loss of his ability to move spontaneously, Murphy suggests that he also had lost aspects of his self:

> I could go nowhere without a driver, usually Yolanda [Murphy's wife] or Bob [his son], and every trip entailed logistics. If we wanted to eat at a restaurant or go to the movies, we had to call first to make sure there were no steps. And if we wanted to stay at a motel, we had to measure the width of the bathroom door, for my wheelchair is twenty-six inches wide. Whenever we traveled, we needed equipment. Aside from the wheelchair, we had to transport the walker, bedpan, urinal, and assorted accessories. As my condition worsened, the list grew longer. Gone were the days when we would give in to a sudden urge to go somewhere or do something. But gone also were the days when I could wander into the kitchen for a snack or outside for a breath of fresh air. This loss of spontaneity invaded my entire assessment of time. It rigidified my short-range perspectives and introduced a calculating quality into an existence that formerly had been pleasantly disordered. (1987, p. 76)

Home Care, Family Dynamics, and Rehabilitation Policy

The personal meaning of self-care is shaped, also, by the resources of the family or household. Who gives care, what kind, and how much, is important to the meaning of self-care activities. Within marriages, or with people who live together, the couple typically works as a unit to manage the disability (Corbin & Strauss, 1988). One partner may help perform the self-care activities of the other. Consequently, the meaning of the activity for the individual receiving care stands in a reciprocal and dynamic relation to that of the caretaker.

The division of labor in the family can become unbalanced as a spouse or children take responsibility for another's basic needs. Feelings of exhaustion, depression, anxiety about money, self-pity, resentment, and secondary reactions of guilt are common. In a study about couples managing chronic illness at home, one woman described her exhaustion over the physical work she did to help her ill spouse:

> All night long he would say, "Get me water, put me on the commode." I would tell K., "Let me sleep; let me rest. I don't mind waiting on you hand and foot during the day, but at night let me sleep". . . . He got out of bed one night and urinated all over the floor. I had to get up and clean him up and put him back to bed. I didn't realize he was taking up so much of my energy. That twenty-four hour stuff was getting to me . . . . After he died, I was so exhausted. . . . I am still. . . . God was good to me in a way. Had [my husband] been sick any longer, it would have broken me physically and financially. (Corbin & Strauss, 1988, pp. 293–294)

Women, whether or not they work outside the home, continue to shoulder the primary responsibility for caring for family members with chronic illnesses and disabilities (Abel & Nelson, 1990). Studies suggest that it is more common for a wife to remain married to and help with the activities of self-care for her partner with a chronic illness or disability than the reverse (Asch & Fine, 1988).

In an important sense, the meaning of self-care is shaped by public policy (Fisher & Tronto, 1990; Strauss & Corbin, 1988). The slogan of the women's movement, "The personal is political," applies. Access to health insurance, coverage for rehabilitation, and the availability and quality of nursing homes, attendant care, and respite care all contribute to the meaning of self-care within relationships between caregivers and those cared for.

When men help their partners or children with self-care activities, they experience the same pressures, of course, that women do. How men learn to provide primary care needs to be better documented, as traditional gender roles for men give way for some to more egalitarian life-styles (Hochschild, 1989). An older man explained his resentment in the role of caregiver for his wife:

> I am a bundle of nerves because I can't get out and play handball anymore. I have to give up my sex life. I am a healthy physical man. It is a toughie. You can't masturbate at seventy-three; it isn't going to do you any good. I'll be honest with you, there isn't a dame that I miss when I go out shopping or anywhere. . . . Sometimes I get impatient. She pushes me pretty hard in the morning: "I want my cereal. You didn't do this." I say, "Give me a chance. If you were in the hospital, you would have three or four attendants." I lift her out of the bed onto the commode. I have to make sure of the catheter. I say, "Honey, I only have two legs, two arms, and one mind." I can't afford to have someone living here full time. I would have to mortgage my house. Some of the bills I have received from the doctors are unbelievable. It has been a year now and I am still paying on some. . . . She gets depressed and so do I. . . . Some of my friends are going to Reno on a bus. I wish I could climb on the bus and go with them. (Corbin & Strauss, 1988, p. 296)

The father of a child with emotional disabilities, Josh Greenfeld (1972), writes about his fear that he always will have to take care of his son Noah's toileting needs. Greenfeld's fears about the future amplify the unpleasantness of his present situation:

> What a night! Noah was up all of it. Two urinations, two b.m.'s, four diaper changes in all. And the period in between, he bounced and jumped and chirped.
>
> Obviously Noah isn't making much headway; he has become more and more lax in his toilet training. And when I project, all I see is a sleepy life of never-ending diaper-changing for us all. (pp. 106-107)

A family schedule oversaturated with maternal responsibility explains Helen Featherstone's (1980) outrage when a practitioner suggested a small addition to her son Jody's home program. It was recommended that she brush Jody's teeth three times a day, for 5 minutes, with an electric toothbrush to counteract gum overgrowth caused by his antiseizure medication. Featherstone, mother of three children, was handling so many demands already that she exploded:

> Jody, I thought, is blind, cerebral-palsied, and retarded. We do his physical therapy daily and work with him on sounds and communication. We feed him each meal on our laps, bottle him, change him, bathe him, dry him, put him in a body cast to sleep, launder his bed linens daily, and go through a variety of routines designed to minimize his miseries and enhance his joys and his development. (All this in addition to trying to care for and enjoy our other young children and making time for each other and our careers.) Now you tell me that I should spend fifteen minutes every day on something that Jody will hate, an activity that will not help him to walk or even defecate, but one that is directed at the health of his gums. This activity is not for a finite time but forever. It is not guaranteed to make the overgrowth go away but may retard it. Well, it's too much. Where is that fifteen minutes going to come from? What am I supposed to give up? Taking the kids to the park? Reading a bedtime story to my eldest? Washing the breakfast dishes? Sorting the laundry? Grading students' papers? Sleeping? Because there is no time in my life that hasn't been spoken for, and for every fifteen-minute activity that is added, one has to be taken away. (pp. 77–78)

Those who are cared for at home are frequently conscious of the sacrifices made for them and try to avoid demanding too much. While visiting the independent living community at Het Dorp, Irving Kenneth Zola (1982) noted that residents frequently commented on how much freer they felt there than elsewhere, even at home. This triggered a childhood memory for Zola. He remembered trying to avoid bothering his parents rather than dealing with the consequent feelings of guilt and childishness:

> I recalled the experience of confinement at home after my accident. As much as my parents assured me of their love, I could not help but feel that I was a burden. So gradually I tried to adjust: to eat, to sleep, to defecate when it was convenient for them. They never asked for that adjustment, but I knew that if I made them stay up later, or get out of bed to fetch something, I would feel not only more like a little child, but guilty for making demands! (p. 126)

Hospitals and Institutional Care

Viewed sociologically, the "physician's workshop" is a factory for the sick (Rosenberg, 1987). Standardized procedures of the hospital make depersonalization of patients a common risk. One depends for care on strangers. Routines dictate not only when eating and grooming, but toileting, will occur.

> If dinner is scheduled for 4:30 p.m., as it was on a floor in which I once spent two months, then that's when you eat. And if your bowels don't move often enough to suit the nursing staff, laxatives are the answer. The infamous routine that demands that all temperatures be taken at 6:00 a.m. is well known to all who have been patients. I even spent five weeks on one floor where I was bathed at 5:30 every morning because the daytime nurses were too busy to do it. (Murphy, 1987, pp. 20–21)

For Arnold Beisser (1989), hospitalized for 3 years beginning in 1950 after becoming paralyzed by polio, alienation from his own failed body ("more like a sack of flour than a human being," [p. 21]) was exacerbated by depersonalizing care. Beisser's first year and a half was spent entirely on his back in an iron lung. In his mid-20s, a medical school graduate and national tennis champion, he could no longer perform formerly automatic functions. This included his bladder and bowel functions, in spite of the urges he felt. Thus he had to depend on strangers to help him:

> Intermittently people would open one or another of the portholes of my new metal skin and invade my private space. They would enter the most personal and private parts of me as they reached inside to move a leg or arm, or insert a needle or a bedpan. There was not even the pretense that my new space belonged to me, and entry beneath my new metal skin was at the discretion of others. (p. 18)

Beisser's body boundary was now the iron lung; his head, which extruded, was the only part of him that remained recognizably human. From Beisser's vulnerable position, lying on his back, people with whom he came into contact felt like attackers:

> I would often see their shadows before I saw them. They came at me from above like great condors, diving toward my exposed soft parts. People would capriciously and suddenly enter my most private spaces to do what was "best" for me. Since they did not ask my permission before doing things to me, they were like hostile invasions, and I felt violated. (1989, p. 23)

Beisser discovered that his caregivers treated his body as an object. He would become enraged to find that they made judgments for him, even about his sensations of heat and cold. But he quickly learned to smile patiently and try to explain to his nurses why he might need the blanket despite their perception that he didn't. He dared not express his anger for fear of being punished by being ignored or handled roughly:

You cannot get mad in hospitals. If you do, you may be in trouble. The next time you call for something, there may be a long delay in the nurses' response, or no response at all. There is always more than enough for the nurses to do in hospitals, so some things come first and some are left unattended. Angry patients come last. (1989, p. 19)

Mature patients who depend on others for help with bowel and bladder functions are frequently infantilized. Beisser realized that he was seen as a baby. He noticed a range of attitudes among his caregivers toward that image—some were concerned with controlling what they considered the unruly child, others with nurturing a helpless infant:

Nurses and attendants often talked to me as if I were a baby. If I became soiled through no fault of my own, they were likely to say, "Naughty, naughty," or "You've been a bad boy." Some people were so perplexed that they simply fled in despair. None of these attitudes helped clarify my confusion about how I thought of myself. (1989, p. 22)

Institutional routines relegated Beisser's survival needs to "just a job" for some of his caregivers. A nurse or attendant could leave him suspended midair in a lift, or in some other awkward position, to go on a coffee break. Getting help during the nurses' change of the shift was impossible, no matter how urgent the problem. Beisser felt completely humiliated by these callous helpers, who earned such nicknames as "Leona the Late," "Ed the Reluctant," and "Ivan the Terrible." He felt robbed of his sense of himself as a person and made to feel like "an undeserving outsider" (1989, p. 37).

However, several compassionate and willing helpers on the hospital staff provided Beisser with a completely different set of experiences. With them, he learned about the life-enhancing effects of care that is generously given and felt "returned from exile" and "a pariah forgiven for his crime" (1989, p. 38). It had been dehumanizing to concentrate anxiously on his basic needs. Simply knowing that compassionate helpers were present made it possible for Beisser to relax and tolerate otherwise unbearable urges:

Getting enough air, being able to go to the bathroom when necessary, having enough food and rest are urgent needs, and I could do none of these elemental things for myself. When those needs were not met, I could not be compassionate to someone else. There is no opportunity for higher levels of human function when you are short of air, and all that you can think of is getting the next breath. I am not good for anything else unless these needs are met.

But here is the remarkable thing. The urgency with which I experience my needs depends on the confidence I have that they *can* be met, whether they are or not. They are not so urgent when I am surrounded by people who willingly help me if called upon. (p. 39)

Feeding, Eating...and Dining

Physical limitations, the availability of helpers, and institutional routines shape the meaning of eating, just as they affect toileting. The general rubric of body performance failures that provoke frustration and anger therefore frames Robert F. Murphy's (1987) discussion of his inability to feed himself:

A paralytic may struggle to walk and become enraged when he cannot move his leg. Or a quadriplegic may pick up a cup of coffee with stiffened hands and drop it on his lap, precipitating an angry outburst. I had to give up spaghetti because I could no longer twirl it on my fork, and dinner would end for me in a sloppy mess. This would so upset me that I would lose my appetite. (pp. 106–107)

Differences in the social organization of eating and toileting frame the meanings of these self-care activities further. Excretory functions are the most private and unseen of activities. Toileting evokes profound shame when body failures become visible. Eating is the most social of activities. Ideally, meals are shared. To partake in them means to be involved in social relations, to be a recognizable member of the human community and of family life.

Feeding Oneself—Shame and Pride

Irish author Christopher Nolan (1987), writes about his "agony" as a 15-year-old schoolboy sitting through a science lesson trying to control his bowels while dosed with a laxative. Born with cerebral palsy, he was accustomed to asking for assistance, except in this area of function. "He knew he cast roles of responsibility on his fresh-faced friends, but bringing him to the toilet was a chore he would never ask them to do for him" (p. 117).

Comments by Diane DeVries, a woman born in 1950 with quadrilateral limb deficiencies, suggest that people with disabilities may experience deep shame about failures to eat normally in public. People with even severe congenital disabilities may impose strict standards of table behavior upon themselves and others:

> Whatever I did, like feed myself, drink, I was able to do it without any sloppiness. You know, I've even seen a girl at camp with no arms that bent down and lapped her food up like a dog. . . . And I knew her. And I went up to her and says: "Why in the hell do you do that?" And I said, "They asked if you wanted a feeder or your arms on. You could have done either one, but you had to do that." She said, "Well, it was easy for me." To me that was gross. She finally started wearing arms, and she started feeding herself. But that to me was just stupid, because people wouldn't even want to eat at the same table as her. (Frank, 1986, p. 209)

DeVries (Frank, 1986) goes on to express great pride in her own ability to eat and drink independently and avoid making a mess. The ability to feed oneself, like bowel and bladder control, is an important developmental milestone. The self-concept and social acceptance of children with disabilities depends in part on their ability to find alternative means of attaining such abilities (Gliedman & Roth, 1980).

Diane DeVries' (1992) discovery of a way to feed herself, using her above-elbow stumps, became an important foundation for developing a sense of herself as a competent person:

> I have been [feeding myself] for so long that I cannot recall when I took my first independent mouthful of food. According to Irene [Diane's mother], this memorable event occurred one morning when she left me sitting in my highchair before a bowl of cereal, as she went to prepare dishwater over at the sink. When she returned I was balancing a spoonful of food on the rim of the bowl, and by applying pressure to the spoon's handle, I was able to raise the food-laden spoon high enough for it and my mouth to meet. I was about three years old. (p. 112)

Food Choices—Preferences and Limitations

In addition to the frustrations derived from limitations in mobility and dexterity in getting food to one's mouth, a sense of profound deprivation can be evoked by the need for new food habits. For most people, food has associations deeply rooted in infancy as a form of comfort associated with being fed and cared for by one's mother (Erikson, 1968; Buckley, 1986). Frustrations can be particularly severe that involve getting food into one's mouth, adjusting to being fed by others, and losing the power to make food choices. For a person who develops a metabolic disorder, such as diabetes, changing eating habits can become a life and death struggle.

In a study aimed at uncovering social factors in the deaths of 40 patients on dialysis, for example, researchers found that 11 deaths mainly from cardiac arrest could be reclassified as due primarily to dietary indiscretions (Plough, 1986; Plough & Salem,

1982). These included consumption of large quantities of restricted foods, such as potato chips and beer, and disregard for fluid restrictions. A conclusion is that some people would rather risk dying than change their oral gratifications.

Institutions not only schedule meals without regard to individual preferences, but often provide nutrition in unpalatable forms. In her personal narrative concerning reproductive and disability rights, Anne Finger (1990) portrays herself as someone whose idea of a snack is a bran muffin and some fresh-squeezed orange juice. From her vantage, in the hospital after giving birth, an only routinely unappetizing institutional meal was virtually inedible:

> My breakfast tray arrives. Since I am on a liquid diet, I get a carton of milk—which I can't drink because I am lactose intolerant—a plastic container of reconstituted orange juice, a cup of beef broth and a square of red jello on a white plastic plate. I drink the orange juice. (p. 123)

Among the middle classes in the late 20th century in North America, as in most societies, what one eats is a marker of social identity. In Western societies during the 19th century, the period of capitalist accumulation, corpulent bodies were a sign of wealth and health. Our culturally ideal body type and related food preferences have changed. In the 1950s and 1960s, the "meat and potatoes" man was exalted. Today he is a dying breed in every sense.

More recently, *abstaining* from food has become a marker of status, along with the slim "hard" body (Bordo, 1990). Suddenly there has been a new awareness in popular culture of widespread eating disorders, such as bulimia and anorexia. Not that anorexia is new, it has probably always existed, but it has different social configurations (Bell, 1985).

Social and personal meanings tend to converge in food choices. Pizza and beer mean something different on a date than filet mignon and cabernet sauvignon. It is even possible to "be" what one eats: A person may say, "I am vegetarian" or "I am kosher." Individuals may take delight and pride in eating spicy Szechewan, Indian, Thai, or Mexican food. They may need to eat Oreo cookies at least once a day. People with disabilities may experience less freedom and choice in pleasurable consumption and self-expression, due to low income, lack of mobility, and lack of public access.

A Louis Harris (1986) survey indicates that Americans with disabilities participate much less often in a host of social activities that other Americans regularly enjoy, including going to restaurants. People with disabilities are 3 times more likely than people without disabilities never to eat in restaurants. As many as 13% of people with disabilities never shop for groceries, as compared with only 2% of the non-disabled population. Since a disproportionate number of people with disabilities are poor, nutrition may be severely compromised for the homeless mentally ill population, many elderly and sometimes house-bound women and men, people with developmental disabilities and mental illness in board and care facilities, and others.

Meals as the Enactment of Social Relationships

Food sharing is the most basic form of reciprocity or exchange. There is no society that does not define what possible foods are edible and that does not prescribe appropriate eating behaviors. Life cycle ceremonies everywhere involve sharing food across households. Almost all holidays, secular and religious, involve some kind of feasting. In religious contexts, food often symbolizes the holiest of states, whether eaten in communion with the divine or offered to the ancestors.

In addition to meeting survival needs, the most important thing about food may be the social relations embedded within meals—that is, the act of dining. "The dining room is concerned, of course, with food," writes Agnes de Mille (1981), "and therefore had been the focal point of my life as a child. It was the place of family interchanges" (p. 197). Although de Mille claims that the dining room is concerned with food, she goes on to talk neither about bread and soup, nor pheasant and soufflés, but about the faces, manners, and emotions associated with the changing roles of the family members who have sat in the various seats.

For de Mille's 32nd wedding anniversary, 1 month after her stroke, her husband Walter brought together a party at the hospital of the people she loved, including her son Jonathan. It prompted memories of many happy celebrations in the past and gave her the sense that she could overcome her disability. The food provided was evidently more for symbol than substance:

> The celebration was topped by the hospital's present, a great big beautiful wedding cake, very rich and delicious. (The wedding cake Walter and Jonathan had brought was later given to the nurses.) And I knew that my friends and Walter were glad that I was alive, glad for me, glad for Walter. Glad for what I was beginning to be able to do. And there was happiness there because I was going to live. And we had toasts, many of them. They did. I had only a thimbleful of the champagne (de Mille, 1981, p. 79).

The celebration strengthened de Mille's resolve to recover. At 8:00 she found herself in bed; her husband leaned over the pillow. "I'm going to live," she whispered. "I'm going to make it. I'll be out of here soon" (1981, p. 80).

For people living at home, enjoyable family meals may mean sacrificing rehabilitation goals of independence. The mother of a small child who is blind continued to spoon-feed her child to preserve quality of life for the family:

> Rosalyn Gibson...told the group that she still spoon-fed her blind three-year-old because the alternatives created such chaos. Meanwhile, the teachers encouraged Nancy to feed herself at school and urged Rosalyn to follow their lead. . . . they spoke of time saved in the long run. Rosalyn thought about the family meals ruined by flying food and recrimination, and the long hours of clean-up. (Featherstone, 1980, p. 29)

To introduce oral feeding successfully to a 22-month-old with Hirschsprung disease, occupational therapist Esther Huecker had to engage the child, Timmy, in a social relationship. Huecker's use of self—her emotions, empathy, judgment—was the lure to reduce Timmy's total dependence on intravenous feeding. Her task was to get him to enjoy food despite his unfamiliarity with hunger and reluctance to put objects in his mouth. After months of treatment, a successful meal became like a "dance" between them:

> His mother had saved his food tray so that we could have dinner together. We began our usual rituals. He brushed his teeth, washed his face, opened all of the containers, and began to smell and name what was on his plate. Timmy picked up a green bean and dipped it into the gravy to lick. I talked about putting gravy on his potatoes, but there was no hole to keep it from spilling. He gingerly poked a hole with his finger and licked the potatoes. He helped to mince some chicken in a grinder and then took small tastes from a spoon. The meal felt like a well-choreographed dance. I could anticipate his needs and prepare him for his risk-taking actions. His success generated more risk taking. After exploring and tasting everything on his tray several times, Timmy announced he was "all done." Picking him up from the high chair, I felt exhilarated that the experience had been so satisfying. Timmy put his arms around my neck and gave me a kiss, something that had never occurred in a spontaneous moment. (Frank et al., 1991, p. 258)

Eating together is a profoundly social act. In this culture and many others when people lack autonomy and cannot reciprocate their dependence on others, anthropologist Murphy (1987) writes, their status is lowered. He describes two young women living together in a wheelchair-adapted apartment in a retirement housing project, whose meals together challenged that potential debasement:

> One is a spinal cord–damaged quadriplegic with good upper body strength, although she has considerable atrophy of the hands. The other has cerebral palsy; she has moderate speech impairment and very limited arm and hand use. Both women use wheelchairs. Nevertheless, they both completed college, where they lived in dorms, and now were sharing an apartment. Each had a van, and the two did their own cooking and shopping, taking care of all their needs. The woman with cerebral palsy was unable to hold and use eating implements, so she was hand-fed by the other. (pp. 201–202)

In the mutual relationship of these two women, one helping the other takes place within a larger context of reciprocity. Together they appear to transform one's "feeding" the other into eating together. In occupational therapy, even when the treatment goal is focused narrowly on helping a person get food to his or her mouth with built-up utensils, eating retains its character as a vehicle for the expression of social membership, cultural aesthetics, and personal preferences.

Grooming and Dressing as Self-Expression

For people with chronic illnesses and disabilities, grooming and dressing present functional problems that vary, depending on the kind of impairment, its severity, access to helpers, architectural barriers, and the availability of suitable clothes and equipment. In addition, as for people everywhere, dress and adornment mark social identity in terms of gender, age grade, occupation, achieved and acquired statuses, ethnicity, and class (Storm, 1987). Ultimately, functional issues affect the display of one's place in society through personal appearance.

Hospital gowns, pajamas or nightgown and slippers worn as daytime attire, and wheelchairs or other adaptive equipment serve to announce: "Here is a sick person!" Disheveled hair and strong body odors, from the standpoint of mainstream North American society, also serve to mark social marginality. They are "stigma symbols" (Goffman, 1963), inviting others to question the individual's social competence, on either a temporary or a permanent basis.

Chronic illnesses and disabilities are stigmatizing, however, only when perceptible or known to others. Grooming and dressing can reveal and conceal information about personal and social identity. Thus, maintaining or achieving control over the presentation of self helps define the meaning of a disability for oneself and to others.

Stigma and Deviance Disavowal

An approach known as social interactionism, developed by the Chicago school of sociologists in the 1930s, holds that people learn to regard themselves according to the reactions they elicit from others (Mead, 1934). The autobiography of Jane Addams, a Progressive Era leader of the settlement movement and co-founder of Hull House, provides a famous example. Although Addams was born with a spinal deformity, her father's supportive regard helped her to internalize a sense of self-worth:

> As a child, Jane Addams imagined herself to be a grotesque outsider: "I prayed with all my heart that the ugly, pigeon-toed little girl, whose crooked back obliged her to walk with her head held very much upon one side, would never be pointed out to the visitors as the daughter of this fine man." The tender gallantry of Mr. Addams bowing

to his little girl and tipping his "high and shining silk hat" in public recognition, a charming fairy-tale picture the older autobiographer remembers with abiding gratitude, prevents a morbid self-hatred from festering in her mind. She could, at least inwardly, hold her head high. (Liebowitz, 1989, p. 119)

The term *stigma* refers to negative social evaluations attached to particular national or ethnic groups, engagement in morally disapproved behaviors, or physical differences of various kinds (Goffman, 1963). To escape from being viewed as inferior, individuals may hide what can be discredited and try to "pass" as normal. Those whose disabilities are highly noticeable may try to "cover" their stigma to minimize its impact.

Scholars in the social interactionist tradition study how people with stigmatized conditions present themselves in daily life to manage the impression they make upon others. Even when they cannot hide their difference, people with disabilities and chronic illnesses do not passively adopt negative evaluations made by others. Instead, they act strategically to influence how they are perceived and treated.

They may vigorously reject the "sick role" (Parsons, 1951), which temporarily exempts individuals from customary social expectations, such as going to work, in return for a loss of status and autonomy while they are getting well. For people who have chronic illnesses or disabilities, the "sick role" threatens to become a permanent trap they must actively struggle against.

One form of resistance is to adopt a militant stance. Activists pointedly display their "stigma symbols" to challenge stereotypes of social inferiority and to combat discrimination. Like blacks, gays, and women, Independent Living and Disability Rights Movement activists have effected changes in laws, policies, and social awareness through strategic exposure of highly stigmatized conditions and oppressive situations (Berkowitz, 1987).

In everyday life, style allows men and women with disabilities—including militants—to reject or "disavow" social deviance (Davis, 1964). The clothing, makeup, and hair styles of a particular period create a language or cultural code (Barthes, 1967; Sahlins, 1976) that individuals use to communicate information about themselves. Like everyone else, people with disabilities use clothing and cosmetics to conceal a perceivable defect, deflect attention from it, or compensate for it (Kaiser, Freeman, & Wingate, 1990). Agnes de Mille (1981) used all three strategies after her stroke:

I bought Chinese suits with long coats and the brace was hidden in my pants [concealment] and I was told I looked very smart. . . . indulging myself with the loveliest tunics and Indian Benares silk pants of contrasting or complementary tones and little colored slippers [deflecting attention]. The more decrepit my body, the more dashing my dress [compensation]—plain but très gai, très daring. Another flag went up the mast to signal my recovering and making my new life a happy one. (p. 223)

Publications by poet and essayist Nancy Mairs (1987, 1989) likewise describe the effective use of clothes to manage the impact of an impairment upon her self-presentation. Diagnosed with multiple sclerosis at about age 30, Mairs lost some ability to groom and dress herself:

With only one usable hand, I have to select my clothing with care not so much for style as for ease of ingress and egress, and even so, dressing can be laborious. I can no longer do fine stitchery, pick up babies, play the piano, braid my hair. (p. 121)

The photo of Mairs on the dust jacket of her memoir *Remembering the Bone House* (1989) shows an attractive woman. Mairs is dressed in a simple shift. Her straight hair cut to chin length and the tilt of her shoulders draw attention to Mair's incisive yet kind dark eyes and generous mouth. A touch of cosmetics (nail polish and lipstick) and a bit of jewelry (long earrings, a wide bangle bracelet, a glimpse of narrow gold chains about her neck and wrist, plain gold wedding ring) add to the effect of a woman in the mainstream. Sensuality and elegance (rather than plainness or disability) are communicated in this portrait.

Not all people want to invest themselves and their resources in grooming and dress, nor is everybody capable. But grooming and dress serve expressive functions regardless, as in the case of Billy, a NICU (Neo-natal Intensive Care Unit) patient born with multiple handicaps, ventilator-dependent, and fed through a gastrostomy tube (Pierce & Frank, 1992). Occupational therapist Doris Pierce writes: "When Billy was dressed in his first baby outfit, his oldest brother, who had refused to see Billy since his first visit, stayed with him all day" (Pierce & Frank, p. 974). In her field notes, Pierce recorded the brother's comment, "He looks like a real baby!"

Finally, there are circumstances in which the display of stigmatizing behaviors, such as those associated with the mentally ill homeless population, may be either self-protective or involuntary. Anthropologist Paul Koegel (1987) writes about homeless women in Los Angeles:

> Were they chronically mentally ill or were they simply reacting very sanely to the enormous stress of an insane situation? Was the fact that they wore four pairs of pants during the summer a reflection of an inability to properly identify weather-appropriate clothing or was it a highly conscious strategy aimed at frustrating potential rapists?...Was their poor hygiene the result of poor self-management skills or their restricted access to sinks and showers? (p. 30).

Occupational therapist Sandra Greene (1992), who studied a day shelter for women in the Los Angeles area, found a wide range of strategies related to grooming and dress among its homeless clients. A few were able to maintain a normal appearance, taking pride in their personal cleanliness and dress. Some rented storage spaces to protect their clothing from theft. They were aware that carrying suitcases or bundles of possessions were stigma symbols marking them as homeless. For others, just taking a shower remained important, even when they made no attempt in their dress to conceal their homelessness:

> For women who value passing as a non-homeless woman, the availability of a place to keep clean is extremely important so that they don't "look like one of these filthy women." For some women who do not seem to take steps to pass as a non-homeless woman, this service is still considered important and is often mentioned as one of the services they like to use at the shelter. (p. 168)

Cultural Stereotypes of Beauty and Fashion as Cultural Code

Stigma is always relative to the dominant values of a particular culture. Anthropologist Nora Groce (1985) studied the population on Martha's Vineyard, where there had been, since the early 17th century, a strikingly high incidence of hereditary deafness due to the small gene pool and frequent intermarriage of families on the island. She discovered that hearing impairments were not stigmatized there:

> I thought to ask Gale what the hearing people in town had thought of the deaf people.
>
> "Oh," he said, "they didn't think anything about them, they were just like everyone else."
>
> "But how did people communicate with them—by writing everything down?"
>
> "No," said Gale, surprised that I should ask such an obvious question, "You see, everyone here spoke sign language."
>
> "You mean the deaf people's families and such?" I inquired.
>
> "Sure," Gale replied, as he wandered into the kitchen to refill his glass and find some more matches, "and everybody else in town too—I used to speak it, my mother did, everybody." (pp. 2–3)

Today, writers in the Disabilities Rights Movement are challenging the dominant standards of beauty and sexuality in society. Research shows that people attribute positive personal traits to persons who are physically attractive and negative traits to those who are seen as abnormal or different (Kaiser et al., 1985). Negative stereotypes of disabled men and women have been perpetuated in television and films, fiction, and drama (Kent, 1987; Longmore, 1987).

Political scientist Harlan Hahn (1988), a polio survivor, poses the question, "Can disability be beautiful?" Hahn suggests that, when confronted with disability, the dominant able-bodied response is to experience an "existential" anxiety (the projected threat of the loss of physical capabilities) and an "aesthetic" anxiety (fear of others whose traits are perceived as disturbing or unpleasant). His historical research indicates, however, that Western cultures have eroticized as well as stigmatized people with physical differences. People with disabilities, he argues, have had a "subversive" sensual appeal.

Hahn urges people with disabilities to speak out as cultural critics of rigid, conformist ideals of the body beautiful. The culturally shared "language" of grooming and dress provides a vocabulary to do so. Some students with disabilities, for example, wear T-shirts with disability rights mottos and humorous slogans that display their social uniqueness and suggest a desire for more attention from society: "I'm no quad; I'm just tired of walking," "High level quads do it with a 'joy stick,'" "I'm accessible," and "If I prove I'm better, will you admit I'm equal?" (Kaiser et al., 1990, p. 42). A printed T-shirt itself is a fashion statement that "reads" differently, depending on the wearer's age, sex, status, occupation (student, account executive), and context (college campus, wedding party).

Growing up without legs and arms except for above-elbow stumps, Diane DeVries has made choices since childhood about her grooming and dress. Her choices embodied cultural ideals of attractiveness *and* challenged negative stereotypes about the handicapped. As a child, Diane wore shift dresses over a three-wheeled "scooter" used with a crutch. In puberty, she began to regard the scooter as strange-looking and decided to use an electric wheelchair instead.

While any adaptive equipment is normally a "stigma symbol," a wheelchair was more appropriate for Diane than her three-wheeled scooter, especially at the county rehabilitation facility where she then resided. Living among teenagers and young adults with disabilities, Diane participated in a peer culture of disability and modeled herself after a young women with a spinal cord injury who encouraged her to use her feminine assets to look "together." For Diane, this has meant:

> …to go around in whatever you're in, your wheelchair, or your braces, or whatever, and not look clumsy. It's not looking "self-assured" either. I keep wanting to say that, but I don't think that's the word. I mean, people are already looking at you. You know, any crip's going to be looked at. But at least if they look at you, at least they'll say: "Wow, look at that person in the wheelchair. Hey, but you know, not too bad!" (Frank, 1986, p. 208)

Some individuals with amputations choose to wear long sleeves or full skirts to conceal their missing limbs:

> — I get a different response from people when I wear short sleeves so I very seldom wear short sleeves. It camouflages my disability (missing arm) when I wear long sleeves.

> — Because of my amputation at the hip, I prefer dresses without a waist or gathering at the bodice of the dress. Dresses that flare out more at the tail are more attractive. (Kaiser et al., 1990, p. 39)

Diane prefers, however, to wear form-fitting clothes that accentuate her assets.

Displaying what she *does* have has been a better strategy for her than attempting to conceal her multiple limb deficiencies:

> Like when I was a kid, I hated wearing skirts and dresses, because with a skirt you could notice even more that there are legs missing than when you wore shorts and a top. Shorts and a top fitted your body and that made the fact that no legs were there not look so bad. (Frank, 1986, p. 209)

Overcoming Barriers to Self-Expression

Dependence upon "helpers"—family members, professionals, and attendants—can hinder or facilitate the ability of people with disabilities to project an authentic self through their appearance. Diane DeVries liked dresses with narrow straps that she could slip into by herself and that allowed her the greatest freedom of movement. Her clothing preferences were opposed, however, by members of her rehabilitation team:

> Diane prefers wearing spaghetti strap or other low cut sun dresses because she feels less encumbered and can also undress more easily. Those present felt that this is somewhat unattractive and possibly disturbing. It has been suggested to the family that she wear unbuttoned bolero jackets over the dresses but this has not been carried through. The subject of Diane's appearance to those present and to those around her was discussed at length. This seems to be a definite problem. Some felt that the cart [which Diane uses for mobility] is disturbing to behold. Some felt that they prefer seeing her with the prosthesis and others dissented. This area might be explored further as this seems to be a somewhat problematic area. (Frank, 1986, p. 207)

Diane suggests that people with handicaps need to be assertive with helpers to take control of their grooming and dress:

> Like me, I would never wear a skirt, a long skirt, like they used to. I've even seen some people with no arms wearing long sleeves pinned up or rolled clumsily so they're *this* fat. You can find a lot of clothes that fit you. It's not hard. If they have someone take care of them, they won't tell them: "No. I want my hair this way." They'll just let them do it. That's dumb. It's *your* body. They're helping *you* out. (Frank, 1986, p. 210)

At conventions of Little People of America (LPA), a self-help organization for people of profound short stature, one of the most best-attended events is the annual fashion show (Ablon, 1984). Although most little people could wear children's clothing with minor alterations and children's shoes, children's styles are inappropriate for mature people. The fashion show displays clothing made by the models themselves or made for them, and adult-size clothing adapted with major alterations. Women model elegant suits, dresses, and sports clothes, while men usually model formal suits. LPA members also attend sewing workshops and patronize representatives of tailoring firms who fit them and take custom orders. Women sometimes order shoes from Hong Kong, where average sizes are smaller than in the United States.

When a person with a disability reclaims his or her appearance as an essential feature of self-expression and social identity, it can be a deeply affirming experience. Ernestine Amani Patterson (1985) had an intense desire to wear her hair braided in cornrows, African-style, with colorful beads and tinkling bells. Her blindness limited her. After discouragement from beauticians and others, her desire was gratified by a woman from Liberia, owner of "a most exotic African artifacts shop." It was an important means for Patterson to reject the stigma of disability and claim her identity as a Black sister:

> Of course, people are still the same—inevitable and specific in their cruelty—"Your hair is pretty," or "Your dress is pretty." The lines between womanhood and blindness are never supposed to meet. And with Blackness on top of that, what must people be

seeing! And although I seldom hear: "*You* are looking nice," I am not the same, even if they are. Since that Saturday in the shop with the wooden floor and squeaky steps, where the heater had to be turned on against the chilly morning, I have always looked forward to the bus ride and short walk there. Mrs. Younger [her Liberian friend] has not only increased her clientele, other girlfriends of hers from Africa help out with the hair. So it's lovely talking to all of them. And since most of these women are used to me now, we relate as Black sisters. And though this was not a first step in my growth, mine is actually a case wherein the style of my hair altered the shape of my head within. How many women can say that with satisfaction about *any* beauty treatment they try? (p. 243)

Conclusion

The personal meanings of self-care are based in society. Diseases and impairments take on specific, shared meanings in particular historical contexts. Cultural factors, such as the dominant values promoted in national, ethnic, and local traditions; the division of labor by age and sex within a specific family; and class relations, all contribute to the framework for individual experiences through which personal meanings emerge.

Narratives of people with chronic illnesses and disabilities in the mainstream of the United States and other developed countries emphasize that, after survival needs are met, the central problems of disability are occupational. Impairments prevent people from learning or maintaining the performance of customary activities that give their lives substance and meaning. The potential for fundamental self-esteem or profound shame is embedded in the successes or failures people experience in even the most mundane aspects of self-care. Personal identity and social relations are at stake.

Occupational therapists can assist people with disabilities first by recognizing that mundane activities of self-care are deeply meaningful. People must cope with feelings of frustration when their performance of customary activities breaks down. They experience anger and depression over losses of control, temporal distortion in everyday routines, feelings of infantilization and dehumanization related to helplessness and dependence on others, reconfigurations of familial relations that promote distress and guilt, and various other situational anxieties.

Rehabilitation issues such as adjustment to the losses of function and to social stigma have long been considered psychological. But the meaning of impairments is equally social, cultural, and occupational. Resources based in social policy are essential: basic health care, rehabilitation services, attendant care, equipment, employment opportunities, and income supports. Caregivers make a significant difference.

Perhaps most important, from the standpoint of the individual, is the process of adaptation over time. The meaning of symptoms depends in part on their timing within an overall illness or disability trajectory. Abilities and contexts change. The ability to reevaluate cultural rules about "the right way" to do things can make impairments, at any point, less handicapping and less stigmatizing. Experience over time, and practice, can result in methods and models of self-care that enhance, rather than limit, personal and social identity. ◆

References

Abel, E.K., & Nelson M. (1990). Circles of care: An introductory essay. In E.K. Abel & M.K. Nelson (Eds.), *Circles of care: Work and identity in women's lives* (pp. 4–34). Albany, NY: State University of New York Press.

Ablon, J. (1984). *Little people in America: The social dimensions of dwarfism.* New York: Praeger.

Asch, A., & Fine, M. (1988). Introduction: Beyond pedestals. In M. Fine & A. Asch (Eds.), *Women with disabilities: Essays in psychology, culture, and politics* (pp. 1–37). Philadelphia: Temple University Press.

Barthes, R. (1967). *Système de la mode.* Paris: Seuil.

Bayer, R. (1989). *Private acts, social consequences: AIDS and the politics of public health.* New York: Free Press.

Beisser, A.R. (1989). *Flying without wings: Personal reflections on being disabled.* New York: Doubleday.

Bell, R. (1985). *Holy anorexia.* Chicago: University of Chicago Press.

Berkowitz, E.D. (1987). *Disabled policy: America's programs for the handicapped.* New York: Cambridge University Press.

Bordo, S. (1990). Reading the slender body. In M. Jacobus, E.F. Keller, & S. Shuttleworth (Eds.), *Body/politics: Women and the discourses of science* (pp. 83–112). New York: Routledge & Kegan Paul.

Brandt, A.M. (1988). AIDS: From social history to social policy. In E. Fee & D.M. Fox, (Eds.), *AIDS: The burdens of history* (pp. 147–171). Berkeley: University of California Press.

Buckley, P. (Ed.). (1986). *Essential papers on object relations.* New York: New York University.

Clark, F.A., Parham, D., Carlson, M.E., Frank, G., Jackson, J., Pierce, D., Wolfe, R.J., & Zemke, R. (1991). Occupational science: Academic innovation in the service of occupational therapy's future. *American Journal of Occupational Therapy, 45,* 300–310.

Corbin, J.M., & Strauss, A. (1988). *Unending work and care: Managing chronic illness at home.* San Francisco: Jossey-Bass.

Davis, F. (1964). Deviance disavowal: The management of strained interaction by the visibly handicapped. In H. Becker (Ed.), *The other side: Perspectives on deviance* (pp. 119–137). New York: Free Press.

de Mille, A. (1981). *Reprieve: A memoir.* New York: Doubleday.

DeVries, D. (1992). *Autobiography.* Unpublished manuscript.

Eisenberg, L. (1977). Disease and illness: Distinctions between professional and popular ideas of sickness. *Culture, Medicine, and Psychiatry, 1,* 9–23.

Ekman, P. (1980). Biological and cultural contributions to body and facial movement in the expression of emotion. In A.O. Rorty (Ed.), *Explaining emotions* (pp. 73–201). Berkeley: University of California Press.

Erikson, E. (1968). The life cycle: Epigenesis of identity. In *Identity: Youth and Crisis* (pp. 91–141). New York: Norton.

Featherstone, H. (1980). *A difference in the family: Living with a disabled child.* New York: Penguin.

Fee, E. (1988). Sin versus science: Venereal disease in twentieth-century Baltimore. In E. Fee & D.M. Fox (Eds.), *AIDS: The burdens of history* (pp. 121–146). Berkeley: University of California Press.

Finger, A. (1990). *Past due: A story of disability, pregnancy and birth.* Seattle, WA: Seal Press.

Fisher, B. & Tronto, J. (1990). Toward a feminist theory of caring. In E.K. Abel & M.K. Nelson (Eds.), *Circles of care: Work and identity in women's lives* (pp. 35–62). Albany, New York: State University of New York Press.

Frank, G. (1986). On embodiment: A case study of congenital limb deficiency in American culture. *Culture, Medicine and Psychiatry, 10,* 189–219.

Frank, G., Huecker, E., Segal, R., Forwell, S., & Bagatell, N. (1991). Assessment and treatment of a pediatric patient in chronic care: Ethnographic methods applied to occupational therapy practice. *American Journal of Occupational Therapy, 45,* 252–263.

Gliedman, J., & Roth, W. (1980). *The unexpected minority: Handicapped children in America.* New York: Harcourt Brace Jovanovich.

Goffman, E. (1963). *Stigma: Notes on the management of spoiled identity.* Englewood Cliffs, NJ: Prentice Hall.

Greene, S.L. (1992). *An ethnographic study of homeless mentally ill women: Adaptive strategies, needs and services.* Unpublished master's thesis, University of Southern California, Los Angeles.

Greenfeld, J. (1972). *A child called Noah.* New York: Holt, Rinehart & Winston.

Groce, N.E. (1985). *Everyone here spoke sign language: Hereditary deafness on Martha's Vineyard.* Cambridge, MA: Harvard University Press.

Hahn, H. (1988). Can disability be beautiful? *Social Policy, 18,* 26–32.

Harris, Louis, & Associates. (1986). *The ICD survey of disabled Americans: Bringing disabled Americans into the mainstream.* New York: International Center for the Disabled.

Hochschild, A. (1989). *The second shift: Working parents and the revolution at home.* New York: Viking.

Kaiser, S.B., Freeman, C.M., & Wingate, S.B. (1990). Stigmata and negotiated outcomes: Management of appearance by persons with physical disabilities. In M. Nagler (Ed.), *Perspectives on disability* (pp. 33–45). Palo Alto, CA: Health Markets Research. (Reprinted from *Deviant Behavior, 6,* 205–224).

Kent, D. (1987). Disabled women: Portraits in fiction and drama. In A. Gartner & T. Joe (Eds.), *Images of the disabled, disabling images* (pp. 47–63). New York: Praeger.

Kleinman, A. (1988). *The illness narratives: Suffering, healing, and the human condition.* New York: Basic Books.

Koegel, P. (1987). Ethnographic perspectives on homeless and homeless mentally ill women. In P. Koegel (Ed.), *Proceedings of a two-day workshop sponsored by the Division of Education and Service Systems Liaison.* Bethesda, MD: National Institute of Mental Health.

Leibowitz, H. (1989). The sheltering self: Jane Addams's *Twenty Years at Hull-House.* In *Fabricating lives: Explorations in American autobiography* (pp. 115–156). New York: Knopf.

Lipton, J.A., & Marbach, J.J. (1984). Ethnicity and the pain experience. *Social Science and Medicine, 19,* 1279–1298.

Longmore, P.K. (1987). Screening stereotypes: Images of disabled people in television and motion pictures. In A. Gartner & T. Joe (Eds.), *Images of the disabled, disabling images* (pp. 65–78). New York: Praeger.

Lorde, A. (1980). *The cancer journals.* San Francisco: Spinsters Ink.

Mairs, N. (1987). On being a cripple. In M. Saxton & F. Howe (Eds.), *With Wings: An anthology of literature by and about women with disabilities* (pp. 118–127). New York: The Feminist Press.

Mairs, N. (1989). *Remembering the bone house: An erotics of place and space.* New York: Harper & Row.

Mead, G.H. (1934). *Mind, self, and society: From the standpoint of a social behaviorist.* Chicago: The University of Chicago Press.

Murphy, R.F. (1987). *The body silent.* New York: Henry Holt.

Nolan, C. (1987). *Under the eye of the clock: The life story of Christopher Nolan.* New York: St. Martin's Press.

Parsons, T. (1951). Illness and the role of the physician: A sociological perspective. *American Journal of Orthopsychiatry, 21,* 452–460.

Patterson, E.A. (1985). Glimpse into transformation. In S.E. Browne, D. Connors, & N. Stern (Eds.), *With the power of each breath: A disabled women's anthology* (pp. 240–243). Pittsburgh, PA: Cleis Press.

Pierce, D., & Frank, G. (1992). A mother's work: Feminist perspectives on family-centered care. *American Journal of Occupational Therapy, 46,* 972–980.

Plough, A.L. (1986). *Borrowed time: Artificial organs and the politics of extending lives.* Philadelphia: Temple University Press.

Plough, A.L., & Salem, S.R. (1982). Social and contextual factors in the analysis of mortality in end-stage renal disease patients. *American Journal of Public Health, 72,* 1293–1295.

Rosenberg, C.E. (1987). *The care of strangers: The rise of American's hospital system.* New York: Basic Books.

Rosenberg, C.E. (1988). Disease and social order in America: Perceptions and expectations. In E. Fee & D.M. Fox (Eds.), *AIDS: The burdens of history* (pp. 12–32). Berkeley: University of California Press.

Sahlins, M. (1976). La pensee bourgeoise: Western society as culture. In *Culture and practical reasons* (pp. 166–204). Chicago: University of Chicago Press.

Scheper-Hughes, N., & Lock, M.M. (1987). The mindful body: A prolegomenon to future work in medical anthropology. *Medical Anthropology Quarterly, 1,* 6–41.

Sontag, S. (1978). *Illness as metaphor.* New York: Farrar, Straus and Giroux.

Strauss, A., & Corbin, J.M. (1988). *Shaping a new health care system: The explosion of chronic illness as a catalyst for change.* San Francisco: Jossey-Bass.

Storm, P. (1987). *Functions of dress: Tool of culture and the individual.* Englewood Cliffs, NJ: Prentice Hall.

Treichler, P.A. (1988). AIDS, gender, and biomedical discourse: Current contests for meaning. In E. Fee & D.M. Fox (Eds.), *AIDS: The burdens of history* (pp. 109–266). Berkeley: University of California Press.

Webster, B.D. (1989). *All of a piece: A life with multiple sclerosis.* Baltimore: Johns Hopkins University Press.

Wolff, B.B., & Langley, S. (1968). Cultural factors and the response to pain: A review. *American Anthropologist, 70,* 494–500.

Wright, B.A. (1983). *Physical disability—A psychosocial approach* (2nd ed.). New York: Harper & Row.

Yerxa, E.J., Clark, F., Frank, G., Jackson, J., Parham, D., Pierce, D., Stein, C., & Zemke, R. (1990). An introduction to occupational science, A foundation for occupational therapy in the 21st century. *Occupational Therapy in Health Care, 6,* 1–17.

Zborowski, M. (1969). *People in pain.* San Francisco: Jossey-Bass.

Zola, I.K. (1982). *Missing pieces: A chronicle of living with a disability.* Philadelphia: Temple University Press.

3

Assessment of Self-Care Skills

Catherine Backman

Catherine Backman, MS, OT(C), *is a Senior Instructor in the Division of Occupational Therapy at the School of Rehabilitation Sciences at the University of British Columbia, Vancouver, Canada.*

Chapter 3 Outline

Purpose of Self-Care Assessment

Client-Centered Assessment

The Relationship Between Self-Care Performance and Performance Components

Self-Report Versus Observation of Actual Performance

A Strategy for Assessing Self-Care

Client Priorities

Selecting Instruments

Validate and Communicate

Instruments for Assessing Self-Care

Characteristics

A Review

Conclusion

References

*"Functional assessment is
the measurement of purposeful behavior in interaction with the environment,
which is interpreted according to the assessment's intended uses."*
(Halpern & Fuhrer, 1984, p. 3)

The purpose of this chapter is to describe and discuss ways of assessing self-care. The literature refers to many instruments and recommendations for evaluating self-care and activities of daily living (Law & Letts, 1989). The challenge to the occupational therapist is to develop an effective strategy to evaluate self-care ability and to select the appropriate instrument(s) for specific clients. Some instruments are standardized, many are not; some are diagnosis specific; few are based in theory (McDowell & Newell, 1987) or adequately validated (Law & Usher, 1988). In practice, "most occupational therapists use homegrown evaluation tools that lack known validity or reliability" (Fisher, 1992b, p. 278). It is time to change this practice.

Before proceeding, it is useful to clarify some of the terms as they tend to be used in the literature. *Functional*, as used in the terms *functional assessment, functional status*, and *functional performance*, usually describes a broad range of activities, including self- and home maintenance, and participation in work and leisure pursuits. Most authors use *activities of daily living* (ADL) to refer to self-care and mobility, rather than to the vast array of activities implied by the phrase. ADL and self-care are synonymous terms for the purpose of citations from the literature in this chapter. The typical activities included under the term *self-care* are eating, drinking, bathing, toileting, dressing, mobility, medication management, and functional communication. *Instrumental activities of daily living* (IADL) refers to those activities beyond self-care that one requires for independent living, such as meal preparation, housekeeping chores, and transportation within the local community. IADL is not addressed in this chapter, but the literature pertinent to self-care refers to those activities from time to time. *Assessment* broadly refers to the process of collecting, interpreting, and documenting data about a client's current status. An assessment may include the use of one or more *tools, instruments*, or *scales* that categorize or quantify a skill or behavior of interest.

Purpose of Self-Care Assessment

There are at least four reasons for assessing self-care ability (Alexander & Fuhrer, 1984; Donaldson, Wagner, & Gresham, 1973):

1. *To describe self-care status.* An objective description of a client's self-care ability at a given point in time can be useful to identify problems, goals, and plans for therapy. It will indicate if, or how much, personal assistance is required to complete self-care tasks, and assist in discharge planning. A description of status may be required to determine compensation for clients who sustained temporary or permanent injuries attributed to the negligence of others.

2. *To measure change and monitor progress.* Periodic assessment will help monitor the effects of therapy by detecting improvement or changes in performance that can guide further intervention.

3. *To facilitate communication and decision making.* The results of a self-care assessment will enhance communication among the therapist, client, team members, family, and others involved in treatment or providing assistance in self-care tasks. Assessment results also guide decision making on the part of the

client, especially when it comes to prioritizing goals for therapy, or choosing between independence and personal assistance in managing self-care.

4. *To evaluate programs and conduct research.* Use of standardized instruments helps promote comparability in research or evaluation of outcomes attributed to therapeutic programs.

Occupational therapists involved in one or more of the above activities need to offer credible assessment results to contribute meaningfully to these activities. Client-centered assessment, the relationship between performance of self-care and performance components (or skill constituents), and the use of self-report versus observation of actual performance all warrant consideration. After discussing these issues, a strategy for assessment will be described and selected instruments reviewed.

Readers unfamiliar with a cited instrument title may wish to refer to the description in the review section at the end of this chapter before continuing.

Client-Centered Assessment

Client-centered assessment refers to acknowledgment of the client's roles, values, and priorities, so the client's important tasks or activities focus the assessment process. Self-care, as one of three occupational performance areas, is rarely assessed in isolation. While self-care skills are fundamental to an individual's independence, they represent only a portion of a comprehensive approach to rehabilitation, and the "repertoire of behaviors required to lead a meaningful existence is obviously much broader" (Keith, 1984, p. 75). The relevance or importance to a given client of performing self-care activities should be evaluated before the occupational therapist selects a self-care evaluation tool. The shift toward the client's active participation in the assessment process, and evaluating that which the client needs or wants to do, has been documented by several sources (Alexander & Fuhrer, 1984; Canadian Association of Occupational Therapists & Health Services Directorate [CAOT & HSD], Health & Welfare Canada, 1991; Fisher, 1992a; Law et al., 1991; Tugwell et al., 1987). Alexander and Fuhrer suggest that the rehabilitation field should expand opportunities to investigate the array of activities that match the client's personal goals, stressing the importance of measuring how well the client performs in his or her customary environment, rather than in the hospital or clinic. "Anderson, for example, found that the usual brand of rehabilitation does not prepare individuals to live in an urban ghetto" (Keith, p. 75). This train of thought begins to build a case against the use of standardized self-care instruments because these instruments have an inadequate number of items to cover all situations, and normative data would have little meaning in individual contexts. On the other hand, a seemingly endless list of self-care tasks may help to describe the individual situation, but serves little purpose as an instrument to measure change or the effectiveness of occupational therapy intervention. Accordingly, both standardized and non-standardized instruments have a place in assessing function.

Functional assessments need to relate to an overall rehabilitation goal that is environment-specific; that is, clients should be assessed in the environments in which they choose to live and seek success (Cohen & Anthony, 1984). The demands of the environment, and the interaction between client and environment, need to be considered as part of the self-care assessment. Effective assessments are always individualized and capture the uniqueness of the client, regardless of the use of standardized instruments in the process. Cohen and Anthony suggest that an assessment always begins and ends with the client; that is, the client identifies what needs to be assessed, and the occupational therapist shares the resulting assessment data with the client for validation. Only then will the information be meaningful in planning an intervention strategy. The relative importance of independence in self-care varies with the individual. A frequently cited example is that of a person who accepts being dependent in personal hygiene or dressing because this permits spending a greater amount of time at work (Alexander & Fuhrer, 1984). It is therefore critical to be aware of the client's goals throughout the assessment and intervention process. This does not imply that the occupational therapist should withhold an informed opinion that could modify client goals, but suggests that negotiation among health care providers, client, and family should direct the assessment and intervention plans. One way to operationalize a client-centered approach is described by Tugwell et al. (1987), who assessed physical disabilities among people with arthritis. They began with the statement, "Please tell me which activities are affected by your arthritis," and then ranked the top five activities by asking, "Which of these activities would you most like to be able to do?" until they identified five priority activities. They propose that this approach may make an instrument more responsive to change, assuming intervention focuses on the client's priorities as determined in the rank-ordered list.

A number of important decisions are made based on a person's ability to perform self-care requirements. An individual who cannot eat, bathe, or dress independently requires some type of personal assistance. Previous occupational roles and social and physical environments may change. A possible outcome following evaluation of self-care activities is the determination of if, and how much, care or assistance is necessary. This contributes to decisions regarding discharge from acute and rehabilitation facilities back to the preadmission environment or into long-term care, nursing, or supported home care environments. A meaningful assessment employs a collaborative process and gives the client the opportunity to choose the tasks that require evaluation (Fisher, 1992a), based on the environment in which he or she chooses to live.

The Relationship Between Self-Care Performance and Performance Components

Occupational performance is supported by performance components, specifically the interaction among the physical, mental, sociocultural, and spiritual aspects of the individual (CAOT & HSD, 1991). Understanding the relationship between occupational performance areas, such as self-care, and performance components, is important when evaluating the causes of dysfunction and subsequent intervention plans.

Standardized assessments are sometimes helpful in identifying who is in need of therapeutic services, but give little information on how to target intervention (Fisher, 1992b). "That is, they tell us what a person can and cannot do (e.g., dress, eat), but not why or why not (e.g., limited dexterity, memory loss, apraxia) or whether the client wants or needs to do the task" (Fisher, p. 278). Further, pathology or impairment does not necessarily mean the client is unable to achieve a goal that was formerly achieved without the pathology or impairment. For example, decreased hand strength resulting from arthritis does not necessarily mean one can no longer open a can of tomatoes (Lawton, 1990). Understanding the relationship between performance areas and performance components or constituent skills will help occupational therapists target interventions to the particular needs of individual clients. Only a few investigations have begun to examine this relationship as it relates to self-care performance.

In a study of the relationship between cognitive skills performance and activities of daily living, Carter, Oliveira, Duponte, and Lynch (1988) evaluated the effect of 3 weeks of cognitive skills training on a group of adults who had recently sustained a stroke. The control group of 16 subjects received the setting's usual occupational therapy, physical therapy, and speech therapy services, and the experimental group of 17 subjects received the same services plus cognitive retraining (defined as completion of *The Thinking Skills Workbook*). The Barthel Index[1] was administered to all subjects on admission and discharge. Although the experimental group had, on average, higher mean scores on the Barthel Index, this was not statistically significant (see Figure 1 for a discussion on significance). When ceiling scores representing complete independence were excluded from analysis, there were significant differences in hygiene, bathing, and toileting, with the experimental group performing better than the control group ($p < .05$) (Carter et al.). The same investigators conducted a second study of 21 adults, each of whom had sustained a stroke. The Kenny Self-Care Evaluation was administered prior to commencing the cognitive training and again 3 to 4 weeks afterwards. On average, Kenny Self-Care scores improved 26.2%, and cognitive skills improved 24.26%.

Correlations between specific cognitive skills and ADL skills suggested several relationships (see Figure 2 for a discussion on correlation). For example, hygiene, as measured by the Kenny Self-Care evaluation, correlated with visual-spatial perception ($r = .65$), auditory attention ($r = .63$) and visual scanning ($r = .49$). Dressing correlated with auditory attention ($r = .52$) and visual-spatial perception ($r = .46$). Transfers correlated with auditory attention ($r = .46$) and time judgment ($r = .45$). Correlations do not indicate cause and effect, so it cannot be assumed that remediation of a cognitive deficit, say visual-spatial perception, would improve performance of hygiene activities. However, if the correlation coefficient indicates a strong relationship, changes in one variable (e.g., visual-spatial perception) can help predict changes in the second variable (e.g., performing hygiene activities).

In an investigation with a similar purpose, perceptual-motor performance was found to be significantly related to ADL performance, while visual perception was not (Titus, Gall, Yerxa, Roberson, & Mack, 1991). Twenty-five adult subjects who had sustained a stroke were evaluated with an array of perceptual tests and the Klein-Bell ADL Scale. Significant correlations resulted between a number of perceptual items and upper-extremity hygiene,

Figure 1. Statistical significance.

Statistics are used in group comparison research to assist the investigator in making inferences from the behavior of the sample group to the larger population of interest. A specific statistical test is applied to determine if observed changes in behavior or differences between groups are due to chance or not. Prior to applying the statistical test, a level of confidence or probability is selected as the criterion for statistical significance. A statistically significant result means that the probability value obtained is equal to or less than the level of confidence or probability selected in advance. By convention, .05 and .01 are the more commonly used levels of significance. Even if results reach these levels of statistical significance, there is still a 5% or 1% chance (respectively) of experimental error. Further, statistical significance is influenced by the size and heterogeneity of the sample, and merely indicates a change or difference in behavior that was somewhat consistent across the sample—the change may not have substantial impact on everyday living, and therefore results should be carefully reviewed for their clinical or applied significance to the situation studied (Ottenbacher, 1986).

---

[1]The Barthel Index, and other self-care instruments cited in this discussion, are described in the instrument review at the end of this chapter.

Figure 2. Correlation.

Correlations are statistics used to measure the relationship between a pair of variables. There are a number of different correlation coefficients, the use of which depends on the type of data collected. Commonly used correlation coefficients include the Pearson Product-Moment Correlation Coefficient (r), the Spearman Rank Order Correlation Coefficient (r_s), and the Intra-class Correlation Coefficient (*ICC*). All correlation coefficients vary in value from -1 through 0 to +1. A coefficient of 1 (or -1) indicates a perfect relationship; that is, the change in one variable occurs in direct proportion to the change in the second variable. The sign indicates the direction of the relationship: a positive sign indicates that both variables are changing in the same direction, and a negative relationship indicates that the two variables change in opposition to one another. The value of the correlation indicates the strength of the relationship. Values close to 0 are generally interpreted as poor, and values close to +1 or -1 are considered excellent, with those in the mid-range considered fair. However, the sample size influences the confidence with which correlation coefficients can be interpreted (i.e., lower values are acceptable in larger samples). (Oyster, Hanten, & Llorens, 1987)

eating, and dressing. The strongest relationship with the Klein-Bell total ADL score was with the shape subtest of the Haptic Visual Discrimination Test ($r = .51$, $p = .01$).

Jongbloed, Brighton, and Stacey (1988) examined factors associated with independent meal preparation, self-care, and mobility in a group of 90 clients who had sustained a stroke. The sample was comprised of 49 males and 41 females, with an average age of 71.32 years. Forty-six had a right cerebrovascular accident (CVA) and 44 had a left CVA. There was a relationship between self-care, as measured by the Barthel Index, and meal preparation, as evaluated by an occupational therapist's ratings of independence in preparing soup and a sandwich ($r = .56$). The relationship between motor planning and self-care was poor ($r = .28$).

As part of a project to develop an IADL screening measure, Fillenbaum (1985) performed a factor analysis of ADL and IADL abilities for a sample of 3,751 older adults (> 60 years) from Virginia and Ohio. The OARS questionnaire rated abilities in physical activities of daily living (PADL) and IADL (community living skills, such as cooking, transportation, and home maintenance activities). The PADL items loaded on one factor and the IADL items loaded on two other factors. Four items could not be considered to load on any factor: use of the telephone, taking medications, ability to bathe or shower, and continence. It was suggested, then, that IADL items do measure an activity differently from PADL. This lends some support to the idea that therapists should refrain from making assumptions about how a client will manage IADL tasks based on performance in ADL, and vice versa. Interestingly, continence and the ability to bathe, items found in many self-care instruments, did not load on the same factor as did other PADL tasks.

Self-Report Versus Observation of Actual Performance

Self-care instruments may use interviews, written questionnaires, or direct observation of performance to obtain data. Data may consist of numerical scores intended to quantify the client's performance, or they may be narrative descriptions. Interviews and questionnaires may use the self-report method, where the client responds to the questions, or the proxy report method, where a family member or caregiver provides the information. Some instruments are designed for use by either interview or observation, or a combination of both. Jette (1987) points out major advantages to self-report instruments, including their low cost and relative speed of administration. He also cites their questionable reliability and validity as a major criticism—is it really valid to judge performance based on a person's recollection of what he or she can do, rather than on observing the person performing a task? In his comparison of a self-report instrument (the Functional Status Index) and observations of activities of daily living as made by a physical therapist, the agreement ranged from .71 to .95, suggesting some consistency between the two types of evaluation. The most common discrepancy was patients underreporting their performance when compared to the performance test. However, the patient's report was based on actual behavior in the past week, whereas the performance test consisted of specific tasks done at the request of the physical therapist on the day of the visit. The patients may have been capable of performing the task in isolation as part of the test, but unable to perform at that level in the context of their daily living.

The difference between the client's capability and actual behavior or performance needs careful consideration. An assessment of capability measures the limits of performance, and is a poor indicator of what the client actually does in daily life (Alexander & Fuhrer, 1984). Inquiries about what a client "can do" (i.e., capability) exaggerate healthiness by up to 20%, while asking what tasks the client actually *does* (i.e., behavior) appears to overcome this (McDowell & Newell, 1987). A client may be capable of doing a defined task under contrived circumstances, or on an occasional basis, but unable to do so on a regular basis. Actual behavior, however, can only be measured in the environment in which a person lives day-to-day (Alexander & Fuhrer). Edwards (1990), in a study of the reliability of Lawton and Brody's physical self-maintenance scale (PSMS) and IADL scale, reported that subjects consistently overrated their ability in both self-maintenance and IADL tasks, and subsequently recommended direct observation rather than self-report. Occupational therapists have long been advocates of visiting clients in their own homes, as this is the ideal environment for assessing occupational performance. Given the possibility of inaccurate self-report, therapists working in home health agencies are well advised to select tools that measure actual performance. These therapists can also compare actual performance in the home with self-report tools, in order to investigate further the usefulness of the less expensive self-report format. Therapists "confined" to institutional settings are limited to observing performance under contrived circumstances, and at best make suppositions about performance at home. In this case, interviews about activities at home may supplement the therapist's interpretation of observed assessment data.

The effects of different data sources in functional assessment interviews were examined by comparing the results on the same scale using three different informants: clients (inpatients), a close relative or friend, and the client's nurse (Rubenstein, Schairer, Wieland, & Kane, 1984). A sample of 61 inpatients more than 65 years of age were assessed with Lawton and Brody's PSMS and IADL scale (Lawton, 1971), by interviewing the client, the nurse working with that client, and a close friend or relative (proxy) who lived with or frequently spent time with the client. An analysis of variance (ANOVA) demonstrated a significant effect for data source; that is, there was a significant difference in the data depending on its source. Clients gave the highest scores (most able), followed by nurses, then the proxies. The discrepancy between client and proxy was greatest when the proxy was a spouse. The same investigators compared scores on the Katz Index of ADL obtained from 68 nursing home residents, and their day and night nurses. There was 72.4% agreement between resident and day nurse, and 72.1% agreement between resident and night nurse. When there was disagreement, the nurses tended to rate the resident as requiring more assistance than the resident indicated. Rubenstein et al. (1984) concluded from these two studies that while there is similarity among sources, the similarity is probably not strong enough to use scores from different sources interchangeably.

A Strategy for Assessing Self-Care

The following proposes a strategy for assessing an individual's performance in self-care. It assumes that an assessment will be client-centered and will make use of direct observation of performance where appropriate.

Client Priorities

Identify the client's priorities and only proceed with a self-care evaluation if it is relevant to that client. One instrument based on this orientation is the Canadian Occupational Performance Measure (COPM) (Law et al., 1991). The COPM is an "outcome measure designed for use by occupational therapists to assess clients' perception of their occupational performance" (Law et al., p. 1). It is not limited to the evaluation of self-care, but helps determine if self-care is problematic and should be evaluated in more detail. Based on the model of occupational performance described in *Occupational Therapy Guidelines for Client-Centred Practice* (CAOT & HSD, 1991), the COPM is a semi-structured interview that asks clients if they need to, want to, or are expected to perform activities in the three occupational performance areas of self-care, productivity, and leisure. Once the client identifies performance problems, the problems are weighted on a 10-point scale of importance. Up to five of the most pressing problems are then rated on two scales: a 10-point performance scale representing the client's ability to do the task; and a 10-point scale representing the client's satisfaction with his or her performance. The products of the importance rating multiplied by the performance rating, and the importance rating multiplied by the satisfaction rating, provide scores for measuring change in client status over time. The COPM involves the client in identifying key occupational performance problems, making it an ideal initial assessment tool. In the event that the client identifies one or more self-care problems as priorities, specific evaluation tools can be selected to collect additional data. For example, if the client identifies dressing and bathing as problems, an observational assessment of these self-care activities would be a logical second step.

Selecting Instruments

Select one or more instruments based on the priorities established with the client in step one and on the purpose of the instrument(s). The assessment is most often required to identify problems, goals for intervention, and the intervention's effects. It is important, then, that the occupational therapist select assessment tools that will not only measure change, but that will measure change within the therapist's own domain of practice. It is further recommended that occupational therapists limit the number of instruments they use in their practice (Law & Letts, 1989) in order to learn how the instrument(s) respond and discriminate among clients of differing ability, and to enhance communication with team members. Law (1987) developed a decision tree for guiding the therapist's review and selection of instruments (see Figure 3).

Validate and Communicate

Share the data obtained through the self-care instruments with the client, and use the client to validate the interpretation of findings. Document and communicate the findings with others who need to know, such as the family, team members, or referral

Figure 3. Instrument evaluation process.

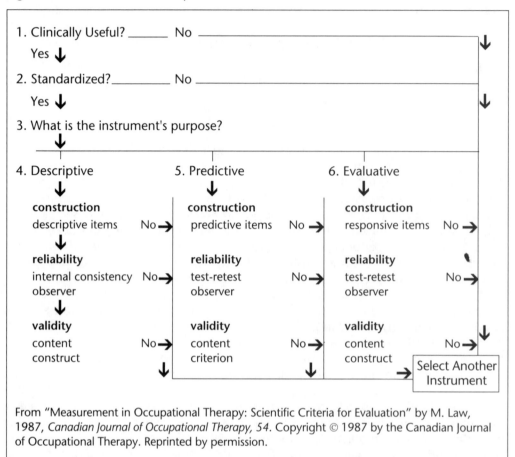

From "Measurement in Occupational Therapy: Scientific Criteria for Evaluation" by M. Law, 1987, *Canadian Journal of Occupational Therapy, 54.* Copyright © 1987 by the Canadian Journal of Occupational Therapy. Reprinted by permission.

sources. Simple graphic displays of data to summarize narrative comments often have a better impact than narrative or numbers alone, and are especially useful to indicate problem areas and to illustrate change over time.

Instruments for Assessing Self-Care

Characteristics

Numerous characteristics must be considered when selecting an instrument to measure any aspect of functional performance, inclusive of self-care. The following describes some of the desirable characteristics and ways instruments may vary.

1. *The breadth of content addressed by the instrument* (Brown, Gordon, & Diller, 1983). Some instruments cover a broad range of functional tasks; others are limited to a few self-care tasks. The extent to which instruments address each self-care task, or the level of function assessed, will also vary. For example, dressing may be evaluated by a single item referring to the complete task, or may be broken down into component parts, such as putting on socks, fastening shirt buttons, and so forth.

2. *The instrument's sensitivity to change in client status* (Brown et al., 1983; Liang &

Jette, 1981). Sensitivity is of particular importance in measuring the effect of intervention. An instrument that lacks sensitivity will not indicate small gains in the client's ability to perform self-care tasks.

3. *The reliability of the test procedures* (Liang & Jette, 1981). The procedures need to be clearly stated in the test manual or protocol. The scores or descriptors obtained with an instrument should be consistent from one test period to another, and among different test administrators (see Figure 4).

4. *The validity of the test* (Liang & Jette, 1981). Validity relates to what behaviors the test measures and how well it does so (see Figure 5). A test that is valid in one situation is not necessarily valid under changed circumstances. For example, a test of mobility that was developed for ambulatory subjects may not be a suitable measure for wheelchair users. In this example, the content validity is not precisely determined by a statistical calculation, but is a judgment call on the part of the potential test user. How well a test measures what it purports to measure may be more precisely measured by comparing performance on the test with another instrument considered to be an accurate indicator of the behavior of interest. This is often expressed as a correlation coefficient, indicating the relationship between two instruments.

Kaufert (1983) identifies four major measurement problems in functional assessment that pose threats to validity: "(1) assessing the impact of aids, adaptations, and helpers; (2) controlling for situational variation and motivational factors; (3) controlling for the professional perspective of the rater; and (4) controlling for the role expectations of the patient in the performance of certain function" (p. 260). As these threats have yet to be resolved in any one instrument, the occupational therapist must be aware of these problems and carefully interpret assessment data.

5. *The resulting data.* On completion, the instrument may provide a detailed profile that describes the client's self-care ability, or it may result in a single code or

Figure 4. Instrument reliability.

Reliability of a test refers to the consistency with which it measures the target behavior. If one is to make decisions based on test results, it is important that the changes in test scores reflect behavior change, and not instability of the test itself. There are two types of reliability commonly reported:

Test-retest reliability refers to the stability of the test over time. To examine an instrument's test-retest reliability, it is administered to a group of subjects on two separate occasions, and the results of the two test sessions are examined by calculating a correlation coefficient. A stable test is expected to have a correlation coefficient that is close to 1. The length of time between test sessions is important, and should be carefully chosen. For example, changes in test scores may occur because the subjects' performance has changed over time if too much time elapses between sessions.

Interrater reliability refers to the consistency of test results between two or more raters administering the test to the same subjects. To examine interrater reliability, two or more raters score the same subjects during the same test session and compare their results. The comparison may be made by calculating the percent agreement, or by using correlation coefficients. (Ottenbacher, 1986; Oyster, Hanten, & Llorens, 1987)

Figure 5. Instrument validity.

The validity of a test is concerned with its accuracy, or the likelihood that it is measuring the behavior of interest. There are three categories of validity.

Content validity refers to the representativeness of the items in the test. Usually the behavior of interest is very broad, and not well defined (as is the case in measuring self-care). To establish content validity, the behavior is defined as thoroughly as possible, and all subsets are identified. The test is then developed with items representing each subset of behavior. Well-developed tests will illustrate content validity with a table of specifications in the test manual. Frequently, expert opinion is relied upon to evaluate the content validity of a test.

Construct validity refers to the instrument's conformation to theoretical constructs. For example, does the test differentiate between adults with hemiplegia and nondisabled adults in their performance of self-care tasks? One of the important constructs examined in self-care tests is the relationship between test scores and the amount of personal assistance required.

Criterion validity refers to the agreement between scores obtained with an instrument and another measure that is known to indicate the target behavior accurately. One of the problems in establishing criterion validity in self-care is the lack of a "gold standard" or precise, accurate measurement for comparison. Concurrent validity refers to the relationship between the test and the criterion measured at the same point in time. Predictive validity refers to the relationship between the test and the criterion at some time in the future. The relationship is usually expressed in terms of a correlation coefficient. (Law, 1987; Oyster, Hanten, & Llorens, 1987)

numerical value that represents a measure of overall function (Brown et al., 1983). Instruments may be descriptive or evaluative (Brown et al.), and the purpose will direct the type of data collected. Liang and Jette (1981) point out that quantification of function is a desirable characteristic of evaluative instruments. The numerical score presumably will change as the subject's status changes at subsequent evaluations, so the instrument must be sensitive to the behavior of interest for the score to be meaningful. However, finding a single global score for something as complex as self-care is wishful thinking (Fisher, 1992b), so caution should be used when interpreting a test score resulting from the sum of several subtests. Most instruments for adults are designed to yield data for evaluative or descriptive purposes that allow one to measure change or to compare performance to normative data. Some tests will have a developmental focus, so that the resulting data indicate the subject's performance in relation to a developmental continuum.

6. *Feasibility.* The time required to administer the test, and the special training and equipment all influence the usefulness of the instrument in any given setting.

Assessments for program evaluations and research purposes have similar desirable characteristics. Bombardier and Tugwell (1987), in their evaluation of some existing functional assessment scales, provide a framework for critically evaluating an instrument before selecting it for use in research. Comprehensiveness, accuracy, sensitivity to change, and feasibility are just some of the issues they suggest one address before making a choice. "Researchers should guard against picking instruments blindly 'off the shelf' simply because they are well known, popular, or have received extensive validation. A less well validated questionnaire may be more appropriate depending on the research question" (Bombardier & Tugwell, p. 10.)

A Review

This section contains a brief description of instruments for assessing self-care. Instruments are discussed in alphabetical order, by test title. Table 1 summarizes the characteristics of the instruments, including the presence of reliability, validity, and sensitivity data; the sample populations tested; and how data may be obtained (observed performance, interview, written self-report). Table 2 identifies the self-care tasks assessed by each instrument.

The *Barthel Index* (Mahoney & Barthel, 1965) was designed to measure independence before and after intervention and to indicate the amount of personal care required. It consists of 10 items: feeding, transferring between wheelchair and bed, personal toileting, transferring on and off the toilet, bathing, walking on level ground, climbing stairs, dressing, bowel control, and bladder control. Items within the index have varied weighting towards the total score. A score of 100 represents a person who is continent; eats, bathes, and dresses independently; is able to rise from a bed, chair, and toilet; walks at least a block; and can go up and down stairs. The authors point out that this individual is not necessarily able to live alone, as the Barthel Index is limited to self-care, but a person scoring 100 would not require a personal attendant. The Barthel Index has been used as a direct observation tool and as a guide for scoring self-care based on interviews or review of medical charts. Good test-retest reliability (.89) and interrater reliability (.95) have been reported (cited in McDowell & Newell, 1987). The Barthel Index was found to be strongly correlated (.91) with the level of support required for self-care and may be useful as a screening device for potential recipients of home support services (Fortinsky, Granger, & Selzter, 1981). Granger, Albrecht, and Hamilton (1979) suggest that scores of less than 60 indicate serious limitations in self-care.

Granger, Dewis, Peters, Sherwood, and Barrett (1979) investigated the ability of the Barthel Index to predict progress in rehabilitation and measured self-care status every 2 weeks in a group of 110 clients who had had strokes. They determined that a score of 60 was pivotal, where assistance was required in dressing, transfers, and ambulation. In a comparison of the Barthel Index, Katz Index of ADL, and Kenny Self-Care scores of 148 clients who had had strokes, all three instruments estimated approximately the same number of clients to be totally independent: 39%, 42%, and 35%, respectively (Gresham, Phillips, & Labi, 1980).

In a group of 41 clients (22 female, 19 male, average age 69 years) receiving rehabilitation services following a stroke, computed tomography (CT) scans and the Barthel Index were administered on a regular basis to determine their value as prognostic indicators (Hertanu, Demopoulos, Yang, Calhoun, & Fenigstein, 1984). The average Barthel score on admission was 45.5, and on discharge (an average 11 weeks later) it was 66. Nine subjects (22%) achieved a score of 100, indicating independence in self-care, and 27% achieved scores between 70 and 100, indicating some assistance required. Half of the group (21 subjects) scored less than 70 and required a great deal of assistance to complete self-care tasks. "Serial functional evaluations proved to be the most reliable method of assessing final outcome; the initial Barthel Index score was the most important variable, explaining 64% of the variability" (Hertanu, et al., p. 507).

Murdock (1992a; 1992b) published a critical evaluation of the Barthel Index and noted that since the Barthel Index is widely used, its reliability tends to be assumed rather than explicitly stated. Further, the Barthel Index was standardized in a hospital environment with an elderly population, so its use in other settings needs further examination.

The *Functional Assessment Inventory* (FAI) (Cairl, Pfeiffer, Keller, Burke, & Samis,

Table 1.
Characteristics of Selected Self-Care Instruments

Instrument	Reliability	Validity	Reported Use With	Data Collected By
Barthel	test-retest = .89 interrater = .95	criterion = .89 (with level of care required) criterion = detects change in parallel with Katz & Kenny	• hospitalized older adults • adults after stroke	• interview • observation • chart review
FAI	test-retest = .71 interrater = .76	criterion = .83 (with OARS) construct √ (differentiated between 3 groups of subjects)	• older males in veterans facilities	• interview
FIM	interrater = .86 to .95	criterion = -.62 to -.84 (with level of help required)	• hospitalized adults • adults in rehab settings	• interview • observation
FSI	test-retest = .40 to .87 interrater = .67 to .89	criterion = .71 to .95 (with physiotherapist ratings of performance)	• adults with arthritis	• interview
Katz	scalability = .74 to .88	criterion = discharge score predicts future personal assistance criterion = detects change in parallel with Barthel & Kenny	• chronically ill • older adults • adults after stroke • adults with hip fractures	• observation
Kenny	interrater = .67 to .74	criterion = detects change in parallel with Barthel & Katz	• adults in rehab settings	• observation

Klein-Bell	interrater = 92%
	(agreement/
	adult subjects)
	
	interrater = .99
	
	test-retest = .98
	(child subjects)
		criterion = .86
		(with hours of
		personal care
		required)
		construct √
		(differentiated
		between 2 groups of
		children)
			• adults in rehab
			  settings
			• children with
			  cerebral palsy
			  and no disability
				• observation

(continued)

Table 1. (continued)

Instrument	Reliability	Validity	Reported Use With	Data Collected By
MEDLS	interrater = .40 to 1.0	content √ (panel of experts)	• adults in long-term psychiatric settings	• observation • interview
OARS-PSMS	interrater = .87 interrater = .96 test-retest = .50	criterion = .62 (with physician ratings of health)	• older adults	• interview • self-report question-naire
PULSES	test-retest = .87 interrater = .90	criterion √ (with Barthel)	• adults in rehab settings	• interview • observation
RTI	not tested	not tested	• adults with psychiatric conditions	• observation
SSCE (personal care subscale)	test-retest = .05 interrater = .50 to .96	not tested	• nondisabled teens and adults	• observation

1983) is a streamlined version of the Older Americans Resource Service (OARS) Multidimensional Functional Assessment Questionnaire. It has 11 sections, ranging from mental status to ADL, with 90 fewer items than the OARS questionnaire. A trained interviewer administers the questionnaire. Sections are rated on a scale of 1 (excellent) to 6 (totally impaired). Its reliability and validity were assessed with a group of 157 patients (mostly male, mean age 67.5 years) from two affiliated Veterans' Administration facilities: a nursing home and a domiciliary institution. With a subgroup of this sample (N = 58) the ADL section demonstrated good test-retest reliability (ICC = .71, $p < .001$) and good concurrent validity with the parent OARS instrument (ICC = .83, $p < .001$). The ADL section's interrater reliability with a subgroup of 26 patients was .76 ($p < .001$). It took 30 to 40 minutes to administer; about 10 to 15 minutes less time than the OARS.

Robinson, Lund, Keller, and Cuervo (1986) validated the FAI against the opinion of a multidisciplinary home care team seeing 30 veterans over 60 years of age. The FAI was administered by an independent rater 1 week before team members conducted their own evaluations. Robinson et al. compared the FAI ratings to a rating assigned by the team as a whole (which included an occupational therapist). There was agreement between FAI scores and team ratings for all sections of the FAI *except* the ADL section, where the FAI score was greater, indicating more impairment than the team's rating. Whether this resulted from invalid ADL items on the FAI that are poor predictors of self-care, team members overestimating the client's abilities, or other factors, is unknown.

The FAI was used to distinguish among the elderly residents of three different settings in a rural community (Pfeiffer, McClelland, & Lawson, 1989). Three investigators were trained in administration and achieved interrater reliability of .98 (coefficient alpha)

Table 2.
Summary of Selected Self-Care Instruments (By Number of Items in Each Category)

Instrument:	Barthel	FIM	FSI*	Katz	Kenny	Klein-Bell	MEDLS*	OARS*/PSMS	RTI	SSCE* (personal care subscale)
Feeding	1	1	0	1	1	15	1	1	1	0
Grooming	1	1	0	0	0	18	5	1	1	1
Bathing	1	1	1	1	3	12	2	1	1	0
Toileting	1	1	0	1	1	19	0	1	1	0
Continence	2	2	0	1	2	4	0	0	0	0
Dressing	1	2	3	1	3	65	2	1	1	0
Mobility	3	5	3	1	7	30	0	1	1	0
Medication Management	0	0	0	0	0	1	1	0	1	0
Functional Communication	0	2	2	0	0	6	2	0	1	2

Note: * indicates additional items beyond self-care tasks

with a sample of six interviews. They interviewed 125 elderly people, and the FAI scores resulted in three clusters that were statistically substantiated by ANOVA. One cluster included those residents of a state mental health facility and a nursing home; a second cluster consisted of people receiving visiting nurse home care; and the third cluster included well elderly, recruited from a seniors' center as a control group. This suggests that the FAI can discriminate among people of varying levels of ability.

The conceptual basis for the *Functional Independence Measure* (FIM) is that the level of disability should indicate a burden of care (Heineman et al., 1991). That is, the individual and society pay a certain cost when that individual is not functionally independent. Therefore, the basis for scoring the FIM is the presence of a helper. There are 18 items in six categories. *Self-care* includes eating, grooming, bathing, dressing upper body, dressing lower body, and toileting. *Sphincter control* includes bladder management and bowel management. *Mobility* addresses three transferring skills: bed/chair/wheelchair, toilet, and tub/shower. *Locomotion* refers to either walking or using a wheelchair, and using stairs. *Communication* includes comprehension and expression. And the final category, *social cognition*, includes social interaction, problem solving, and memory. Items are weighted equally, and each item is scored on a 7-point scale, where 7 and 6 indicate the absence of a helper, and 5 through 1 represent increasing levels of assistance from a helper. A score of 7 is complete independence that is judged to be timely and safe, while 6 indicates independence with the use of one or more devices. Scores for the 18 items are summed to obtain a total FIM score.

The FIM demonstrates good interrater reliability, with coefficients ranging from .86 to .95 (Heineman et al., 1991). It has been suggested that the FIM is a valid predictor of assistance required by persons with a disability. In a group of 24 adults with multiple sclerosis (mean age = 45.7 years) the help required, in minutes per day, was highly correlated with FIM scores. The highest correlations were obtained between minutes per day and FIM tub transfers scores (-.84), FIM bed transfers scores (-.82), and FIM bathing scores (-.81) (Granger, Cotter, Hamilton, Fiedler, & Hens, 1990).

The *Functional Status Index* (FSI) (Jette, 1987) is a self-report instrument developed for use with people who have arthritis. The FSI has 18 items in five categories: gross mobility, hand activities, personal care, home chores, and social/role activities. A trained interviewer administers it in approximately 30 minutes. The client ranks the degree of assistance required in the past 7 days on a 5-point functional dependence scale:

0 = independent,

1 = uses equipment,

2 = uses human assistance,

3 = uses equipment and assistance, and

4 = unable to do or unsafe.

The individual also rates the pain and difficulty associated with the tasks on a 4-point scale ranging from none (a value of 1), to mild, moderate, and severe (a value of 4). In a sample of 141 adults with rheumatoid arthritis, the reliability of the FSI, as estimated with intraclass correlation coefficients, was moderate to good, depending on the category:

	functional dependence	pain/difficulty
test-retest	.40–.87	.69–.88
interrater	.67–.89	.71–.82

Concurrent validity was examined in a sample of 41 clients recovering from hip fractures, by comparing FSI scores with ratings of performance of selected activities of daily living made by a physical therapist. The agreement between the self-report and the therapist's opinion ranged from .71 to .95, indicating reasonable agreement between the two sources.

The *Katz Index of ADL* (Katz, Downs, Cash, & Grotz, 1970; Katz, Ford, Moskowitz, Jackson, & Jaffe, 1963) was developed to measure function in the chronically ill and aging populations. It summarizes self-care ability in six areas: bathing, dressing, toileting, transferring, continence, and feeding. Performance can be observed, or questions asked of the client, and the rater checks one of three descriptors for each of the six areas: independent, some assistance required, or dependent. The criteria for the three descriptors is operationalized for each of the six areas. The ratings are then transformed into a global score represented by letters:

A = independent in all six functions,

B = independent in any five functions,

C = independent in all but bathing and one other,

D = independent in all but bathing, dressing, and one other,

E = independent in all but bathing, dressing, toileting, and one other,

F = independent in all but bathing, dressing, toileting, transfers and one other,

G = dependent, and

OTHER = cannot be classified in A–G, dependent on two or more functions.

The letter scores represent a hierarchy of returning function during rehabilitation that closely resembles a developmental sequence. The authors noted that feeding and continence tended to return earlier than transferring and toileting ability, which returned before dressing and bathing skills. Katz and Stroud (1989) reported that this same hierarchy was observed in primitive societies, and suggested that this ordered profile of independence is reliable and valid. Guttman analyses on Katz ADL scores for 100 subjects yielded a coefficient of scalability ranging from .74 to .88, suggesting that it is a successful cumulative scale (McDowell & Newell, 1987).

The *Kenny Self-Care Evaluation* (Schoening et al., 1965; Schoening & Iverson, 1968) was developed as an instrument to evaluate actual performance and to estimate the ability of clients to live at home. It has seven categories: bed activities, transfers, locomotion, dressing, personal hygiene, bowel and bladder control, and feeding. Each category contains one to four activities, each divided into tasks. In all, there are 17 activities and 85 tasks. Ratings are summed for a total score. Interrater reliability among 43 raters ranged from .67 to .74 (cited in McDowell & Newell, 1987). McDowell and Newell noted that although the Kenny Self-Care Evaluation contains more detail than some instruments, it doesn't seem to discriminate any better than others; however, the details may have some clinical utility in enhancing descriptions of client function.

The *Klein-Bell ADL Scale* (Klein & Bell, 1982) is comprised of easily observable components of activities of daily living in all people, regardless of diagnosis or disability. It consists of 170 items that a rater scores as "achieved" or "failed," with full credit given for independence with the use of assistive devices. Items are assigned a point value corresponding to their level of difficulty, as determined by a group of 10 occupational therapists, physical therapists, and nurses experienced in rehabilitation. The more difficult items are worth 3 points, less difficult items 2 points, and the easier items 1 point. If the individual achieves the item, full points are given; no points are given for failed items. The scores are summed for an overall independence score. Three pairs of occupational therapists and three pairs of nurses rated 20 subjects and achieved 92% agreement overall. Predictive validity was assessed by contacting 21 former patients and inquiring about the number of hours per week of assistance they required to complete activities of daily living, and comparing this with the predischarge Klein-Bell ADL scores. The resulting Pearson correlation coefficient was -.86 ($p < .01$), indicating that subjects with lower Klein-Bell scores subsequently required more hours of personal assistance. Scores for two subjects were compared over time with the Barthel Index and Katz Index of ADL, and the Klein-Bell ADL scale appeared to have greater sensitivity to change.

Law and Usher (1988) conducted a pilot study to validate the use of the Klein-Bell ADL scale with children. They first searched the literature to determine the age at which children normally achieve each Klein-Bell ADL item. A panel of four pediatric occupational therapists reviewed the proposed ages, judged discrepancies, and agreed upon appropriate age ranges. A score range was calculated for developmental levels: "For example, a child of two years should achieve a score of 109 on the scale out of a possible score of complete independence of 310 which should be achieved by age seven" (Law & Usher, p. 65). The Klein-Bell ADL scale was then administered to 20 children, 10 with cerebral palsy and 10 nondisabled, who were matched as closely as possible by age and gender. They ranged in age from 13 months to 6 years. ADL were evaluated at baseline and at 9 months, with five subjects tested at 1 week to examine test-retest reliability, and five subjects were scored by two raters to examine interrater reliability. Parents were interviewed at the end of the study for their opinions about their children's change in ADL skills. Because of the small sample, results need to be interpreted with caution. However, the Klein-Bell ADL scale demonstrated very good test-retest reliability (ICC = .98) and interrater reliability (ICC = .99). It distinguished between nondisabled children and those with cerebral palsy (mean difference of 95 points, $p < .0001$), demonstrating construct validity. An occupational therapist, blind to the subjects' identities, categorized children as "normal" or having cerebral palsy based on the ADL scores, with 100% accuracy. The scale did not demonstrate statistically significant responsiveness in this sample; however, the nondisabled children's scores increased 21 points on average, and the children with cerebral palsy changed an average of 11 points. It was suggested that a ceiling effect with the scores for three nondisabled children contributed to the lack of statistical significance.

The *Milwaukee Evaluation of Daily Living Skills* (MEDLS) (Leonardelli, 1988a; 1988b) was designed to measure performance of long-term psychiatric clients. A broad range of self-care tasks are assessed in 20 subtests. The self-care areas for inclusion in the MEDLS were based on a survey of 56 occupational therapists and occupational therapy assistants from a pool of 300 AOTA members indicating full-time employment in settings with the chronically mentally ill (Leonardelli, 1989). The subtests may be used individually or in any combination, and a screening form is provided in the manual to assist in selecting the subtests applicable to any one client. It takes approximately 80 minutes to administer 18 subtests at one time. Tasks are observed by the occupational therapist, preferably as part of the client's routine. There is no cumulative score; each subtest is scored separately based on performance in that area. The manual provides a description of the method, skill list, key words for observing each skill, and scoring criteria for each subtest. Initial interrater reliability has been assessed with a group of 26 men who were residents in a psychiatric facility, resulting in moderate to good results, depending on the subtest ($r = .40$ for shaving, which was not significant; other subtests ranged from .60 to 1.00 and were significant at $p < .001$). Leonardelli (1988a) found the MEDLS to be particularly compatible with the model of human occupation in practice, as a measure of the performance subsystem.

Lawton (1971) described a functional assessment of the elderly that included physical ADL, instrumental ADL, mental status, social roles and activities, attitudes, morale and life satisfaction, and psychiatric status. Its conceptual basis stems from the belief that human behavior can be ordered in a hierarchy of complexity, from physical self-maintenance through instrumental activities of daily living and motivation, to social interaction. This eventually became a structured interview known as the *Older Americans Resource Service (OARS) Multidimensional Functional Assessment Questionnaire* (McDowell & Newell, 1987). The *Physical Self-Maintenance Scale (PSMS)* and *Instrumental Activities of Daily Living Scale (IADL)* developed by Lawton and Brody (1969) comprise the physical ADL and instrumental ADL sections of the OARS. The PSMS, which addresses self-care, has six sections: toileting, feeding, dressing, grooming, physical ambulation, and bathing. Two nurses rating 36 subjects achieved interrater reliability of .87 (Pearson r). Its correlation with physician ratings of health in 130 subjects was .62.

Edwards (1990) examined the reliability and validity of Lawton and Brody's PSMS and IADL scales in a group of 30 subjects recruited from two geriatric specialty units. The interrater reliability for the PSMS was very good (ICC = .96), and the test-retest reliability was fair (ICC = .59). Subjects were observed performing two ADL and two IADL tasks in order to investigate the relationship between self-report (PSMS and IADL scores) and direct observation. The results indicated poor correlations, ranging from .17 to .45. Without exception, the subjects consistently overrated their ability in both self-maintenance and IADL tasks, and Edwards subsequently recommends the use of direct observation in order to obtain a valid description of a client's performance abilities.

Morris and Boutelle (1985) compared agreement between interview and self-administered protocols with the OARS with 22 residents of a low-income-housing project

(12 females, 10 males, aged 63 to 89 years). The sample was divided into two groups of 11. Group 1 was interviewed, then 2 weeks later the entire sample received the self-administered questionnaire in a group setting. Group 2 was interviewed 2 weeks later. Four judges scored the interview and self-administered data. There was general agreement between the two data sources, with intraclass correlation coefficients ranging from .82 to .95. There was no significant difference between the judges' ratings or the sequence of administration.

The *PULSES Profile* (Granger, Albrecht, & Hamilton, 1979) has been used to measure independence in self-care. PULSES is an acronym for physical condition, upper limb function in self-care, lower-limb function in mobility, sensory components (seeing, hearing), excretory function, and support factors (emotional, family, and social). Each of the six components has equal weight, scored on a scale of 4 levels of impairment, from 1 = intact, independent; to 4 = fully dependent. The component scores are summed. The scores range from 6 to 24, with higher scores representing greater dependence. McDowell and Newell (1987) recommend that the summed score not be used; rather, the score for each category should be presented separately, so as not to obscure any one section. For example, a numerical score would be listed for each letter in the acronym: L-3 refers to someone who walks with supervision (L = lower extremity, 3 = supervision). The test-retest reliability was .87, and interrater reliability exceeded .95 (cited in McDowell & Newell). In a group of 307 adults (mean age 50 years) receiving rehabilitation services, the PULSES and Barthel Index correlated well, suggesting reasonable concurrent validity between the two instruments (Granger, Albrecht, & Hamilton, 1979). It was noted, however, that the Barthel scores at admission indicated less dependence than did the PULSES. It has been suggested that scores higher than 12 reflect serious limitations in function (Granger, Albrecht, & Hamilton, 1979; McDowell & Newell) and scores higher than 16 indicate severe disability (McDowell & Newell).

The *Routine Task Inventory* (RTI) (Allen, 1985) describes the functional severity of a person's disability. Interviewing the client and a caregiver, and direct observation, can be used to obtain data. The RTI is essentially an observation guide of 14 tasks, each with descriptors that correspond to Allen's six cognitive levels. It is based on the physical self-maintenance and instrumental activities of daily living scales developed by Lawton for use with the elderly. The self-care inventory describes six areas: grooming, dressing, bathing, walking, feeding, and toileting. A new instrument, it has not yet been subjected to rigorous reliability or validity testing, so its use as a tool to measure change in behavior is limited. Its development, however, is grounded in the theoretical framework of Allen's cognitive model. Therapists applying Allen's cognitive model to their practice may find the inventory useful in describing their clients' self-care ability.

The *Satisfaction With Performance Scaled Questionnaire (SPSQ)* (Yerxa, Burnett-Beaulieu, Stocking, & Azen, 1988) was designed to measure individuals' satisfaction with their performance of independent living skills. Satisfaction was defined as being pleased or content with one's performance. An original 137 items were tested with a sample of 24 adults with physical disabilities, and achieved good split-half reliability. Item and factor analyses with the questionnaires from 50 subjects eliminated many items, reducing the total number to 46, in two scales: home management and social/community problem solving. The split-half reliability for the revised SPSQ was .97 for the home management scale and .93 for the social/community problem solving scale. The authors suggest that the SPSQ can be useful in creating a contractual, rather than a prescriptive, basis for planning occupational therapy intervention. The SPSQ addresses instrumental activities of daily living, but is included here as an approach that involves the client's perceptions and priorities.

The *Scorable Self-Care Evaluation (SSCE)* (Clark & Peters, 1984) is a standardized self-care evaluation instrument designed to assess comprehensively and quantifiably the client's performance of self-care tasks. In this case the term *self-care* describes a broader set of tasks than it does in most self-care instruments. The SSCE contains four subscales: personal care, housekeeping, work and leisure, and financial management. Within the subscales there are 18 tasks, each with varying point values. The rater assigns points based on responses to questions and the appearance of the client, not actual performance. Points reflect the *in*ability to do a task. The authors of the manual report data collected from a group of 67 subjects (30 male, 37 female), 13 to 62 years of age, who had no known disability and who were employed or attending school. The personal care subscale has a focus that is different from the majority of self-care instruments available. It evaluates initial appearance, orientation, hygiene, communication, and first aid. Of the 51 points that could be assigned to personal care, 24 relate to responses to first aid questions. The personal care subscale had poor test-retest reliability (Pearson $r = .05$), although the other subscales performed better. The reliability was assessed only on a subset of 10 subjects. For these reasons, the SSCE is not yet ready to be used as a reliable measure of performance in self-care.

The *Unified ADL Form* (Donaldson et al., 1973) was developed after an examination of 25 ADL scales published from 1950 to 1970. Only those scales that were scorable, used in research, and applicable to a general population were considered. All ADL variables that were found in two-thirds or more of the scales were organized into a coded form. The new form was used to evaluate 100 patients on admission and 1 month after discharge. The data was entered into a computer and transformed into Barthel Index, Katz Index of ADL, and Kenny Self-Care scores, and examined for changes in patient scores. Of the 100 subjects, 68 moved in parallel fashion across the three indexes, while divergences were demonstrated for 32 patients:

- 19 demonstrated no change on the Katz, but did change on the Kenny and Barthel scores;
- 5 demonstrated no change on the Katz or Barthel, but did change on the Kenny; and
- 8 demonstrated no pattern.

The advantage to using the Unified ADL form is that it provides comprehensive data that are easily convertible to three standard indexes from the single format. The items on the Unified ADL form are scored using a general rating criteria ranging from 1= able to do the task and does it; to 8 = does not perform any part of the task. The investigators suggested that the Kenny Self-Care evaluation is more detailed and sensitive to change than the Barthel Index and Katz Index of ADL; that the Katz Index is the least sensitive to change; and that the Barthel Index is intermediate to the other two.

Conclusion

In 1971, Lawton noted that "the tradition that each institution makes its own ADL schedule has resulted in instruments of similar content that vary widely in psychometric sophistication" (p. 469). The preceding review of instruments indicates the availability of several that should discourage this practice. McAvoy (1991) found 200 or more ADL indexes reported in the literature, yet her own survey of occupational therapy departments in Northern Ireland indicated that none of the departments used published, standardized assessments of ADL. "Self-care and mobility are included in most functional assessment scales, so agreement on an instrument for measuring these functions would be an important first step" (Keith, 1984, p.74). Unfortunately, the rehabilitation community has yet to reach agreement, and there is no "gold standard" for the evaluation of self-care. Adoption of a few select instruments in any one setting would facilitate communication among the health care team in that setting (Law & Letts, 1989) and would encourage the further development of the instruments selected. In a discussion of the standardization, reliability, and validity of several instruments, Keith calls for a move toward agreement on how to evaluate self-care and recommends the Katz Index of ADL and the Barthel Index. In their review of 13 ADL scales, Law and Letts recommend adopting the PULSES or Katz Index of ADL when the evaluation seeks to describe self-care function, and the Klein-Bell ADL scale for prediction and evaluative purposes.

In making these recommendations, the authors support the further development and validation of existing scales and discourage the practice of department-specific, "homemade" evaluations. Most homemade assessments of self-care address the same tasks as do existing scales, so the reasons for not using existing instruments are not clear. There is a great need for more clinician reports of how existing scales perform in varied settings and with different populations. Are they sensitive to change? Do they predict future occupational performance at home? Can existing interview and self-report instruments be modified to include observation of performance rather than reported performance? Occupational therapists have expertise in performance evaluation, and should be at the forefront of the development of performance-based assessments (Fisher, 1992b). ◆

References

Alexander, J.L., & Fuhrer, M.J. (1984). Functional assessment of individuals with physical impairments. In A.S. Halpern & M.J. Fuhrer (Eds.), *Functional assessment in rehabilitation* (pp. 45–59). Baltimore: Paul H. Brookes.

Allen, C.K. (1985). *Occupational therapy in psychiatric diseases*. Boston: Little, Brown.

Bombardier, C., & Tugwell, P. (1987). Methodological considerations in functional assessment. *Journal of Rheumatology, 14*(Suppl. 15), 6–10.

Brown, M., Gordon, W.A., & Diller, L. (1983). Functional assessment and outcome measurement: An integrative review. *Annual Review of Rehabilitation, 3*, 93–120.

Cairl, R.E., Pfeiffer, E., Keller, D.M., Burke, H., & Samis, H.V. (1983). An evaluation of the reliability and validity of the functional assessment inventory. *Journal of the American Geriatrics Society, 31*, 607–612.

Canadian Association of Occupational Therapists and Health Services Directorate (CAOT & HSD), Health and Welfare Canada. (1991). *Occupational therapy guidelines for client-centred practice*. Toronto: CAOT Publications.

Carter, L.T., Oliveira, D.O., Duponte, J., & Lynch, S.V. (1988). The relationship of cognitive skills performance to activities of daily living in stroke patients. *American Journal of Occupational Therapy, 42*, 449–455.

Clark, E.N., & Peters, M. (1984). *Scorable self-care evaluation*. Thorofare, NJ: Slack.

Cohen, B.F., & Anthony, W.A. (1984). Functional assessment in psychiatric rehabilitation. In A.S. Halpern & M.J. Fuhrer (Eds.), *Functional assessment in rehabilitation* (pp. 79–100). Baltimore: Paul H. Brookes.

Donaldson, S.W., Wagner, C.C., & Gresham, G.E. (1973). A unified ADL evaluation form. *Archives of Physical Medicine and Rehabilitation, 54*, 175–179.

Edwards, M.M. (1990). The reliability and validity of self-report activities of daily living scales. *Canadian Journal of Occupational Therapy, 57,* 273–278.

Fillenbaum, G. (1985). Screening the elderly: A brief instrumental activities of daily living measure. *Journal of the American Geriatrics Society, 33,* 698–706.

Fisher, A.G. (1992a). Functional measures, part I: What is function, what should we measure and how should we measure it? *American Journal of Occupational Therapy, 46,* 183–185.

Fisher, A.G. (1992b). Functional measures, part II: Selecting the right test, minimizing the limitations. *American Journal of Occupational Therapy, 46,* 278–281.

Fortinsky, R.H., Granger, C.V., & Selzter, G.B. (1981). The use of functional assessment in understanding home care needs. *Medical Care, 19,* 489–497.

Granger, C.V., Albrecht, G.L., & Hamilton, B.B. (1979). Outcome of comprehensive medical rehabilitation by PULSES profile and Barthel Index. *Archives of Physical Medicine and Rehabilitation, 60,* 145–154.

Granger, C.V., Cotter, A.C., Hamilton, B.C., Fiedler, R.C., & Hens, M.M. (1990). Functional assessment scales: A study of persons with multiple sclerosis. *Archives of Physical Medicine and Rehabilitation, 71,* 870–875.

Granger, C.V., Dewis, L.S., Peters, N.C., Sherwood, C.C., & Barrett, J.E. (1979). Stroke rehabilitation: Analysis of repeated Barthel Index measures. *Archives of Physical Medicine and Rehabilitation, 60,* 14–17.

Gresham, G.E., Phillips, T.F., & Labi, M.L.C. (1980). ADL status in stroke: Relative merits of three standard indexes. *Archives of Physical Medicine and Rehabilitation, 61,* 355–358.

Halpern, A.S., & Fuhrer, M.J. (Eds.). (1984). *Functional assessment in rehabilitation.* Baltimore: Paul H. Brookes Publishing.

Heineman, A.W., Hamilton, B.B., Wright, B.D., Betts, H.B., Aguda, B., & Mamott, B.D. (1991). *Rating scale analysis of functional assessment measures.* Chicago: Rehabilitation Institute of Chicago. [Final Report to the National Institute on Disability and Rehabilitation Research.]

Hertanu, J.S., Demopoulos, J.T., Yang, W.C., Calhoun, W.F., & Fenigstein, H.A. (1984). Stroke rehabilitation: Correlation and prognostic value of computerized tomography and sequential functional assessments. *Archives of Physical Medicine and Rehabilitation, 65,* 505–508.

Jette, A.M. (1987). The functional status index: Reliability and validity of a self-report functional disability measure. *Journal of Rheumatology 14*(Suppl. 15), 15–19.

Jongbloed, L., Brighton, C., & Stacey, S. (1988). Factors associated with independent meal preparation, self-care and mobility in CVA clients. *Canadian Journal of Occupational Therapy, 55,* 259–263.

Katz, S., Downs, T.D., Cash, H.R., & Grotz, R.C. (1970). Progress in development of an index of ADL. *Gerontologist, 10,* 20–30.

Katz, S., Ford, A.B., Moskowitz, R.W., Jackson, B.A., & Jaffe, M.W. (1963). Studies of illness in the aged. The index of ADL: A standardized measure of biological and psychosocial function. *Journal of the American Medical Association, 185,* 914–919.

Katz, S., & Stroud, M.W. (1989). Functional assessment in geriatrics: A review of progress and directions. *Journal of the American Geriatrics Society, 37,* 267–271.

Kaufert, J.M. (1983). Functional ability indices: Measurement problems in assessing their validity. *Archives of Physical Medicine and Rehabilitation, 64,* 260–267.

Keith, R. A. (1984). Functional assessment measures in medical rehabilitation: Current status. *Archives of Physical Medicine and Rehabilitation, 65,* 74–78.

Klein, R.M., & Bell, B. (1982). Self-care skills: Behavioral measurement with Klein-Bell ADL scale. *Archives of Physical Medicine and Rehabilitation, 63*, 335–338.

Law, M. (1987). Measurement in occupational therapy: Scientific criteria for evaluation. *Canadian Journal of Occupational Therapy, 54*, 133–138.

Law, M., Baptiste, S., Carswell-Opzoomer, A., McColl, M.A., Polatajko, H., & Pollock, N. (1991). *Canadian occupational performance measure.* Toronto: CAOT Publications.

Law, M., & Letts, L. (1989). A critical review of scales of activities of daily living. *American Journal of Occupational Therapy, 43*, 522–528.

Law, M., & Usher, P. (1988). Validation of the Klein-Bell activities of daily living scale for children. *Canadian Journal of Occupational Therapy, 55*, 63–68.

Lawton, M.P. (1971). The functional assessment of elderly people. *Journal of the American Geriatrics Society, 19*, 465–481.

Lawton, M.P. (1990). Aging and performance of home tasks. *Human Factors, 32*, 527–536.

Lawton, M.P., & Brody, E.M. (1969). Assessment of older people: Self-maintaining and instrumental activities of daily living. *Gerontologist, 9*, 179–186.

Leonardelli, C.A. (1988a). *The Milwaukee evaluation of daily living skills: Evaluation in long-term psychiatric care.* Thorofare, NJ: Slack.

Leonardelli, C.A. (1988b). The Milwaukee evaluation of daily living skills (MEDLS). In B.J. Hemphill (Ed.), *Mental health assessment in occupational therapy: An integrative approach to the evaluative process* (pp. 149–162). Thorofare, NJ: Slack.

Leonardelli, C.A. (1989). Specification of daily living skills for persons with chronic mental illness. *Occupational Therapy Journal of Research, 9*, 323–333.

Liang, M.H., & Jette, A.M. (1981). Measuring functional ability in chronic arthritis: A critical review. *Arthritis and Rheumatism, 24*, 80–86.

Mahoney, F.I., & Barthel, D.W. (1965). Functional evaluation: The Barthel Index. *Maryland State Medical Journal, 14*, 61–65.

McAvoy, E. (1991). The use of ADL indices by occupational therapists. *British Journal of Occupational Therapy, 54*, 383–385.

McDowell, I., & Newell, C. (1987). Measuring health: A guide to rating scales and questionnaires. New York: Oxford University Press.

Morris, W.W., & Boutelle, S. (1985). Multidimensional functional assessment in two modes. *Gerontologist, 25*, 638–643.

Murdock, C. (1992a). A critical evaluation of the Barthel Index, part 1. *British Journal of Occupational Therapy, 55*, 109–111.

Murdock, C. (1992b). A critical evaluation of the Barthel Index, part 2. *British Journal of Occupational Therapy, 55*, 153–156.

Ottenbacher, K.J. (1986). *Evaluating clinical change: Strategies for occupational therapists and physical therapists.* Baltimore: Williams & Wilkins.

Oyster, C.K., Hanten, W.P., & Llorens, L.A. (1987). *Introduction to research: A guide for the health science professional.* Philadelphia: Lippincott.

Pfeiffer, B.A., McClelland, T., & Lawson, J. (1989). Use of the functional assessment inventory to distinguish among the rural elderly in five service settings. *Journal of the American Geriatrics Society, 37*, 243–248.

Robinson, B.E., Lund, C.A., Keller, D., & Cuervo, C.A. (1986). Validation of the functional assessment inventory against a multidisciplinary home care team. *Journal of the American Geriatrics Society, 34*, 851–854.

Rubenstein, L.Z., Schairer, C., Wieland, G.D., & Kane, R. (1984). Systematic biases in functional status assessment of elderly adults: Effects of different data sources. *Journal of the American Geriatrics Society, 39*, 686–691.

Schoening, H.A., Anderegg, L., Bergstrom, D., Fonda, M., Steinke, N., & Ulrich, P. (1965). Numerical scoring of self-care status of patients. *Archives of Physical Medicine and Rehabilitation, 46*, 689–697.

Schoening, H.A., & Iverson, I.A. (1968). Numerical scoring of self-care status: Study of Kenny Self-Care Evaluation. *Archives of Physical Medicine and Rehabilitation, 49*, 221–229.

Titus, M.N.D., Gall, N.G., Yerxa, E.J., Roberson, T.A., & Mack, W. (1991). Correlation of perceptual performance and activities of daily living in stroke patients. *American Journal of Occupational Therapy, 45*, 410–418.

Tugwell, P., Bombardier, C., Buchanan, W.W., Goldsmith, C.H., Grace, E., & Hanna, B. (1987). The MACTAR patient preference disability questionnaire: An individualized functional priority approach for assessing improvement in physical disability in clinical trials in rheumatoid arthritis. *Journal of Rheumatology, 14*, 446–451.

Yerxa, E.J., Burnett-Beaulieu, S., Stocking, S., & Azen, S.P. (1988). Development of the satisfaction with performance scaled questionnaire (SPSQ). *American Journal of Occupational Therapy, 42*, 215–221.

4

Principles for Teaching Self-Care Skills

Martha E. Snell

Martha E. Snell, PhD, *is Professor of Special Education at the Curry School of Education, University of Virginia, Charlottesville, VA.*

Chapter 4 Outline

Initial Planning of Instruction
    Guiding Principles
        Age Appropriate and Functional
        Ecological Inventories
    Stage of Learning

Direct Assessment of Skills
    Assessment Data
        Observational Data
        Test and Training Data
    Types of Tasks
        Discrete and Chained Behaviors
        Task Analyses

Teaching Strategies
    Artificial and Natural Prompts and Feedback
    Antecedents: Instructional Cues
    Antecedents: Prompts
        System of Least Prompts
        Graduated Guidance
        Time Delay
    Consequences
        Following Correct or Approximate Responses
        Following Errors

Evaluation of Learning and Teaching
    Baseline and Probe Data
    Training Data
    Using Data

Summary

References

Regardless of who or what is being taught, there are some general principles and methods of good instruction. When the learner has cognitive limitations, several other principles should be reflected in teaching, and additional methods should be considered. The purpose of this chapter is to describe these principles and methods for an audience of occupational therapists. The chapter is organized into four sections: (a) initial planning of instruction; (b) direct assessment of skills; (c) teaching strategies; and (d) evaluation of learning and teaching.

Initial Planning of Instruction

Guiding Principles

Age Appropriate and Functional

Perhaps the most important aspect of teaching involves decisions about what to teach. While it is possible to devise methods to teach just about any skill, if unneeded or inappropriate skills are targeted, the learner's and the instructor's time are wasted. There are several principles that therapists should consider when selecting target skills:

1. Skills taught need to suit a person's chronological age;

2. Skills should be useful to the person now and in the future;

3. Skills taught should be ones the individual and/or the family prefer and deem important;

4. Skills should enable the person to accomplish desirable, normalized outcomes such as self-management, mobility, leisure, employment, and so forth; and

5. Even if partial, rather than independent, participation is the goal, realistic objectives should be selected.

With individuals who have cognitive disabilities, the first principle often is violated by teaching skills that suit individuals younger than the person to whom they are being taught. Sometimes the skill targeted is valid (useful and age appropriate) but the activities or materials used to teach the skills are not. For example, teenagers with movement limitations may be asked to toss bean bags into a wooden frog's mouth to improve eye-hand coordination, when an adapted pool game or a TV computer game would be better.

The second through the fifth principles address different aspects of functionality. Functional or useful skills are likely to be used, not forgotten through disuse, and will promote less dependence on others. Functional skills have purpose and thus are valued by others. Learning to perform skills that are valued improve the way an individual is viewed by others and by him- or herself. Targeting skills that cannot be realistically accomplished by the individual, in part or in full, means that the skills will not be used.

For many individuals it is appropriate to be taught to participate partially in a skill, rather than to perform the entire skill or to perform the skill in typical ways. This practice is known as *partial participation* (Baumgart et al., 1982), and includes: (a) help from others on difficult steps (e.g., the therapist brushes Anne's teeth, but Anne learns to open her mouth, hold it open, and close it) (Snell, Lewis, & Houghton, 1989); (b) changing the order of the task performance (e.g., putting a bathing suit on before getting to the pool); (c) changing the rules (e.g., letting another student bat for John, then pushing John in his wheelchair to the bases); or (d) adding adaptations (e.g., Carla can use the computer with a large joystick switch). Skills that include partial participation should be carefully planned so they will be functional and thus used. Reassessment at later ages also is important, because the individual may be able to learn more or all of the skills or the adaptation may need adjustment (Ferguson & Baumgart, 1991).

Functional skills often involve activities or routines and thus may require related skills in addition to the primary skills an occupational therapist addresses. Fredda Brown (Brown, Evans, Weed, & Owen, 1987) describes two types of related abilities that add to the core portion of a skill: extension and enrichment. Extension skills include the ability to initiate a routine, prepare for the task, monitor the speed and quality of the task, problem-solve, and terminate the task or clean up when done. Enrichment skills involve expressive communication (nonsymbolic or symbolic), social behavior, and choice. Figure 1 illustrates how this component model is applied to the task of grooming one's nails. If target skills are viewed in this comprehensive manner, therapists need to work actively as part of a team and avoid "dividing up" the client into parts that reflect each team member's specialty.

Ecological Inventories

How does one determine which skills are functional for a particular person? Skill checklists, typically developmentally sequenced, are often used to assess current abilities and to identify target skills. While these checklists sometimes can help determine if a person has the obvious prerequisite skills, they may also lead instructors to teach skills that are not needed or that are less needed than others. Sometimes the sequencing nature of a checklist causes instructors to regard earlier skills as prerequisites to later skills, when they may not be. In the field of special education, the terms *ecological inventory* and *environmental assessment* refer to an indirect method of assessment (Brown & Snell, 1993; Ford et al., 1989; Giangreco, Cloninger, & Iverson, 1993). Therapists interview those who know most about the individual's current skill needs: parents and family members, past teachers, peers, and therapists; and those who are familiar with upcoming skill needs: the next teacher or therapist, peers, vocational trainers, and so forth. The learner's preferences for target skills also are assessed through interview or by observation. "Informants" are asked questions such as:

- What skills do you think are important for ＿＿ to learn?
- What skills are required of ＿＿that he or she does not know or that others must perform regularly?
- Are there some skills critical to ＿＿ 's safety and health that he or she might learn partially or totally?
- What skills are expected of ＿＿ 's peers in the same activities and places?
- Could ＿＿ learn to assist with this skill (partial participation) or to perform the skill with adaptations? Without adaptations?

Therapists also may examine program entry requirements, or visit programs, desired places of employment, or residences to understand what skills are needed for the person to participate and to consider creative accommodations. Once information is obtained from those who know the client best, therapists work with the client's team to set priorities. They consider other assessment information at this time as well. The skills that seem most needed and functional for the person typically become intervention objectives or habilitation targets.

80

Figure 1. Task analysis: Illustrating the component model.

Student:_____

Age:_____ Date:_____

Domain:_____

Routine:_____

	Yes	No	NA	With Adaptations	Comments
1. Grooms or indicates to another the need to groom nails when nails are dirty, jagged, or long. (Initiate)					
2. Finds and selects needed materials, such as clippers, scissors, or file. (Prepare)					
3. Cleans and trims nails. (Core)					
4. Checks nails for cleanliness and neatness. (Monitor quality)					
5. Grooms nails within acceptable amount of time. (Monitor tempo)					
6. If a problem arises, such as being unable to find materials or has a hangnail, takes action to address the problem. (Problem solve)					
7. Puts trimming supplies away, throws nail clippings in trash. (Terminate)					
8. Communicates about any aspect of nail grooming, such as nail care, length, and materials used. (Communicate)					
9. Makes choices concerning nail grooming, such as length of nails and color of polish. (Choice)					
10. Performs routine at appropriate time and place. (Social)					

Adapted from "Making Functional Skills Function: A Component Model" by F. Brown, I.M. Evans, K. Weed, and V. Owen, 1987. *Journal of the Association for Persons With Severe Handicaps, 12*, p. 122. Copyright © 1987 by the Association for Persons With Severe Handicaps. Adapted by permission.

Stage of Learning

Learning is often viewed as occurring in stages or phases, from initial instruction or acquisition to expanded instruction or generalized skills (Farlow & Snell, in press). During the initial phase of instruction, learners receive assistance and more feedback (reinforcement and error correction) as they progress to the stage of understood knowledge or self-regulated, developed skills. *Scaffolding* refers to the assistance provided to move a learner from initial learning to mastery. Others call this assistance *prompting*. Regardless of the term, most agree that assistance should be provided to decrease a learner's frustration with new or difficult tasks and to facilitate success while reducing errors. As the learner's competence increases, assistance is reduced. Figure 2 illustrates the relationship among the following four stages of learning (Snell & Brown, 1993).

1. Acquisition learning concerns initial learning of a skill. In this stage, learners perform the target skill with roughly 0 to 60% accuracy.

2. Maintenance learning concerns the routine use of a skill and improving its accuracy under fairly stable and familiar conditions. Learners perform the target skill with roughly 60% or better accuracy during maintenance.

3. Fluency learning concerns improving the accuracy, quality, and speed of performance. In the fluency stage, learners perform the skill with roughly 60% or better accuracy.

4. Generalization learning concerns performance under changing conditions (location, materials, time, task variation, etc.). Learners perform the skill with roughly 60% or better accuracy during generalization.

Based on this brief description, it becomes clear that teaching approaches and criteria should vary somewhat to match the different stages of learning.

While skills proceed from acquisition to later stages, instruction can focus concur-

Figure 2. Four stages of learning.

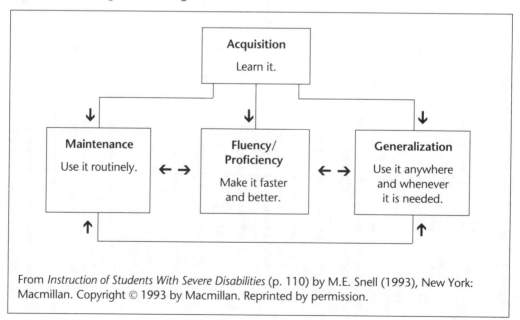

From *Instruction of Students With Severe Disabilities* (p. 110) by M.E. Snell (1993), New York: Macmillan. Copyright © 1993 by Macmillan. Reprinted by permission.

rently on stages 2 through 4 if instructors are clear about their goals, instruction does not get too complex, and performance data are kept to evaluate whether learning is occurring.

Maintenance and generalization are promoted even during initial learning (acquisition) when therapists select skills that are functional, needed, or valued by others, because these skills will be routinely required over multiple settings. By targeting skills suited to the individual's age, he or she may be more inclined to use them, and peers, family members, or therapists will tend to encourage the skills more than they would if the skills stigmatized the person in some way. Additionally, when skills are not fluent or proficient, other people are not likely to encourage their use. For example, consider a child who dresses so slowly that the parents always do it; a boy who self-feeds but will only eat blended fruits, so is rarely taken to restaurants and requires supplemental nutrition to be healthy; or a young adult who cannot work in a motel because after making the beds all of the sheets and blankets are draped unevenly and none of the wrinkles are smoothed. These are fluency and generalization problems, and unless instruction addresses them, learning does not produce skills that others value. Stated another way, those skills that are not learned to a reasonable speed, degree of accuracy, quality, and generalization are not socially valid.

During the acquisition stage of learning, therapists can also build some elements into the intervention plan that will promote generalization from early on. Ways to do this include:

1. Teaching under natural or as close to natural conditions as possible;

2. Using "real," not simulated, materials that are appropriate to the task (e.g., real shoes to teach dressing and shoe tying, though larger clothes may be used during early instruction);

3. Involving multiple teaching examples (therapists, locations, materials, etc.); and

4. Selecting the multiple examples carefully, starting with those that best sample the range of variation (e.g., a turtleneck, tank top, and T-shirt are taught first because they best sample the range of variations in collar, sleeve length, fit, and fabric from a group of eight shirts) (Day & Horner, 1986). This practice teaches individuals a generalized skill that is durable across changing stimulus conditions and response requirements.

Target objectives must specify the behavior, the criterion for performance, and the conditions under which the behavior or skill will be performed. The conditions for performing a skill concern issues of when and where the task is performed, who is present, what materials are involved, and what assistance or adaptations are allowed or possible. A general rule to follow is to let the individual learner's reality dictate the conditions for learning. If the individual shows little or no learning under natural conditions, then the conditions may be simplified; for example, with fewer variations in materials, location, times, and therapists; less noise and distraction, and so forth. Eventually, the individual must learn to perform the skill under natural conditions or the skill will not be useful.

Direct Assessment of Skills

Often I have referred to testing and data collection as an "evil necessity." They are "evil" for several reasons: Individuals seldom learn during testing; and many therapists find data collection tedious and time-consuming, then do not know how to use the data meaningfully to justify the effort. But some performance data are necessary, because only data relevant to the performance of the target behavior can provide the objective information required to judge the instruction's success. For instruction to be efficient and effective, therapists need to gather and analyze student performance data related to its objective. When data indicate minimal or not as expected progress, the program can be improved. Likewise, if the data indicate that the objective has been met, then instruction can be directed toward other objectives, as well as toward the same skill in a different stage of learning. For example, if an adolescent has learned to assist on targeted steps with 60% accuracy while moving in and out of a wheelchair, then the therapist might continue to improve accuracy but shift the focus of instruction toward several new goals: (a) *maintaining* use of the skill in all the situations where training has occurred; (b) improving the speed with which the transfer is made (*fluency*); and (c) adding more new transfer situations to the training sessions and involving the family (*generalization*).

Assessment Data

Observational Data

There are many kinds of data pertinent to skill instruction. This discussion primarily addresses learner performance data; that is, data that measure some aspect of skill performance relevant to the instructional objective. These data are mainly collected through direct observation of the learner during performance of the skill. However, valuable data can be collected *after* the skill has been performed by measuring the "permanent products" resulting from the performance (e.g., checking to see if Josh fastens all of his pajama buttons correctly after bathing; estimating the spillage on the table and floor after Sam finishes eating). Another source of data relevant to assessing progress is the opinions of peers on the success of instruction of a skill they regularly see (e.g., is Sam's eating neat enough?), or the comparative performance of peers on the same skill (e.g., how fast and how neatly do Sam's peers eat?). These data from peers use two different approaches to validate Sam's program outcomes socially: (a) obtaining the subjective opinions of peers, and (b) comparing the student's performance to the peers' performance.

Test and Training Data

Observational data on skill performance are collected under either training or test conditions. Both types of data (training and test) can be useful to therapists. *Training data* reflect student performance during training or instructional conditions (e.g., when assistance, corrective feedback, and reinforcement are provided according to the teaching plan), and *test data* reflect performance during test or nontraining conditions (also referred to as criterion conditions) when little or no assistance or feedback is available other than that naturally occurring in the environment. Test data often show lower performance than do training data.

Types of Tasks

Discrete and Chained Behaviors

Target behaviors can be thought of as either *discrete behaviors* (individually distinctive behaviors that stand alone) or *chained behaviors* (a routine or skill involving a sequence of discrete behaviors). Therapists target many types of discrete behaviors, including lip closure, steps taken during walking, grasping objects with finger and thumb, and release of held objects. Discrete behavior targets are typically defined in observable terms, then counted during a fixed period of time or over a set number of opportunities. For example, a therapist defines what constitutes the form of grasping that is targeted for Muriel (correct response) and what does not (incorrect response). Then the daily activities during which grasping occurs and can be measured are defined, along with the length of the observation. Data gathered might be rate data: the number of correct and error grasps Muriel makes during 10 minutes of toy and block play with peers in kindergarten. Because this example might be highly variable due to changing opportunities during play, a better measurement procedure might be to count her correct (and error) grasps during the first 10 opportunities to grasp during playtime.

Chained behaviors are often thought of as task analyses. Examples include dressing tasks; standing and transfer tasks; some vocational skills; and most grooming, housekeeping, and cooking tasks. Frequently, task analyses serve as the guide for teaching and testing because they list the behaviors and the sequence involved in performing target skills.

Task Analyses

Many of the skills therapists teach can be broken into smaller steps or component behaviors referred to as *task analyses*. Commercially available task analyses may seem to be time-savers but are not recommended, because they fail to individualize the task to the person and the situation. Instead, to develop good task analyses, several steps are important: (a) spend time observing the individual and others performing the task; (b) develop the best approaches for completing the task; (c) ask others' opinions about the task performance (including the person who will learn it and/or family members who will support it); and (d) field-test the task analyses and revise them with needed improvements. To promote skill generalization, develop a task analysis that is relatively generic or suits a number of situations where the learner will need to perform the skill (see Figure 3).

I have found the following guidelines valuable in the development of task analyses:

1. Use steps of fairly even "size";
2. Be sure each step is observable and results in a visible change in behavior;
3. Order the steps in a logical sequence, but indicate when the sequence is optional;
4. Distinguish any "teacher/therapist" steps or those parts of the task performed by individuals other than the student or client;
5. Write the task steps in second-person singular (so they can be used as verbal prompts);
6. Use words that are meaningful to the student or client with whom they will be used, and place in parentheses any additional information that may be difficult for the client to understand, but that is needed for the observer (e.g., "using a pincer grasp"); and
7. Place the steps on a task analytic data sheet, which allows one to record step-by-step data over a number of days (see Figure 4) (Snell & Brown, 1993).

Once a good task analysis is prepared, the therapist uses this as a guide for observing and measuring the skill, and for teaching. Much like measuring discrete behaviors, the learner is asked to perform the skill, then each behavior or step in the task analysis is observed and scored as correct or incorrect. For example, Figure 5 contains the teaching objective and task analysis for the routine tasks Chris needs to gain independence in sitting down on a chair. Chris is 3½ years old and attends a preschool five mornings a

Figure 3. Task analysis for teaching spoon, cup, and napkin use.

Behavior	Discriminitive Stimuli	Response
Spoon	"Eat"	Grasp spoon
	Spoon in hand	Scoop food
	Food in spoon	Raise spoon to lips
	Spoon touching lips	Open mouth
	Mouth open	Put spoon in mouth
	Food in mouth	Remove spoon
	Spoon out of mouth	Lower spoon
	Spoon on table	Release grasp
Cup	"Drink"	Grasp cup
	Cup in hand	Raise cup to lips
	Cup touches lips	Tilt cup to mouth
	Liquid in mouth	Close mouth and drink
	Liquid swallowed	Lower cup to table
	Cup on table	Release grasp
Napkin	"Wipe"	Grasp napkin
	Napkin in hand	Raise hand to face
	Napkin touching face	Wipe face
	Face wiped	Lower napkin
	Napkin on table	Release grasp

From "Using Constant Time Delay to Teach Self-Feeding to Young Students With Severe/ Profound Handicaps: Evidence of Limited Effectiveness" by B.C. Collins, D.L. Gast, M. Wolery, A. Halcombe, and J. Letherby, 1991. *Journal of Developmental and Physical Difficulties, 3*, p. 163. Copyright © 1991 by Plenum Publishing. Reprinted by permission.

week, where he receives his therapy integrated into daily activities. Prior to being taught this skill, Chris waited for help to sit down and stand up from a chair, as his balance was unsteady and he sometimes fell when not assisted. His teachers planned to use a total task approach to teach both sitting and standing up from a chair, so that whenever training occurred each step would be performed in order, with the needed assistance provided. His teachers used the task analysis to guide their observation of his performance on each step.

Two general methods of task analytic observation can be used:

1. During single opportunity task analytic assessment the learner is asked to perform the task. Testing stops after the first error, with all remaining steps scored as errors. Errors include performing the wrong step, making a mistake on a step, taking too long (if time is important), or not performing.

2. During multiple opportunity task analytic assessment, the learner is asked to perform the task. Each step is observed. Whenever an error occurs it is recorded, and the tester positions the student for the next step. Positioning for testing a step is done without comment or instruction—it is not teaching!

Chris's teacher and therapist decided to use a multiple opportunity task analytic assessment approach so they could observe his performance on all steps during each test. Figure 5 displays his baseline performance over 5 days of assessment; he consistently missed the first five steps, but was successful on the last three, though inconsistently and

Figure 4. Task analysis data sheet for Chris's objective of sitting down in a chair.

Name: Chris
Instructor: Maura
Instructional Cue: "Find your chair"
Program: Sitting
Method: Least to Most/4-second latency

Objective: Given a natural opportunity or a request to sit in a preschool cube chair for an activity and a reponse latency of 4 seconds, Chris will perform correctly on at least 88% (7 of 8 steps) of the task analysis without assistance for 3 consecutive training opportunities and one probe.

Date	Baseline*					Training																		Probe
	2/27*	3/4*	3/5*	3/6*	3/7*	3/18	3/19	3/20	3/21	3/22	3/25	4/8	4/11	4/12	4/16	4/17	4/18	4/22	4/23	4/26	4/29	4/30	5/1	5/2*
1. Face cube chair	−	−	−	−	−	P	P	P	P	P	V	+	+	+	+	+	+	+	+	+	+	+	+	+
2. Bend forward	−	−	−	−	−	P	P	P	P	P	V	+	+	+	+	+	+	+	+	+	+	+	+	+
3. Grip arm handles	−	−	−	−	−	G	+	G	G	G	V	+	+	+	+	+	+	V	+	+	+	+	+	+
4. Shift right arm to left arm handle	−	−	−	−	−	P	P	P	P	P	P	+	+	+	+	+	G	+	+	+	+	+	+	+
5. Twist trunk and hips	−	−	−	−	−	P	P	P	+	+	V	+	+	V	V	+	+	+	+	+	+	+	+	+
6. Lower bottom to chair	−	−	−	−	+	+	+	+	+	+	+	+	+	+	+	+	+	+	+	+	+	+	+	+
7. Reposition hands and feet	+	−	+	+	+	+	+	+	+	+	+	+	+	+	+	+	+	+	+	P	+	+	+	+
8. Push bottom to back of chair using feet and hands	+	+	+	+	+	+	+	+	+	+	+	+	+	+	+	+	+	+	+	P	+	+	+	+
	25	13	25	25	38	58	50	38	50	50	38	100	100	88	88	100	88	88	100	75	100	100	100	100*

Key:

Baseline*
(+) independent
(—) error

Training
(+) independent
(V) verbal prompt
(G) gestural prompt
(P) physical prompt

Created by Maura Burke. Used by permission.

Figure 5. Chris's performance during baseline and training of sitting.

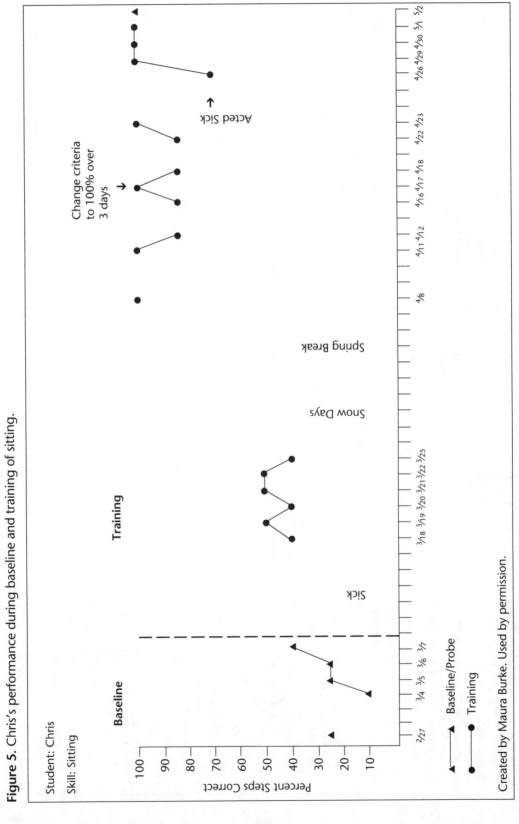

Created by Maura Burke. Used by permission.

with slightly improving performance over the 5 days. His baseline performance seems to indicate that Chris did not know the skill and that targeting the skill was appropriate. His parents and teacher also indicated independent sitting and standing as much needed skills for many daily activities at home and at school.

When related or enrichment target skills are addressed at the same time as core skills, these can simply be placed on the task analysis sheet. For example, if the teacher and therapist want to include choice-making or use of a picture communication wallet in Lynn's task analysis for eating neatly in the cafeteria, these can go directly into the task sequence (if that can be predicted) or these related skills can simply be listed at the end of the task analysis with frequency count entered for each meal. If teachers want a record of any problem behaviors (spitting food), the behaviors can be defined and added to the end of the task steps as well. When graphing these related behaviors it may be best to separate them from the core skill steps. Problem behaviors also need to be analyzed separately, because the intended goal is to decrease their frequency by replacing them with skills. The use of data and graphing is discussed further in the last section of this chapter.

Teaching Strategies

Before discussing general teaching strategies, it might be helpful to review Figure 6, which portrays the arrangement of events that may occur before and after the targeted behavior. Antecedent events are those things that happen before the behavior; some events are intentionally arranged and others that may or may not be under the teacher's or therapist's control simply happen. For example, just prior to learning spoon, cup, and napkin use at lunch (see the task analysis in Figure 3), Sam is hungry. The internal stimuli are setting events, or antecedents. In school, the bell ringing at lunchtime and classmates rushing to their lockers to get packed lunches are also stimuli that set the occasion for lunchtime. Once the children are seated in the lunchroom, more specific stimuli are present: the therapist's request to Sam to "eat" and all the discriminative stimuli (S^D) that are created by performing each response in the chain of taking a spoonful of food. As shown in Figure 3, performance of each response (right hand column) creates antecedent discriminative stimuli (middle column) relevant to the upcoming response in the chain. To teach Sam these skills, his teachers and therapists decided to use physical prompts, or planned antecedent events; they used only as much hand-over-hand assistance as was needed to get him to demonstrate each behavior in the three targeted chains. The physical prompt worked for Sam; that is, the physical assistance prompts controlled his behavior, but the discriminative stimuli that resulted from performing each step of the task did not yet control the responses that they preceded. When the teacher placed the spoon in Sam's hand, he seemed to know he needed to scoop some food, but he did not yet respond in a way that got food on the spoon. One major goal of instruction was to fade out the controlling antecedents that were provided by teachers or therapists (i.e., requests to "eat" and physical prompts), while teaching Sam to attend to the relevant antecedent stimuli (i.e., food on his plate with a spoon, napkin, and filled glass beside it; spoon in hand, food on spoon, spoon touching lips, etc.).

Also portrayed in Figure 6 are consequences, or the events (planned or unplanned) that follow a response. During teaching situations, these general events include comments or information given about the accuracy of the response (confirmation of accuracy—"that's right," or feedback about an error—"You forgot to hold the bottom of the zipper" while pointing to the end of the zipper); reinforcement (praise, activity choice); and correction. While punishing consequences (withholding reinforcement or

Figure 6. Antecedents and consequences to the target response.

Antecedent Events		Response	Consequences
New stimuli "To be Learned"	Controlling Stimuli or Prompts	Correct response	Confirmation
Teacher's request	*Response prompts:*	Approximation	Praise
Task materials	Specific verbal instructions	Incorrect response	Tangible reinforcement
Time	Model	Error	Activity reinforcement
Setting stimuli	Gesture	No response	Choice
Internal stimuli	Physical assistance		Withhold reinforcement
	Stimulus prompts:		Correction
	Color coding		Wait for self-correction
	Pictures		Ignore
	Materials		

giving sharp criticism) are also possible, they do not contribute to good learning conditions and are not regarded as socially valid methods.

Artificial and Natural Prompts and Feedback

Antecedents and consequences can be naturally occurring or artificially arranged. They also can either help or hinder learning. As learners advance into different stages of learning, artificial antecedents and consequences should be faded out, leaving only those that are natural. The teaching task becomes one of directing learners to attend to things in the environment that assist them in performing skills. In many cases, natural cues should be emphasized as prompts from the very beginning of learning. Sam, who is learning to use a spoon and napkin, will benefit from having his teachers call attention to his peers, who sit nearby and can remind him to wipe his face clean. When Rose, an older woman described in Chapter 8 who has recently had a stroke, is relearning many of the daily living skills she once performed with ease, the therapist's verbal, gestural, and physical assists will be helpful, as will the confirmations about her performance and the help with her errors. However, Rose must learn to pay attention to the visual and tactile cues from the left side of her body and the cues of material placement, so she can self-regulate and recognize whether her body is moving as it should be while she is dressing or helping her daughter with meal preparation (e.g., patting lettuce dry, putting salad in a bowl). In place of the therapist's consequences, the comments and reactions of others that naturally occur will become the corrective and reinforcing consequences. For younger children, the natural antecedents of peer modeling and the consequences of peer approval provide important means for learners to judge their own performance.

Antecedents: Instructional Cues

One common error in teaching is saying too much. What is given as an instructional cue should be stated once in a way that the learner understands, which may mean that the cue is accompanied by gestures if symbolic communication is less meaningful, or by signs if the learner is deaf. When the student does not make the desired response, assistance or prompts are given to encourage his or her performance, rather than just repeating the cue. When the objective is functional, the conditions for teaching will be activity-based, thus providing many natural cues to the learner (e.g., location, task materials, time of day, others performing a similar task, and the need for the task to be completed). For Chris, who is learning to sit and stand by himself during preschool activities, the natural cues include his peers getting cube chairs, the teacher calling for circle time, and others sitting. If the instructional cue, "Find your chair" does not result in Chris's performance of the first task step, then the teacher and therapist will use one of three prompts given in order of increasing assistance, but only as needed.

Antecedents: Prompts

As shown in Figure 6, there are two types of prompts: response and stimulus. Response prompts, which are more commonly used, are directed toward the learner's response and thus include verbal instructions; gestures, such as pointing to needed materials, models, or demonstrations of the response; and physical assistance, either partial or full. Stimulus prompts are directed toward the stimuli associated with the task (materials; symbols, like words or numbers; body parts, etc.) and often are used with multiple choice discrimination tasks (e.g., "Find your jacket"). Stimulus prompts include color coding; position or placement (e.g., moving the correct choice closer); and showing the learner miniatures, pictures, or photos of the correct choice. Prompts can be given singly (e.g., verbal request to pick up the soap in a hand-washing task or a photo of the first step in a job), in combinations (e.g., verbal request plus pointing to the soap; back of shirt marked with color tag plus therapist's gesture to tag), or as part of a planned hierarchy of prompts given one at a time as needed.

Prompts must be selected to fit the student and the task. For example, some learners with cerebral palsy may understand the task and the order of its steps, but need to learn the associated muscle control and movement. For these learners, prompts of deep pressure on the required muscles may be far more effective than verbal or model prompts. For example, in Chris's three-step task analysis of standing up from sitting, the therapist provides support at the knees after Chris scoots to the edge of the chair and positions his hands on the arm rests. At this point, Chris can push up to stand. Some prompts depend on the learner having certain skills before they can be used; such prompts are not "controlling stimuli" for a given response. For example, if Rose's therapist uses task step photos to prompt her completion of daily living tasks, but Rose has very limited vision or does not readily associate pictured items with three-dimensional items, the photos will not elicit the required response.

Some assistance may be more permanently added to the task on the steps learners cannot master independently. This version of partial participation is called personal assistance and may include various facilitative therapy techniques, such as tone reduction during a movement, support at a point of control (the hips, elbow, etc.), or even the performance of one or several entire steps. For example, a therapist may apply a tone-reduction technique, such as firm vibration at the forearm and wrist during dressing, as a form of assistance that is not meant to be faded out because it allows the individual to move his or her arm forward (L.K. Vogtle, personal communication, April 5, 1993). In the same dressing task, the therapist may complete several nontarget steps (place the shirt over the student's head, hold one sleeve out), but teach the remaining task steps.

91

System of Least Prompts

Because Chris, the preschooler learning to sit in a chair and stand up did not readily perform the steps in these tasks, his teacher planned to use a prompting procedure. There are many ways to prompt or provide help to someone who does not know the steps in a particular task. Since all prompts will need to be *faded out* for the person to achieve complete independence, Chris's teacher chose a prompting procedure which has a "built-in" means for fading. A *system of least intrusive prompts*, also called *least prompts* for short, involves a hierarchy of prompts that work for the learner and the task and are used one at a time, starting with less assistance and moving to more. Therapists first select a *latency period* or a short time when no assistance is given and the learner initiates the response with no help or with no additional help. For Chris, who has some high tone due to cerebral palsy, a slightly long latency of 4 seconds is chosen; thus, his therapist will pause for 4 seconds following her instructional cue to let him initiate the first step in a task and before giving any assistance (unless he begins making an error, at which point she will interrupt the error with the least intrusive level of assistance). She will pause for the latency (4 seconds) after giving any type of assistance or prompt, again to allow him to initiate the step with a certain amount of assistance. Typically, there are three levels of prompts:

1. Verbal instructions (simple statements for each task step);
2. Verbal instructions plus a gesture (depending on the step, the therapist will point to the materials needed; for other tasks a brief, partial model or demonstration of the movement required may be used); and
3. Verbal instructions plus physical assistance (the therapist provides only as much guidance as is needed, placing a hand on the person's hand, wrist, forearm, or elbow, or at control points such as the knees, shoulders, waist, or hips).

The therapist starts with the least intrusive prompt but proceeds to more intrusive prompts if Chris cannot complete a particular step of the task or if he makes an error and needs more help. For each step of the task the therapist will initially wait for Chris's initiation during the latency before giving any help, and then if he does not initiate (or makes an error) she will offer a verbal prompt and wait. If he does not initiate the response (or makes an error) she will provide a verbal prompt and gesture, and wait during the latency again. Finally, if Chris does not complete the step within 4 seconds following the gesture, the therapist will move to the most intrusive prompt and physically help him to complete the step.

A least-prompts system is adaptable to many tasks and individuals; it has been demonstrated to be effective for persons with mental retardation and other disabilities across many daily living tasks (Snell & Brown, 1993). On the negative side, this system is initially a bit complex for therapists to learn; employs artificial, instructor prompts rather than natural ones; and can appear to be quite intrusive to learners (e.g., physically helping a person move through the step of grasping a box of cereal in the grocery store). A least-prompt system that uses model and physical prompts is better during the early phases of learning, while more subtle prompts are better during later stages of learning. Examples of subtle prompts include an initial nod to confirm a hesitant learner to keep going, followed by a nonspecific verbal prompt of "What's next?," followed finally, if needed, by gestures toward relevant stimuli cues.

Some individuals do not like to be touched; others cannot use certain prompts due to skill limitations (e.g., not everyone can imitate a model prompt or follow verbal instructions). Therefore, the therapist needs to select prompts that work with a particular person, or, like simple verbal instructions, that could be learned after being associated with meaningful prompts. Least-prompts systems require that at least two levels of prompts be selected, that they be arranged in a hierarchy from least to most intrusive, and that prompts be preceded by a latency. Given these basic characteristics, the least-prompts system can be adapted to suit many different learners and tasks.

Graduated Guidance

Therapists using this prompting approach apply more intrusive physical prompts first, then fade them out. Several variations of graduated guidance have been applied when teaching self-care procedures to individuals with disabilities. In the hand-to-shoulder approach therapists initially provide full hand-over-hand guidance throughout the task, but give only the amount of assistance that is needed for the learner to complete the task. This requirement—"give only as much help as is needed"—means that therapists must become highly sensitive to the pressure cues learners give back as they are being assisted. If the learner's hands move in the desired direction during a dressing task, the therapist tries to "back off" and give less guidance. But if the student stops forward movement before he or she should, the therapist provides the movement. The general order of fading assistance is from the learner's hands upward to the shoulder, and then to omit physical assistance altogether. This approach has been used to teach eating and dressing skills (Arzin & Armstrong, 1973; Arzin, Schaeffer, & Wesolowski, 1976; Richman, Sonderby, & Kahn, 1980).

One difficulty with graduated guidance is knowing when to reduce assistance. The best approach is to try reducing assistance periodically while encouraging the learner's attempts at performing with less assistance. The learner's own movements are the best guides to where less assistance is needed. Another approach is to use a response latency before physically assisting each step (or some steps) in the task, thus giving the student opportunities to initiate each step before prompting. Probe data can also help determine what steps may need less assistance.

A second general graduated guidance approach involves using three different levels of physical assistance, varying again from more assistance to less assistance during training:

1. full hand-over-hand assist,
2. two-finger assist, and
3. "shadowing" the person's hand from about 1 to 2 inches.

This approach has been used with dressing skills (Reese & Snell, 1991), to teach adults leisure skills (Demchak, 1989), and with exercising in physical education (Moon, Renzaglia, Ruth, & Talarico, 1981). In both graduated guidance approaches, if the learner resists the prompted movement, the therapist may maintain contact with the learner but simply wait until there is no resistance before continuing to assist. When the therapist has successfully reduced assistance, praise for the learner's increased effort should be increased. When the learner seems to require more assistance, more assistance can be given. Graduated guidance allows the learner to "get the feel" of the movement required by a skill and gradually to take more responsibility for making the movement without the therapist's guidance. This method does not work for individuals who do not like to be touched or guided, nor will it work for those who become dependent on physical assistance.

Time Delay

Besides moving across a hierarchy of prompts, another way to fade prompts is to add time or to delay giving a prompt. During delay periods, the learner may either wait for assistance or try the response on his or her own. If the learner tries, the response may be correct or incorrect. Consider Sam, who is learning some basic self-eating skills (Figure 3). His therapists decide that a physical prompt is best for him and plan to fade the prompt using time delay. They start teaching each skill using a no-delay (zero seconds) period between the discriminative stimulus (S^D) and the prompt, so Sam gets physical prompts continuously through each spoon, napkin, and cup cycle for several meals. Then his therapist inserts a 4-second pause between each S^D and the prompt, allowing Sam time to attempt the response without help. For some steps in the tasks, Sam waits for assistance (prompted correct responses); for others, he completes the steps (independent responses). On a few steps he tries on his own he makes errors, and the therapist immediately repeats that step with help. Because Sam can eat faster when he tries on his own rather than waiting out the delay for help, time delay seems to motivate him to initiate without help; but, because help is forthcoming at the end of a delay period, uncertain learners can simply wait.

Therapists using time delay may adopt the simpler *constant delay approach* (e.g., no delay or 0-second delay followed by delays of 4 seconds) or they may use a *progressive delay approach*, where a delay is gradually increased from 0 to 6 or 8 seconds or longer depending on the learner's natural response latency (e.g., 0, 2, 4, 6, or 8 seconds) (Schuster & Griffen, 1990; Snell & Brown, 1993). When using a delay, the therapist needs to select a single or a combined prompt (verbal plus physical) rather than a hierarchy of prompts and should plan how or when to increase the delay. The best guide is to increase the delay only after a period (several sessions or several trials, depending on the student and the task) of successful waiting responses (the learner does not make an error but allows him- or herself to be prompted) or correct responses (the learner makes the response during the delay without help). If the learner makes errors before the prompt, the delay might be shortened for several trials. If the learner makes an error after the prompt, the prompt may not work for that person. If this happens repeatedly, another prompt should be considered. The delay should not be increased following errors; instead, the therapist should determine what type of error has occurred and address it accordingly.

Prompt systems, especially least prompts and time delay, offer the advantage of a "built-in" plan for fading out assistance, and research has demonstrated their effectiveness. When therapists rely only on consequences to teach new skills, students may become discouraged by their errors and fail to make progress. The combined use of antecedent-prompt strategies with planned consequences is the best teaching approach.

Consequences

Following Correct or Approximate Responses

Figure 6 shows some of the consequences that adults and peers can offer to a learner after a target response. The following practices for using positive consequences are recommended for most learners.

1. *Schedule*. During early learning or acquisition, reinforcement following correct and approximate responses (even when they were prompted) facilitates learning. The reinforcement will occur more frequently during acquisition than during later stages of learning, but should be "thinned" to an intermittent frequency so the student learns to perform without continuous reinforcement from others. If continuous schedules are not reduced over time, students may fail to use the skill under natural conditions when little reinforcement is forthcoming.

2. *Appropriate to learner.* Reinforcing consequences should suit the learner's chronological age, preferences, level of understanding, and the learning situation. Some learners find simple confirmation to be reinforcing ("That's right") while others like and benefit more from task specific praise ("Good job sweeping in the corner"). While tangibles (toys, stickers, food) or preferred activities can be provided at the end of a relatively long task during the acquisition stage, it is best to let the learner have a choice about the consequence rather than trying to anticipate what the individual might find enjoyable.

3. *Natural reinforcers.* During later stages of learning, it is good to teach the learner to self-monitor his or her performance by asking and answering, "How well did I do this time?" It is also helpful to teach learners to look to more natural forms of self-reinforcement, such as taking a mid-morning break at the completion of cleanup tasks or participating in the next activity once seated in circle at preschool.

Consequences are also part of prompt systems. For least prompts and graduated guidance and when single prompts are used (with time delay or simply with a fixed latency), praise is the typical consequence given for completing a step. Only if more concrete reinforcers are needed should they be added, and then they should meet the "appropriateness" criteria. Early in learning, praise can be given following the completion of every step whether or not the step was prompted. As learning progresses, the reinforcing consequences need to be decreased, so praise (and other reinforcing consequences) is reserved for progress made on more difficult steps, and is not given for steps completed with the most intrusive prompts.

Following Errors

When learners make errors, there are many different ways to respond. The stage of learning and the type of error made will influence the consequence, as will many of the learner's characteristics (e.g., age, disabilities, skills). Consider Chris, the preschooler who is learning to sit and stand up from sitting. Before he has learned these tasks to about 60% accuracy, the therapist will need to correct any errors (e.g., "Grip the arms right here," while pointing to the chair arms). Corrections typically involve assistance given following mistakes. Some prompt systems provide clear ways to respond to errors. For example, in a least-prompts approach the therapist interrupts any mistakes with the next prompt in the hierarchy. However, if the incorrect response is simply a failure to respond, then the next prompt in the hierarchy is given following the latency. In graduated guidance, the teacher also responds to errors by giving more assistance, but typically more physical assistance. So, if Linda, who is learning to brush her teeth, fails to remove the cap before squeezing the tube of toothpaste, the therapist may move her guiding hand away from Linda's elbow (a point of less assistance) to the wrist or hand (both points of greater assistance) and ask Linda to repeat the missed step.

Using the same example, once Linda has learned more of the toothbrushing task, the therapist might ask her, "What's next?" (nonspecific verbal prompt) when Linda hesitates on a step she has done before without help. Alternately, the therapist may simply wait longer, giving Linda time to self-correct. Both of these approaches encourage more thinking and independence by the learner, something that is especially desirable during the later stages of learning. Learners at this stage of acquiring a skill may simply check with the therapist when they've completed the task; if it has not been done adequately, the therapist might withhold approval or ask them to try again.

Unfortunately, many of us have learned to provide punitive consequences in an effort to reduce errors or undesirable interfering behaviors. For example, using time-out or reprimands as consequences with some individuals *may* decrease certain behaviors, but they may not, or they may have undesirable effects. The use of punitive consequences may create many problems. First, punishment does not teach skills, it is simply meant to reduce certain behaviors and does not always have the expected outcomes. Second, the therapist is put into a position of control, emphasizing the negative aspects of the teaching environment, which may hinder the therapist's effectiveness as a teacher. Third, punitive methods often are socially invalid or unacceptable to professionals, peers, or care providers, and may violate the learner's basic rights. The best approach to problem behavior is to ignore it unless it harms the learner, others, or task materials, in which case a careful study of the situation is called for. When a problem behavior exists that is not serious, it is best to ignore it and focus on teaching needed skills or alternate replacement skills. This chapter cannot deal adequately with this important topic, and the reader is referred to a variety of useful references on problem behavior (Durand, 1990; Meyer & Evans, 1989; Zirpoli & Melloy, 1993).

Evaluation of Learning and Teaching

Student performance data (test and training) are used in a number of ways. Test data help teachers and therapists

1. make decisions about what to target, depending upon the learner's baseline data (performance before instruction begins), and

2. judge progress once training has begun (probe data) by monitoring the learner's progress under criterion or test conditions.

Baseline and Probe Data

Baseline data should be collected over several days until it is fairly stable, not varying by 40% or more in either direction. When these data are relatively representative of the learner's performance, then instruction can begin with baseline performance serving as a comparative guide for judging progress made during training. Chris's baseline performance in Figure 5 was measured over a week and indicated some improvement. Probe data involve repeating the test observation after teaching has begun. I have found that probe observations need not be taken more than once every 5 training days unless progress is poor. Even then, training data, rather than probe data, are more useful when analyzing the reasons for lack of progress (see Farlow & Snell, in press). Test data (both baseline and probe) typically are recorded using symbols for correct and incorrect responses. Test data may be summarized as the percent or number correct out of the total opportunities. It is useful to record these data on the same graph as training data but to use different symbols to distinguish between them (see Figure 5). Furthermore, the ungraphed or step-by-step task analytic data should be saved and dated because this record shows which steps were correct and which were missed. Chris's trial-by-trial data are shown in Figure 4 and his percent correct performance is graphed in Figure 5.

Training Data

Training data are collected during the training session. Typically, learners perform a given skill better during training than during test conditions. When recording training data, use symbols for correct responses and for the types and amounts of assistance needed by the learner to complete the behavior or step in the task. Thus, steps in the three tasks in Figure

3 (spoon, cup, and napkin use) could either be rated "correct" or noted with a *P* to indicate that a physical prompt was given (see Figure 4). If several prompts are possible, different symbols may indicate which prompt obtained the response (e.g., *V* for verbal, *G* for gestural, *M* for model, *P* for physical assist). Training data provide the therapist with objective information about how the learner responded to the teaching program. Like test data, training data should be both preserved in an ungraphed form (so the information on individual steps is not lost) and graphed using the percent correct or the number of steps correct. Note that in Figure 4, Chris's baseline and probe data are indicated with an asterisk.

Using Data

Besides simply scanning graphs for the trend in progress and for variability, teachers or therapists can examine "raw" or ungraphed (step-by-step) data for specific error patterns that provide clues to needed changes if progress is poor. Dated anecdotal records about student behavior, interfering circumstances, and illnesses will also help resolve why progress may be inadequate. Chris's data in Figure 4 indicate steady progress with less and less assistance on the first five steps of the task during March and April; on April 26 he did require some physical assistance on steps he usually got correct, and the teacher noted on the graph that he did not appear to feel well that day. Since his performance was soon back to its higher level, the teachers made no changes in the program.

Farlow and Snell (in press) provide a detailed method for using data effectively; Brown and Snell (1993) also give some guidelines for this approach. Several general steps are involved in analyzing data to improve instructional programming:

1. Collect data relevant to the instructional objective. Collect training data several times per week, and probe data periodically.

2. Preserve step-by step data by graphing it, indicating dates and baseline, intervention, test, and training data. In addition, note (and date) any relevant anecdotal comments pertinent to the performance data on the back or front of the graph. Use graphs that show all school or program dates so absences, vacations, and other missed days are clear (see Figure 5). Connect data that are from continuous periods of time.

3. If the data seem to be reliable and representative of the learner's performance, determine their trend after graphing 6 to 8 data points: ascending, flat, or descending. If the data are not representative (i.e., the learner has been sick) or not reliable (e.g., for 3 of the data points the aide "recalled" the performance rather than recording the data during the performance), examine the trend after more data have been collected. Note that Chris's initial flat progress in March was followed after spring break by perfect performance during training. This higher-than-criterion performance caused the therapist and teacher to increase the criterion to 100% (see Figure 5).

4. If the trend is ascending, continue the program unless the criterion has been met, whereupon the objective needs to be changed.

5. If the trend is flat or descending, work with the learner's team to determine the possible reason(s) for the lack of progress:

    a. Is there a cyclical variability related to time—some days or sessions are worse due to a weekend, the trainer, medication, and so forth?

    b. Are test data better than training data? If so, what are the differences between the two situations?

    c.   Does the learner have difficulty with the same step(s) across sessions?

    d.   What are the reasons for errors? Is it a specific step? Are the errors setting, time, or staff specific? Are they due to the learner not attempting the task or performing incorrectly? Is the learner reinforced after making errors?

6. Compare performance on other skills and behaviors with this performance. Are the errors similar? Does the target behavior interact with other behaviors (e.g., interfering behavior)? Are problem behaviors increasing? Does the program prevent access to more interactions and activities?

7. Working with the learner's team, develop a hypothesis about the lack of progress.

8. As a team, decide on instructional changes that will address the hypothesis. If more than one hypothesis is developed, determine which one(s) should dictate program change, perhaps by making more observations.

Consider the example of Millie, an adolescent who is working on improving her use of a walker at school. Millie's lack of progress on walking seems cyclical or related to sessions that isolate her from peers, but she is improving during training sessions held during physical education class with peers and at lunchtime in the cafeteria. Anecdotal records state that Millie often refuses to try walking during these sessions where no progress is being made and has cried several times. Two hypotheses could be developed:

- During these time periods when there is progress, Millie's trainers are doing something different (and more effective) than are her trainers at other times.

- Millie enjoys instruction in the context of her peers—perhaps it's the cheering they sometimes give her when she tries harder at walking.

The first hypothesis was ruled out after team members realized that instructors during physical education and lunch were rotated and not specific to those times. Millie's team then decided to focus on the second hypothesis. They asked Millie if she might prefer to have a peer volunteer help during the times of the day when peers had not been present. When Millie indicated she would like this, they recruited volunteers and included them in all training sessions where little progress was occurring. Data collected after this change indicated that her progress showed ascending trends in all sessions.

Therapists must collect and organize student performance data to follow these program evaluation steps. Relevant data include intermittent test data (during baseline and probes of training progress) and training data which are supplemented with anecdotal notes about the learner's performance and social validation of the progress attained. To validate learners' progress socially, one can: (a) query learners themselves, their peers or family members, and teachers and therapists to obtain subjective opinions about progress, or (b) compare learners' performance to their peers'. Though learning evaluation is never simple, it need not be overly complex to provide information pertinent to the effectiveness of a teaching program. The evaluation process should be ongoing, not applied at the conclusion of a program or a school year. Ongoing evaluation means that if the data indicate the client's progress is below expectations, the data are analyzed to clarify the reasons and to design the needed program changes. The data are then used to monitor whether program changes actually lead to performance improvements.

Summary

The goal of most occupational therapy includes teaching individuals in ways that promote learning and encourage their normalized performance. To accomplish these ends, therapists need to target skills that will be useful to an individual learner, use methods that are effective and respect the learner, and evaluate the learner's progress on an ongoing basis. ◆

References

Arzin, N.H., & Armstrong, P.M. (1973). The "mini-meal": A method for teaching eating skills to the profoundly retarded. *Mental Retardation, 11*(1), 9–11.

Arzin, N.H., Schaeffer, R.M., & Wesolowski, M.D. (1976). A rapid method of teaching profoundly retarded persons to dress by a reinforcement-guidance method. *Mental Retardation, 14*(6), 29–33.

Baumgart, D., Brown, L., Pumpian, I., Nisbet, J., Ford, A., Sweet, M., Messina, R., & Schroeder, J. (1982). Principle of partial participation and individualized adaptations in educational programs for severely handicapped students. *Journal of the Association for the Severely Handicapped, 7*, 17–27.

Brown, F., Evans, I., Weed, K., & Owen, V. (1987). Delineating functional competency: A component model. *Journal of the Association for Persons with Severe Handicaps, 12*, 117–124.

Brown, F., & Snell, M.E. (1993). Meaningful assessment. In M.E. Snell (Ed.), *Instruction of students with severe disabilities* (4th ed.) (pp. 61–98). New York: Macmillan.

Collins, B.C., Gast, D.L., Wolery, M., Holcombe, A., & Letherby, J. (1991). Using constant time delay to teach self-feeding to young students with severe/profound handicaps: Evidence of limited effectiveness. *Journal of Developmental and Physical Disabilities, 3*, 157–179.

Day, H.H., & Horner, R.H. (1986). Response variation and the generalization of a dressing skill: Comparison of single instance and general case instruction. *Applied Research in Mental Retardation, 7*, 189–202.

Demchak, M.A. (1989). A comparison of graduated guidance and increasing assistance in teaching adults with severe handicaps leisure skills. *Education and Training in Mental Retardation, 24*, 45–55.

Durand, V.M. (1990). *Severe behavior problems: A functional communication training approach.* New York: Guilford.

Farlow, L., & Snell, M.E. (in press). Effective and efficient use of student performance data. *AAMR Research to Practice Series.* Washington, DC: American Association on Mental Retardation.

Ferguson, D.L., & Baumgart, D. (1991). Partial participation revisited. *Journal of the Association for Persons with Severe Handicaps, 16*, 218-227.

Ford, A., Schnorr, R., Meyer, L., Davern, L., Black, J., & Dempsey, P. (1989). *The Syracuse community-referenced curriculum guide for students with moderate and severe disabilities.* Baltimore: Paul H. Brookes.

Giangreco, M.F., Cloninger, C.J., & Iverson, V.S. (1993). *C.O.A.C.H.: Choosing options and accommodations for children.* Baltimore: Paul H. Brookes.

Meyer, L.H., & Evans, I.H. (1989). *Nonaversive intervention for behavior problems: A manual for home and community.* Baltimore: Paul H. Brookes.

Moon, S., Renzaglia, A., Ruth, B., & Talarico, D. (1981). *Increasing the physical fitness of the severely mentally retarded: A comparison of graduated guidance and hierarchy of prompts.* Unpublished manuscript, University of Virginia.

Reese, G.M., & Snell, M.E. (1991). Putting on and removing coats and jackets: The acquisition and maintenance of skills by children with severe multiple disabilities. *Education and Training in Mental Retardation, 26*, 398–410.

Richman, J.S., Sonderby, T., & Kahn, J.V. (1980). Prerequisite vs. in vivo acquisition of self-feeding skill. *Behaviour Research and Therapy, 18*, 327–332.

Schuster, J.W., & Griffen, A.K. (1990). Using time delay with task analyses. *Teaching Exceptional Children, 22*(4), 49–53.

Snell, M.E., Lewis, A.P., & Houghton, A. (1989). Acquisition and maintenance of toothbrushing skills by students with cerebral palsy and mental retardation. *Journal of the Association for Persons with Severe Handicaps, 14*, 216–226.

Snell, M.E., & Brown, F. (1993). Instructional planning and implementation. In M.E. Snell (Ed.), *Instruction of students with severe disabilities* (4th ed.) (pp. 99–151). New York: Macmillan.

Zirpoli, T.J., & Melloy, K.J. (1993). *Behavior management: Application for teachers and parents*. New York: Macmillan.

5

Self-Care Strategies for Children With Developmental Deficits

Jane Case-Smith

Jane Case-Smith, EdD, OTR, FAOTA, is an Assistant Professor in the Division of Occupational Therapy at the School of Allied Medical Professions, The Ohio State University, Columbus, OH.

Chapter 5 Outline

Self-Care Development

Child and Family Variables Related to Self-Care
Child Variables
Family Variables
Interaction of Parent-Child Variables
Family Life Cycle

Feeding
Typical Development of Oral Feeding
Feeding Problems in Children With Developmental Disabilities
Feeding Intervention
    Nutritional Considerations
    Feeding as a Social Event
    Parent-Child Interaction
    Family Mealtime
Intervention Approaches for Children With Motor Delays
    Positioning
    Handling Techniques
    Jaw and Tongue Support
        Facilitation and Inhibition
        Appropriate Application of Handling Techniques
    Sensory Aspects of Food
Interventions for Children With Tactile Defensiveness
Children Who are Non-Oral Feeders
    Recommending Non-Oral Feeding
    The Transition From Non-Oral to Oral Feeding
Children With Behavior Problems

Self-Feeding
Typical Development of Self-Feeding
Intervention Approaches

Positioning

Handling Techniques

Adaptive Equipment

Dressing

Typical Developmental Sequence of Dressing

Children With Delays in Dressing Skills

Interventions for Dressing Children

Children With Motor Impairments

Infants and Young Children

Older Children

Children With Tactile Defensiveness

Intervention Approaches to Improve Self-Dressing

Children With Motor Impairments

Motor Analysis

Activities to Improve Self-Dressing Skills

Adapted Techniques

Appropriate Clothing

Adapted Equipment

Children With Tactile Defensiveness

Children With Dyspraxia

Bathing Skills

Typical Sequence of Bathing Skill Development

Issues Related to Developing Bathing Skills

Intervention for Bathing Young Children

Infants With Motor Delays

Safety Issues

Bath Time Therapy

Infants With Tactile Defensiveness

Bath Time as Play

Interventions to Improve Self-Bathing in the Child
With Motor Delays

       Adapted Equipment

       Other Intervention Approaches for
       Improving Self-Bathing

Functional Communication

       Children Who Benefit From Augmentative Communication

       Selecting Augmentative Communication for Children

              Direct Selection

              Scanning Mode

              Encoding

       Mounting and Positioning for Optimal Use of the System

              Mounting

              Positioning

       Enhancing the Child's Skills to Use a Device

       Integrating the Augmentative Communication System
       Into the Home and Classroom

Functional Mobility

       Typical Development of Mobility

       Children Who Require Assisted Mobility

              Selecting a Wheelchair and Wheelchair Components

                     Transport Chairs

                     Self-Propelled Wheelchairs

                     Powered Chairs

                     Scooters

                     Standard Powered Chairs

       Positioning and Fitting the Child to the Chair

       Functional Use of the Mobility Device in the Child's
       Daily Activities

Conclusion

References

Most children with developmental disabilities experience delays or difficulties in accomplishing self-care skills. The level of independence in self-care that the child achieves relates to the nature of the disability, the child's strengths and resources in compensating for the disability, the home environment, and the caregiving support of the family. The child develops self-care skills in the context of the family's daily life activities; therefore, these two variables cannot be separated. As a result, family resources and concerns, as well as the child's needs and strengths, guide the direction of occupational therapy and determine the strategies selected. Self-care skills are a basic family function (Turnbull & Turnbull, 1986) and, as such, they are inevitably affected by the family's values and cultural background. For example, a family may hold very strong beliefs in how and what a child should be fed. The family's culture can also influence clothing selection, bathing regularity, and other areas of self-care.

While the family and home environment are important, the child's self-care development is equally influenced by how the disabling condition has compromised functional skill development. Achievement of each feeding, dressing, bathing, or mobility milestone is determined by the child's sensory system function, motor skills, perceptual skills, cognitive level, social interaction, motivation, attention span, and communication, and other aspects of development.

In this chapter, a framework is presented for assisting children in developing self-care skills. Specific sensory-motor-perceptual problems are addressed while considering the whole child in the context of the family. The influences of family variables, such as family values and resources, are discussed as they relate to the child's care and self-care.

This chapter is divided into sections that describe typical development and problems in feeding, dressing, bathing, and functional communication and mobility. Interventions to improve and promote the development of these self-care skills are presented as solutions to specific problems. Compensation techniques and adapted equipment to increase the child's self-care independence are described.

Self-Care Development

Knowledge about typical self-care development helps the occupational therapist identify delays and problems, and creates appropriate goals for the child. The step-by-step sequence of self-care skill development has been documented by Coley (1978), Finnie (1975), Klein (1988), Morris and Klein (1987), and others. Self-care is also a domain of most developmental curricula. Examples are the Hawaii Early Learning Profile (Furuno et al., 1984) and the Carolina Curriculum (Johnson-Martin, Jens, & Attermeier, 1986). These curricula guide the therapist assisting the child to develop step-by-step achievement of self-care; however, many children do not follow the typical developmental sequence. For example, a preschooler with severe oral tactile sensitivity may be totally independent in self-feeding, but may have immature chewing ability and need assistance in developing basic oral motor skills. A child with spastic diplegia may learn to button and tie (a 4-year-old skill) prior to learning to put on pants (a 2-year-old skill). Because children with disabilities do not always follow the typical sequence of development, the normal self-care development model guides, rather than determines, the intervention goals. Within this frame of reference, the unique strengths and limitations of the child, family, and environment form the basis of the intervention plan.

The occupational therapist approaches self-care problems in children with disabilities after comprehensive assessment of the child, task, and environment. Information regarding the following variables is synthesized to develop plans and strategies to facilitate the child's independence in self-care.

Child and Family Variables Related to Self-Care

Child Variables

The child's self-care skills are determined by his or her sensory, motor, perceptual, cognitive, social-emotional, and communication skills. A developmental disability may affect any or all of these functional domains. When creating an intervention plan, the therapist identifies the developmental skills inherent in each self-care function. The self-care skills targeted as intervention goals are then matched to the child's developmental skills and individual strengths and needs. For example, children with cerebral palsy may have postural instability and limitations in sensorimotor skills, and have strengths in cognitive and psychosocial skills. The skills that the child demonstrates, those that are missing, and those that are emerging, determine which intervention strategies are used in therapy and what recommendations are made to the caregivers and teachers involved in the child's self-care. The therapist builds on the child's strengths and helps the child develop or compensate for limitations. In each section of this chapter, strengths (skill areas) and limitations (skills that are missing or require assistance) that are associated with different developmental disabilities are discussed relative to intervention to improve self-care skills.

Interaction skills, motivation, attention span, initiative, and temperament are other characteristics that influence the accomplishment of self-care tasks. High levels of motivation and initiative in developing self-care independence are important assets toward achieving self-care goals. Children with seemingly mild disabilities—for example, tactile defensiveness or difficulty in motor planning—may have repeated failures, resulting in decreased motivation and initiative (Brinker & Lewis, 1982; Kielhofner, 1985). Significant delays in self-care achievement may result. These delays can be major problems for parents who must deal every day with feeding, dressing, and bathing the child. Frustrations and stress increase when the parents have high expectations for independence and limited understanding of the basis of the problem.

Self-care skills can also exceed expectations or become one of the highest levels of achievement in children with severe disabilities. With adaptive equipment for feeding or dressing, a child with severe motor limitations can achieve independence. When self-care tasks are structured into the everyday routine, the regular repetition enables children with mental retardation to learn the steps in dressing and bathing or to achieve mobility within the home environment. In these examples, self-care skills may be a source of mastery and achievement important to the child's self esteem. The child's independence in daily living skills is equally important to the family's daily function.

Family Variables

The child learns self-care in the context of his or her home. Based on the child's cognitive, social, and motor readiness, he or she progresses through a continuum from total care by the parents to self-care independence. As the child's skills increase, the parents engage less in "doing for" the child and more in promoting self-care independence. This gradual process does not involve teaching self-care skills as much as it involves providing opportunities for the child, encouraging the child, and adapting the activity to enable the child to participate. As mentioned above, this process is important to the child's sense of mastery as well as to the family's daily function and balance of family activities.

Children with developmental disabilities may never achieve complete independence in self-care. A child with multiple and severe disabilities may always need to be fed, bathed, and dressed. As a result, not only do these daily living tasks remain the total responsibility of the caregivers, but they become more difficult. Because the older child is heavier and may have increased physical problems (e.g., contractures), the total care of a child with severe cerebral palsy becomes more time consuming and more difficult as he or she reaches adolescence. Mild behavior problems in the infant can, in the older child, become major behavior problems that negatively affect the family. Self-abusive or controlling behaviors may be exhibited, compounding the daily work of the caregivers. The therapist helps the family develop adapted methods to manage the daily care of the child when self-care independence is not a goal. This chapter describes methods used to help family members manage the child's daily care and enhance the child's self-care skill development using therapeutic and compensatory approaches.

Families are an important part of intervention with children with developmental disabilities (Case-Smith, 1991). Intervention programs for children involve the family's participation in assessment, program planning, implementation, and evaluation of the program's effect (see Figure 1).

The child's self-care skills cannot be separated from the family's daily function. Therefore, the occupational therapist becomes quite involved with all the family members in therapy related to self-care issues. The family's characteristics determine the

Figure 1. Family roles in occupational therapy with the child.

Therapy Processes	Family Roles
Assessment	• Provide information • Verify child's performance • Give history of development • State concerns and priorities
Planning	• Assist in problem solving • Give priorities • Make decisions regarding preferred goals • When possible, select therapy settings • Contribute ideas to plan
Implementation	• Communicate child's progress • Communicate concerns, resources, priorities • Practice activities at home • Try new methods and strategies • Make decisions regarding changing goals or beginning new goals • Help monitor child's progress • Communicate therapy strategies to other family members • Provide feedback to therapist

strategies used by the therapist and influence the effectiveness of the methods selected. Examples of some family variables that affect the child's self-care development are:

1. *Culture.* Does the family value self-care independence? Is assistive technology accepted in the home? Are family traditions and rituals important?

2. *Time.* Do family members have time for each other and for the daily care of a child who is dependent in self-care?

3. *Commitment.* Is the family committed to the effort needed to promote self-care independence? When the child's behavior is an issue, self-care independence may require consistency, behavior management, and discipline.

4. *Communication.* Do family members communicate daily problems and successes with the therapists, and do they communicate new strategies or ideas to each other? Often intervention strategies require that family roles become flexible (i.e., the siblings and father help with child care) and that family members are able to ask for each other's help.

The therapist needs to consider the parents' communication and learning styles when designing a program (Turnbull & Turnbull, 1986; Winton, 1988). The parents' methods of learning will determine if written, verbal, or visual methods are selected for instructing them. Parents often choose their own methods for facilitating and adapting the child's self-care activities and may only need reassurance and an occasional new idea. Parents with developmental disabilities themselves may need more assistance in problem solving around feeding, bathing, and dressing of their children. However, with guidance from the therapist, all parents, including those with special needs (such as those with mental retardation) should make decisions about their child's care (Espe-Sherwindt & Kerlin, 1990).

Interaction of Parent-Child Variables

It is the interaction of parent and child variables that guides the occupational therapist's intervention and determines the child's progress. When the family is highly flexible and seems able to accept and adapt to the child's disability, self-care development may progress quickly, following a sequence similar to that of a typically developing child. Even children with severe problems can fit well into a family's daily routine when members have a caring commitment toward each other and have external social supports.

Family structures that are chaotic, and family members who do not support each other, can compound the child's self-care problems. The lack of self-feeding skills and poor oral motor control may result in the child's failure to thrive if the family is unable to spend the hours needed consistently to feed the child. When the caregiver lacks self-esteem and an inner sense of control, he or she may feel that therapeutic methods will not change the child's problem, and may abandon attempts to increase the child's self-care skills. For example, an adolescent single mother may resent the time and energy required to care for a child who is difficult to feed, dress, and bathe. The child senses the mother's resentment and stress, which decreases his or her own sense of control and self-esteem. In such an instance, support for the mother and her ability to care for the child is as important as teaching the child new self-care skills.

Family Life Cycle

Self-care issues change as the child develops and matures (Turnbull, Summers, & Brotherson, 1986). Early issues in learning to chew solid food and drink from a cup are often resolved as issues in independent mobility and dressing become more important.

When the child enters school, independent feeding, dressing, and mobility may become increasingly challenging in the new environment. Adaptive equipment may be acquired to assist the child in independent function. The typically developing child gains new independence from the family when he or she enters school. The child with disabilities may remain quite dependent in all areas of self-care and mobility, which could affect social interactions with peers and adults. The child's level of self-care independence can determine classroom placement and level of supervision needed throughout the day.

Self-care independence becomes critically important when the issue of independent living is evaluated by the young adult and his or her family. As the child becomes an adolescent and prepares for work and independent living, additional self-care skills may be needed and new levels of independence must be achieved (Barber, Turnbull, Behr, & Kerns, 1988; Case-Smith, 1991). Whether it is to function in the home, school, or an independent living situation, self-care skills are critical to the child's ability to adapt to and become independent in those environments.

Feeding

Typical Development of Oral Feeding

Feeding is essential to life and is initially accomplished in the neonate by reflexive sucking. The typical child is equipped with all the reflexes needed to consume liquids successfully by mouth (i.e., rooting and sucking reflexes, a gag, and automatic cough). As these early reflexes are integrated at 2 to 3 months of age, the infant develops rhythmic suckling movements in which the tongue moves in extension-retraction, stroking the nipple while the jaw moves up and down. True sucking, which involves an up-and-down movement of the tongue, develops by age 6 months. The sucking tongue movement is a more effective method for expressing liquids from a nipple than the suckle response. At this age the infant no longer loses liquid from the mouth during sucking, and cup drinking may be introduced. The infant uses wide jaw excursions and suckling tongue movements with the cup, and significant amounts of liquids are lost. Lip activity is minimal, and the tongue moves using a combination of suckling and sucking.

The child usually spoon-feeds by 6 months of age. At this time, the lips do not actively participate in obtaining the food. The tongue moves backwards and forwards in a suckling pattern. Lip coordination and pressure continue to improve, and by age 9 months the child demonstrates active lip control. By this time the wide jaw excursions are graded so that the amount of mouth opening begins to match the amount of food on the spoon. Gradually, tongue tip elevation and lip closure occur during swallowing. Tongue and lip movements become separated from jaw movements, and an increasing variety of movement patterns are observed.

The development of chewing occurs simultaneously with the refinement of sucking behaviors. The infant has a bite reflex at birth that becomes integrated with the development of an active, controlled bite. Chewing begins as a munching pattern at about 5 months of age. Soon after this up-and-down jaw pattern is established, the child demonstrates tongue lateralization and elevation. At first the food is mashed against the upper palate in a sucking movement. True chewing develops gradually as the tongue becomes more active and the jaw begins to move in diagonal, and then rotary, patterns. Rotary chewing requires smooth interaction of all of the muscles that surround the mouth. Quite often, refined chewing is not observed until the child is 18 months old.

At age 18 months, the child is also more proficient in cup drinking. The jaw stabilizes on the rim of the cup, and lip seal has improved, so less liquid is lost. At age 24 months, the child has developed internal jaw stability and can rest the rim of the cup between his or her teeth while controlling the intake of liquid with the lips. In spoon feeding and cup drinking, the child opens the mouth only as much as is required for the intake of food. Chewing movements are smooth and rotary, and the child is capable of grinding jaw movements and transferring food to all areas of the mouth (Morris, 1978; Morris & Klein, 1987).

Feeding Problems in Children With Developmental Disabilities

Feeding problems may be associated with various developmental disabilities. Children with cerebral palsy and other neuromotor impairments often have delays in oral motor development and benefit from assistance in developing control of oral movements (see Figure 2).

Children with a wide range of feeding problems may benefit from occupational therapy. Those receiving services range from non-oral feeders with only reflexive oral movements, to semi-independent feeders with mild delays associated with decreased sensory tolerance of food textures and consistencies. The continuum of oral motor problems can be associated with primary sensory, motor, or behavior problems. The occupational therapist selects a frame of reference and corresponding strategies that match the underlying basis of the feeding problem.

Feeding Intervention

Nutritional Considerations

Many children with cerebral palsy are underweight. Children with severe cerebral palsy who have limited oral motor control are particularly at risk for poor weight gain and growth (Pipes & Pritkin, 1989). When oral motor control is limited, and abnormal oral reflexes are present, feeding requires long periods of time and at best is inefficient. As a result, the child may lose as much food from the mouth as he or she consumes, and chewing and swallowing may require a great amount of energy. The child can become fatigued during feeding before being satiated. Interventions must be carefully selected for a child whose oral motor control problem has resulted in slow growth and possible malnutrition (Palmer & Elkvall, 1985).

For the infant who is at risk for growth and nutrition problems, mealtime may not be an optimal time for implementing oral motor intervention (e.g., practice of chewing and tongue lateralization). Therapy activities to enhance oral motor control can be implemented in between meals and at less critical eating times. Perhaps an additional snack can be instituted in the child's day, specifically to work on oral motor skills. For example, the cold stimulation of an ice cream snack tends to increase the suck-swallow response and to reduce a swallow delay. A snack of crunchy foods can facilitate chewing and increase tongue movements in the child who has tactile discrimination problems.

When intervention to improve oral motor skills involves changing the child's diet, a nutritionist should be consulted. Increasing the texture of the food consumed, such as recommending soft, instead of pureed, food texture, requires that a nutritionist evaluate how the change will affect the child's overall diet. A change in food texture can greatly enhance tongue movement and chewing skill, but it can also reduce the total number of calories and change the nutritional balance consumed. Planning such dietary changes with the nutritionist and family results in diet changes that increase both oral motor skills and the health and nutrition of the child.

Figure 2. Functional problems in feeding associated with developmental disabilities.

Condition	Functional Problems That May be Emphasized in Feeding Intervention
Cerebral palsy	• Oral movement patterns (sucking, chewing) • Oral reflexes • Oral muscle tone • Sequence in chew/suck/swallow • Lip, tongue, and jaw mobility • Trunk, neck, and jaw stability • Postural control • General mobility
Sensory integration dysfunction	• Oral sensory perception • Tolerance of tactile input • Chewing and biting skills • Oral praxis • High activity level • Sensory defensiveness
Autism	• Tolerance of specific tastes • Sensory defensiveness • Interaction skills
Respiratory or cardiac problems	• Endurance • Coordination between swallowing and breathing • Coughing strength
Severe sensorimotor disabilities	• Stability and mobility of oral structures • Control of oral phase of chewing and drinking • Control of swallow • Coordination of suck/swallow/breathe
Failure to thrive	• Negative behaviors • Interactions between parent and child

Note: Behavior and interaction issues may accompany any of the oral motor programs listed above.

Feeding as a Social Event

Feeding almost always involves interaction with others. Initially, feeding is an intimate experience between mother and child (Humphry, 1991; Humphry & Rourk, 1991). This is particularly true if the infant is breast fed. As the child develops and begins to eat solid foods, family mealtimes become the context for feeding. When the child enters school and eats with his or her peers, feeding is accomplished in a larger social context.

Parent-Child Interaction

When feeding is a problem, all of these interactions are affected. For the child who has great difficulty eating, typically enjoyable, pleasant interactions can become unpleasant and stressful. When the child is a young infant, the parents are probably the sole feeders. Barnard and Kelly (1990); Brazelton, Koslowski, and Main (1974); Vietze, Abernathy, Ashe, and Stich (1978) and others, discuss the essential nature of these early parent-child interactions. Feeding is a time for responsive give-and-take between parent and child (Barnard & Kelly, 1990). The child gives the parent cues regarding hunger and satiation, and the parent responds with appropriate amounts of food. Holding the child close to the body, patting and stroking, and eye contact are important elements in feeding. In the rhythmic, turn-taking interaction, the mother feels competent and gains satisfaction in nourishing the child. When the child struggles to eat, spits, chokes, or gags, the experience quickly becomes anxiety-producing, rather than pleasurable. The parent seldom feels competent, and the satisfaction of the feeding interaction is lost. Reading and appropriately responding to the infant's cues become more difficult, and the synchrony and rhythm of the interaction are lost. When feeding interactions are stressful over time, the relationship between parent and child can be negatively affected (Chamberlin, Henry, Roberts, Sapsford, & Courtney, 1991; Humphry, 1991).

The occupational therapist's recommendations regarding feeding must always consider the importance of the feeding interaction. Strategies to promote the child's feeding skills should not add to the stress experienced by the dyad. The methods suggested should increase, rather than decrease, the parent's confidence and sense of competence in feeding the child. Therefore, the therapist should carefully select recommendations that match the parents' skills. Complicated handling techniques that involve icing or vibration should only be given to parents who express interest in such methods. Simple methods for improving feeding skills are most likely to be implemented and to affect the feeding interaction positively. Helpful strategies include all of the elements that comprise positive interactions between caregivers and children: eye contact, sensitivity to the child's cues, gentle touch, verbal/nonverbal communication, and turn-taking (Barnard & Kelly, 1990). Affectionate touch is part of any feeding intervention. If the therapist reminds parents about these "most important" aspects of feeding, the specific handling and recommended techniques do not dominate the activity. When recommending specific methods, such as spoon placement and downward pressure with external jaw control, the therapist must demonstrate how such techniques can be integrated into the natural interaction. It is critical that the mother feel comfortable with these techniques so she can communicate with the child in a positive manner. The mother's comfort level can be increased with modeling and practicing the techniques during therapy, followed by positive encouragement.

Family Mealtime

By 12 months of age, the child sits with the family at mealtime. The family congregates at this time to share and communicate and to enjoy each other. This social occasion is as important to the child with disabilities as it is to the other family members, but a number of factors may limit the child's participation.

1. The child may require 100% of the attention of one family member in order to be fed.
2. The child may become excited and distracted when sitting with the family and may be less able to eat.
3. The child's feeding may be extremely messy and may negatively affect the family's interaction.

After consulting with the occupational therapist, the family selects specific methods and techniques that will facilitate management of mealtimes and provide positive family experiences. They have several options, and the occupational therapist may offer consultation regarding which might work for the family. If the child cannot sit at the table, placing the wheelchair near it will include him or her in the family circle. The child may be fed prior to the family mealtime and then spend time at the dinner table playing with small amounts of food placed on the high chair or wheelchair tray. The participation of the child who is a non-oral feeder in the family's meal helps to normalize his or her daily experiences and provides an optimal time for communication and interaction. The family's enjoyment of mealtime can help the child who has oral sensory defensiveness to approach feeding with a more positive attitude and to demonstrate greater tolerance of oral stimulation.

The family mealtime may not be the optimal time for feeding a child with severe oral motor problems, and if inclusion of the child is impractical, or if family mealtimes are chaotic, the therapist should advocate that other family times be established as a routine occurrence. Family meals may best serve as a time to experience food texture in hand play or to practice finger or spoon self-feeding. Parents should learn to tolerate "messy" food play and implement efficient ways to clean up food spillage. The concept of mealtime as a social routine is important to maintain.

Intervention Approaches for Children With Motor Delays

The occupational therapist approaches feeding problems holistically, considering factors in the environment, family, and the child that seem to influence the child's feeding skills. With the input of the parents and other team members, the occupational therapist recommends and uses a number of strategies to increase feeding abilities. These strategies have been described in detail by Case-Smith (1989); Farber (1982); Glass and Wolf (1993); Hunter (1990); Morris, (1978); Morris and Klein (1987); Mueller (1975); and Wolf and Glass (1992); and are briefly outlined below.

Positioning

The child's postural alignment and control are essential aspects of feeding. Stability of the head, shoulders, and pelvis need to be adequate to support oral motor control. When the child's postural stability is low, external support must be provided. High-back chairs with lateral supports and straps are examples of devices that provide maximal amounts of postural stability and offer the child the best opportunity to demonstrate oral motor control.

When head control is an issue, lateral head supports are beneficial. Slightly reclining the chair while maintaining 90° of hip flexion may assist the child in head control and improve oral movements and feeding. A slightly reclined position (30°) also enables the child to use gravity to assist in the suck-swallow sequence (Morris & Klein, 1987). When the chair is tilted backwards, it is important that the neck alignment remain neutral or in slight neck flexion.

A slightly forward position of the head appears to aid in the child's swallow by decreasing the distance the larynx must elevate during this activity (Wolf & Glass, 1992). If the child appears at risk for aspiration, a videofluoroscope can reveal the head and neck position in which this seems least likely to occur (Fox, 1990).

Handling Techniques

Handling techniques to support and improve oral motor function have been developed by therapists using the neurodevelopmental treatment approach. These methods are appropriate for children who have cerebral palsy. Jaw and tongue support and facilitation and inhibition techniques are described.

Jaw and Tongue Support

The therapist's or parent's fingers, or a cupped hand, can be placed under or around the child's chin to increase head and jaw stability (see Figure 3). To promote chin tuck, pressure is applied with the fingers backwards from the front of the chin and upwards under the chin. Holding under the chin supports the movement of the tongue rather than moving the jaw. Continuous application of the hand may be more easily tolerated than frequent on-and-off application. The flat parts of the hand and fingers, rather than the fingertips, should be applied, and the therapist's or parent's hand should be a stabilizing, not a mobilizing, force for the jaw and tongue.

Facilitation and Inhibition

Downward pressure on the tongue with the bowl of the spoon or the nipple can inhibit tongue retraction or protraction and facilitate sucking. This gentle pressure with a spoon promotes a normal tongue position and organized, rhythmic sucking.

Increasing muscle tone can be accomplished prior to the meal by a quick stretch to the masseter and buccinator muscles (Glass & Wolf, 1993). Some techniques should be applied carefully, since they can easily cause an aversive response when applied inappropriately or without preparing the child.

Appropriate Application of Handling Techniques

All of the handling methods should be weighed for their cost-benefit ratio to the child and family. Techniques performed by the therapist once or twice a week that are not carried over into the school and home environments are of limited value to the child who feeds four or five times per day. Simple handling techniques may be selected over complex inhibition and facilitation techniques (e.g., use of ice, lemon swabs, or vibration), when persons other than the therapist usually implement them. The effects of techniques that improve the quality of oral movements, but increase the time and effort that feeding requires, should be carefully assessed prior to recommending implementation. When oral motor techniques reduce the efficiency of feeding and less food is consumed at increased energy cost, the techniques should be judiciously limited in application. For example, the therapist and parent may implement techniques to inhibit tongue thrust and facilitate lip closure only during snack times if the handling methods include several minutes of preparation to the mouth area and longer intervals between each spoonful of food. Some techniques to promote swallowing (i.e., bits of ice given between bites of food) significantly increase the length of the meal and should only be used at snack time.

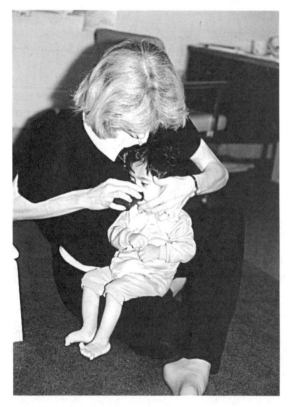

Figure 3. Use of jaw control during cup drinking.

Sensory Aspects of Food

Altering the sensory aspects of food is another way to improve oral motor skill (Case-Smith, 1989; Morris & Klein, 1987). The tongue moves primarily in response to the texture of food or to a sensory stimulus in the mouth (e.g., a nipple or spoon). As such, some textures overpower the child and decrease oral motor control, resulting in disorganized tongue movements. Foods that are smooth and cohesive may facilitate organized tongue responses. Thick, heavy, and cohesive foods (e.g., oatmeal or puddings) tend to facilitate an efficient suck-swallow pattern. In general, highly textured foods result in increased tongue movement.

To promote more mature oral movements, the occupational therapist carefully selects appropriate textures to use in therapy and to recommend to the family. In selecting the optimal food textures for the child, consideration is given to the child's present level of jaw-and-tongue movement patterns as well as sensory acceptance. Some guidelines for texture selection follow.

1. Pureed, smooth foods will elicit a suck-swallow response and should be used primarily if no lateral tongue movements or munching patterns are present.

2. Thin liquids are the most difficult consistency to control in the mouth and should be thickened when the child has poor tongue control and an inefficient suck-swallow pattern.

3. Soft foods that have cohesion when masticated offer increased sensory experiences. These foods (cheeses, chicken, well-cooked vegetables with no skins) increase chewing when placed in between the teeth.

4. Graham crackers, butter cookies, and some cereals (e.g., Cheerios) are good foods for chewing because they dissolve very quickly once inside the mouth, presenting less danger of choking.

5. If the family uses a food grinder to puree the child's food, food texture can easily be altered by changing the food grinder setting.

6. Grainy breads are better than soft white breads, which tend to stick to the upper pallet in a ball.

7. It may be helpful to introduce textured foods that require some chewing by mixing them in foods that are familiar to the child and that add cohesion to the

food bolus. For example, mashed potatoes can be mixed with other vegetables and soft meats to help hold those foods together. This sensory experience may be more acceptable to the child than the new food alone, which becomes a collection of discrete bits after chewing. Parents should be alerted to adding the right amount of moisture to food to make it more manageable in the mouth. For example, oatmeal should be not too watery or too thick. Thicker foods may stay in the mouth longer and increase the work of the tongue, but they are easier to control. Foods that are too thick may present a danger for choking. Peanut butter is an example of a food that is generally too thick when consumed by itself. When it is placed on a cracker with a small amount of jelly, the consistency becomes much easier to handle.

8. Some foods can increase muscle tone and chewing. Fruit Rollups promote rotary chewing and graded jaw movements, but at the same time dissolve fairly quickly to minimize the risk of choking. Some dried fruits (e.g., apricots, apples) can be used to increase chewing. The therapist may decide to encourage the child to chew the dried fruit or Rollup while holding onto it, if aspiration is a concern. Tough or fibrous meats are contraindicated.

9. A long piece of vegetable or meat can be held between the side teeth to promote graded biting. Strips of soft cheese, chicken, or long green beans may initially be used. Soft cookies and crackers placed to the side can also promote controlled biting. Pretzels and apple slices require more jaw strength and can be tried as a next step in biting skill.

A combination of the above strategies can be more successful than selecting any one method. Foods that are contraindicated for a child with severe oral motor problems are those that break apart into small pieces that are difficult to manage (e.g., raw carrots, crisp cookies) and those that are tough and require a grinding motion to masticate.

Interventions for Children With Tactile Defensiveness

Oral motor delays and limited feeding skills may be associated with tactile defensiveness and the child's aversion to textured food. In children with cerebral palsy, prematurity, or other medical problems that result in an extended period of non-oral feeding, sensory defensiveness may result from a lack of appropriate oral experiences. In children with such a medical history, oral hypersensitivity clearly is the predominate problem interfering with feeding.

Sensory defensiveness can be identified through observation and parent interview. The sensory defensive child exhibits discomfort when different textures are placed in his or her mouth or may swallow them quickly without chewing. In evaluating this problem, repeated attempts should be made to give the child different food textures and sensory experiences. Some children exhibit defensiveness at the first bite, but acclimate quickly to the stimulation after several spoonfuls. Other children express discomfort with every mouthful and frequently clamp their lips on the spoon or exhibit a tonic bite. Some children refuse food, even when they are not yet satiated, because they can no longer tolerate the sensory experience.

When the child has oral tactile defensiveness, sensory preparation for feeding may improve acceptance and tolerance of food in the mouth. The most appropriate preparation is determined by the child's responses to touch. Children with autism often cannot tolerate tactile stimulation applied by another, but may imitate self-stimulation of the mouth with a toothbrush or washcloth. In other children with severe tactile defensiveness, the therapist can apply stimulation, beginning outside the mouth with deep pressure and then entering the mouth, rubbing the child's gums and upper palette. The stroking and rubbing may be done with the finger or a washcloth. Tooth brushing, with extra input to the gums and sides of the tongue, can help prepare the child for feeding. Rhythmic deep stroking is often more accepted by the child (Farber, 1982). If the parent or therapist establishes the same routine for desensitization each time (e.g., begins around the mouth and then rubs along the gum line), the child generally demonstrates more tolerance of the stimulation.

Sensory experiences should be offered to the child at times other than meals. Chewing on a washcloth seems to be an acceptable, even enjoyable, experience for some children. Rubber toys are also beneficial in promoting tongue and jaw movements, while desensitizing the mouth.

Sometimes parents report that their child chews on everything, yet the child has obvious aversive responses to food inside the mouth. These two observations, one of craving oral sensory input and one of avoiding it, seem to be contradictory. However both may indicate a need for additional oral stimulation. The stimulation from chewing on one place in the mouth (involving deep pressure to one area) is quite different from sensory stimulation throughout the mouth (involving light touch on all mouth surfaces). This child needs to expand his or her sensory experiences. The parent can build on the self-stimulating behaviors by encouraging the child to chew on safe objects in different places in the mouth, or the parent and child can play a turn-taking game, in which the parent rubs the toy or cloth on the child's gums, tongue, and upper palate, then the child holds and controls the object in self-stimulation.

Brushing with a regular or NUK toothbrush can be very helpful in desensitizing the child's mouth and may be among the least stressful methods for the parent; it is also more methodical than the oral play described above. The parents should be offered a variety of methods for stimulating the mouth from which they can choose one that best fits into their daily routine (see Figure 4).

The guidelines for introducing food textures to the child with sensory defensiveness are similar to the sequence of textures used to promote oral motor skills. Probably the most

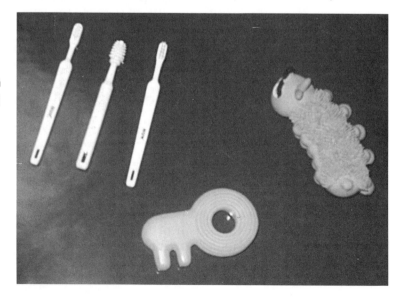

Figure 4. A NUK toothbrush set and rubber toys. These help desensitize the mouth, and children often enjoy chewing them.

difficult textures to tolerate are small, discrete bits of food, such as Cheerios, small pieces of meat, or other hard, dry substances. With some children, hiding textured food in smooth food substances like pudding or applesauce makes the texture tolerable; in other children, any discrete bit of food is expelled from the mouth. A sequential progression of textures of food is described in Figure 5.

Understanding the basis of the child's oral defensiveness is important when planning an intervention program. Tactile defensiveness may be related to a neurological impairment; due to a history of offensive oral sensory experiences, such as oral tube feeding or oral intubation; or due to a lack of oral sensory experiences, such as the child with a gastrostomy tube who has not been orally fed. Understanding the factors that seem to be associated with the defensiveness gives the therapist direction regarding appropriate techniques. The child with neurological impairments may need more specific sensory input for desensitization (e.g., deep touch, firm rubbing). A child whose primary problem is lack of sensory experience may rapidly improve when given graded sensory input, such as that suggested in Figure 5. Although the same guidelines apply to all types of children, every child is unique and has individual preferences for oral sensory experiences, food textures, and tastes.

Children Who are Non-Oral Feeders

Occupational therapists can make important contributions to decisions regarding whether a child should be fed through oral or non-oral means. They are also members of the health care team who help the children in the transition from non-oral to oral feeding.

Recommending Non-Oral Feeding

The occupational therapist may be one of the first professionals to recognize that the child with severe disabilities is at risk for aspiration—all children with severely limited oral motor control are in danger of aspiration of some amount of food. The therapist assesses the degree of control the child has with different food consistencies. If swallowing is delayed or out of sync with the sucking movements, breathing sounds raspy after eating, or the child continually has upper respiratory infections, the possibility of aspiration should be investigated. The child without a strong cough is particularly at risk. A clinical evaluation of the swallowing mechanism reveals only a limited amount of information. A videoflouroscope is indicated if aspiration is suspected or if oral motor delays are severe (Fox, 1990; Wolf & Glass, 1992).

A number of different recommendations may be given based on the results of videofluoroscopy (Fox, 1990; Glass & Wolf, 1993). If the child aspirates when ingesting a variety of textures and consistencies, then the family is advised to allow placement of the gastrostomy tube. If the child aspirates when given a few specific food consistencies, the therapist may recommend that these consistencies be altered or eliminated from the diet. If the child aspirates only in specific positions, others can be recommended.

Many parents have difficulty accepting the idea of a gastrostomy tube. They may be reluctant to discontinue feeding the child by mouth because this activity is their primary opportunity for one-on-one interaction with the child, or feeding may appear to be the only pleasure the child has during the day. Frank discussions with the parents about the benefits of gastrostomy tube placement, especially in relation to the health and nutritional status of the child, can help them decide to approve the surgery. The therapist can explain that placement of the gastrostomy tube does not preclude some oral feeding, and that oral motor stimulation and food play are strongly recommended for children with gastrostomies. Other opportunities for parent-child interaction can be discussed.

Figure 5. Food texture progression.

Recommendations	Examples	Nutritional Value	Precautions
1. To facilitate sucking and swallowing, use pureed or soft foods.	Gelatin	High sugar Limited protein value	Avoid gelatin with fruit pieces.
	Pureed meats and vegetables	Good variety of vitamins and protein	Avoid using baby foods for extended periods of time.
	Pudding/custard	High carbohydrates; milk provides calcium and protein	Tapioca pudding can be very offensive to hypersensitive children, and may provide extra stimulus to hyposensitive children.
	Applesauce	Low calorie; high fluid content	
2. To facilitate sucking and swallowing, use a heavy food that forms a bolus easily and gives proprioceptive input.	Mashed potatoes (excellent consistency for providing proprioceptive input)	High carbohydrate; adding margarine provides calories; adding powdered milk adds protein and calcium	Mixing firm bits of food with mashed potatoes may not be tolerated by sensitive children; inconsistency in texture may cause choking.
	Oatmeal	High carbohydrate; milk adds calcium and protein	
3. Liquids may need to be thickened to improve and facilitate swallowing.	Liquids may be thickened with yogurt, wheat germ, gelatin, cereal, carageen	Yogurt: protein and calcium Wheat germ: carbohydrates and fiber Gelatin: see above Cereal: carbohydrates, vitamins (depends on the type of cereal)	Avoid high carbohydrates to thicken liquids; when food pools in the back of mouth, alternate with thinner liquids; avoid cornstarch.
4. To promote chewing initially, use chewy or gummy foods that hold together to make a bolus.	Bananas; cheese; progress to chicken, lunch meat, marshmallows, soft vegetables, crackers, dried fruit, apples, zwieback toast, graham crackers	Fruits: carbohydrates and vitamins Cheese: protein and calcium Meat: protein Vegetables: vitamins and complex carbohydrates	Avoid foods and meats that break apart; avoid vegetables with skins unless well cooked.
5. To promote chewing when jaw is more stable but movement is primitive, use crispy or harder solids.	Crackers; graham crackers; dried fruit	Crackers: complex carbohydrates Graham crackers: complex carbohydrates and fiber Dried fruit: high-calorie carbohydrates	If you use carrots or beef jerky, avoid allowing child to bite off pieces. Use of tough meat my increase abnormal postures.
6. To densensitize the mouth, grade the texture of the food; use a blender if possible to make small variations in texture.	Begin with pureed, then progress to soft foods, then lumpy or solid.	Different nutrients can be provided in a variety of textures.	Do not begin with lumpy foods—a hypersensitive child will be intolerant of these. When blending foods, avoid mixing all foods together.
Use a variety of tastes, textures, and temperatures.	Be creative, given the above guidelines.	Variety should improve the nutritional balance.	Consult nutritionist and occupational or speech therapist for advice.

The Transition from Non-Oral to Oral Feeding

Occupational therapists also assist in the transition from non-oral to oral feeding (Blackman & Nelson, 1985; Chamberlin et al., 1991). Children who are fed through gastrostomy may develop a number of conditions secondary to non-oral feeding. First, they may have strong tactile defensiveness, due usually to a lack of experience and neurological impairment. Second, they often have delayed or abnormal oral motor skills. Poor oral motor skills may have been the reason for the original tube placement; if the child was not orally fed after the gastrostomy, then it is unlikely that these skills have improved. The child may also have gastro-esophageal reflux, which causes constant irritation to the esophagus, thus reducing the desire to feed by mouth due to the discomfort.

The transition from non-oral to oral feeding is initiated with a physician's recommendation based on the child's medical status and an evaluation of the child's oral motor skills by an occupational or speech therapist. After considering the health care team's recommendations, the family decides whether or not this transition is desirable and, if so, when they might best initiate the process.

A program to transition a young child from non-oral to oral feeding typically includes four components. The first is *oral motor intervention*. The child must demonstrate that he or she is capable of oral feeding. The therapist works with the child to desensitize the surfaces around and in the mouth. Specific oral motor skills are facilitated during sensory play (Morris & Klein, 1987). A focus may be the development of chewing and increased control of tongue and jaw movement using rubber toys and textured cloth. Small amounts of food textures are gradually offered to the child, usually while he or she is fed through the gastrostomy tube. The therapist may offer the child pureed food on the finger tip as a first step (Morris & Klein; Hunter, 1990). Other activities can increase oral motor skills. Engaging the child in making sounds, blowing bubbles, and giving kisses can provide oral motor exercise for better chewing and swallowing. Tooth brushing and oral play with toys are emphasized. It is important that the parent see small steps of progress, and that offensive and unacceptable oral experiences for the child are avoided. Usually the first food experiences are introduced as play, and whatever the child chooses to do with the food is praised and rewarded.

The second component is *behavior intervention*. Almost universally the child has adopted manipulative behaviors during feeding, generally in relationship to long-standing sensory defensiveness. Behavior problems also relate to the parents' anxiety about feeding and the child's growth and nutritional status. Behavior interventions are discussed in the following section.

The third component is *manipulation of the gastrostomy feeding* to emulate a meal schedule. Bolus feedings are given 4 to 5 times per day instead of continuously through the night or during other long periods. The bolus feedings enable the child to experience being full and hungry at different times during the day. In order to expect the child to take in significant amounts of food by mouth, the gastrostomy feeding must be reduced. This reduction requires consultation with a nutritionist, and both physician and parent approval. Often these children are not medically and nutritionally stable enough to reduce their caloric intake; therefore, this transitional stage is lengthy. Some weight loss is almost inevitable during the transition from non-oral to oral feeding, so children who cannot tolerate any weight loss are not candidates for the transition process.

The fourth component of successful transition to oral feeding is the *therapist's support and encouragement*. The longer the child has been on non-oral feeding, the more difficult the transition. Continual support to the family is needed; therefore, regular communication with the family is critical. The parents need encouragement for the small steps of progress and during the frequent steps backwards. Since it is important that the parents remain positive and supportive of the child, the therapist's encouragement helps maintain their energy and focus on the goal of oral feeding.

Parents who experience feeding problems with their children can provide mutual support and assist each other in problem solving. Parent-to-parent support has been reported to strengthen their abilities to cope with stressful problems on a day-to-day basis (Chamberlin et al., 1991). This approach seems particularly appropriate for difficult feeding problems that include sensory, motor, and behavioral issues.

Children With Behavior Problems

Feeding problems almost invariably are associated with behavior problems. Initially, feeding may be uncomfortable and stressful for the child, which leads to negative interactions that may become established between the caregiver and child. The caregiver becomes anxious about the child's limited nutritional intake and negative behaviors. The child is reinforced by the parent's or caregiver's increased attention and may try to sustain this type of response. Some children retain the behaviors associated with oral defensiveness (e.g., avoidance, rejection of food) after the sensory defensiveness has improved, because these behaviors result in increased attention from the parents and others.

Other avoidance behaviors may result from inappropriate feeding methods (Morris & Klein, 1987). When the child is fed textures and/or amounts that exceed oral capabilities, he or she responds with negative behaviors (e.g., spitting or crying) to indicate displeasure. These behaviors most often result when the parent is insensitive to the child's cues. The child may indicate satiation or discomfort with texture without an appropriate response from the parent. The child then exhibits more obvious negative behaviors that generally disrupt the feeding interaction.

Behavior problems are prevalent during feeding for several reasons. First, for a child with severe impairments and minimal motor control, feeding may be the only opportunity to exercise control over his or her environment. The child may be held and handled all day according to the needs of others, but no one can force the child to eat. Furthermore, refusal to eat or rejection of food almost always causes a reaction in the caregiver or feeder; thus, the child feels in control of the situation as well as in control of his or her own body.

Second, the child quickly becomes aware that the parent is concerned about this issue and that refusal to eat usually results in an emotional response. The child receives increased attention when he or she exhibits negative behaviors at meal time (e.g., crying, refusing food, spitting or rejecting food).

Behavior problems during feeding are not easily solved. Usually the child's behavior reflects a greater issue of negative interactions and a history of problems in feeding. The following are some guidelines for therapists to improve the child's behavior during feeding.

1. Encourage positive and pleasant interactions during feeding. Positive interaction between the child and parent or other family members should have priority over other goals (e.g., intake of a specific amount of food).
2. Assist the parent in reading the child's cues. The child may only subtly indicate that he or she is satiated or needs more time between bites. If the parent is sensitive to all the child's cues, then smooth, reciprocal turn-taking results.
3. Give the child choices to enable participation in positive decision making if the

issue is the child's need for control. The child can select which food to eat or indicate when a bite is desired. The child should direct the pace and sequence of the meal, for example choosing a drink versus solid food, or meat versus a vegetable, as much as is reasonable.

4. Give praise and positive touches for encouragement, especially if the child has great difficulty eating due to sensory defensiveness or poor motor control. When the positive nature of interaction is emphasized, both child and parent maintain a higher level of communication and sensitivity.

5. Use behavior management when the child uses feeding as a time to control and to demonstrate behaviors that are disruptive to the family. Consultation with a psychologist may be helpful. A regime can be established in which limits to the child's behavior are defined, and there is a specified consequence when the child exceeds these limits. The discipline is applied consistently so that the child learns which behaviors are allowed and which are not. The punishment enforced is usually "time out" or elimination of something desired, like the parent's attention.

Behavior management is most effective when consistently applied across caregivers and environments. The decisions regarding types of behavior to target and methods of reinforcement to use should be made by the parents. By observing the parent-child feeding interaction, the occupational therapist can identify the behaviors to be targeted and recommend possible reinforcement strategies. A successful behavior modification program involves all caregivers of the child who may be involved in feeding, including teachers, therapists, and other family members.

Self-Feeding

Typical Development of Self-Feeding

Self-feeding, like other self-care skills, develops over an extended period of time. Hand to mouth is one of the first motor behaviors the infant demonstrates, and he or she may hold a bottle by age 6 months. Finger feeding with a cracker or soft cookie is accomplished by age 8 months.

By 7 to 8 months of age, the child usually sits in a high chair with the family at the dinner table. While observing the other family members, he or she engages in food play or finger feeding. The infant may play with a spoon by banging it on the high chair tray. Dried cereal or small bits of soft foods provide entertainment and multiple opportunities to practice pincer grasp and finger skills. The selection of finger foods should match the child's oral motor skills. Nuts, hard candy, popcorn, grapes, and hot dogs cut width-wise are contraindicated, as these can totally occlude the airway if aspirated. Soft foods that dissolve in the mouth or require minimal chewing and are not as large as the airway are appropriate for first finger feeding.

Independent spoon feeding develops between 15 and 18 months of age. At this time, shoulder and wrist stability are adequate for holding the spoon to scoop the food and bring it to the mouth with minimal spillage. The child holds the spoon in a pronated gross grasp and brings the spoon to the mouth using exaggerated shoulder and elbow movements. By age 24 months the child uses a supinated grasp of the spoon, holding it in the radial fingers. The subtle movements at the wrist and forearm needed to obtain the food and efficiently enter the spoon into the mouth also emerge at this age. With this increased control, the child may begin to use a fork and to eat from a spoon foods that are more difficult to handle (e.g., peas, corn, rice, cold cereal).

Between 12 and 18 months of age the child learns cup drinking, initially with a cup that has a lid and a spout. Some children can best manage a cup with handles; others prefer a small plastic cup without handles. Spillage is considerable when using a cup without a lid until 24 months of age, when jaw stability and hand control increase (Morris & Klein, 1987).

Intervention Approaches

When children have motor limitations or delays that interfere with self-feeding, a variety of therapeutic interventions may be needed to increase their skills. Interventions to improve self-feeding may be categorized as positioning, assistive handling, and adaptive equipment. These interventions are described in the following sections.

Positioning

Correct alignment and adequate support for stable posture, described as important to oral feeding skills, are equally important to the development of eye-hand coordination for self-feeding. The mid-range movement of the hand and arm through space requires either well-developed trunk stability or external support of the trunk. Children with cerebral palsy often lack adequate postural stability as a base of control for smooth, active range of the arm at midline. The child must feel secure and relaxed during self-feeding to utilize the strength, control, and endurance needed to eat an entire meal. Positioning with the head, neck, and trunk in correct alignment (the chin tucked, the shoulders depressed and slightly forward, and the pelvis in neutral alignment) is similar to the positioning previously described for feeding the child. In order to self-feed, the chair and child must be completely upright (Mueller, 1975). This position may be maintained with pelvic and hip abductor straps. Lateral trunk supports may also be helpful. When the child tends to retract his or her shoulders, padded humeral "wings" on the back of the chair or on the wheelchair tray can maintain the arms in a forward protracted position. These "wings" help increase arm stability and maintain the child's hands at midline for self-feeding (Bergen & Colangelo, 1985).

Another wheelchair tray adaptation that helps increase arm stability and improve the arm's position for feeding is a small (short) bolster that can be placed under the arm. By separating the elbow from the trunk, the shoulder is abducted into a normal feeding position and the elbow is stabilized at a height that enables the child to scoop food onto the spoon and reach the mouth with minimal movement of the shoulder and elbow. The bolster serves as a lever from which the child can effectively move the forearm from the tray surface to his or her mouth.

For children who need a greater degree of proximal arm stability in order to bring their hand to their mouth, the tray may be elevated. Raising the tray promotes upright sitting and humeral abduction (Bergen & Colangelo, 1985) for increased hand-to-mouth control. The child stabilizes the elbow on the tray and then scoops the food and brings it to the mouth in a simple elbow flexion and extension motion. Feeding when positioned with an elevated, well-fitting tray enables the child with cerebral palsy to gain the postural control needed to self-feed independently when given easily managed foods (see Figure 6).

Handling Techniques

Self-feeding is a challenge for children with cerebral palsy, particularly those who have athetoid movements and limited control of mid-range movements. Occupational

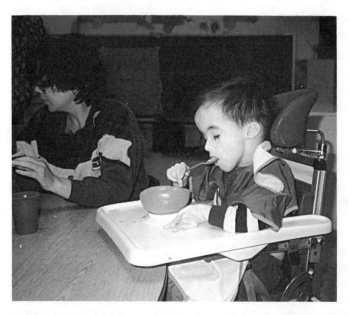

Figure 6. A boy feeds himself, with his elbow resting on an elevated tray.

therapy with the child with athetosis or poor postural control emphasizes developing postural stability as a base for control of the arm in space (Boehme, 1988). Handling during self-feeding often involves facilitation of shoulder depression and protraction and scapular stability to increase the child's control of distal arm movement. The therapist may place his or her hand on top of the child's shoulders or scapula. Support and/or guidance of the humerus may be needed to establish a smooth hand-to-mouth pattern. The handling by the therapist should stabilize the arm in space rather than move it through the range. Hand-over-hand methods tend to make the child passive, rather than an active participant in the feeding process. Therefore, hand-over-hand methods do not promote skills as effectively as supporting the child's shoulder and eliciting the child's active participation.

Boehme (1982) recommends a technique in which the therapist holds the spoon handle between extended index and third fingers. The therapist slips these fingers into the child's palm with a thumb on the dorsum of the child's hand. The child holds onto the fingers and spoon using a gross grasp, and the therapist facilitates a self-feeding pattern using subtle and natural facilitation from within the child's hand. This technique is particularly successful with a child who has developed a basic hand-to-mouth pattern, but spills frequently. The therapist's fingers inside the child's hand guide small ranges of supination, wrist extension, and radial deviation, increasing hand control and reducing spillage.

The disadvantages of these handling techniques are that they require the therapist, teacher, or parent to be seated behind the child. Communication is limited without face-to-face interaction, which reduces the social aspects of feeding. The position required to use these techniques is difficult to implement at family mealtimes; frequently, only the therapist uses these handling methods.

Such techniques are generally most effective when regularly applied. The therapist's goal is to provide the least amount of support that will facilitate the child's success in self-feeding. Therefore, the therapist continually works to decrease the amount of physical assistance, while increasing the child's efficiency in self-feeding.

Adaptive Equipment

Adaptive equipment is often helpful, if not necessary, for the child learning to self-feed. Parents have frequently remarked about the benefits of adapted utensils, plates, and cups to increase the child's ability to self-feed and to decrease spillage and frustration.

Scherzer and Tscharnuter (1982) recommend built-up handles, plates with high curved rims, and nonskid pads. Morris and Klein (1987) provide numerous examples of utensils, cups, and bowls that enable the child to self-feed successfully. Plates or bowls should have raised edges and resistive surfaces so they are stable on the table's surface (see Figure 7).

Characteristics of spoons that assist the child in self-feeding are enlarged handles, latex-covered spoon bowls, and angled handles. Cups with lids reduce spillage. Lids without spouts may be helpful when the child exhibits suckling tongue movements (extension-retraction). Straws can promote the child's ability to suck and can allow the child to drink without lifting the cup from the table surface. More sophisticated adapted equipment, such as the electric feeder, may enable a child to self-feed without using the arms. Criteria for selecting adaptive equipment to improve the child's independence in self-feeding include durability, ease of cleaning and use, and developmental appropriateness (Coley & Procter, 1989).

Dressing

The age at which children develop dressing skills varies according to their experiences and the types of clothing they wear. It also relates to how much the family members value self-dressing skills and whether or not the family's daily routine provides opportunities for the child to practice self-dressing. The child's initiative and motivation to be independent are important variables in learning to dress.

Typical Developmental Sequence of Dressing

The development of dressing skills takes 4 to 5 years. The child first begins to participate in dressing at about 12 months of age. It is not until 5 or 6 years of age that the child can accomplish the most difficult fasteners. Table 1, based on the work of Coley (1978) and Klein (1988), provides some guidelines as to the sequence and typical ages that specific dressing skills are accomplished.

Children With Delays in Dressing Skills

As in oral- and self-feeding, children can experience delays in developing dressing skills,

Figure 7. A bowl with a high rim and suction cup at its base enables the child to eat independently.

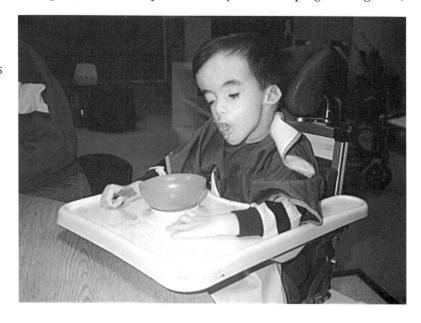

Table 1.
Sequence of Typical Dressing Skills

Age (in years)	Self-Dressing Skills
1	• Cooperates with dressing (holds out arms and feet) • Pulls off shoes, removes socks • Pushes arms through sleeves and legs through pants
2	• Removes unfastened coat • Removes shoes if laces are untied • Helps pull down pants • Finds armholes in over-the-head shirt
2½	• Removes pull-down pants with elastic waist • Assists in pulling on socks • Puts on front-button coat, shirt • Unbuttons large buttons
3	• Puts on over-the-head shirt with minimal assistance • Puts on shoes without fasteners (may be on wrong foot) • Puts on socks (may be with heel on top) • Independent in pulling down pants • Zips and unzips jacket once on track • Needs assistance to remove over-the-head shirt • Buttons large front buttons
3½	• Finds front of clothing • Snaps or hooks front fastener • Unzips front zipper on jacket, separating zipper • Puts on mittens • Buttons series of three or four buttons • Unbuckles shoe or belt • Dresses with supervision (help with front and back)
4	• Removes pullover garment independently • Buckles shoes or belt • Zips jacket zipper • Puts on socks correctly • Puts on shoes with assistance in tying laces • Laces shoes • Consistently identifies the front and back of garments
4½	• Puts belt in loops
5	• Ties and unties knots • Dresses unsupervised
6	• Closes back zipper • Ties bow knot • Buttons back buttons • Snaps back snaps

Adapted from *Pre-Dressing Skills* by M.D. Klein, 1988. Tucson, AZ: Therapy Skill Builders.

miss specific skills, or have problems with specific skills. Problems that interfere with dressing skills include limitations in motor control, muscle strength, motor planning, sensory perception, and cognition (see Figure 8).

Interventions for Dressing Children

Prior to when the child begins to develop self-dressing skills, the occupational therapist assists the parents or caregivers with adapted or specialized handling methods for dressing the child. The goals of the therapist when consulting with a parent on adapted methods for dressing are (a) to increase the efficiency of the task for the parent, and (b) to provide therapeutic handling of the child. Expected outcomes from using adapted dressing techniques are less time spent in dressing, less stress during this activity, and specific goals for the child (e.g., increased range of motion, or improved head or trunk control).

Children With Motor Impairments

Infants and Young Children

For the young infant who has cerebral palsy, dressing may be difficult. Dressing can particularly be a challenge (e.g., fitting arms through tight sleeves or changing diapers) with the child with hypertonicity and limited range of motion. Typically the child with spasticity holds his or her arms close to the body and holds his or her legs in adduction and internal rotation. For children whose extensor muscle tone is increased when lying on the back, the typical supine dressing position is not appropriate.

Therapeutic handling during dressing accomplishes several objectives. First, it relaxes the child and reduces muscle tone, facilitating much of the dressing task. With the child's muscle tone reduced, the legs easily separate and the arms move overhead. The task becomes less difficult for the parent and more comfortable for the child. Second, intervention goals, such as improved active shoulder flexion, increased control of legs and hips, and

Figure 8. Considerations in facilitating dressing skills in children with specific conditions.

Condition	Possible Areas of Strength	Possible Areas That Require Assistance
Cerebral palsy	• Motivation • Interaction skills • Ability to imitate • Receptive language • Memory	• Range of motion • Sensory perception • Postural stability • Manipulation, dexterity • Strength • Endurance
Sensory defensiveness	• Motor skills • Postural stability • Problem solving • Strength • Energy	• Tactile perception • Interaction • Tolerance of clothing • Motivation to dress • Organization
Dyspraxia	• Postural stability • Muscle strength • Problem solving • Visual perception	• Coordination/dexterity • Motor planning and sequencing • Sensory integration

sitting balance can be included in dressing activities. During dressing is a convenient time to employ therapeutic activities, because it is a daily routine for the child. Twice-daily handling during dressing provides regular, consistent input at a low cost to the parent, especially when inhibition techniques seem to facilitate accomplishment of the task.

Examples of inhibition and facilitation techniques during dressing of the infant with increased muscle tone include:

1. Elongation of the spine prior to dressing by gently lifting the pelvis while the child is supine. The hips are slowly abducted with the parent's hands to prepare the infant for diaper changing.

2. Slow rotation of the trunk by tilting the pelvis from side to side. This activity may be done prior to dressing. Trunk rotation, from right side lying to left side lying to back, can be incorporated into the task of donning pants or shirts.

3. Dressing the child in the prone position. After play in the supine position and twisting of the trunk from side to side, the child can roll (or be rolled) to the prone position (see Figure 9).

4. Holding the child prone over the parent's thighs and stretching the arms over the head. The child's extensor tone is inhibited in this position and flexor tone is facilitated (see Figure 10). Pullover shirts are easily donned. Pants can be donned by rolling the child from side to side. The parent should support the infant well under the abdomen if the infant has a tendency to arch the trunk (Scherzer & Tscharnuter, 1982).

5. Completing the dressing activity in side-lying by rolling from one side to the other until the child is dressed (Finnie, 1975). Rolling should include some trunk rotation with the arms over the head. A small pillow might be used if head control is poor.

6. Dressing the older infant, who has some trunk control, in a supported sitting position. The infant sits between the parent's legs, so the pelvis and lower trunk are supported. Sitting behind the child, the parent guides the infant's movements as he or she pushes the arms and legs through the sleeves and pant legs. This activity allows the infant to practice bilateral movements while sitting and is an effective method of upper extremity dressing for infants of differing motor skill levels. Pulling socks on and off becomes enjoyable play in this position and reinforces sensory motor skills in the child. To bring the pants completely

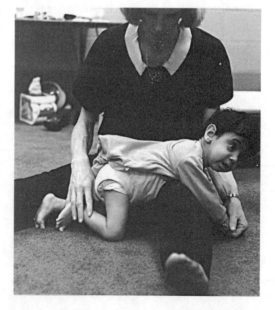

Figure 9. Dressing the child with extensor tone in the prone position.

Figure 10 (right). A father dresses his son in prone position. Note that the body is well-supported under the chest, with the shoulders higher than the pelvis.

Figure 11 (below). Dressing the child in a supported sitting position can help elicit the child's participation.

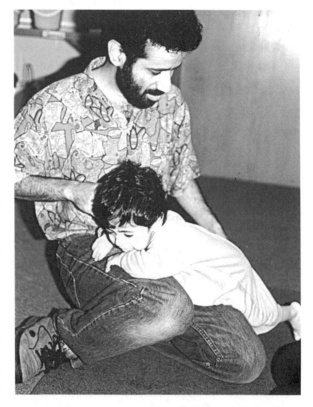

over the buttocks, the infant is moved from supported sitting to supported quadruped, with the infant's abdomen gently resting on the parent's thigh.

These techniques are continually upgraded to require more participation from the child. Supine, prone, and side-lying positions are selected first for the infant. Sitting enables greater participation of the child in the dressing activity, but is not used until the child has adequate head and trunk control (see Figure 11).

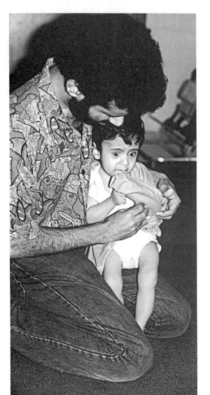

Older Children

Dressing becomes more difficult for the caregiver as the child with multiple or severe disabilities who does not attain dressing skills approaches adolescence. The dressing activities usually require more strength and energy from the caregiver because the older child is larger and heavier and may also have increased muscle tone and joint contractures. Due to the child's increasing size, a number of adaptations may need to be made in the dressing techniques used by the family members. In some families, the father takes responsibility for dressing tasks once the child is an adolescent, if he is the physically stronger parent.

For the child whose motor control remains low, the side lying and supine positions may remain the dressing positions of choice. Side lying is selected for the child whose increased extensor tone is inhibited when in a semi-flexed sideling position. Dressing of both upper and lower body may be completed on one side prior to rolling the child onto the other side.

When the child is dressed in a supine position, a firm pillow under the head may inhibit neck and trunk extension so that the child is better able to bring the head and arms forward during dressing.

It is important that the parent dress a heavy child on a surface at an appropriate height for reaching that does not require bending over and lifting. Continually bending over the child to pull on pants and lift the buttocks is stressful to the parent's lower back, even when good body mechanics are used. A large crib or high bed that positions the child between waist and chest height reduces the amount of energy and lower back stress incurred in dressing.

The characteristics of the clothing selected can increase the ease of dressing. Loose-fitting clothing is easily donned. Front opening garments, donned using side-to-side rolling, are preferable to over the head shirts. Coley and Proctor (1989) offer additional suggestions for clothing selection.

Children With Tactile Defensiveness

Adapted dressing methods are needed for children with sensory, as well as motor, problems. Young children with tactile defensiveness can resist wearing any clothes, express a dislike of certain clothing materials that create discomfort, and demonstrate aversive responses to the repetitive light touches associated with the dressing task. Wilbarger and Wilbarger (1991) propose a model of intervention for children with sensory defensiveness. The role of the occupational therapist is three-fold. First, the therapist provides the parents with information about tactile defensiveness and its associated behaviors, which helps the parents to understand their infant's behaviors. Second, the occupational therapist recommends methods for dressing and selecting clothing that decrease the child's aversive responses. Holding the child firmly and providing intermittent deep pressure or joint compression as part of the dressing activity can help modulate the child's sensory systems and make him or her more comfortable and accepting of touch during dressing. Third, the occupational therapists suggests direct intervention to improve the child's ability to receive and integrate tactile input. The therapist may recommend and/or implement a program in which the child receives rapid brushing of the extremities and back followed by deep touch, deep pressure, and joint compression (Wilbarger & Wilbarger). The intervention activities should immediately proceed the dressing task and are performed regularly throughout the day. In this child, as in the child with cerebral palsy, the dressing activity can be transformed from a frustrating, stressful, interaction to a therapeutic and playful one.

Intervention Approaches to Improve Self-Dressing

As the child reaches preschool and school age, self-dressing should be encouraged. While some participation in dressing is usually achieved by all children with developmental disabilities, the level of independence the child accomplishes depends on the developmental level of sensory motor skills, cognition, language, perception and, to an extent, social-emotional skills.

Dressing independence becomes important to the child during the preschool years. At this age, the child is striving for independence in many daily activities. The accomplishment of independent dressing strengthens the child's self-esteem and sense of mastery. When the child's disability delays the acquisition of full-dressing independence, it is nonetheless important that the child continue to receive positive reinforcement by achieving some parts of the task. Due to the relationship of dressing skill to self-esteem, as well as the importance of self-dressing in the child's and family's daily routine, dressing skills are an important area of focus for the occupational therapist.

The strategies selected by the therapist to assist in the development of dressing skills depends on the child's problems and strengths. The therapist works with the family, and possibly the teacher, to identify the child's specific skills and limitations related to dressing. While much of the dressing evaluation can be accomplished through interview, the therapist also observes the child undressing and dressing and assesses sensory, motor, and perceptual skills using standardized tests and/or structured observations. Once the performance limitations are identified (e.g., motor control or tactile defensiveness) those areas are more specifically evaluated. With this information, the occupational therapist, in collaboration with the intervention team, develops a program for the child that focuses on the specific skills needed to improve dressing independence. The therapist's role includes assisting the child, family, and team in identifying and understanding the child's problems related to dressing; providing intervention activities that remediate the problem(s); and instructing in adapted techniques. Adapted techniques may include teaching methods, clothing, or equipment.

Children With Motor Impairments

The child who has poor motor control and abnormal muscle tone may always require some dressing assistance. To establish a focus and strategies for the intervention, the therapist completes a motor analysis of the dressing task.

Motor Analysis

This provides specific information about skills that are present, missing, and emerging. It is accomplished by observing the child performing the targeted task (see Figure 12).

Activities to Improve Self-Dressing Skills

Through the motor analysis of each task, the therapist identifies which components of movement interfere with accomplishing dressing independence. Those skills that are emerging but require physical assistance of another become the focus of therapy. If reduced active range of motion is an identified problem, the therapist provides activities to enhance shoulder strength and controlled mobility. These activities may require weight bearing on the hands in prone and sitting positions, reaching forward and overhead, and forcefully pushing large objects with the hands at shoulder height (Boehme, 1988).

Dressing practice is integrated into therapy sessions. The motor components of the task are facilitated through handling by the therapist. The therapist may sit behind and straddle the child, who is sitting on a low bench. The therapist's trunk and legs support and guide the child's trunk during the weight shifts required in the activity, and the therapist's hands can stabilize the scapula when reaching forward and overhead. Handling reinforces the postural symmetry of this particular activity and facilitates the overhead arm and hand movements.

Lower extremity dressing requires well-developed trunk control and sitting equilibrium. Reaching forward and across the midline with the arms extended is required to place the feet through the pant legs. Handling the child at the pelvis reinforces neutral pelvic alignment, backward weight shift, and trunk rotation for reaching to the feet. In addition to having sufficient sitting balance to reach the feet, the child must demonstrate sufficient trunk control to rise to a standing position to pull the pants over the buttocks. Therapeutic activities that require the child's dynamic balance in the sit-to-stand transition are

Figure 12. Motor analysis for donning a T-shirt.

Donning a T-Shirt	Observe
Reach for shirt	• Shoulder stability in directed reach • Trunk control in forward weight shift • Quality of reach—smooth and directed • Symmetry of bilateral reach
Grasp of shirt	• Hand opening • Grasping pattern and control • Use of two hands together • Isolated distal finger prehension
Bring T-shirt over head	• Use of two hands together • Ability to maintain grasp during active movement of shoulder and elbow • Adequate shoulder range for bringing shirt over top of head • Smooth bilateral shoulder flexion with elbow flexion • Maintenance of head and trunk stability • Resistive grasp and arm flexion during forceful movement of shirt opening over head
Right arm through sleeve	• Ability to locate arm opening (using visual and/or tactile perception) • Ability to stabilize shirt with left hand • Shoulder extension with elbow flexion to position arm • Shoulder abduction with elbow extension to push arm through sleeve
Left arm through sleeve	• Same, location of the sleeve is usually easier • May require slightly greater arm strength to push through sleeve if the T-shirt fits tightly

emphasized. As the child prepares to stand to pull up the pants, forward weight shift and trunk and hip extension are facilitated. Standing balance adequate to allow the child to lean forward and pull the pants over the buttocks can also become an intervention program goal. While the specific sensory motor skills are a focus of intervention, adapted techniques and equipment are also important for increasing the child's dressing independence.

Adapted Techniques

Adapted techniques for dressing with children have been described by Coley and Procter (1989), Finnie (1975), Klein (1988), and others. Examples of techniques appropriate for children with cerebral palsy include dressing in supported-sitting or side-lying positions; placing shirts on the lap and pushing the arms through, then bringing the shirt overhead; and altering the typical sequence of dressing.

Appropriate Clothing

Clothing design is a consideration for every child who has difficulty dressing. Clothing that is easy to don and doff saves the parents and the child time and energy. Clothing for children with emerging dressing skills has easy-to-secure fasteners (VELCRO®), is loose fitting, has elastic waistbands and oversized openings for the head, and is made of stretchy material. Examples are sweat shirts and pants, oversized T-shirts, and elastic-waist shorts and skirts. Shoes with touch fasteners are available in most shoe stores in a range of styles. Buttons should be avoided until the child is learning buttoning skills; zippers should glide easily and have large pull rings. Easy-to-don clothes are available in most children's clothing stores.

Adapted Equipment

Button hooks, long shoe horns, long-reach zipper aids, and adapted shoe ties are examples of equipment that can increase the child's dressing independence (Klein, 1988). When recommending equipment, the therapist should weigh the cost of the device with the likelihood that the family and child will actually use it and how long it is likely to be needed. Most dressing aids are inexpensive and are well worth the investment if they increase dressing independence. Use of devices for dressing independence may become more important when dressing is required outside the home environment (i.e., at school or in independent living situations).

Children With Tactile Defensiveness

Behaviors such as tantrums at dressing time and undressing at every opportunity can be associated with tactile defensiveness. Since the child with tactile defensiveness usually demonstrates more positive responses to active, rather than passive, touch, self-dressing may be more tolerable to the child than being dressed (Royeen & Lane, 1991). The same considerations discussed for the infant are appropriate for the older child. Brushing and joint compression, and possibly vestibular activities, may be helpful for the child and increase attention to the task. The parents may begin the child's day with rocking and sustained hugging for 2 to 3 minutes prior to dressing activities (Wilbarger & Wilbarger, 1991).

While supporting the child's modulation of the sensory systems, behavior modification principles are also appropriate when the original cause of the dressing problem, tactile defensiveness, has improved, and the child continues to refuse to dress because he or she has learned that this behavior results in increased attention from the parents. Since behavior management and sensory integration are based on different theoretical approaches, careful planning is important to ensure that recommendations complement each other and work in concert toward the same goals. The approaches might be combined by using sensory preparation prior to the dressing to prepare the child to make his or her best effort, then implementing a system of positive and negative reinforcement for specific behaviors.

Finally, the child should be allowed to wear clothes that "feel good" to him or her. When appropriate, the child should have input into the purchase of new clothing. Clothes with easy fasteners should be used with children with delayed finger skills.

Children With Dyspraxia

Although the child with dyspraxia may achieve early motor milestones at approximately the same rate as other children, the skills associated with dressing are inevitably delayed (Cermak, 1985). The child's struggle to manipulate clothing may be the first indication to the parents of a motor problem. The parents may not understand why their child, who has learned to run and jump, cannot perform simple dressing tasks without assistance. As the child approaches school age, the delays in manipulation skills become more apparent. The child may be referred to occupational therapy at this time.

The occupational therapist completes an evaluation that includes analysis of sensory integration function as a possible causative factor in the child's dyspraxia. The evaluation also assesses the mechanisms and sensory systems through which the child best learns (e.g., by visual or verbal cuing).

Again, a primary role of the therapist is reframing for the parents why the child has difficulty learning to dress and accomplishing new motor tasks. The motor planning problem is explained as it relates to underlying sensory integration and cognitive skills. Dyspraxia may result in secondary body-image and self-esteem problems, as well as self-care delays (Cermak, 1991), so it is important that the parents understand the problem and its basis. Once the child's difficulty in dressing is understood as a sensory integration or praxis problem, the parents no longer associate the reluctance to dress with purposeful negative behavior, poor motivation, or lack of cooperation. This understanding helps them approach the dressing issue with greater patience and a more positive attitude.

Therapy to improve dressing skills for a child with dyspraxia may include activities that use a sensory integration approach, backward chaining to teach the tasks, and practice with positive reinforcement. Sensory integration activities might provide the child with selected tactile and vestibular input that evokes specific adapted responses. The sensory input is graded according to the child's needs, and integrative activities are made available to the child (Ayres, 1981; Clark, Parham, & Malloux, 1989).

Various training strategies can be used to achieve success in acquiring dressing skills (see Chapter 4, "Principles for Teaching Self-Care Skills"). Backward chaining methods for teaching dressing skills as described by Klein (1988) are often successful for teaching the child to dress with a minimum sense of failure and a genuine sense of accomplishment because the child performs the final steps that complete the task. Backward chaining provides a strategy for teaching the task one step at a time. This repetitive, low-failure method holds many advantages for the child with dyspraxia.

Practice of the dressing tasks is a simple, but important, part of the intervention program. This child needs repetitive practice in order to learn and then generalize the skills. Practice should involve the same methods in the same environment, as the introduction of new methods presents a great challenge (Cermak, 1991).

Bathing Skills

Bathing is a relaxing and pleasurable activity for most children and parents. The evening (or morning) bath is a time for play and interaction, as well as hygiene. For children with developmental disabilities, bathing may be a difficult struggle, but it has the potential to become a playful, social time when adaptations are made to increase the child's and parent's comfort and the child's safety. As with other self-care skills, independence in bathing becomes important to the child's sense of mastery and self-esteem.

Typical Sequence of Bathing Skill Development

Coley (1978) suggests that bathing skills develop after feeding and dressing skills. The child should be able to self-wash and -dry with supervision by 4 years of age. Complete independence in bathing cannot be expected until 8 years of age. At this time the child can wash all body parts and prepare the bath and shower water.

Issues Related to Developing Bathing Skills

Cultural values influence how the family defines bathing, how often bathing is performed, and the importance of hygiene. While the therapist may stress the importance of good hygiene to the family for health reasons, the family's cultural norms regarding cleanliness and bathing must be accepted.

Due to the personal nature of bathing and the logistics of the bath, the therapist usually does not observe the child and parent in bathing. When observation of bathing is possible through a home visit, the therapist is able to recommend specific intervention activities (it also provides an opportunity to develop rapport with the parent and child). See Figure 13 for some of the issues in bathing for children with different diagnoses.

Intervention for Bathing Young Children

Infants With Motor Delays

Prior to the age when the emergence of independent bathing skills are expected, the occupational therapist may make suggestions to the parent for bathing the infant. The focus of the therapist may be categorized into safety issues, bath time therapy, and bath time play.

Safety Issues

Safety becomes a focus for the child whose sitting balance and motor control are delayed. The therapist can recommend methods for lifting the child and holding him or her in the tub to increase the sense of security. Finnie (1975) describes methods for placing the infant with cerebral palsy in the tub. The child should be held symmetrically in slight trunk and neck flexion. This method of securely holding reduces the possibility of the child exhibiting a startle response or increased trunk extensor tone.

Nonslip bath mats or rubber appliques are essential. The young infant can be positioned on a sponge insert in an infant tub or in the regular bathtub. The sponge insert is slightly higher at the head and provides additional security and comfort.

Figure 13. Issues in the development of bathing skills in children with developmental disabilities.

Condition	Issues
Cerebral palsy	• Sitting balance in tub • Safety • Reach to all body parts • Reaching and washing hair • Lifting the child in and out of tub • Transferring in and out of tub
Spina bifida	• Sitting balance • Lower extremity sensation
Tactile defensiveness	• Aversion to bathing; may have tantrum at bath time
Dyspraxia	• Dexterity in bathing skills • Thoroughly washing specific body parts
Mentally retarded	• Sequencing task and thoroughly bathing all areas • Dexterity and bathing skills

A variety of bath chairs are commercially available. Hammock chairs made of plastic netting stretched over PVC piping support the child's head and trunk in a semi-reclined position. The hammock chairs, which are commercially available or can be fabricated, offer the child stability and safety and raise the child in the tub to ease the bathing task for the parent. When the child develops head control, and sitting balance is emerging, commercially available bathtub rings increase the sense of security in the tub (Coley & Proctor, 1989).

Bath Time Therapy

Activities during bathing often have therapeutic value. The therapist may suggest specific tasks for bath time to inhibit hypertonicity, increase range of motion, and enhance the child's mobility. Warm water tends to relax the child and inhibit muscle tone. The water also provides some buoyancy to the extremities, facilitating movement in general.

Since the bath is a time for one-on-one interaction and is part of the family's daily routine, it is an ideal opportunity to incorporate therapeutic exercises. Most of the therapist's recommendations are adaptations to the normal bathing activities.

With the infant reclined in the tub and supported on a sponge insert (cushion), the arms can be gently brought over the head, holding near the shoulders. The hips can be ranged in flexion, abduction, or pelvic rotation. Providing range of motion to the extremities in the water is advantageous because the child is relaxed and muscle tone is inhibited. Mobilizing tight joints at the beginning of the bath enables the child to move in greater active ranges during the bath. For the child with minimal movement who does not experience success or mastery in interacting with the environment, the sensation of extremity movement through the water offers immediate reinforcement of his or her smallest movements. Splashing is delightful for most children. Adding bubbles and floating toys to the water can increase the child's motivation to move.

Infants With Tactile Defensiveness

Infants with tactile defensiveness may enjoy bathing or may be uncomfortable with its associated tactile experiences. These children tend to withdraw from the tactile input of the washcloth and soap when the parent uses disorganized, quick touches to multiple body parts. This type of tactile input is associated with increased tactile defensive behaviors. When the child consistently withdraws from the parent, and the parent persists in approaching the child, both are frustrated and stressed by the bathing experience.

The occupational therapist can assist in increasing the child's tolerance of bathing and in the social interaction during bathing by explaining the child's problem to the parents. By reframing the child's negative behaviors, the parents can adopt a more positive, confident approach. The therapist may also recommend that the washcloth and towel be used with deep pressure in rhythmic, organized strokes. The extremities and back should be washed prior to the stomach and face. After bathing, the child can be wrapped tightly in a towel and held snugly in the mother's lap. This procedure can be followed by deep rubbing of all extremities, perhaps beyond the point of becoming dry. The child and parent may enjoy application of lotion to the extremities and trunk as an additional and different source of tactile stimulation. This opportunity for rubbing is a natural and convenient time for the parent to provide the child with additional tactile and proprioceptive input. Rubbing may be combined with slow rocking to increase sensory integration. The parent continues and/or repeats the stimulation according to the response of the child.

Bath Time Play

Due to the sensory and pleasurable nature of the bath, it can be established as a play time. Once the child and parent feel secure and comfortable, the bath offers many opportunities for turn-taking, sensory play, and imaginative play. Play may include body exploration or splashing (Finnie, 1975). Rubbing with the washcloth can become a turn-taking game for the child with tactile perception problems. Bath toys with suction cups that adhere to the sides of the tub are appropriate for the child with poor arm and hand control. Rubber toys are favorites for mouthing and bilateral manipulation. The opportunities for interaction between the parent and child should be emphasized by suggesting sensory and nonfail activities that offer opportunities for turn-taking.

Interventions to Improve Self-Bathing in the Child With Motor Delays

Self-bathing becomes an issue after the child is 4 years old and the parent has difficulty handling the child in the tub.

Adapted Equipment

Options for adapted equipment change as the child grows to adult size. Many of these options are described in detail elsewhere in this book. As the child with cerebral palsy approaches school age and continues to require assistance in bathing, use of a shower chair with locking wheels is considered. The chair provides back support and comfort during the shower. It requires a shower stall accessible to a chair on wheels and an adjustable shower head. When the family does not have an accessible shower, the bathtub can be adapted to increase the child's independence in self-bathing. Bathtub bars may be installed to assist the child entering the tub, and bathtub benches provide support to the trunk during the child's transfer to, and while sitting in, the tub.

A hand-held showerhead may enable independent hair washing and is useful for wetting and rinsing the back and other areas that are difficult for the child to reach. A long-handled bath sponge can also help reach these body areas.

Other Intervention Approaches for Improving Self-Bathing

Through a motor analysis of the bathing tasks, specific motor skills are identified to become a focus of intervention activities. Typically, the movements that limit bathing independence are reaching to the feet, back, and head. Intervention activities that improve reach to various body parts are directed toward improving range of motion, strength, and postural stability.

In the child with cerebral palsy, the ability to reach to the feet may be limited by tight hamstrings and postural instability. In coordination with physical therapy, activities to increase range of motion at the hips are implemented. Reaching to the top of the head and the back are also difficult for the child with cerebral palsy. Postural stability with scapular stability and mobility are essential. The child also rotates the shoulders and forearm. During these arm movements, the child grasps the washcloth or soap, so bathing the head and back may be practiced in activities that require carrying objects in wide-range movements. Activities involving reaching overhead and behind can build the motor skills required in self-bathing. Facilitation of postural stability may be another emphasis of therapy.

Both adapted equipment and activities to improve postural stability and motor skills are recommended to the parents. Because bathing involves safety and comfort issues, adapted equipment ensuring these things should be used while motor control develops.

The equipment allows the child and parent to be comfortably positioned while practicing bathing skills.

Functional Communication

Communication skills are essential to the child's ability to function. When the child has no or minimal verbal communication ability, augmentative communication methods are employed. These methods are selected through ongoing assessment of the child's skills, his or her developmental and educational goals, and the environment. Using this information, the parents and professional interdisciplinary team select an appropriate augmentative communication system that enhances the child's ability to interact meaningfully with others. The occupational therapist, as one of the professionals on the team, assists in selecting, positioning for, training in, and using augmentative communication. (For general information regarding the selection of technology, see Chapter 14, "Technology for Self-Care.")

Augmentative communication includes a wide range of methods, and often the child uses more than one to communicate (for example, combining sign language and an electronic device). Unaided augmentative communication refers to the use of gestures, facial expressions, and vocal sounds (Lloyds & Fuller, 1986). Everyone uses some of these nonverbal means to communicate. While these means do not require equipment or devices, they often require sophisticated hand and body movements (e.g., American Sign Language). Assistive communication systems use a device, computer, or aid. They usually employ symbol systems other than traditional orthography. A wide range of input and output devices are available to adapt the system to the individual's unique skills and needs.

This section describes the types of children who benefit from using augmentative communication devices, the role of the occupational therapist in selecting systems, mounting and positioning systems for optimal function, enhancing the child's skills to use the system successfully, and integrating the augmentative communication system into the child's natural environments.

Children Who Benefit From Augmentative Communication

Augmentative communication is appropriate for all individuals who are non-speaking and who have a desire to communicate. Children with severe disabilities who exhibit severely delayed cognitive and motor skills may use a simple method for communicating, such as eye gaze to one of four objects to indicate a desired activity. Another candidate is someone who does not have delays in cognitive or receptive language skills, but has severe limitations in oral-motor skills. Examples of children who benefit from augmentative communication are described below.

The child with spastic or athetoid cerebral palsy often has oral motor delays that interfere with speech production. Usually the child with cerebral palsy is not a candidate for a completely unaided communication system, such as sign language, because gestures are difficult to produce reliably. A variety of aided augmentative communication systems may be selected, including those that use scanning with a manual, head, or light switch, or direct selection using a keyboard or adapted keyboard.

Children with autism often have communication limitations. They may have strengths in motor skills and specific academic tasks (e.g., reading or math) but frequently have extreme difficulty in social interaction and verbal communication. Eye contact and nonverbal communication are delayed as well. Children with autism can successfully use alternative or augmentative communication to increase dramatically their ability to communicate with others. Interaction with a device seems to be a more acceptable and comfortable means of communication than speech directed to another individual. Children with autism exhibit a wide range of skills when using such a device and may be capable of using a standard keyboard.

The child with extreme intellectual disabilities may also benefit from alternative and augmentative communication systems. Individuals with severely limited cognitive skills often exhibit accompanying disabilities, such as cerebral palsy, sensory impairments, and maladaptive behaviors (Snell, 1987). Such individuals can communicate their basic needs and make simple decisions with well-designed communication systems (McNaughton & Light, 1989).

Selecting Augmentative Communication for Children

Many individuals who use augmentative communication have severe motor disabilities. The team selects an augmentative communication system that will match the child's sensory, motor, and perceptual skills, as well as his or her communication needs.

Occupational therapists are particularly helpful to the team that is selecting an augmentative communication system. The occupational therapist is most involved in the following decisions related to assessment of the individual:

1. What type of system is most appropriate for the child, given current developmental skills and present and future communication needs?

2. How will the child access the system?

3. What skills must be supported and/or developed for the child to use the system successfully?

4. What strategies should be used to develop the skills and endurance needed to use the system?

5. What are the training needs of the other individuals in the home and school environments who use the system with the child? (See Chapter 14, "Technology for Self-Care.")

The range of aids available can be adapted to meet the specific needs and strengths of individual children. Nonelectric devices, such as picture boards and books, may be most appropriate as a first choice for a new user (Musselwhite & St. Louis, 1988). In general, the advantages of nonelectric devices are that they are: (a) low cost, (b) easily transported, (c) easily changed and adapted, and (d) nonthreatening and comfortable for the communication partners to use. The child may use a head pointer, mouth stick, or hand to select the pictures. Some disadvantages of these systems are: (a) there is no audible output (requiring the communication partner to attend visually as the child creates the message), (b) there is no record or memory of the message—it is not displayed on a computer screen, and (c) there is a limited ability to expand the vocabulary. Electronic devices include systems that use computers and dedicated systems that operate as a single unit. A recent trend is toward systems that use or act like computers and are easily adapted and expanded to meet the user's evolving needs.

Kraat (1986) suggests that assessment for matching an augmentative system to the individual involves three phases. First the child's skills, needs, postural stability, and fine motor (or head) control are assessed. Visual and visual perception are evaluated. Cognitive and language skills are determined.

Second, a variety of aids are considered and, when possible, one or two are selected for trial use. Features to consider in device selection are:

1. The child's technique for accessing. (Is direct selection or scanning used?)
2. The method of input. (Are symbols or written words used?)
3. The type of output. (Does the device produce speech or printed words?)
4. Portability of the device. (Is a computer versus dedicated device used?)
5. Special features of the device. (Are special features available? Is special training required?) (Musselwhite & St. Louis, 1988).

Third, the fit of the device to the needs of the child in the everyday environment is considered.

1. Does the device offer versatility?
2. Does it have the features (e.g., language and accessibility) that the child needs?
3. Does it work in the child's environment and with the child's communication partners?
4. Are there support services available for maintenance and training?

A primary focus of the occupational therapist is how the child will access the device and what methods of input will be used. When selecting the optimal input method, consider the variables in Figure 14.

Three basic methods of accessing a communication system are available with unlimited adaptations that can be made to meet specific needs.

Direct Selection

In direct selection, the child selects a message through pointing to a picture, photograph, word, or letter. The child uses the body part (finger, hand, head, or foot) that has the greatest amount of control and that can be used with the least amount of fatigue. In order to use direct selection, the child must have accuracy and speed with that body part. The child must also have the range of motion, strength, and reliability to use the input device. Examples of direct selection devices are a computer keyboard, unicorn board, touch talker, and picture board. Direct selection may be the easiest and most straightforward mode of communication if the child has the motor skills and control to use these systems (see Figure 15).

If the child appears to have the potential for a direct selection device but is not completely reliable, adaptations may be made to improve accuracy or endurance.

Figure 14. Evaluation criteria for selecting input methods.

1. What method (e.g., pointing with head, hand, or other body part) is most accurate?
2. Which method provides optimal speed in communication?
3. How much effort or energy is required, and how quickly does the child fatigue using this method?
4. What cognitive level is required to use the access method (scanning versus direct selection; pictures or symbols versus letters)?
5. What visual perceptual skills are required to use the device?
6. Does the device produce methods that are understood by all communication partners?

Increasing the child's postural support, adjusting the height or angle of the device, or using a variety of tools for access (e.g., a head stick, light beam, or hand stick) may enable the child to use this method successfully.

Scanning Mode

In this method, the child selects a message by scanning numerous messages, pictures, or symbols that are presented on the screen. The child uses a switch to indicate the correct choice when it is pointed to or underlined by the cursor. If letters are used, they are not arranged alphabetically, but according to patterns of use. The advantage of scanning is that the user only needs to master one or two movements with a switch to select a message (or the elements of a message). The primary disadvantage is that it is quite slow, and the users must be able to visualize clearly and attend to the screen in order to select a message. The listener or communication partner must also attend for relatively long periods of time and must be of the cognitive level to interpret the message.

Encoding

In the third type of message selection, messages are encoded in symbols or partial words and are placed on a matrix presented to the child. The child uses scanning or direct selection to choose a specific level of symbols (often a row or an overlay) that allows access to a selected number of message choices. One symbol can represent a specific message or a group of messages. Use of a code allows the individual to indicate a small number of items that correspond to a much larger vocabulary. Encoding methods require the child to have the cognitive ability to remember the meaning of symbols and the pattern for accessing specific messages. The motor skills involved depend on whether direct selection or scanning are used.

A wide range of input devices is available, from which the most appropriate mode must be selected for a specific child. Direct selection may be made with the eyes, head, mouth, hand, or fingers; a light pointer or stick may be used (Cummings, 1989). The ability of the child to target a precise area and to point or push determines what size keyboard or picture board can be used. The keyboard may require varying degrees of range of motion and strength (touch pressure). Direct selection requires greater motor control than scanning.

Scanning (and encoding with scanning) offers the child with severe motor

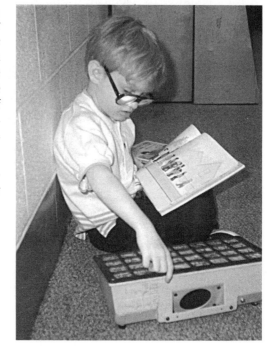

Figure 15. The Introtalker communication device uses direct selection (the child touches the appropriate cell, and the device emits a word or phrase).
Note: For more information contact Prentke-Romich, Wooster, OH 44691.

limitations the greatest access to communication, because a single switch is required. A wide variety of switches are available. Musselwhite and St. Louis (1988) list features that should be considered in selecting a switch for a child.

1. The type and size of activating surface.
2. Resistance and pressure required.
3. Range of motion required.
4. Type of movement required.
5. Position of the device.
6. The sensory feedback the switch provides.

Examples of switches that can be used with augmentative communication systems are sip and puffs, joysticks, and those that are pressure sensitive, infrared, light sensitive, and movement- or sound-activated (Brandenburg & Vanderheiden, 1987; Smith, 1991). Switch selection should be based on what the child can use reliably with a minimal effort for long periods of time (see Figure 16).

Mounting and Positioning for Optimal Use of the System

Mounting

Once a device has been selected, the occupational therapist can help determine its optimal position. If the child spends much of the day in a wheelchair that has a tray, it may be appropriate to mount the device and switch on the tray or wheelchair. The mounting of the device can determine whether or not the child is able to use it efficiently or independently. The mounting can include hardware such as clamps, couplings, rods, or goosenecks. The device should be mounted so that the child has adequate range of motion, strength, visual field, and motor control to operate it. For the child with asymmetrical involvement, the device may be positioned to one side. Mounting the device at an angle can assist the child in gaining control by stabilizing the hands at its base surface. Mounting at an angle can also improve visualization of the device and can promote upright positioning, since the child does not need to bend over it to use it. A swing-away mounting is desirable for when the device is not in use. Mounting of switches for head or foot control may involve adapting the chair and compensating for postural instability.

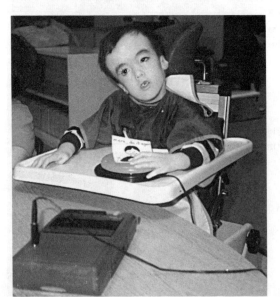

Positioning

Positioning is an important issue in the child's access to the augmentative communication device, and more than one

Figure 16. Before introducing a child to a scanning communicator, it is important to establish that the input switch can be used consistently. Here the child practices with a press switch connected to a tape recorder. His movements start and stop appropriate music.

Figure 17. Options for positioning when using an augmentative communication device include (counterclockwise from top): (a) a prone stander; (b) a corner chair; and (c) a Rifton child's chair.

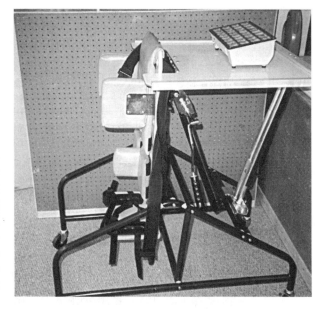

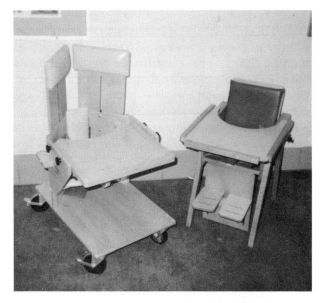

position should be used. An upright position may be ideal for communication purposes but is not always possible or desirable throughout the day. As discussed in the section on feeding, an optimal seating position offers maximum postural stability and alignment. The feet should be flat, with the pelvis flexed at 90° and in alignment with the hips, knees, ankles, and buttocks. After correct trunk alignment has been obtained, stability can be maintained with straps, trays, and footrests. Correct pelvic and trunk positioning facilitates optimal hand and head control. Head stability is important for visual motor control for scanning and direct selection methods. Trunk alignment and stability increase the child's control, strength, and endurance of arm and hand precision movements (see Figure 17).

The occupational therapist can help the team determine an optimal position and then several other positions that are appropriate for accessing the device. The child who spends a significant amount of time on the floor can use the device at that level, but may need external support during use and may need the device supported on a higher surface (e.g., a bench) and at an angle.

Enhancing the Child's Skills to Use a Device

The skills needed to access the device are developed in a number of contexts, with and without the device, using a variety of therapeutic activities. Posture, fine motor, cognitive, and language skills should be encouraged as the child learns to use an augmentative communication system. Switch and keyboard skills can be developed through the use of a computer and switch-activated toys. Play with adapted toys may initially be more motivating than a communication device. Numerous computer programs are available to teach children cause-effect, scanning, and symbol use. Most of these programs are accessed with a switch. To reinforce the needed visual, fine motor, and cognitive skills, the occupational therapist selects switches that elicit motivating and reinforcing activities. From simple plate switches, the child progresses to the use of toggle switches and joysticks. Computer games that use the power pad or unicorn board simulate the direct selection skills needed to use a keyboard. Computers also offer voice output or synthesized speech and therefore can emulate an augmentative communication dedicated system. Use of programs with synthesized speech not only reinforce the motor and perceptual skills needed for device use, but can increase the user's motivation to communicate.

While a focus on switch access and fine motor skills is essential, often the limiting factors in device use are the child's visual attention, visual perception, and cognitive skills. For example, to use an augmentative communication system, the child must demonstrate sustained attention and the visual ability to scan and focus on one item in a confusing background (i.e., figure ground skills). The therapist may engage the child in turn-taking during play and other activities demanding attention to reinforce the skills necessary for using a device. They become a focus of the occupational therapist's recommendations for the child who is a candidate for an augmentative communication system (see Figure 18).

Integrating the Augmentative Communication System Into the Home and Classroom

Once a device has been selected and programmed, and positioning and mounting allow for easy access, the team should focus on integrating its use into the child's life. In the past, training efforts have concentrated on the child's use of augmentative communication, but it has become increasingly apparent that the child's communication partners (teachers, parents, and therapists) also need training in using the systems (Light, 1989). The communication partners of the children are critical to the child's success in using the device, and they need to ensure access or the development of effective strategies and communication opportunities (McNaughton & Light, 1989). Because use of a device slows communi-

Figure 18. A dual switch can be introduced to facilitate decision making and turn-taking.

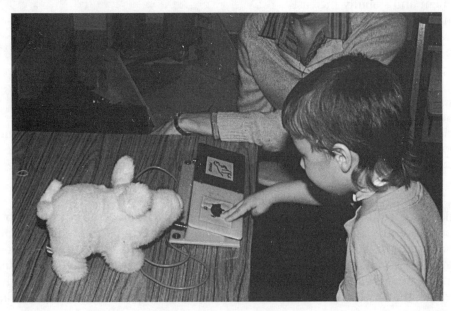

cation, the partners must adapt the pace and rhythm of the natural turn-taking interaction. Patience and attentiveness beyond that required in normal conversation is necessary. It may be tempting to speak for the child rather than allowing him or her to use the device. But when the use of augmentative communication is preempted or interrupted, the child becomes discouraged and is no longer motivated to use it. The device may be used in artificial situations to practice and increase the child's skills; however, skills developed in these situations may not generalize to natural conversation use. The occupational therapist can encourage and support functional use of augmentative communication in the child's natural environments (i.e., school and the home). If the device is to become an integral part of the child's life, individuals with whom the child communicates must learn to use it efficiently and consistently. The case study illustrates the types of outcomes that can be realized when augmentative communication is successfully implemented.

Case Study. Amy: A case in augmentative communication.

> Amy was 4 years old when an augmentative device was contemplated. She had multiple disabilities, including total blindness, cerebral palsy, and cognitive delays. She was fed via a gastrostomy tube and used only three or four sounds to indicate pleasure or displeasure. She did not sustain interaction with any of the preschool staff. She rolled from place to place, primarily away from those who attempted to hold her, as she was severely tactually defensive. She had no opportunities for decision making, but did have approximately six signs that she had developed to interact with her family. Her signs included "love," "mom," "dad," "sis," "bye-bye," and "no." In addition, she uttered "ma," and "da" appropriate for her mother and father.
>
> After an evaluation by an augmentative communication team, an Introtalker with four programmed messages was introduced. The keys were identified by different textures, such as corduroy, a coin, and sandpaper. Quickly Amy became consistent in locating the message keys. Whenever she rolled to her Introtalker, she immediately began using it. She began to request it with grunts and to use the messages appropriately. Within months, Amy was using 12 spaces covered with 12 different textures. She indicated "want," "down," "stop," "want music," "want mom," "want up," "love," and "want sis." The classroom staff was thrilled at her ability to communicate, which had been essentially nonexistent just months earlier. Amy clearly indicated for the first time that she understood language and could make simple choices. The amount of time that she spent interacting with others increased tenfold.
>
> Amy became a different child with her new communication ability, and more willingly participated in other classroom activities. She maintained a more positive affect and began to seek interaction. She began to laugh and giggle in the classroom and to participate more in the circle and group time. The Introtalker was always by her side, and peers became interested in using it with her. By the time Amy entered school, she was using a Touch Talker with more than 30 messages programmed on different overlays.

Functional Mobility

Functional mobility refers to the child's ability to move within the home, school, and community. All children who are nonambulatory are candidates for mobility devices. While the wheelchair is the most common solution to mobility limitations in individuals with developmental disabilities, a range of devices should be considered for the young child. Play toys on wheels (e.g., carts or scooter boards) and strollers may be the first transportation devices for the child (Swinth, in press). Powered mobility is considered at any age when the child is unable to self-propel a wheelchair manually, or it can be an appropriate additional chair when the child has long distances to travel, as in changing classrooms in high school or college. The occupational therapist is a member of the educational or health team that makes recommendations about the range of mobility devices the family should consider and what are most appropriate for the child. The occupational therapist has specific input regarding seating and positioning to support the child's optimal function, adapting the environment to accommodate the device and integrating the wheelchair or device into the child's daily life. The latter objective may involve assisting the child in developing transfer and self-propulsion skills, and in directing the chair in his or her environment.

Typical Development of Mobility

Children become mobile at an early age. Purposeful rolling may begin at age 5 months, and crawling or pivoting on the abdomen by age 6 months. With these first forms of mobility the child begins to explore the environment in order to gain a new understanding of depth, direction, space, and of his or her own body. As children become mobile, they learn about the properties of space and develop rules about their own (Robinson, 1977). Studies have demonstrated that the development of mobility is related to the development of cognitive and social skills (Butler, 1986). The development of independent mobility seems to provide the infant with a sense of mastery over the environment that is critical to self-esteem and self-image.

Children Who Require Assisted Mobility

Children who have sensory motor disabilities often require devices to achieve independent mobility. The mobility device may be used for all travel, only for long distance travel, or for travel within specific environments, like school. Wheelchair mobility is appropriate for children with limitations in strength (muscular dystrophy, myotonia) paralysis (myelomeningocele), and/or poor motor control (cerebral palsy). The child with limited lower extremity strength and control and adequate upper extremity strength and control may be a candidate for a self-propelled chair. When a child lacks upper extremity control and the visual or cognitive skills to self-propel the wheelchair, a travel chair or stroller becomes necessary. Children with severe or multiple disabilities or limited strength and endurance may benefit from transport or travel chairs that provide postural stabilization and alignment. The child with limited motor strength and control, but visual, perceptual, and cognitive skills sufficient for driving a chair, may be a candidate for powered mobility.

Selecting a Wheelchair and Wheelchair Components

The type of mobility device that best matches the child's skills and needs is a team and family decision. The critical variables are: (a) the child's developmental and functional skills and needs, and (b) the family's resources and concerns and the child's environments. These variables are discussed below as they relate to the available selection of mobility devices.

Transport Chairs

Child Considerations. The first mobility device of the young child is usually a stroller, as it is lightweight and practical for community travel. While the umbrella stroller is convenient for young children, it becomes inappropriate for older children due to its soft contours, especially when the child has poor postural control and abnormal muscle tone. Strollers with firm seats and backs that can be adjusted to different angles provide greater postural support and are appropriate for young children with trunk instability. Large, sturdy strollers offer a convenient means for transportation. If the child has poor trunk and head control, a seat insert can fit into the stroller to provide additional external support. Commercial seat inserts have secure strapping systems, footrests, and lateral supports if needed.

When the child reaches the age and size when a stroller is no longer appropriate or no longer offers adequate support, another mobility device is considered. If the child is unable to self-propel, a travel chair is recommended (see Figure 19). Travel chairs can be customized to fit the needs of the child by selecting optional features that assist in maintaining postural stability and alignment. The options available include head and trunk supports, wedged or contoured seats, various strapping systems, and lap trays. Complete modular systems with replaceable and adjustable components can be modified to assist the child. These features allow for correct trunk and pelvic alignment and for postural stability (Bergen, 1990). The entire seat tilts from upright to various reclining angles, offering the child a variety of functional positions. Upright is selected for most fine-motor activities. Semi-reclined may be appropriate for feeding and can be used intermittently throughout the day to provide the child with rest in a relaxed position. All parts of the chair can be adjusted to improve the fit and to increase the child's function. Refer to the section titled, "Positioning and Fitting the Child to the Chair."

Family and Environmental Considerations. Parents may prefer strollers because a child in a stroller appears "normal" and does not carry the stigma of a child in a wheelchair. A stroller is also less expensive and more lightweight than a wheelchair. If the stroller provides security and good positioning, it can be a temporary option for the family prior to considering purchase of a wheelchair.

A stroller collapses easily and can be transported in a car, making it ideal for shopping, public events, or appointments away from home. The stiff structure of the stroller base does not allow for a smooth and comfortable ride over rough terrain, however. Rough terrain may also cause damage to its structure and wheel base. The stroller is most appropriate for use outdoors on smooth surfaces. Because strollers do not support trays and are usually fixed in a semi-reclined position, they cannot be converted into functional chairs for use in the classroom or home.

While travel chairs are much more expensive than strollers, they are more durable, more versatile, and can grow with the child. These chairs and their special features allow for adaptation to the child's postural and functional needs. They also offer the child security and stability during feeding and fine motor activities, freeing the parents from the need to provide postural support.

While these chairs are now lighter than the first models, they remain fairly heavy,

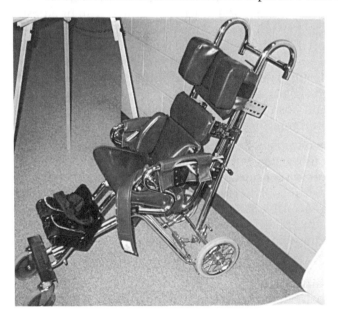

Figure 19. A travel chair can tilt at its base.

which may present a problem for a parent with back pain and/or weakness. Yet because the chair fits the child well and provides optimal postural support, the older child can stay in it for extended periods of time. This may be helpful during social and meal times, especially if the tilting feature is used to help the child shift his or her weight on the buttocks. Travel chairs can be placed in most cars' front seats by collapsing the wheel base; however, they do not always fit into small compact cars. They are also difficult to lift into jeeps and vans. The family should evaluate the fit of the chair in their car prior to purchase.

Travel chairs provide transport for short and long distances and serve as functional chairs within the home and classroom. As such, they are quite versatile. They are usually sturdy, and provide smooth riding over rough terrain. However due to the slanting base of four small wheels, the chair requires more space in the classroom and is more difficult to maneuver than the small wheelchairs. The tilting feature offers the child an optimal view of the room based on his or her visual field, and although the travel chair's frame does not easily fit at a table, it is routinely ordered with a tray. Large trays with bordering rims make ideal surfaces for play, but are sometimes awkward in small spaces.

Self-Propelled Wheelchairs

Child considerations. The range of manual wheelchairs available has dramatically increased in recent years. A manual wheelchair is considered for children who have the arm strength, control, and endurance for self-propulsion, and who have the cognitive and visual skills to direct a chair within their environment. Most manual wheelchairs are lightweight, and easily handled and transported. Small chairs that are low to the ground match the needs of the young child to be at the height of his or her peers. These small wheelchairs may not have the maneuverability of larger chairs, but they are most appropriate for the classroom environments of young children.

Regular-size wheelchairs offer a choice of seat and back sizes and shapes, and should be ordered to fit the child with projected growth considered. Manual sport or ultra-light wheelchairs are about half the weight of a standard chair (Mann & Lane, 1991). The amount of support the chair provides can be adjusted by adding or eliminating lateral supports, trays, and strapping. Footrests, a firm back and seat, and armrests are standard items, and are available with different features and functions. Armrests can be adjusted to change the height of the lap tray for various activities. For example, the tray may be raised during self-feeding to support the hand-to-mouth movement. Most manufacturers also offer a variety of back and seat designs and dimensions. Seating may also be customized by companies specializing in designing and fabricating contour seating and wheelchair equipment. Ultra-light chairs do not have as many seating options, and typically do not have armrests and push handles. Other important considerations in selecting a wheelchair are listed in Figure 20.

Family and Environment Considerations. Self-propelled wheelchairs, as with travel chairs and strollers, come in various weights, but are typically lightweight and are easily collapsed and lifted into a car. Cost is a consideration, particularly when evaluating the purchase of optional features. Appearance of the chair is important, and the current chairs (such as the Sports wheelchairs) are available in a range of colors and styles (see Figure 21). The space available in the home, the child care center, and the school may be factors in wheelchair choice should any of these environments lack wheelchair accessibility.

Powered Chairs

Child considerations. In general, children who do not have the upper extremity strength or control necessary to propel a chair but have the cognitive and perceptual skills to plan

Figure 20. Wheelchair variations.

Wheelchair Feature	Options	Considerations
Seat	• Width and depth • Seat firmness • Contours • Wedge seat • Cushion	• Child's size • Skin integrity • Spine or pelvic alignment/ deformity • Trunk stability • Asymmetry
Strapping	• Strapping fasteners • Pelvic strap • Thigh straps • Chest straps • Upper body support/harness	• Who fastens the belt • Angle, type of fastener • Trunk stability

Foot supports	• Foot plate
	• Footrests with and
	  without straps
	• Swing-away footrests
		• Sensation in lower extremities
		• Lower extremity tone, control,
		  and strength
		• Foot size
		• Does child transfer
		  independently?

Back	• Height and width • Contoured back	• Head and trunk control and stability • Pelvic alignment • Asymmetries
Armrests	• Fixed armrest • Detachable armrest • Adjustable arms	• Transfer techniques • Surface needed for tray • Postural control
Wheels	• Size • Durability	• Type of terrain • Indoor/outdoor • Self-propel
Rim	• Chrome handrims	• Arm and hand strength • Arm and hand size • Asymmetrical strength

and direct chair movement from one location to another are candidates for powered mobility. Advancements in technology allow children with severe physical and cognitive disabilities to use this option.

Powered mobility can also be appropriate for children who can walk or propel a chair short distances, but who have limited strength and endurance and cannot independently manage long distances. Powered mobility may be a choice for the older child who, on entrance to high school or college, has long distances to cover daily, sometimes over rough terrain. Below are several options for the child who would benefit from powered mobility.

Scooters

Motorized scooters are typically used as additional systems for long distances by ambulators

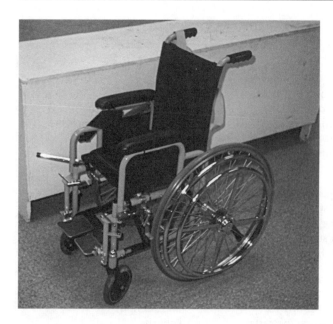

Figure 21. A wheelchair with a left-arm drive. The long extension on the brake enables the child to reach with his or her left hand to the opposite side to lock the wheels.

who have adequate upper body control to sit with minimal trunk support. While the scooter is usually considered a vehicle for community travel, it is available in a front wheel drive, lightweight model that has enhanced maneuverability for indoor use (Long, 1992).

Standard Powered Chairs

Standard powered chairs are usually equipped with proportional joysticks, but can be adapted with alternative input controls. Electronic programming varies: The chair may be direct-drive or belt-driven and may have one of several different types of braking systems. The occupational therapist is instrumental in evaluating whether or not the child's visual perceptual and cognitive skills support introduction of a powered chair, and for implementing an intervention program to develop the prerequisite skills needed for powered mobility.

If visual and cognitive skills are adequate, there are numerous input devices to choose from to offer the child the greatest control. The most typical input device is the proportional joystick. The child moves the joystick in the direction he or she wants the chair to go. The chair's speed is proportional to the amount of joystick deflection. Digital control, using a microswitch, provides the child with less control over direction and starting/stopping the chair than the proportional joystick, but speed is usually programmed into the switch system. While switch systems offer less control, they also require less control. These systems include a press pad, arm slot, and individual switches (Long, 1992). Switches enable the child to control the chair through sip and puff, or by the head, knee, arm, foot, or other body parts using different mounting of switches. The child with fair control, but poor strength and endurance, can easily operate and direct a chair using microswitch control. When the child has poor control and forceful movement, the switch can also correct for the degree of force by responding with a programmed speed and a limited choice of directions.

Family and Environmental Considerations. While powered chairs may offer the child the first and only opportunity for independent mobility, a number of variables must be considered by the family prior to investing in this expensive endeavor. If the powered chair is an additional mobility device for the child who already has a travel chair, its cost may not be covered by insurance. The chairs are heavy, and even when the battery pack can be detached and lifted separately, transportation of a powered chair requires a van and a lift. Therefore, the expense of powered mobility may be unmanageable for the family. The home environment must be accessible, with wide spaces to accommodate the chair's limited maneuverability.

Recent literature has advocated use of powered mobility for the young child (i.e., ages 18 to 24 months) who is immobile (Butler, 1986; Trefler & Taylor, 1988). If the occupational therapist and other team members feel that a recommendation for powered mobility at age 2 is appropriate, they need to consider the implications for the family. At this early age the family may be reluctant to accept a major, "permanent" symbol of the child's disability. In addition, given the expense of the chair, the growth and development of the child should be considered when ordering the size and features. The powered chair needs ongoing maintenance and may require relatively frequent repair. The family must be willing to undertake this ongoing responsibility.

Positioning and Fitting the Child to the Chair

Functional use of self-propelled or powered-mobility travel chairs requires correct positioning and seating. Occupational therapists and other team members evaluate the child's neuromotor, sensory, and orthopedic status in order to make recommendations regarding seating (Taylor, 1987). The goals when recommending and selecting seating are to promote normal muscle tone while inhibiting abnormal or primitive reflexes, to prevent the development or progression of orthopedic deformities, to increase functional skills, to accommodate impaired sensation, and to provide comfort. An extensive range of commercial seating systems are available (Mann & Lane, 1991).

Taylor (1987) describes three components of evaluation for seating and positioning:

1. functional assessment of the child that includes his or her daily activities and educational goals;
2. evaluation of specific positions by observing the child in different positions or on a seating simulator; and
3. selection of a seating system that is the appropriate material, size, angle, and shape.

Trunk support and pelvic alignment are critical to positioning in the chair. In order to maintain the pelvis in neutral alignment with the hips flexed at 90°, strapping at a 45° angle is recommended. Additional straps for the trunk can provide support and stability when the child lacks internal control. Straps that cross the chest in a *V, H,* or *X* design can assist with alignment, upright posture, and maintenance of posture when fatigue becomes a factor. Straps that originate on the chair back below the level of the shoulders and fit over the top of the shoulders effectively maintain postural alignment. Rigid supports are also available to maintain the trunk in a symmetrical position (Bergen & Colangelo, 1985).

The lower extremities should be well supported, with neutral rotation at the hips and 90° of flexion at the hips, knees, and ankles. This promotes neutral pelvic alignment, preventing posterior pelvic tilt and lower extremity extension. Seating angles of less than 90° at the hips may be needed with clients who have excessive extensor tone.

Additional features may be added to the chair when shoulder retraction and head control are issues. Shoulder protraction wings encourage midline positioning of the upper extremities. Head supports can assist the child in maintaining his or her head at midline. When head control is poor and frequently pulls into flexion, head straps or a cervical collar can be considered; however, these devices must be selected and used with care as the head often slips into an undesirable position, reinforcing, rather than helping, poor neck alignment. Stabilization of the head may not be as important as neck alignment for swallowing and as head tilt that allows optimal visualization of the environment.

Strapping of the head may feel restrictive and uncomfortable. A better choice may be to tilt the seating unit backwards, allowing gravity to assist in maintaining head alignment against the chair's back.

Functional Use of the Mobility Device in the Child's Daily Activities

Occupational therapists often focus on improving the child's function while in the chair (Deitz, Jaffe, Wolf, Massagli, & Anson, 1991). One primary method is to give the child a functional surface. Wheelchair trays are used with travel chairs and some powered chairs. Self-propelled chairs may come with desk arms to accommodate sitting at a table.

Wheelchair trays can provide a surface for eating, working on school or vocational tasks, or play. The tray may also provide a surface for a communication device or computer. Augmentative communication devices must remain with the child; therefore, mounting them on the wheelchair tray is ideal. The tray has the additional benefits of helping the child maintain an upright posture by supporting the midtrunk and maintaining the upper extremities in a functional position (Bergen & Colangelo, 1985). Other functional issues to be assessed with the child in his or her chair are:

1. Can the child reach with adequate range to manage the environment (e.g., turn faucets on and off; write on the blackboard; and reach shelves, the floor, and a light switch)?

2. Can the child turn the chair and maneuver it through rooms and hallways?

3. Can the child propel or drive up to a table or desk and position him- or herself comfortably for tabletop activities?

4. Can the child propel or drive the chair over grass, rough terrain, and other outdoor surfaces in his or her environment (Wolf, Massagli, Jaffe, & Deitz, 1991)?

5. Can the child transfer in and out of the chair independently?

The family and therapist can identify the areas that require assistance. Together, they help the child to remediate or compensate for the functional limitations. In some cases the environment can be adapted; for example, table heights can be adjusted and home or school modifications can be made. The child may become independent in transferring into the chair with adapted environmental supports and modified techniques. (Features on the chair itself must accommodate the child's ability to step out of and into the chair and to stand and pivot next to the seat.) Other interventions may include improving sitting balance and arm strength, and increasing arm range and arm and hand control.

Conclusion

Children with developmental disabilities usually require assistance in self-care and daily living skills. The child's ability to achieve independence and mastery in self-care is important to self-esteem. Autonomy in self-care also enhances the child's interaction within the family unit. Occupational therapists are particularly skilled and resourceful in enhancing the child's daily living skills using sensorimotor analysis, an understanding of development and occupation, and therapeutic skills that promote sensorimotor-perceptual performance. Occupational therapists work closely with family members and other disciplines to ensure that a consistent, comprehensive approach is implemented that places the family's priorities first, enables the child, and draws on the appropriate community resources. Occupational therapists recognize that the self-care issues of the child with developmental disabilities are often long-term and sometimes even life-long. Methods appropriate for the young child are adapted and expanded for older children.

This chapter described some of the variables in the child's home and school environments that can affect development of self-care independence. The holistic approach of the occupational therapist enables him or her to assimilate these variables into a therapeutic approach that offers the family new understanding of the child and provides the child with increased mastery of the environment. ◆

References

Ayres, J.A. (1981). *Sensory integration and the child.* Los Angeles: Western Psychological Corporation.

Barber, P.A., Turnbull, A.P., Behr, S.K., & Kerns, G.M. (1988). A family systems perspective on early childhood special education. In S.L. Odom & M.B. Karnes (Eds.), *Early intervention for infants and children with handicaps* (pp. 179–198). Baltimore: Paul H. Brookes.

Barnard, K.E., & Kelly, J.F. (1990). Assessment of parent-child interaction. In S. Meisels & J. Shonkoff (Eds.), *Handbook of early childhood intervention* (pp. 278–302). Boston, MA: Cambridge University Press.

Bergen, A.F. (1990). *Positioning for function: Wheelchairs and other assistive devices.* Valhalla, NY: Valhalla Rehabilitation Publications.

Bergen, A.F., & Colangelo, C. (1985). *Positioning the client with CNS deficits: The wheelchair and other adapted equipment* (2nd ed.). Valhalla, NY: Valhalla Rehabilitation Publications.

Blackman, J.A., & Nelson, C.L.A. (1985). Reinstituting oral feedings in children fed by gastrostomy tube. *Clinical Pediatrics, 24,* 434–438.

Boehme, R. (1982). *Neurodevelopmental treatment.* Eight-week certification course sponsored by NDTA, Inc., Augusta, GA.

Boehme, R. (1988). *Improving upper body control.* Tucson, AZ: Therapy Skill Builders.

Brandenburg, S., & Vanderheiden, G. (1987). *Communication, control, and computer access for disabled and elderly individuals. Resource Book 2: Switches and environmental controls.* San Diego: College-Hill Press.

Brazelton, T.B., Koslowski, B., & Main, M. (1974). The origins of reciprocity: The early mother-infant interaction. In M. Lewis & L.R. Rosenblum (Eds.), *The effect of the infant on its caregiver* (pp. 49–76). New York: Wiley-Interscience.

Brinker, R.P., & Lewis, M. (1982). Discovering the competent handicapped infant: A process approach to assessment and intervention. *Topics in Early Childhood Special Education, 2*(12), 1–15.

Butler, C. (1986). Effects of powered mobility on self-initiated behaviors of very young children with locomotor disability. *Developmental Medicine and Child Neurology, 28,* 325–332.

Case-Smith, J. (1989). Intervention strategies for promoting feeding skills in infants with sensory deficits. *OT in Health Care, 6*(2/3), 129–141.

Case-Smith, J. (1991). The family perspective. In W. Dunn (Ed.)., *Pediatric occupational therapy: Facilitating effective service delivery.* Thorofare, NJ: Slack.

Cermak, S. (1985). Developmental dyspraxia. In E.A. Roy (Ed.), *Neuropsychological studies of apraxia and related disorders* (pp. 225–248). New York: North-Holland.

Cermak, S. (1991). Somatodyspraxia. In A. Fisher, E. Murray, & A. Bundy, (Eds.), *Sensory integration: Theory and practice*. Philadelphia: F.A. Davis.

Chamberlin, J., Henry, M.M., Roberts, J.D, Sapsford, A.L., & Courtney, S.E. (1991). An infant and toddler feeding group program. *American Journal of Occupational Therapy, 45,* 907–911.

Clark, F., Parham, D., & Malloux, Z. (1989). Sensory integration and children with learning disabilities. In P. Pratt & A. Allen (Eds.), *Occupational therapy for children* (pp. 457–509). St. Louis: Mosby.

Coley, I. (1978). *Pediatric assessment of self-care activities*. St. Louis: Mosby .

Coley, I.L., & Procter, S.A. (1989). Self-maintenance activities. In P. Pratt & A. Allen (Eds.), *Occupational therapy for children* (p. 260–294). St. Louis: Mosby.

Cummings, F.J. (1989). Children with communicative impairment. In P. Pratt & A. Allen (Eds.), *Occupational therapy for children* (pp. 442–456). St. Louis: Mosby.

Deitz, J., Jaffe, K.M., Wolf, L.S., Massagli, T.L., & Anson, D. (1991). Pediatric power wheelchairs: Evaluation of function in the home and school environments. *Assistive Technology, 3,* 24–31.

Espe-Sherwindt, M., & Kerlin, S.L. (1990). Early intervention with parents with mental retardation: Do we empower or impair? *Infants and Young Children, 2*(4), 21–28.

Farber, S.D. (1982). *A multisensory approach to neurorehabilitation*. Philadelphia: W.B. Saunders.

Finnie, N. (1975). *Handling the young cerebral palsied child at home* (2nd ed.). New York: Dutton-Sunrise.

Fox, C.A. (1990). Implementing the modified barium swallow evaluation in children who have multiple disabilities. *Infants and Young Children, 3*(2), 67–77.

Furuno, S., O'Reilly, K., Hosaka, C.M., Zeisloft, B., & Allman, T. (1984). Hawaii early learning profile. Palo Alto, CA: VORT.

Glass, R.P., & Wolf, L.S. (1993). Feeding and oral-motor skills. In J. Case-Smith (Ed.), *Pediatric occupational therapy and early intervention* (pp. 225–288). Andover, MA: Andover Medical Publishers.

Humphry, R. (1991). Impact of feeding problems on the parent-infant relationship. *Infants and Young Children, 3*(3), 30–38.

Humphry, R., & Rourk, M.H. (1991). When an infant has a feeding problem. *Occupational Therapy Journal of Research, 11*(2), 106–120.

Hunter, J. (1990). Pediatric feeding dysfunction. In C. Semmler & J.G. Hunter (Eds.), *Early occupational therapy intervention: Neonates to three years*. Rockville, MD: Aspen Publishers.

Johnson-Martin, N., Jens, K.G., & Attermeier, S.M. (1986). *The Carolina Curriculum for handicapped infants and infants at risk*. Baltimore: Paul H. Brookes.

Kielhofner, G. (1985). *A model of human occupation: Theory and application*. Baltimore: Williams & Wilkins.

Klein, M.D. (1988). *Pre-dressing skills*. Tucson, AZ: Therapy Skill Builders.

Kraat, A.W. (1986). Developing intervention goals. In S.W. Blackstone (Ed.), *Augmentative communication: An introduction* (pp. 197–266). Rockville, MD: American Speech-Language-Hearing Association.

Light, J. (1989). Toward a definition of communicative competence for individuals using augmentative and alternative communication systems. *Augmentative and Alternative Communication, 5,* 137–144.

Lloyds, L.L., & Fuller, D. (1986). Toward an augmentative and alternative communication symbol taxonomy: A proposed superordinate classification. *Augmentative and Alternative Communication, 2,* 165–171.

Long, S. (1992). Introducing powered mobility to students with multiple disabilities. *Technology Special Interest Section Newsletter, 2*(1), 2–4.

Mann, W.C., & Lane, J.P. (1991). *Assistive technology for persons with disabilities: The role of occupational therapy* (pp. 37–128). Rockville, MD: American Occupational Therapy Association.

McNaughton, D., & Light, J. (1989). Teaching facilitators to support the communication skills of an adult with severe cognitive disabilities: A case study. *Augmentative and Alternative Communication, 5,* 35–41

Morris, S.E. (1978). Oral-motor development: Normal and abnormal. In J. Wilson (Ed.), *Oral-motor function and dysfunction in children* (pp. 106–186). Chapel Hill: University of North Carolina at Chapel Hill.

Morris, S.E., & Klein, M.D. (1987). *Pre-feeding skills.* Tucson, AZ: Therapy Skill Builders.

Mueller, H. (1975). Feeding. In N. Finnie (Ed.), *Handling the young cerebral palsied child at home* (2nd ed.) (pp. 113–140). New York: Dutton-Sunrise.

Musselwhite, C., & St. Louis, K. (1988). *Communication programming for persons with severe handicaps: Vocal and augmentative strategies.* Boston: College-Hill.

Palmer, S., & Elkvall, S. (1985). *Pediatric nutrition in developmental disorders.* Springfield, IL: Charles C. Thomas.

Pipes, P.L., & Pritkin, R. (1989). Nutrition and feeding of children with developmental delays and related problems. In P.L. Pipes (Ed.), *Nutrition in infancy and childhood* (3rd ed.) pp. 347–371. St. Louis: Mosby.

Robinson, A.L. (1977). Play: The arena for acquisition of rules for competent behavior. *American Journal of Occupational Therapy, 31,* 248–253.

Royeen, C.B., & Lane, S. (1991). Tactile processing and sensory defensiveness. In A.G. Fisher, E.A. Murray, & A.C. Bundy (Eds.). *Sensory integration: Theory and practice* (pp. 108–136). Philadelphia: F.A. Davis.

Scherzer, A., & Tscharnuter, I. (1982). *Early diagnosis and therapy in cerebral palsy.* New York: Marcel Dekker.

Smith, R.O. (1991). Technological approaches to performance enhancement. In C. Christiansen & C. Baum, (Eds.), *Occupational therapy: Overcoming human performance deficits* (pp. 747–788). Thorofare, NJ: Slack.

Snell, M. (1987). *Systematic instruction of persons with severe handicaps.* Columbus, OH: Charles E. Merrill.

Swinth, Y. (in press). Technology for young children with disabilities. In J. Case-Smith (Ed.), *Pediatric occupational therapy and early intervention.* Andover, MA: Andover Medical Publishers.

Taylor, S.J. (1987). Evaluating the client with physical disabilities for wheelchair seating. *American Journal of Occupational Therapy, 41,* 711–716.

Trefler, E., & Taylor, S.J. (1988). Power mobility for severely physically disabled children: Evaluation and provision practices. In K.M. Jaffe (Ed.), *Childhood power mobility: Developmental, technical and clinical perspectives* (pp. 117–126). Washington, DC: RESNA.

Turnbull, A.P., Summers, J.A., & Brotherson, M.J. (1986). Family life cycle: Theoretical and empirical implications and future directions for families with mentally retarded members. In J.J. Gallagher & P. Vietze (Eds.), *Families of handicapped persons: Current research, treatment and policy issues* (pp. 45–66). Baltimore: Paul H. Brookes.

Turnbull, A., & Turnbull, H.R. (1986). *Families, professionals, and exceptionalities.* Columbus, OH: Merrill.

Vietze, P.M., Abernathy, S.R., Ashe, M.L., & Stich, F. (1978). Contingent interaction between mothers and their developmentally delayed infants. In G.P. Sackett (Eds.), *Observing behavior: Vol. 1* (pp. 115–132). Baltimore: University Park Press.

Wilbarger, P., & Wilbarger, J. (1991). *Sensory defensiveness in children aged 2–12: An intervention guide for parents and other caretakers.* Santa Barbara, CA: Avanti Educational Programs.

Winton, P. (1988). Effective communication between parents and professionals. In D.B. Bailey & R.J. Simeonsson (Eds.), *Family assessment in early intervention* (pp. 207–228). Columbus, OH: Merrill.

Wolf, L.S., & Glass, R.P. (1992). *Feeding and swallowing disorders in infancy: Assessment and management.* Tucson, AZ: Therapy Skill Builders.

Wolf, L.S., Massagli, T.L., Jaffe, K.M., & Deitz, J. (1991). Functional assessment of the Joncare Hi-Lo Master power wheelchair for children. *Physical and Occupational Therapy in Pediatrics, 11*(3), 57–72.

6

Self-Care Strategies for Persons With Arthritis and Connective Tissue Diseases

Jeanne L. Melvin

Jeanne L. Melvin, MS, OTR, FAOTA is Clinical Director of the Pain Management Program at the Daniel Freeman Memorial Hospital, Inglewood, CA.

Chapter 6 Outline

Major Rheumatic Diseases

Osteoarthritis (Degenerative Joint Disease)

Hand Involvement

Other Joint Limitations

Rheumatoid Arthritis

Hand Involvement

Intervention for Non-Hand Joints

Psoriatic Arthritis

Ankylosing Spondylitis

Systemic Lupus Erythematosus (SLE)

Systemic Sclerosis (SSc)

Juvenile Rheumatoid Arthritis (JRA)

Self-Care Assessment and Intervention for People With Arthritis

Special Factors to Consider in the Self-Care Assessment

Medications

Morning Stiffness

Fatigue and Endurance

Disease Variability

American College of Rheumatology Functional Classification

Joint Protection Techniques

Equipment Recommendations—Factors to Consider

Assistive Devices for People With Rheumatic Diseases

Aids for Hand Impairment

Aids for Elbow Impairment

Aids for Shoulder Impairment

Aids for Neck Impairment

Aids for Knee Impairment

Aids for Hip Impairment

Aids for Limitations in Dressing

Aids for Limitations in Grooming

Aids for Limitations in Bathing

Aids for Limitations in Toileting

Aids for Limitations in Housekeeping

Aids for Limitations in Meal Preparation

Aids for Limitations in Eating

Summary

References

Suggestions for Further Reading

This chapter emphasizes the unique differences between assessing and remediating self-care limitations in people with arthritis and other rheumatic diseases. Rheumatic disease includes diseases that have muscle or joint pain as a primary symptom. Thus, it is important to realize that *arthritis*, which means joint inflammation, is not a specific disease but a symptom of more than 100 different diseases.

The most common rheumatic diseases that limit a person's ability for self-care are: osteoarthritis (OA), rheumatoid arthritis (RA), psoriatic arthritis (PA), ankylosing spondylitis (AS), systemic lupus erythematosus (SLE), systemic sclerosis (SSc), and juvenile rheumatoid arthritis (JRA). Rheumatoid arthritis is a particularly important disease to understand because it provides a model for treating chronic inflammation of all the extremity joints. In other words, if you know how to treat inflammation of the wrist in an adult with RA, you will know how to treat inflammation of the wrist in any other disease.

Rheumatic diseases are excellent examples of conditions that affect an individual at multiple system levels. That is, while the inflammatory processes associated with the rheumatic diseases produce pain and swelling in the joints and may result in pathology in other organ systems, they restrict function through the resulting pain, limitation of strength or movement, fatigue, or flu-like symptoms. In turn, these restrictions in function interfere with role performance. Studies (Affleck, Pfeffier, Tennen, & Fifield, 1988) have shown that patients with arthritis view limitations of activity and mobility as more difficult to cope with than the pain associated with the disease.

Although little research has been done that examines the relationship of symptoms and physical problems associated with arthritis and engagement in self-care activities, a study by Gerber and Furst (1992) is notable in this regard. In this study, patients were asked to log their daily activities, including self-care, and to assign ratings of these activities according to the degree of pain, fatigue, meaningfulness, enjoyment, competence, and difficulty they experienced during each activity. In addition, patients were asked to complete measures of pain and disability, undergo an articular examination, and complete an assessment of psychological adjustment to illness. The findings of the study showed that pain, fatigue, and joint tenderness were correlated with activity engagement as well as with the subject's satisfaction with the activity.

Major Rheumatic Diseases

Osteoarthritis (Degenerative Joint Disease)

Osteoarthritis (OA) is the most common rheumatic disease, affecting both men and women equally during middle age and beyond (ages 45–90), with its prevalence increasing with age (Hicks & Gerber, 1988). The progression of OA involves a two-stage process. First, a wearing down or deterioration of the articular cartilage occurs, and second, the build-up of bone around the margin of the joint creates the lumpy, enlarged appearance. This two-stage process is frequently painless, with stiffness and limited range of movement (ROM) as the primary problems, although there may be inflammation and associated pain and swelling. Joints frequently affected by osteoarthritis include the hands, spine, knees, hips, and large-toe metatarsal phalangeal (MTP) joint (Bland & Stulberg, 1985).

Hand Involvement

Osteoarthritis of the hands typically affects the finger distal interphalangeal (DIP) and proximal interphalangeal (PIP) joints; the thumb carpometacarpal (CMC) and interphalangeal (IP) joints; and the trapezial intercarpal joints (Swanson & deGroot Swanson, 1985). It generally does not affect the metacarpophalangeal (MCP), radiocarpal or radioulnar joints. *In the hand, ROM limitations are due to bony block from osteophyte formation around the joint.* This may result in the inability to make a full grip to hold onto objects or the inability to extend the digits fully. Specific ROM exercises are not necessary or helpful when the limitation is due to bony block, as people use their full available ROM during daily activities (Melvin, 1989). Therapeutic intervention for hand conditions primarily includes orthotics to stabilize joints or treat inflammation, assistive devices, adaptive methods, and Joint Protection Techniques (JPT).

Other Joint Limitations

Limitations in hand, arm, shoulder, or neck function due to pain and stiffness can have a significant effect on the performance of self-care skills. Figure 1 provides a list of common joint limitations experienced with osteoarthritis and the intervention approaches often recommended by occupational therapists and other health care providers.

Rheumatoid Arthritis

Rheumatoid arthritis (RA) is a systemic disease with inflammation of the synovia, which lines the joint capsules and tendon sheaths, as a primary symptom. Primarily affecting women between the ages of 20 and 50 (but also affecting men and adolescents ages 16 to 20), the course of RA is often characterized by exacerbations and remissions. It primarily affects the extremity joints and the neck (the back and trunk joints are often spared). For many people with RA, joint disease is the sole problem. However, a minority of people develop extra-articular manifestations; that is, disease of the lungs, blood vessels (vasculitis), heart, and eyes (Krane & Simon, 1986). Because it is a "systemic" disease it affects every cell in the body, even if obvious pathology can only be identified in the joints. When these patients have a "flare" of their arthritis they feel terrible all over, and as if they have the flu. Symptoms include joint pain and swelling, fatigue, malaise or flu-like feelings, muscle atrophy, and pain inhibition of muscle strength.

Hand Involvement

Most people with RA have bilateral or symmetrical hand involvement. The disease may only involve the wrists or the MCP joints or any and all of the joints and tendon sheaths. It may be mild or severe, slowly or rapidly progressive, with or without remissions. Acute involvement includes warm, swollen, painful joints, and swelling in the flexor and extensor tendon sheaths (this tenosynovitis may be painless or painful). As synovitis persists, the synovia in the joints and tendon sheaths grows and thickens (pannus), damaging and distending the joint capsules and supporting ligaments and eroding the cartilage in the joints. The damage to these structures is both biochemical and mechanical.

During active inflammation, therapy focuses on reducing it with orthotic treatment, cold modalities, JPT, assistive devices, and adaptive methods to reduce stress to the joints and prevent contractures. During periods of remission, soft tissue contractures can be corrected with exercise and orthotics.

Patients with end-stage rheumatoid arthritis frequently have severe fixed deformities, but no pain or inflammation. Treatment in these cases primarily focuses on adaptive devices and methods, and thumb or digit stabilization orthotics (Melvin, 1989).

Figure 1. Osteoarthritis: Common limitations and interventions.

Limitation	Treatment
1. Severe stiffness in morning	Thermoelastic gloves at night or active ROM in warm water
2. Inability for full grip 2° to decreased finger ROM	Enlarged or nonslip handles on equipment/devices
3. Inability to hold objects 2° to pain	Joint protection techniques, enlarged handles, adaptive methods, patient education on optimal treatment for inflammation
4. Inability to open hand flat to neutral	Assistive devices
5. Inability to apply pinch due to CMC/pantrapezial pain	MP-CMC orthosis to restrict CMC motion during activities (Pantrapezial arthritis also requires wrist immobilization)
6. Inability to hold objects due to thumb metacarpal adduction contracture (the most common thumb deformity)	Reduce handles to accommodate diminished web space
7. Inability to apply pinch due to thumb IP, MP*, or CMC instability	Thumb orthosis to stabilize IP joint alone, MP joint alone, MP-CMC or CMC-MP-IP joints combined
8. Shoulder pain: decreased upper extremity dressing and bathing	Adaptive methods and assistive devices (see Figure 6)
9. Back pain: decreased toilet/tub/low seat transfer, lower extremity dressing/bathing	Assistive devices to don pants, shoes, and socks, and to tie shoes; transfer bars, bathing aids, adapted seats (see Figures 4–14)
10. Decreased hip flexion: decreased lower extremity dressing, toilet or low seat transfer	Assistive devices to don pants, shoes, and socks and to tie shoes (see Figure 9)
11. Decreased hip abduction: decreased perineal care	Adaptive bathing and toileting devices
12. Decreased knee flexion or pain: decreased lower extremity dressing, low seat transfer	Same as #2, plus walker adaptions if necessary
13. Cervical pain and decreased ROM (Nerve root compression: decreased hand strength)	JPT, assistive devices, soft collar for positioning (not immobilization)
14. First MTP joint pain/stiffness: limit ambulation endurance	Foot orthotics, lightweight shoes with cushioned soles
15. Decreased ambulation and coordination; risk of falling	Home safety evaluation and education/adaptation

*metacarpal phalangeal

Figure 2 lists common limitations associated with involvement to joints of the hand with rheumatoid arthritis and the types of intervention commonly associated with these limitations. Measures to reduce swelling and pain are frequently coupled with the use of assistive devices and orthotics to increase function, provide joint protection, and stabilize joints. Figure 3 lists other levels or forms of joint involvement and their functional consequences, which can interfere with the performance of self-care tasks.

Intervention for Non-Hand Joints

A combination of therapeutic strategies is required to decrease joint stress and inflammation. These include joint protection techniques, proper body mechanics, energy conservation strategies, thermal modalities, adaptive methods, and assistive devices.

Proper body mechanics can serve the person with arthritis in two ways: by reducing the stress on the joints during activities; and by reducing the work load on the muscles, thus increasing efficiency and conserving energy. It is helpful to incorporate the principles of body mechanics relevant to a person with RA into the joint protection instruction. Most literature on body mechanics is directed toward the back pain patient, who has healthy hands, arms, and knees.

Maintaining normal body weight can play an important role in reducing stress to the hips, knees, ankles, and toes. For example, in gait stride, force exerted per square inch over the joint surface in the hip is four times the body weight. Consequently, for every pound of weight loss, there is a 4-pound reduction of force, per square inch, on the hip joint.

Some specific measures for the problems described in Figure 3 include padded elbow sleeves to reduce pressure on elbow nodules; soft neck collars to improve postural alignment during activities; swivel chairs to accommodate restricted neck rotation; and

Figure 2. Rheumatoid arthritis: Hand limitations for self-care and interventions.

Limitations	Treatment
1. Swollen, painful joints: limited ROM, inhibited strength, decreased function in all activities	Cold modalities to decrease swelling, inflammation; JPT, adaptive devices, and orthotics
2. Joint contractures diminish grip.	Adaptive handles, devices, and methods (some soft tissue contractures can be reduced with serial splinting)
3. Joint instability in thumb or finger: decreased function and prehension strength	Individual joint orthosis to stabilize joint
4. Severe MCP ulnar drift decreases function.	MCP ulnar drift positioning orthosis (static or dynamic)
5. Active ROM is limited due to flexor tenosynovitis.	Cold modalities to decrease swelling (if not effective, a steroid injection is the next treatment of choice)
6. Limited wrist flexion or wrist orthotics: limited ability to manage proximal dressing, fasteners, toileting, hygiene	Adaptive methods or equipment, or flexible orthosis

Figure 3. Rheumatoid arthritis: Other joint involvement. Limitations to self-care and ADL.

Condition	Functional Consequences
1. Radioulnar synovitis, proximal or distal	Decreased supination or pronation.
2. Elbow synovitis	Decreased extension limits ability for transfer push off, lower extremity dressing, desk activities; decreased flexion limits ability for feeding, and face and upper body care.
3. Elbow nodules	Pain that limits bed mobility, chair transfer at a table.
4. Shoulder synovitis	Decreased shoulder ROM (less than 90°) limits ability to reach and dress. Pain results in decreased ability for lifting, carrying, pushing, and grip.
5. Neck pain or limited ROM	Reduced visual field for safety and interpersonal communication, requires person to turn his or her whole body to see.
6. Hip and knee pain and limitations cause the same functional problems as OA (see Figure 1).	OA limitations are due to bony block, whereas RA limitations are due to inflammation, swelling, soft tissue damage, or contracture.

proper positioning during sleep, work, and leisure activities, which is critical in the treatment of cervical arthritis (Melvin, 1989).

Psoriatic Arthritis (PA)

Psoriatic arthritis is a distinct systemic disease in which psoriasis is associated with inflammatory arthritis and a negative serologic test for rheumatoid factor. Psoriasis is a chronic dermatitis consisting of discrete pink or dull-red lesions surrounded by a characteristic silvery scaling. There are five distinct subgroups based on clinical patterns: (a) predominant involvement of the DIP joints of the hands, associated with psoriatic nail involvement and asymmetric peripheral joint arthritis; (b) arthritis mutilans (osteolysis of the bones in involved joints) creating floppy joints, which may be associated with spinal arthritis; (c) symmetrical polyarthritis similar to the pattern seen in RA, in which rapid ankylosis can occur; (d) asymmetric, oligo-articular arthritis (affecting a single or few joints) of the fingers or toes (this pattern accounts for 70% of all PA); and (e) ankylosing spondylitis similar to idiopathic AS or associated with severe peripheral joint disease (Moll & Wright, 1973).

Occupational therapy for psoriatic arthritis is essentially the same as for RA for peripheral involvement and AS for axial involvement, in terms of joint limitations and methods for improving self-care and ADL. However, treatment of the arthritis and skin require the following specific considerations (Melvin, 1989, p. 278).

1. The diffuse digital (sausage) swelling seen in PA is extremely difficult to treat. It is resistant to mechanical methods for edema reduction such as Coban wrapping, string wrapping, stretch gloves, and compression sleeves. Cold modalities can help reduce joint swelling, but they are generally ineffective for treating the sausage swelling. Even drug therapy may not help manage this problem.

2. Patients with severe, acute, PA are prone to developing rapid contractures, as well as having a tendency for bony ankylosis. These patients need to have their range of motion carefully monitored. Proper bed positioning, especially for the neck, wrists, knees, and ankles is critical. Hand and ankle orthoses may be the only effective means of preventing dysfunctional contractures.

3. Psoriatic skin lesions may restrict options in orthotic treatment. Plastic orthoses should not be applied directly to involved skin—a cotton (not nylon) stockinet can be used to protect it. All orthoses and liners should be washed daily. Moleskin and soft foam liners should not be used.

4. The hand assessment should include PIP and DIP lateral stability testing to detect mutilans deformity (osteolysis of the joint). Mutilans can be stopped with surgical fusion (Nalebuff & Garrett, 1976). If the patient is not a surgical candidate, the joint can be stabilized with a Silver Ring Splint Orthosis.[1]

Ankylosing Spondylitis (AS)

Ankylosing Spondylitis is a chronic systemic disease in which the primary sites of inflammation are the ligamentous, capsular, and tendinous insertions into the bone (the entheses). AS primarily involves the sacroiliac, spinal apophyseal, and axial joints. Other symptoms may include asymmetric or peripheral arthritis or ocular, cardiac, or pulmonary involvement (Calin, 1985).

Hand involvement in ankylosing spondylitis tends to be mild and episodic, usually involving one or a few joints in an asymmetrical pattern. Shoulder involvement is more common than elbow or hand synovitis. Treatment for limitations in these areas is the same as for rheumatoid arthritis.

Spinal involvement in AS creates a stiff or "poker" spine. The goal of rehabilitation is to educate the patient early regarding posture so the spine becomes stiff or ankylosed in a straight, upright posture (Wright & Moll, 1976). Positioning during leisure activities, work, and bed rest is critical to this goal. People who have not had adequate posture education use multiple pillows to support their head and knees, resulting in spinal kyphosis with a bent-over, rigid posture with their face toward the ground, rendering them unable to see ahead of them. In some cases fixed ankylosis can occur in a few days (Melvin, 1989).

Spinal rigidity and pain can restrict bed mobility, lower extremity dressing, bathing, transferring, driving, and vocational skills. Safety precautions against falling require special attention. People with fused backs can lose their balance and fall during activities requiring bending, resulting in a cervical fracture and quadriplegia (Melvin, 1989).

Systemic Lupus Erythematosus (SLE)

Systemic lupus erythematosus, occurring mostly in women, is a systemic inflammatory disease characterized by small vessel vasculitis with a diverse clinical picture. Manifestations of the disease depend on the organ systems involved and may include any or all of the following: fever; erythematous rash; polyarthritis; pneumonitis; polyserositis (especially pleurisy and pericarditis); myositis; anemia; thrombocytopenia; and renal, neurological, psychological, and cardiac abnormalities (Rothfield, 1981). Stroke, psychosis, depression, and memory difficulties can occur as central nervous system manifestations of the disease (Liang, Roger, & Larson, 1984).

---

[1]Silver Ring Splint Co., P.O. Box 2856, Charlottesville, VA 22902

Hand involvement may look like RA, but the deformities are usually due to soft tissue damage rather than bone erosions. The arthritis has the same pattern of involvement as in RA; only a small percentage of SLE patients develop severe arthritis limitations (Dray, Millender, Nalebuff, & Phillips, 1981; Melvin, 1989).

This disease is treated with moderate- to high-dose corticosteroids. Patients on this medication are often slightly euphoric or "spacey," making retention of verbal instructions difficult. All instructions for patients in this situation need to be given in writing and reviewed in a follow-up session when possible (Melvin, 1989).

Systemic Sclerosis (SSc)

Sometimes referred to as scleroderma, systemic sclerosis is a generalized disorder of the small blood vessels and connective tissues characterized by fibrotic, ischemic, and degenerative changes in the skin and internal organs. The skin and underlying tissues (fascia, muscles, tendons, capsules) become tight, hard, and restricted. There is frequent involvement of the alimentary tract, synovia, lungs, heart, and kidneys. When it is associated with calcinosis, Raynaud's phenomenon, esophageal dysfunction, sclerodactylia, and telangiectasis, it is called CREST syndrome (LeRoy, 1981).

Systemic sclerosis may stay confined to the hands and face or spread to the entire body. The characteristic hand deformity includes restriction of the wrist to mid-range, loss of thumb palmar abduction, loss of MCP flexion, and severe flexion contractures of the PIP joints, resulting in a claw deformity pattern. In the early stages it is crucial to maintain thumb abduction and MCP flexion, as well as to prevent wrist flexion contractures. Some patients have severe resorption of the ends of their distal phalanges, thus shortening their digits; and a few develop gangrene from severe Raynaud's phenomenon. These patients can develop joint restrictions in any body region affected (Medsger, 1985). Self-care assessment is a key part of all occupational therapy for these patients.

In addition to hand and face ROM therapy, these patients need deep breathing to maintain rib cage excursion, full body range of motion, and fitness. They also require instruction to maximize gravity assist to esophageal motility and instruction for managing Raynaud's phenomenon (Melvin, 1989; Melvin, Brannan, & LeRoy, 1984).

Juvenile Rheumatoid Arthritis (JRA)

Juvenile rheumatoid arthritis is delineated into three major types and seven subtypes, defined by the symptoms present during the first 6 months following onset. The major types are systemic-onset, polyarticular-onset, and pauciarticular-onset. These have been further divided according to the type of course the disease follows. All forms of JRA are systemic in nature and have an element of fatigue, fever, and malaise associated with active disease (Jacobs, 1982).

In children with young-age onset, polyarticular disease is the most severe. The type of hand involvement they get is totally different from that in adult RA. These children tend to have flexion contractures of the wrists and digit joints, with ulnar deviation at the wrist and secondary radial drift at the digits. It is not uncommon for lateral pinch to be their main prehension pattern. Children with late-age onset (13 to 16 years) may develop hand problems similar to those in adults with RA (Melvin, 1989).

Self-care training is a critical part of treating JRA, and is correlated to developmental ages. For older children, the activities of daily living (ADL) and self-care assessments must extend into the school. An extensive review of occupational therapy assessment and treatment of JRA has been presented by Melvin (1989).

Self-Care Assessment and Intervention for People With Arthritis

For most disabilities, the ADL or self-care assessment is designed to determine a person's ability or disability. This is also true for arthritis, but how the person performs the activity is critical, for this information provides the data necessary for JPT (Melvin, 1989). Observing patients perform daily activities provides an opportunity to determine if their method causes unnecessary fatigue or puts their safety at risk (Schweidler, 1984).

The self-care assessment should answer the following questions:

Regarding Functional Ability

1. Is the patient performing any daily tasks that are causing pain to or placing potentially deforming stress on his or her involved joints?
2. Are there adaptive methods or equipment that could minimize or eliminate the pain or joint stress in these activities?
3. Is the patient limited in performing any daily tasks that are causing pain to or placing potentially deforming stress on his or her involved joints?
4. Are there adaptive methods, instructions, or equipment that could minimize or eliminate the pain or joint stress in these activities?

Regarding Energy Conservation

5. Is the patient's method of performing activities causing fatigue?
6. Can the activity be done in a more energy efficient manner?

Regarding Safety

7. Is the patient performing the activity safely?
8. Could assistive devices or instruction improve safety?

The need for physical treatment is determined by the musculoskeletal assessment. The purpose of self-care treatment is to: (a) reduce pain and inflammation by reducing stress on the joints; (b) increase functional independence; and (c) eliminate or reduce forces that could cause deformity or unnecessary fatigue, and reduce safety risk factors.

Special Factors To Consider in the Self-Care Assessment

Medications

Have you ever had trouble opening a "child-proof" bottle? Imagine taking medicine at 6:00 a.m., when you are tired, stiff all over, and your hands are so inflexible and sore you can hardly use them. This is the situation for most people with significant hand involvement or severe active disease (Lisberg, Higham, & Jayson, 1983). Many patients wake up early to take their medications then go back to sleep for an hour so they are less stiff when they get up for the day. Others schedule functional activities or exercise in accord with their medications' optimal benefit, which may be 30 minutes to 1 hour after taking them.

It is important to remember that fast-acting medications (e.g., aspirin, nonsteroidal anti-inflammatory drugs [NSAIDs], and analgesics) can alter a patient's performance on objective assessments such as dressing time, grip strength, and ROM, in as little as 30 minutes. Therefore, it is important to note the name and dosage of the medications, and the frequency and regularity of the patient's intake, then determine when medications have been taken prior to the self-care assessment. This is also the ideal time to find out if the patient is taking the medications as prescribed and if he or she can manipulate the bottles and pills without problems. Patients with limited hand function should ask the pharmacist to dispense pills in easy-open bottles (Melvin, 1989).

Effective drug management of inflammation is central to the management of the illness and the person's overall functional ability. The pharmacology and pharmacokinetics of these medications may influence physical, as well as psychological, functioning. If a patient is having trouble with side effects or drug compliance, he or she should be encouraged to discuss this with the physician.

Morning Stiffness

Morning stiffness refers to the prolonged generalized difficulty in joint movement that occurs in association with the inflammatory polyarthritides upon awakening. The stiffness tends to be generalized and may last from 10 minutes to several hours. It is indicative of systemic involvement. This contrasts with the stiffness of osteoarthritis that is localized and occurs only in involved joints after inactivity and tends to disappear within 30 minutes of active motion.

Morning stiffness is an objective indicator of the degree of disease activity present. Patients with uncontrolled or untreated RA may have up to 3 to 5 hours of generalized stiffness in the morning. As the disease becomes controlled by medications or becomes less active, the duration of morning stiffness decreases and may last 15 to 30 minutes. Patients are considered well-controlled if they have less than 30 minutes of morning stiffness. Morning stiffness is distinct and excessive, and wears off at a given point. Patients will often describe the situation thus: "My morning stiffness wears off about 10:00 a.m.; then I have my regular stiffness the rest of the day" (Melvin, 1989, p. 258). Morning stiffness is calculated from the time the patient wakes up until the stiffness wears off, and it is recorded in hours.

How morning stiffness affects functional ability varies from person to person. Many patients feel stiff but are able to get around and to perform self-care functions, whereas others are totally dependent during periods of morning stiffness. Some patients may need assistive devices specifically for this period.

The following questions can assist in determining the patient's duration of morning stiffness (Melvin, 1977, 1989).

1. Are your joints usually stiff in the morning when you awaken?
2. What time do you usually awaken?
3. What time do you usually get out of bed?
4. What time does this morning stiffness wear off, leaving you with the regular stiffness you have during the day? (This may sound awkward, but frequently if you ask patients what time their stiffness wears off, they respond "never," because they have some degree of stiffness all day.)

Fatigue and Endurance

Becoming easily fatigued is one of the complications of all systemic diseases. It can limit a person's ability for bathing, meal preparation, child care, shopping, work, and socializing. For the purpose of planning treatment it is helpful to determine the patient's energy pattern. This would include the following interview questions (Melvin, 1977, 1989).

1. What is the pattern or times of peak and low energy?
2. At what time of day does fatigue occur?

3. What is the duration of the fatigue?

4. How do you handle the fatigue?

5. What do you do to improve endurance or reduce fatigue?

6. What factors, beside illness, contribute to your fatigue or endurance? For example, do you take medications, experience sleep difficulties, or have depression or a poor physical condition that might explain the fatigue or contribute to it?

Disease Variability

We all have "good" days and "bad" days, but when people with arthritis say this they are usually referring to their level of pain and function. It is critical when evaluating a person with arthritis to find out what he or she is like on a "good" and "bad" day, and how many of each are in a typical week. Some people may need assistive devices only on the "bad" days or during a periodic flare. This may be 1 or 2 days a week, or 3 or 4 days a month.

American College of Rheumatology Functional Classification

A general classification system for rheumatoid arthritis (Steinbrocker, Traeger, & Batterman, 1949) was specifically designed for patients with RA, but because it is so general, it can also be used with other rheumatic diseases. This classification system is limited because it is general and can reflect only gross changes in the patient's progression or regression. However, it is often helpful in providing a quick, overall picture of the patient's status. The classification system is commonly used in research (Melvin, 1989) and is presented below.

Class I: Complete functional capacity with ability to carry on all usual duties without handicaps

Class II: Functional capacity adequate to conduct normal activities despite handicap of discomfort or limited mobility of one or more joints

Class III: Functional capacity adequate to perform only a few or none of the duties of the patient's usual occupation or of self-care

Class IV: Largely or wholly incapacitated with patient bedridden or confined to wheelchair, permitting little or no self-care

Joint Protection Techniques

There are two reasons for recommending an assistive device to someone with rheumatic disease: (a) to help him or her become more self-reliant or capable; and (b) to help him or her implement joint protection principles. Because one of the overriding goals in therapy for arthritis is to reduce stress and inflammation in the joints, it is paramount that all self-care instruction incorporate joint protection principles. The concept of joint protection techniques or instruction was developed by Cordery (1965). Major principles include having respect for pain to avoid prolonging activity to the point of exacerbating inflammatory processes, getting sufficient rest, simplifying work, avoiding positions of deformity, using proper body mechanics, and using assistive devices where appropriate. The case examples in the next section illustrate examples of incorporating these principles throughout the care plan.

Equipment Recommendations—Factors to Consider

The determination of the patient's equipment needs is part of the ADL assessment. For people who are employed, the assessment should extend to the workplace. When selecting or designing equipment for a person with arthritis, it is important to keep the following considerations in mind (Melvin, 1989):

1. The patient's equipment needs in the morning may differ from those in the afternoon; they may also differ during periods of exacerbation and remission. Case Example: Mrs. S. is a 53-year-old married woman who has had RA in all of her peripheral joints for 7 years. She has had several remissions, but the inflammation has been steadily active for the last 2 years and particularly bad the past couple of months. Her morning stiffness is severe for 2 hours. Her joints are also very stiff at night, making it difficult for her to use the toilet during the night and early morning. However, after she has showered, taken her medications, and exercised, she is much more limber and has no problem rising from a low seat.

To help her specifically during the night and early morning, the occupational therapist recommended that Mrs. S. raise her bed up 3 inches on custom-made wood blocks that have a well for the bed leg. She also ordered arm bars that attach to the back of the toilet seat, and a lightweight plastic, molded, raised toilet seat (the easiest to clean). Mrs. S. puts it on the toilet before she goes to bed and stores it in a closet during the day, when she no longer needs it. This reduces the inconvenience to other family members. She is also able to take it with her on overnight trips. Next year she plans to remodel her home and install a high toilet, like the ones used in bathrooms that are accessible to wheelchair users. This would be the ideal solution, for it looks the most normal and eliminates an extra cleaning chore.

Her response to this equipment is, "I hate having to use special devices, but it makes it easier to get out of bed to go to the bathroom, knowing I'm not going to have the excruciating pain in my knees and hands trying to get up from a low seat. Raising the bed was also helpful and makes me feel less disabled. I avoided getting a raised toilet seat for years, because I thought they were ugly with clamps that permanently attached, requiring everyone to use it."

2. Activities and equipment involving strong grasp are contraindicated for patients with active metacarpophalangeal joint involvement. Case example: Nancy W. is 40 years old and has had RA for 5 years. She has low-level inflammation in her hands, wrists, shoulders, and knees. Recently, while she was in a general hospital for MTP joint surgery, the occupational therapist gave her a long-handled back brush and squeeze-grip long reachers to facilitate her ability in ADL. But both of these devices hurt her hands. (These devices function as a long lever, increasing the forces on the hand.) When she complained to her rheumatologist, he referred her to an outpatient arthritis treatment program.

The occupational therapist, experienced in arthritis treatment, issued her a long, terry cloth back scrubber with loop handles, which are held with the palms of the hands. Nancy has fragile hands, with active inflammation and beginning joint deformity; consequently all dynamic grip reachers would cause undesirable force to the hand.

The therapist did an extensive ADL assessment, carefully analyzing all reach activities. More than 50% of the activities that Nancy wanted to use the reacher for could be eliminated by reorganizing her cupboards and putting items she did not use in the basement. Many others could be eliminated by using a lightweight step stool (one that rolls on the floor and stabilizes when it is stepped on) in the kitchen.

After the therapist instructed Nancy in joint protection principles and the importance of avoiding strong grip and using her palms bilaterally to lift heavy objects, Nancy actively began to find ways to eliminate grip and stressful reach from her activities. The therapist carefully reviewed how lever forces work and how Nancy could use them to her advantage (for example, using an extended handle on a stiff faucet).

3. The equipment may affect other joints of the body. Case Example: Susan T. is a 30-year-old secretary who has had RA for 1 year. The doctors are still experimenting with different drugs, trying to bring the inflammation under control, but so far nothing has worked. Susan has recently started on gold therapy, which will take 3 to 4 months before it is effective. Her wrists and MCP and finger joints are swollen, as are her toes and left knee. The physical therapist recommended a cane to take the weight-bearing forces off the knee and improve her ability to get around. The occupational therapist was concerned about the stress the cane would put on her right hand. Both grip and the wrist radial deviation required by the cane are powerful forces that can cause MCP ulnar drift. Using a rigid wrist splint with the cane just made the forces on the MCP joints worse. The occupational therapist recommended to the physical therapist that a lightweight forearm crutch with a padded grip be used. This would allow the wrist to be in the desired ulnar deviation or neutral, and reduce much of the force on the hand. The physical therapist agreed, but the patient flatly refused the forearm crutch because it looked too "dorky" and made her appear handicapped. She was reluctant but willing to use the cane. When Susan returned to the occupational therapist with a cane, the therapist listened to all of her concerns about looking disabled and her fears about her boyfriend rejecting her. The therapist acknowledged that these were valid and natural concerns. Then she explained in depth, using pictures to explain, how radial deviation of the wrist and grip can cause the MCP ulnar drift deformity that the patient was also afraid of getting, that deformities occur during periods of swelling, and that the goal of therapy is to protect the joints during periods of inflammation so they will be strong and functional once the medications bring the disease under control or it goes into remission.

The therapist reinforced that the forearm crutch was a short-term measure until the medicines became effective. The patient acknowledged that it would be helpful to be able to tell others that the crutch was only temporary, and that she was more worried about getting hand deformities than what other people might think of the crutch. She walked across the room with the forearm crutch and sheepishly admitted that it did hurt her hands less than the cane.

In the next session, the therapist instructed Susan in joint protection techniques for her MCP joints. This included doing tasks bimanually, using the palms, and adapting handles to keep the MCP joints in extension.

4. Some patients with wrist or hand involvement are unable to grip standard transfer assist equipment. Case Example: Marsha M. is a 55-year-old bookkeeper with severe osteoarthritis in her hands. She is limited in both flexion and extension. She cannot make a full grip; therefore, when she tries to grasp something narrow she "feels" weak because she cannot hold on tight. Her PIP and DIP joints are frequently inflamed and painful, making it difficult to hold onto things. She was referred to occupational therapy for a general activities of daily living (ADL) assessment. One of Marsha's chief concerns was being able to get in and out of the tub safely. She reported that taking a daily hot bath was her "life saver" and the best thing she could do for her arthritis. But she hadn't taken a bath for a month, because the last time she did she almost couldn't get out of the tub. This was particularly scary to her because she lives alone. The occupational therapist had her demonstrate her transfer technique in the clinic model bathroom, and together they problem solved the type and placement of grab bars and the helpfulness of two different kinds of low tub seats. They settled on a chrome grab bar that fits over the tub rail which would allow Marsha to pull herself up by hooking her forearm around it instead of gripping it. Marsha was grateful to the therapist, and reiterated several times how helpful it was to be able to practice with the therapist there, so she could prove to herself that she could do it and that she was doing it correctly or the best way possible.

5. Convenience appliances are not always convenient for patients with arthritis. This principle does not need a case example, as everyone has some personal experience with appliances that are difficult to use. One of the most common examples is electric can openers—both puncturing the can and pressing the lever can be difficult, even for normal hands. Electric knives and toothbrushes can be heavy and often have buttons too small or difficult for some patients to use. It is imperative for therapists to be familiar with the strength and dexterity required to operate an appliance before ordering or recommending it to patients.

6. A change in ambulation aids requires instruction in ADL. Case Example: Leslie T. is a 27-year-old fashion designer who developed severe hip pain. The orthopedist diagnosed it as avascular (aseptic) necrosis of the femoral head and told her the treatment was not to bear weight on the hip for 4 to 6 months. He asked if she knew how to use crutches. She answered yes, and he gave her a brief demonstration. He then gave her a prescription to obtain both crutches and a walker at the local pharmacy. Two days later she called the orthopedist in tears and panic, stating her situation quite graphically: "When I'm using the walker or crutches I feel like a triple amputee, I can't do anything with my hands. Isn't there anything else I can do?" He referred Leslie to physical therapy for functional training, but when the physical therapist heard what the referral was for, it was changed to occupational therapy.

The occupational therapist did an ADL assessment, reviewed transfer techniques, and issued Leslie the following helpful devices: a crutch bag, walker basket, pocket apron, and shower seat. She recommended that Leslie purchase a high stool for the kitchen and reviewed possibilities for having groceries delivered and simplifying meals. She also instructed her in energy conservation techniques to counteract the fatigue of using ambulation aids.

People who are on crutches or walkers for extended periods find it frustrating, as well as exhausting (mentally and physically). Despite this, reliance on these ambulation devices is common. For example, the new cementless total hip replacement surgeries require no or partial weight bearing for 3 months.

7. Lower extremity dressing aids sometimes do more harm than good. Case Example: Dan R. is a 40-year-old computer executive who has had ankylosing spondylitis since age 22. He had extensive rehabilitative services early in the course of his illness. On his last visit to the doctor, he reported having increasing difficulty putting on his socks and shoes. He was referred to occupational therapy specifically for assistive devices for this area of dressing. The occupational therapist had him demonstrate donning and doffing his socks and shoes. He was able to do the tasks with difficulty. The activity did not cause him pain, but he was limited by stiffness in his back and hips. The therapist also ascertained that he had stopped doing his stretching exercises about 1 year ago. She showed Dan the devices available, but would not recommend them for him at this time, because this dressing activity was forcing him to use his available sitting hand-to-floor ROM on a daily basis. Assistive devices would eliminate this daily stretch and encourage a loss of flexibility. She also recommended that he obtain a referral to physical therapy for reevaluation of his home stretching program. She suggested that he be diligent in a daily stretching routine for 2 weeks, to see if this would improve his hand-to-floor range and make dressing and bathing easier. She asked him to call her in 2 weeks with a progress report so she could determine if further therapy was needed.

Note: If the dressing activity was causing hip or back pain and aggravating inflamed joints, then the appropriate treatment would have been to teach an adaptive method that did not cause pain, or to use assistive devices.

Assistive Devices For People With Rheumatic Diseases

Many patients with rheumatic diseases are functionally independent in self-care but need a device to compensate for limitation in a specific joint or to protect a joint from stress. When these patients come to the clinic, therapists tend to think "What can I do for the Hands? Neck? Other areas?" Then there are patients with more severe or total body involvement. For them, it is helpful to analyze needs in terms of functional activities (i.e., what aid will help with dressing, bathing, and other activities of daily living?).

To facilitate working with these two groups of patients, assistive aids have been categorized in this section by joint impairment (see Figures 4 through 9) and by functional activity (see Figures 10 through 17).

A relationship between assistive device training and patient compliance or usage has been demonstrated in a series of studies (Rogers & Holm, 1992). Research in Great Britain has demonstrated that assistive device training programs resulted in higher use rates, improved satisfaction, and safer bathing practices (Chamberlain, Thornley, Stowe, & Wright, 1981; Stowe, Thornley, Chamberlain, & Wright, 1982).

Aids for Hand Impairment

The hand joints are particularly vulnerable to stress because they are small and highly mobile with complex biomechanical forces acting on them. The muscles are used to move the joints, as opposed to stabilizing and supporting them. Moreover, the accumulated force of using the hands over the course of a day is considerable, even if they are used gently.

The activities that tend to cause the greatest pain and damage are those that require tight grip or pinch force. All of the aids recommended in Figure 4 are designed to reduce the force required of the hands in activities.

Aids for Elbow Impairment

Loss of elbow flexion can severely interfere with one's ability to eat, wash, or touch one's face. Loss of extension can interfere with one's ability to touch the feet and perform lower extremity dressing, as well as push off from chairs. Rheumatoid nodules may be aggravated by pressure or repetitive trauma. Severe bilateral limitations are extremely disabling and an indication for surgery (see Figure 5).

Aids for Shoulder Impairment

A considerable amount of shoulder ROM (approximately 50%) can be lost before causing significant restriction to functional activities. People with 90° of shoulder flexion or less generally need some aids to assist with reach or dressing. Painful shoulders can reduce the ability of the upper extremity in all strength tasks such as lifting, carrying, and pushing (see Figure 6).

Aids for Neck Impairment

In the early stages of inflammation, the facet joints can be aggravated by repetitive motion

Figure 4. Aids for hand impairment.

Devices	Comments
Adapted, built-up, or narrowed handles	Adhesive foam, foam tubing, or custom handles made out of orthotic material are the most common methods. On forearm crutches the plastic handle can be removed and the narrow stem lightly padded.
Nonslip pads or plastic sheets (e.g., Dycem mats)	To reduce force required to stabilize items (e.g., when used under a dinner plate); a person only has to cut food, not cut and press down.
Faucet turners	When possible, it is worth investing in lever fixtures for taps or faucets.
House or car key adaptations	Commercial key holders that increase leverage are available. If only one or two keys are a problem, each can be adapted by sealing the end between two pieces of orthotic material. Caution: custom adaptations may not fit the recessed area for ignition keys.
Lamp switch extenders and switches in extension cords	
Soaped runners on kitchen drawers for easier sliding	Silicon spray (e.g., WD 40) can ease operation of sliding doors, locks, and hinges.
Lightwieght kitchen utensils	
Electric can opener	Therapists should be familiar with the strength required to operate openers before ordering.
Jar opener	Wall-hung or under-counter openers that allow bilateral palmer holding of the jar are the best for people with active hand inflammation.
Bowl holders	There are now round bowls with a rubber stabilizing ring that allows the bowl to be positioned at any angle.
Saucepan stabilizers	If a full tea kettle is kept on the stove, the saucepan can be stabilized against it while stirring.
Spring loaded clipping scissors	
Suction bottle/glass brushes	These fit into the bottom of the sink and are very helpful if there is no dishwasher.
Electric scissors	These take practice to learn to use easily.
Cutting boards with stainless steel nails	To stabilize vegetables for cutting.
Strap loops for forearm for oven doors, drawers, sliding doors	Allows one to slip forearm through loop to open door. In the kitchen they can be made out of attractive sturdy ribbon or colored webbing.
Shoulder strap for handbags, suitcases, shopping bags	Commercial shoulder pads for straps are available at luggage stores.
Blanket cradles or ribbon handles sewn on blankets	To make blanket manipulation easier.

(continued)

Figure 4. (continued)

Devices	Comments
Electric blankets	Minimize bulk and aid in reducing morning stiffness.
Sheet tucker (small wooden paddle)	
Universal cuff	To hold brushes, silverware, pencils
Book racks, newspaper holders	To keep books and newspapers at an upright angle without manually holding them. Plastic ones are available for cookbooks.
Pen or pencil holding devices	Many styles are available. My favorite for reducing hand strain is to stick the pen or pencil through the center of a small (2" diameter), firm (not hard), foam ball (usually neon red).
Electric shaver holders	
Cup holders, lightweight mugs, mugs with open handles	Open handle can accommodate deformity.
Button hooks	Again, depending on the hand problem, these may need to be built up or narrowed; padded or firm.
Soap on a roap (for shower or tub)	Prevents soap from falling.
Car door openers	Styles available to open all doors.
Aerosol can holders	Allow grip pressure to press spray knob.
Plastic open handles for milk cartons and large soda bottles	
Pop top and screw cap openers	
Plastic bag and box top openers	
Luggage carrier	Can also be used around the house.

or posture in extremes of range, such as forward flexion while reading. In cases of severe involvement (for example, in JRA or AS), neck immobility restricts visual range. This is particularly critical in activities where safety is a concern, such as driving or child care. An immobile neck also makes it difficult to participate in conversation in a group setting, where speaking may originate from different directions, because the person has to turn his or her entire body to view someone. If ankylosis is inevitable, aids should be considered to help maintain optimal alignment (see Figure 7).

Aids for Knee Impairment

Knee pain inhibits the muscle strength of the knee extensors, reducing ability for rising from a sitting position, standing, and ambulation. Greater than 30° loss of extension can severely limit ambulation. A minimum of 100° of knee flexion is needed to sit in a chair or climb steps comfortably.

Figure 5. Aids for elbow impairment.

Devices	Comments
Elbow sleeve pads	These can be worn to bed to reduce pressure on nodules or sensitive skin. They are made with a loose net sleeve (Diamond®), which is easy to don with weak hands, or with a tighter cotton knit (Heelbo®).
Extended handle tableware for feeding Extended straws	To compensate for loss of elbow flexion and inability to bring hand to mouth.
Lower extremity dressing aids	To compensate for loss of elbow extension.
Chairs, easy to rise from with limited ability to push off	Inability to straighten the elbow limits ability to "push off' during transfer. Higher chairs require less push off with the arms.

Figure 6. Aids for shoulder impairment.

Devices	Comments
Extended handles with enlarged grip on hairbrushes, combs, toothbrushes, tableware, backbrushes	Caution: Extended handles increase the forces on the hand and wrist. Use lightweight devices.
Long cloth back scrubbers (bilateral)	Preferred over backbrushes. Often available at notions counters.
Extended drinking straws	To compensate for severe loss of shoulder flexion.
Coat holders	Available from European companies. Bracket with clips holds coat while donning; foot pedal release.
Lightweight down winter coats	Heavy coats are difficult to take on and off, and the weight hangs on the shoulders.
Reachers	Caution: These may increase forces on the hand and wrist. Use lightweight devices.
Dressing sticks (cup hook on one end, adapted coat hook on other end)	Also helpful for reaching, pulling, or pushing items other than clothing.
Front-opening clothes	Pull-over clothes require considerable shoulder flexion.
Sponges and dustpans with extended handles for floor care	Kneeling to do activities in front of the body requires more shoulder flexion than using extended-handle devices.
One-handed hair rollers	Self-fastening covering holds hair in place without clips, so hair can be rolled without using the affected shoulder.

From *Rheumatic Disease in the Adult and Child: Occupational Therapy and Rehabilitation* (3rd ed.) (pp. 441–448) by J.L. Melvin, 1989, Philadelphia: F.A. Davis. Copyright © 1989 by F.A. Davis. Adapted by permission.

Figure 7. Aids for neck impairment.

Devices	Comments
Chairs that swivel	Neck stiffness or immobility requires turning the entire body to see to the sides. Swivel chairs allow the patient visual range without getting up. Executive office chairs can have the wheels removed and be used in the living room.
Wide-angled rearview mirror	Available at most auto parts stores.
Expandable/mounted mirrors	Allow adjustment to create the correct angle for viewing.
Typing draft holder	Holds typing directly above the typewriter; eliminates the need for repetitive turning to the side.
Adjustable book holders	For students, I recommend using a simple wire holder on top of a stack of books to bring the book to eye level (works well in the library).
Cervical contour pillows (available from medical distributors)	The Jackson Cervipillo® is one recommended example. It also works well in the car against the neck rest.
Telephone receiver holders	For people who work on the telephone, a lightweight headset receiver is a worthy investment. The local telephone company may be able to recommend sources.
Step stool and reachers for upper cabinets	Step stool reduces need to hyperextend the neck.

From *Rheumatic Disease in the Adult and Child: Occupational Therapy and Rehabilitation* (3rd ed.) (pp. 441–448) by J.L. Melvin, 1989, Philadelphia: F.A. Davis. Copyright © 1989 by F.A. Davis. Adapted by permission.

To prevent joint contractures and to reduce joint stiffness, patients with involved knees should be advised to change the position of their legs when sitting, so that the knees are often stretched out. Use of a footstool to support the legs is recommended. It is important to alternate frequently between sitting and standing. Figure 8 lists several devices that can be used to avoid excessive strain on the knees during self-care activities.

Aids for Hip Impairment

A minimal hip flexion contracture can create physical problems, such as encouraging knee flexion contractures or compensatory spinal changes, such as lordosis. These in turn reduce efficiency in gait and movement. An impaired hip may limit or restrict participation in sports but not prevent functional activities. A moderate contracture increases the above problems and makes it difficult for the person to lie supine.

Loss of hip flexion (an extension contracture) creates greater functional limitations. Ninety degrees of hip flexion is necessary to sit in a regular chair comfortably. If a person has less flexion, his or her back will press into the chair (this can become a source of back pain). Severe loss of flexion (e.g., 45°) makes it impossible to sit normally in a chair.

Figure 8. Aids for knee impairment.

Devices	Comments
Elevated chairs in the living room, kitchen, at work (and in the clinic)	Sofas and office waiting room chairs can be adapted by setting them on top of a 3" carpeted platform.
High kitchen stools	It is important that these are lightweight as well as sturdy, so they can be moved easily.
Raised toilet seat	If possible, it is worth having an elevated toilet installed. If it has to be removed frequently, the weight and ease of attachment should be considered.
Arm bars for toilet	These help reduce stress on the knees by transferring some lifting work to the arms.
Shower bench	Benches that block shower curtain closure allow water to get on the floor. The patient's ability to clean up the water must be a consideration. A hand-held shower head may be helpful.
Tub grab bars	Reduce weight bearing and provide stability during transfers.
Walking aids	Canes should have wide rubber tips that are replaced when worn. There are several adaptations for using a cane on icy streets.
"Half step" or short steps	Steps can be adapted so they are half the height of regular steps.
Tea cart for transporting dishes and so forth	If this will be used a lot, a sturdy cart is recommended.
Shopping carts	Eliminate weight bearing required by carrying. Carts should be pushed all the way to the car.

From *Rheumatic Disease in the Adult and Child: Occupational Therapy and Rehabilitation* (3rd ed.) (pp. 441–448) by J.L. Melvin, 1989, Philadelphia: F.A. Davis. Copyright © 1989 by F.A. Davis. Adapted by permission.

Shallow seats or sitting on the edge of a seat may provide an answer in some situations. For any person with this type of problem who is not a candidate for surgery, obtaining comfortable seating is a critical part of therapy. If proper seating would make a difference in employment or attendance in school, rehabilitation agencies may be able to assist in funding for equipment. Equipment for this problem includes specially adapted chairs and toilet seats that allow the patient to sit upright with the hips in less than 90° of flexion.

Figure 9 lists devices that are applicable to restrictions that limit hand-to-foot or hand-to-floor range. They may be used for limited hip flexion as well as for back or elbow restrictions.

Aids for Limitations in Dressing

During dressing, limited range in proximal upper and lower extremity joints may make it difficult to get clothing over the feet or head. Poor grasp strength and loss of fine prehension skills create problems in manipulating fasteners. Upper extremity weakness interferes with putting on coats or jackets.

Figure 9. Aids for hip impairment.

Devices	Comments
Reachers	A wide selection is available.
Sock donners	Also available for pantyhose.
Elastic shoe strings	By replacing regular shoe strings with the elastic variety, shoes can be put on with greater ease, tying is eliminated, and the need for extreme neck flexion is avoided.
Boot jack	This device catches the head of the boot and helps to pull it off.
Dressing sticks Pants dressing poles Extended shoehorns	These devices help compensate for loss of hip flexion. Dressing without aids may be the daily activity necessary for maintaining hip flexion. Use aids only if essential.
Double-faced carpet tape on the end of a stick	To pick up small items like pills or broken glass.

From *Rheumatic Disease in the Adult and Child: Occupational Therapy and Rehabilitation* (3rd ed.) (pp. 441–448) by J.L. Melvin, 1989, Philadelphia: F.A. Davis. Copyright © 1989 by F.A. Davis. Adapted by permission.

It is useful to advise patients that clothing selection is important as part of a management strategy. Clothes should be easy to put on. For example, turtlenecks should be avoided, as should trousers with tight fitting elastic at the waist. Fasteners (buttons and zippers) can be a particular problem, so care should be taken to purchase garments with closures or fasteners in front. For existing clothes, touch fasteners can be used to replace buttons (with the buttons attached permanently to the buttonhole) (Dallas & White, 1982). Alternatively, a button hook device can be useful for managing buttons. Large rings or leather loops are useful aids on zipper tabs.

Dressing sticks are useful for pulling on pants. Stocking devices are valuable for putting on stocks. For women, a useful pantyhose strategy is to dust the thighs with powder before pulling the pantyhose into place. Rolling pantyhose or girdles from top to bottom before putting them on facilitates dressing. The garments can be unrolled once the legs have been inserted.

Shoes should be purchased with care. Desirable characteristics include adjustable closures to accommodate swelling; low heels (less than 1 inch high); cushioned soles; a wide toe area; and soft, stretchable upper materials. Many of the currently manufactured athletic or gym shoes are satisfactory. Adaptations for shoes are also available, and include cushioned inserts and pads. Figure 10 provides a summary of clothing devices.

Aids for Limitations in Grooming

Decreased proximal upper extremity range impedes hair care, applying makeup, shaving, and dental hygiene. The loss of hand dexterity interferes with these tasks, and with nail grooming. Temporomandibular joint disease may complicate dental care (see Figure 11).

Aids for Limitations in Bathing

Limitations in ambulation and transfer skills may make getting in and out of the tub or

Figure 10. Aids for facilitating dressing tasks.

Devices	Comments
Dressing stick Pants dressing poles	These reach-extending devices compensate for loss of hand-to-toe range of motion or loss of shoulder flexion and elbow extension.
Reaching devices	Reachers are appropriate for individuals who have active hand/wrist inflammation. The lightweight passive reacher may solve upper extremity problems.
Shoe/sock aids • Stocking donner • Long-handled shoe horn • Boot jack	Reach extending devices compensate for a lack of hand-to-toe range of motion. The boot jack is used to decrease the force required for removing shoes.

• Adaptive closures
  Elastic shoelaces
  Button hook
  Zipper pull
  Zipper loop or ring
  Zipper tab
	A wide variety of commercial and homemade closures are available. Shoes can be adapted with self-fasteners, zippers, and clip-style closures.

Adapted clothing	Patterns or specially made garments may be purchased. Difficult closures may be replaced with simpler fasteners or self-fastening strips. Clothing may be selected with elasticized waists, front closures, and/or in a wraparound style.

From *Rheumatic Disease in the Adult and Child: Occupational Therapy and Rehabilitation* (3rd ed.) (pp. 441–448) by J.L. Melvin, 1989, Philadelphia: F.A. Davis. Copyright © 1982 by F.A. Davis. Adapted by permission.

shower fatiguing, unsafe, or impossible. Loss of upper extremity strength and range interferes with managing faucets, washcloths, soap, shampoo, and so forth. Limited range in proximal upper and lower extremity joints creates problems in reaching body parts, and fatigue could prevent the person from completing a bath independently. The ability to clean up water that gets on the floor during bathing is a safety concern for many patients, and this problem may deter patients from taking a shower (see Figure 12).

Aids for Limitations in Toileting

Limitations in knee and hip flexion and extension, and in transfer skills, create difficulty getting on and off a toilet. Decreased range in proximal upper and lower extremity joints or loss of hand skills may interfere with managing perineal hygiene as well as cause problems in dressing and undressing for toileting. Figure 13 lists several devices available for facilitating toileting activities.

Aids for Limitations in Housekeeping

Aids and adaptations may be necessary due to limitations in mobility, proximal upper and lower extremity ROM and strength, or hand deformity. It is critical to consider aids that will promote early joint protection and energy conservation. Figure 14 lists devices and approaches for improving the ability to perform housekeeping tasks despite pain, limitations in ROM, or limited strength.

Figure 11. Aids and devices for facilitating grooming.

Devices	Comments
Enlarged or extended handles on toothbrush, comb, razor	Lightweight materials to build up handles include cylindrical foam, adhesive foam, small wooden doweling, and aluminum tubing. Plastic coating or applications of low-temperature plastic splinting materials foster better grip.
Dental hygiene aids • Electric toothbrushes • Water jet appliances • Floss and toothpick holders • Toothpaste tube key	Careful selection of these devices is advised, as some are heavy, have a clumsy grip, or require too much grip.
Nail care devices • Electronic nail files • Buffers	Compensate for weakness and loss of fine pinch. Clippers may be mounted on a wooden block or extensions may be placed on handles.
Adaptations for cosmetic containers	Attachment to aerosol spray can provides a lever to press the spray button. Cosmetics may be selected for accessible containers (push-up lipsticks, deodorants with larger tops).

From *Rheumatic Disease in the Adult and Child: Occupational Therapy and Rehabilitation* (3rd ed.) (pp. 441–448) by J.L. Melvin, 1989, Philadelphia: F.A. Davis. Copyright © 1989 by F.A. Davis. Adapted by permission.

Figure 12. Aids to overcome limitations in the ability to perform bathing activities.

Devices	Comments
Safety Aids • Safety mats • Grab bars	Aid transfer and increase safety. Vertical pole or bars that attach to the tub assist weak grasp because the forearm may be substituted.
Tub shower seats	Aid transfer and increase safety. A wide variety of styles and heights are available.
Lever faucet handles Tap-turning devices	Aid limited upper extremity strength and range. Reduce joint stress.
Bathing supplies • Shower caddies • Tub trays • Soap dispensers	Aid limited strength and range of motion. A wide variety is available.
Washing and drying • Long-handled sponge • Wash mitts • Adapted washcloths • Terry cloth robes	Aid limited range in proximal joints. Long-handled sponges areimpractical if the wrists/hands are involved. Mitts aid limited grasp. A terry cloth robe saves energy required for drying after a bath.

From *Rheumatic Disease in the Adult and Child: Occupational Therapy and Rehabilitation* (3rd ed.) (pp. 441–448) by J.L. Melvin, 1989, Philadelphia: F.A. Davis. Copyright © 1989 by F.A. Davis. Adapted by permission.

Figure 13. Aids to facilitate the performance of toileting activities.

Devices	Comments
Elevated toilet seats	A wide variety of temporary and permanent adaptations are possible.
Commodes Grab bars	Aid transfer and increase safety.
Toilet paper holder	Device holds paper and extends the reach for cleaning after elimination.
Dressing • Adapted clothing • Dressing aids	See section on dressing (Figure 10).

From *Rheumatic Disease in the Adult and Child: Occupational Therapy and Rehabilitation* (3rd ed.) (pp. 441–448) by J.L. Melvin, 1989, Philadelphia: F.A. Davis. Copyright © 1982 by F.A. Davis. Adapted by permission.

Figure 14. Devices and approaches for facilitating housekeeping tasks.

Devices/Approaches	Comments
Kitchen or utility carts	Conserve energy, reduce joint stress, compensate for limited strength. Wheeled carts eliminate lifting and carrying, with many items carried in one trip.
Lightweight sweepers Self-propelled vacuums	Conserve energy. Reduce joint stress. Lightweight sweepers may be used to reduce the frequency of heavier vacuuming.
Adapted handles on broom and dustpan for wheelchair use.	Brooms need to be small and lightweight. Ordinary brooms can be viewed as heavy weights on the end of long levers which increase stress to the wrist joints.
Laundry aids • Platforms to raise washer/dryer height • Lowered clothes racks and lines • Adjustable-height ironing board • Lightweight "travel" iron or plastic regular iron	Compensate for strength and range limitations. Automatic washers and dryers should be selected for accessibility and easy-to-operate controls; clothes should be selected for easy care, little ironing.

From *Rheumatic Disease in the Adult and Child: Occupational Therapy and Rehabilitation* (3rd ed.) (pp. 441–448) by J.L. Melvin, 1989, Philadelphia: F.A. Davis. Copyright © 1982 by F.A. Davis. Adapted by permission.

Aids for Limitations in Meal Preparation

The person with arthritis may need special aids to compensate for impaired mobility, limited range in reaching and bending, or lack of strength and endurance. Because many kitchen tasks are resistive or repetitive, it is especially important to consider joint protection and energy conservation principles. Figure 15 lists several aids and approaches for use with patients who experience difficulty performing meal preparation tasks.

Figure 15. Approaches and devices for facilitating meal preparation tasks.

Devices	Comments
Lightweight utensils, cookware, and dishes	Less strength and energy are required; reduce joint stress. Ceramic plates may range in weight from 11 oz. to 24 oz. each.
Devices to open containers: jar openers, can openers	Compensate for weak grasp and/or loss of fine prehension. Electric appliances must be selected so that the controls are easy to operate.
Aids for cutting, chopping	These compensate for weak grasp and loss of fine hand skills, as well as reduce joint stress. Knives and scissors should be maintained with sharp cutting edges to reduce the force required in cutting. Spring-style scissors are less stressful to joints. A cutting board may be adapted with rustproof nails to hold food.
Labor-saving appliances	Generally lessen joint stress, because less strength and energy are required. Examples include microwave ovens, electric skillets, blenders, and food processors. Appliances should be selected so that controls are easy to operate and parts that must be lifted are lightweight.
Adaptations for storage: pegboard, vertical storage, pull-out shelves.	Conserve energy. May compensate for loss of range and strength. Work areas should be arranged so that tools and equipment are stored where they are first used. Adaptations may be permanent and built-in, or temporary commercially available items.

From *Rheumatic Disease in the Adult and Child: Occupational Therapy and Rehabilitation* (3rd ed.) (pp. 441–448) by J.L. Melvin, 1989, Philadelphia: F.A. Davis. Copyright © 1989 by F.A. Davis. Adapted by permission.

Aids for Limitations in Eating

Limited proximal upper extremity range may impair the person's ability to get food to his or her mouth. Lack of supination or fine prehension may impair the ability to manipulate utensils. Weakness may make it difficult to cut food or lift a glass or cup. Figure 16 lists several devices for making mealtime tasks easier and less painful.

Summary

The common rheumatic diseases reviewed in this chapter all have arthritis or joint inflammation as a common symptom, but have different patterns of joint involvement that can limit the patient's ability to engage in self-care tasks without pain or assistance. It is not enough for people with arthritis to be able to do the activity—they need to be able to perform it in a safe manner that will not cause pain or damage their joints. Because of this, effective occupational therapy intervention in the rheumatic diseases requires knowledge of joint physiology, disease pathology, and joint protection techniques. This is especially important when assisting the patient in managing self-care needs, because these tasks and activities constitute daily regimens that are repeated over weeks and years. The therapist must also be aware that such factors as medications, fatigue, and the duration and severity of morning stiffness can influence the ADL assessment and must be considered when prescribing self-care interventions.

Figure 16. Devices and approaches for making mealtime easier.

Devices	Comments
Adapted utensils • Enlarged or extended handles • Utensil cuffs • Swivel cups and spoons	Attractive utensils with enlarged handles are commercially available. Handles or cuffs of standard utensils may be enlarged with foam or plastic to eliminate tight grasp. Swivel handles compensate for loss of supination.
Aids for drinking • Long straws • Lightweight and spillproof cups • Thermal mugs • Trays • Table height adjustments	Thermal mugs with wide handles allow both hands to be used with MCP joints in a less stressful position. Severely disabled or hospitalized patients may need meals served at a more accessible table height.

From *Rheumatic Disease in the Adult and Child: Occupational Therapy and Rehabilitation* (3rd ed.) (pp. 441–448) by J.L. Melvin, 1989, Philadelphia: F.A. Davis. Copyright © 1989 by F.A. Davis. Adapted by permission.

In the occupational therapy clinic, patients with rheumatic diseases tend to fall into two functional categories. In the first category are those who are essentially independent in self-care and ADL tasks, but may need assistive devices or techniques to compensate for or protect specific joints. Other patients with multiple or total joint involvement specifically seek occupational therapy for help with self-care activities such as grooming, bathing, or dressing. To facilitate clinical problem solving with both types of patients, common assistive devices in this chapter are categorized by functional activity as well as joint impairment.

Assistive devices can represent an effective intervention for reducing stress to joints and improving functional ability. However, people with active inflammation and mobile joints are very vulnerable to external forces, especially long-lever forces, such as those found with brooms and mops. A faucet turner can help a patient use leverage to turn on a tap in a manner that is less stressful to the hands, but lifting an object with a long reacher reverses this process and increases the forces acting on the hand and wrist. This makes aggravated joint inflammation likely and increases the possibility of deformity. It is important to remember that there are specific considerations related to the use of assistive devices for people with arthritis who have dynamic deformities that may not apply to persons with other types of disability who have stable, fixed limitations. Occupational therapy must therefore meet the dual objectives of enabling function to the maximum extent possible and not aggravating joint inflammation or contributing to additional pain and joint deformity. ◆

References

Affleck, G., Pfeffier, C., Tennen, H., & Fifield, J. (1988). Social support and psychosocial adjustment to rheumatoid arthritis: Quantitative and qualitative findings. *Arthritis Care and Research, 1*(2), 71–77.

Bland, J.H., & Stulberg, S.D. (1985). Osteoarthritis: Pathology and clinical patterns. In W.M. Kelly, E.D. Harris Jr., S. Ruddy, & C.B. Sledge (Eds.), *Textbook of rheumatology* (2nd ed.) (pp. 1471–1490). Philadelphia: W.B. Saunders.

Calin, A. (1985). Ankylosing spondylitis. In W.N. Kelly, E.D. Harris Jr., S. Ruddy, & C.B. Sledge (Eds.), *Textbook of rheumatology* (2nd ed.) (pp. 993–1007). Philadelphia: W.B. Saunders.

Chamberlain, M.A., Thornley, G., Stowe, J., & Wright, V. (1981). An evaluation of aids and equipment for the bath, survey II: A possible solution to the problem. *Rheumatology and Rehabilitation, 20*, 38–43.

Cordery, J.C. (1965). Joint protection: A responsibility of the occupational therapist. *American Journal of Occupational Therapy, 19*, 285–294.

Dray, G.L., Millender, L.H., Nalebuff, E.A., & Phillips, C. (1981). The surgical treatment of hand deformities in SLE. *Journal of Hand Surgery, 6*, 339–347.

Dallas, M.J., & White, L.W. (1982). Clothing fasteners for women with arthritis. *American Journal of Occupational Therapy, 36*, 515–518.

Gerber, L.H., & Furst, G.P. (1992). Validation of the NIH activity record: A quantitative measure of life activities. *Arthritis Care and Research, 5*(2), 81–86.

Hicks, J.E., & Gerber, L.H. (1988). Rehabilitation of the patient with arthritis and connective tissue disease. In J.A. Delisa (Ed.), *Rehabilitation medicine: Principles and practice* (pp. 765–794). Philadelphia: J.B. Lippincott.

Jacobs, J. (1982). *Pediatric rheumatology*. New York: Springer-Verlag.

Krane, S.M., & Simon, L.S. (1986). Rheumatoid arthritis: Clinical features and pathogenic mechanisms. *Advances in Rheumatology: Medical Clinics of North America, 70*(2), 263–284.

LeRoy, E.C. (1981). Scleroderma (systemic sclerosis). In W.N. Kelly, E.D. Harris Jr., S. Ruddy, & C.B. Sledge (Eds.), *Textbook of rheumatology* (pp. 1103–1205). Philadelphia: W.B. Saunders.

Liang, M., Roger, M., & Larson, M. (1984). The psychosocial impact of systemic lupus erythematosus and rheumatoid arthritis. *Arthritis and Rheumatism, 27*, 13–21.

Lisberg, R.B., Higham, C., & Jayson, M.I. (1983). Problems for rheumatic patients in opening dispersed drug containers. *British Journal of Rheumatology, 22*(2), 95–98.

Medsger, T.A. Jr. (1985). Systemic sclerosis (scleroderma, eosinophilic fascitis and calcinosis). In D.J. McCarty (Ed.), *Arthritis and allied conditions* (10th ed.)(pp. 994–1036). Philadelphia: Lea and Febiger.

Melvin, J.L. (1977). *Rheumatic disease: Occupational therapy and rehabilitation*. Philadelphia: F.A. Davis.

Melvin, J.L. (1989). *Rheumatic disease in the adult and child: Occupational therapy and rehabilitation* (3rd ed.). Philadelphia: F.A. Davis.

Melvin, J.L., Brannan, K.L., & LeRoy, E.C. (1984). Comprehensive care for the patient with systemic sclerosis. *Clinical Rheumatology in Practice, 2*(3), 112–130.

Moll, J.M.H., & Wright, V. (1973). *Psoriatic arthritis. Seminars in arthritis and rheumatism, 3*, 55–71.

Nalebuff, E.A., & Garrett, J. (1976). Opera-glass hand in rheumatoid arthritis. *Journal of Hand Surgery, 1*(3), 210–221.

Rogers, J.C., & Holm M.B. (1992). Assistive technology device use in patients with rheumatic disease: A literature review. *American Journal of Occupational Therapy, 46*, 120–127.

Rothfield, N. (1981). Clinical features of systemic lupus erythematosus. In W.M. Kelly, E.D. Harris Jr., S. Ruddy, & C.B. Sledge (Eds.), *Textbook of rheumatology* (pp. 1106–1132). Philadelphia: W.B. Saunders.

Schweidler, H. (1984). Assistive devices: Aids to daily living. In G. Riggs & E. Gall (Eds.), *Rheumatic diseases: Rehabilitation and management* (pp 263–276). Stoneham, MA: Butterworth Printers.

Steinbrocker, O., Traeger, C.G., & Batterman, P.C. (1949). Therapeutic criteria in rheumatoid arthritis. *Journal of the American Medical Association, 140*, 659–662.

Stowe, J., Thornley, G., Chamberlain, M.A., & Wright, V. (1982). Evaluation of aids and equipment for the bath and toilet: Survey II. *British Journal of Occupational Therapy, 45*, 92–95.

Swanson, A.B., & deGroot-Swanson, G. (1985). Osteoarthritis in the hand. *Clinics of Rheumatic Disease, 11*, 393–420.

Wright, V., & Moll, J.M.H. (1976). *Seronegative polyarthritis*. Amsterdam: North Holland Publishing Company.

Suggestions for Further Reading

Arthritis Foundation. (1988). *Guide to independent living for people with arthritis* (415 pp.). For purchase information write to: 1314 Spring Street, NW, Atlanta, GA 30309. This is the best single source for identifying assistive devices for people with arthritis.

Arthritis Foundation. (1992). *Using your joints wisely*. (Free pamphlet) Available from the Arthritis Foundation in Atlanta, GA (address above).

Bingham, B. (1985). *Cooking with fragile hands*. Naples, FL: Creative Cuisine. This is an excellent resource for organizing the kitchen.

Coulton, C.J., Milligan, S., Chow, J., & Haug, M. (1990). Ethnicity, self-care, and use of medical care among the elderly with joint symptoms. *Arthritis Care and Research, 3*(1), 19–28.

Furst, G., Gerber, L.H., & Smith, C.P. (1987). A program for improving energy conservation procedures in adults with rheumatoid arthritis. *American Journal of Occupational Therapy, 41*, 102–111.

Feinberg, J.R., & Brandt, K.D. (1984). Allied health team management of rheumatoid arthritic patients. *American Journal of Occupational Therapy, 35*, 613–620.

Gerber, L., Furst, G., Shulman, B., Smith, C., Thornton, B., Liang, M., Colten, K., Stevens, M.B., & Gilbert, N. (1987). Patient education program to teach energy conservation behaviors to patients with rheumatoid arthritis: A pilot study. *Archives of Physical Medicine and Rehabilitation, 68*, 442–445.

Kulp, C.S. (1988). *The use of adaptive equipment by rheumatoid arthritis patients*. Unpublished master's thesis. Richmond, VA: Virginia Commonwealth University.

Lorig, K., & Fries, J. (1986). *Arthritis helpbook*. Reading, MA: Addison-Wesley.

Montgomery, M.A. (1984). Resources of adaptation for daily living: A classification with therapeutic implications for occupational therapy. *Occupational Therapy in Health Care, 1*(4), 9–21.

Pincus, T., Summey, J.A., Soracey, C.A., Wallaston, K.A., & Hummon, N.P. (1983). Assessment of patient satisfaction in activities of daily living using a modified Stanford Health Assessment Questionnaire. *Arthritis & Rheumatism, 26*, 1346–1353.

Pitzele, S. (1985). *We are not alone: Learning to live with chronic illness*. Minneapolis, MN: Thompson & Co.

Rogers, J.C., & Holm, M.B. (1992). Assistive technology device use in patients with rheumatic disease: A literature review. *American Journal of Occupational Therapy, 46*, 120–127.

Sweeney, G.M., & Clarke, A.K. (1992). Easy chairs for people with arthritis and low back pain: Results from an evaluation. *British Journal of Occupational Therapy, 55*(2), 69–72.

U.S. Department of Health, Education and Welfare (1982). *Flexible fashions: Clothing tips for women with arthritis*. Publication No. 1814. Washington, DC: U.S. Government Printing Office.

7

Self-Care Strategies for Persons With Spinal Cord Injuries

Susan L. Garber
Theresa L. Gregorio
Nancy Pumphrey
Pam Lathem

*Susan L. Garber, MA, OTR, FAOTA; Theresa L. Gregorio, MA, OTR; Nancy Pumphrey,
MOT, OTR; and Pam Lathem, OTR, are affiliated with The Institute for Rehabilitation
and Research in the Texas Medical Center, Houston, Texas. **Susan Garber** and
Theresa Gregorio are on the faculty of the Department of Physical Medicine and
Rehabilitation, Bayor College of Medicine, also in Houston.*

Chapter 7 Outline

High-Level Quadriplegia: Levels C-1 Through C-4

Eating and Meal Preparation

    Eating

    Medication

    Meal Preparation

Hygiene and Grooming

    Dental Care

    Bathing

Mobility

    Transfers

    Wheelchair Mobility

    Transportation

Dressing/Undressing

    Upper Extremity

    Lower Extremity

Communication

Bowel and Bladder Care

Quadriplegia: Levels C-5 Through C-8

Eating and Meal Preparation

    Eating

    Medication

    Meal Preparation

Hygiene and Grooming: Levels C-5 Through C-6

    Dental Care

    Combing Hair

    Shaving

Washing Face and Hands

Makeup Application

Bathing

Washing and Drying Hair

Hygiene and Grooming: Levels C-7 Through C-8

Dental Care

Washing Face and Hands, Combing Hair, Shaving, and Makeup Application

Bathing and Hair Washing

Mobility

Transfers

Manual Wheelchair

Motorized Wheelchair

Community Transportation

Dressing/Undressing

Upper Extremities

Lower Extremity

Communication

Writing

Telephone Use

Bowel and Bladder Management

Paraplegia: Levels T-1 Through T-6

Eating and Meal Preparation

Sink Hygiene and Grooming

Bathing

Mobility

Dressing

Communication

Bowel and Bladder

Paraplegia: Levels T-7 Through S-5

Equipment: From Tradition to High Technology

Summary

References

Traumatic spinal cord injury has a history as old as humankind. Perhaps the earliest description of spinal cord injury is found in a 5,000-year-old papyrus in which an Egyptian physician not only characterized the specific symptoms of a complete cervical cord lesion, but also commented on the bleak prognosis of such patients by admonishing that it is "an ailment not to be treated" (Guttmann, 1976, p. 1). Unlike injuries to the extremities, the complexity of the spinal cord injury and the overwhelming loss of function present enormous, often insoluble, problems for patients and practitioners alike. As a consequence, few efforts were made before 1941 to deal effectively with these conditions or their complications.

During World War I, 47% to 65% of those who acquired a spinal cord injury died within a few weeks or months from urinary or respiratory complications or from the effects of pressure ulcers. The mortality rate for this type of injury during the first 3 years after injury was 80% (Guttmann, 1976, p. 5). Even within the last 100 years, while people with other forms of physical disability such as blindness and amputations have benefited from innovative rehabilitation techniques and equipment, spinal cord-injured patients were still considered useless cripples (Guttmann, p. 5).

Because of the large number of spinal cord injuries resulting from World War II, the 1940s saw the development of the first rehabilitation programs for these patients. The efforts of such pioneers as Guttmann, Monroe, Rusk, Kessler, and Covalt, as well as the policies and programs of the United States Veterans Administration, resulted in the creation of a new philosophy of care for people with spinal cord injuries (Clifton, Donovan, & Frankowski, 1985; Monroe, 1943).

The role of the occupational therapist in the treatment of persons with spinal cord injury has evolved into the present concepts of training in activities of daily living, designing and fabricating assistive devices, strengthening upper extremities, exploring avocational and vocational interests and skills, and providing mechanisms to promote maximum independence (Lindberg, 1976; Mosey, 1971). The use of constructive or functional activity to maximize personal independence and economic self-sufficiency was, and continues to be, the central philosophy of occupational therapy in the restoration of physical function (Spackman, 1968).

The effective rehabilitation of spinal cord–injured patients depends on these traditions and identifies new evaluation and treatment efforts in such areas as environmental control systems, pressure ulcer prevention programs, and technology and adaptive skills training (Diasio, 1971). New challenges include reducing the length of hospital stays and developing community-based programs for severely disabled people (Reilly, 1971; Scott, 1984).

There are currently more than 200,000 persons with spinal cord injury in the United States, and it is projected that there will be 7,000 to 8,000 new traumatic spinal cord–injured survivors each year. The mean age of these individuals is 28.7 years, and 82% of them are male. Vehicular accidents are responsible for half of all injuries to the spinal cord;

47% of the injuries result in paraplegia and 53% result in quadriplegia (Fine, Kuhlemeier, & Stover, 1979; Kraus, Franti, Riggins, Richards, & Borhani, 1975; Young, Burns, Bowen, & McCutchen, 1982).

This chapter describes the special self-care issues of persons with spinal cord injuries within the context of levels of injury. Four major categories are presented: high-level quadriplegia C-1 through C-4, quadriplegia C-5 through C-8, paraplegia T-1 through T-6, and paraplegia T-7 through S-5. For some tasks performed by persons with quadriplegia, it was necessary to distinguish between levels C-5 through C-6 and C-7 through C-8. This was necessary because of the differences in use of adapted equipment by these persons.

The functional levels of the spinal cord for the upper and lower extremities are described in Figures 1 and 2. A summary of functional ability by level of injury is presented in Figure 1 and uses the World Health Organization's definitions of impairment, disability, and handicap. Although the functional levels of spinal cord injury form the basis of this chapter, the extent of injury, namely its completeness, warrants a brief description. The American Spinal Cord Injury Association has adopted the Frankel grading system to describe the neurological extent of injury, which is described in Figure 3 (Stover & Fine, 1986).

Figure 1. Functional levels of the cervical spinal cord.

Roots	Muscles	Function
C-2, C-3	Sternocleidomastoid	Neck flexion & head rotation
C-3, C-4	Trapezius	
	Superior	Neck extension & scapular elevation
	Middle	Scapular adduction
	Inferior	Scapular adduction & depression
C-3, C-4, C-5	Diaphragm	Respiration
C-4, C-5	Rhomboids	Scapular medial adduction, retraction, & elevation
C5, C-6	Deltoid	
	Anterior	Shoulder flexion to 90°
	Middle	Shoulder abduction to 90°
	Posterior	Shoulder extension & horizontal abduction
	Supraspinatus	Shoulder abduction
	Intraspinatus	Shoulder lateral rotation
	Teres minor	
	Subscapularis	Shoulder medial rotation
	Teres major	
	Biceps brachii	Elbow flexion & forearm supination
	Brachialis	Elbow flexion
	Brachioradialis	
	Extensor carpi radialis longus	Wrist flexion & abduction
C-5, C-6, C-7	Serratus anterior	Shoulder forward thrust; scapular rotation for shoulder abduction
C-5–T-1	Pectoralis major	Shoulder adduction, flexion, and medial rotation
	Pectoralis minor	Shoulder forward and downward
C-6, C-7	Supinator	Forearm supination
	Pronator teres	Forearm pronation

(continued)

Figure 1. (continued)

Roots	Muscles	Function
C-6, C-7, C-8	Latissimus dorsi	Shoulder medial rotation
	Triceps brachii	Elbow extension
	Extensor digiti communis	MCP extension
	Extensor digiti minimus	Little finger extension
C-7, C-8	Extensor indicis proprius	Index finger MCP extension
	Extensor carpi ulnaris	Wrist extension
	Extensor pollicis longus	Thumb IP extension
	Extensor pollicis brevis	Thumb MCP extension
	Abductor pollicis longus	Thumb abduction
C-7, C-8, T-1	Flexor digitorum superficialis	IP flexion
	Flexor digitorum profundus	DIP flexion
C-8, T-1	Flexor carpi ulnaris	Wrist flexion & adduction
	Interossei	MCP flexion
	Dorsales	Finger abduction
	Palmares	Finger adduction
	Flexor pollicis longus	Thumb IP flexion
	Flexor pollicis brevis	Thumb MCP flexion
	Abductor pollicis	Thumb abduction
	Adductor pollicis brevis	Thumb adduction
	Opponens pollicis	Thumb opposition
	Lumbricales	MCP flexion

There may be some variation among references regarding actual nerve roots and innervated muscles (Burke & Murray, 1975; Chusid, 1985; *Dorland's Medical Dictionary*, 1962; Hoppenfeld, 1977; Sharrard, 1964). From *Specialized Occupational Therapy for Persons With High Level Quadriplegia* by S.L. Garber, P. Lathem, and T.L. Gregorio, 1988, Houston: TIRR. Copyright © 1988 by TIRR. Reprinted by permission.

High-Level Quadriplegia: Levels C-1 Through C-4

High-level quadriplegia refers to the paralysis that results from an injury to the spinal cord at any segmental level between the C-1 and C-4 vertebrae. For the purpose of this chapter, this term describes those individuals with any or all of the following conditions: (a) neurological level of C-4 or above, complete motor and sensory deficits bilaterally; (b) total or partial dependence on respiratory or other breathing aids; (c) long-term medical and personal care needs; and (d) limited expected functional recovery (Garber, Lathem, & Gregorio, 1988).

Although the person with high-level quadriplegia is usually dependent in self-care, learning to give verbal instructions to those who provide assistance returns a measure of control to this individual. There are three major objectives in the rehabilitation of persons with C-1 through C-4 quadriplegia: education regarding their care; exposure to functional activities; and adaptation through the use of high technology. Persons with injuries at the C-1 through C-2 level are ventilator dependent. Primary muscle innervation will be sternocleidomastoid (neck flexion and head rotation). At the C-4 level, the key muscles innervated are the diaphragm and the upper trapezius. The individual may require mechanical ventilation at first but usually is eventually weaned from the ventilator. Movement includes full neck rotation, neck extension and flexion, and some scapular elevation. Little or no scapular depression exists (Trombly, 1989).

Figure 2. Functional levels of the lumbar and sacral spinal cord.

Roots	Muscles	Function
L1–L-3	Iliopsoas	Hip flexion
	Sartorius	Hip flexion & thigh eversion
L-1–L-4	Gracilis	Hip adduction & knee flexion
L-2–L-3	Pectineus	Hip flexion & adduction
L-2–L-4	Adductor longus, brevis, & magnus	Hip adduction
	Quadriceps femoris	Knee extension
L-4–S-1	Tensor faciae latae	Hip flexion & abduction
	Gluteus medius & minimus	Hip abduction & medial rotation
L-5	Tibialis posterior	Ankle plantar flexion & inversion
L-5–S-1	Extensor hallucis longus	Ankle dorsiflexion & great toe extension
	Extensor digitorum longus	Toes II–V extension
	Peroneus brevis	Ankle plantar flexion
	Gastrocnemius	Ankle plantar flexion & knee flexion
L-5–S-2	Gluteus maximus	Hip extension, abduction, & external rotation
L-5–S-3	Biceps femoris	Knee flexion & hip extension
	Soleus	Ankle plantar flexion
S-1–S-2	Flexor hallucis longus & brevis	Great toe flexion
S-1–S-3	Flexor digitorum longus & brevis	Toes II–V flexion
S-2–S-3	Foot intrinsics	Toe abduction, adduction, flexion, & extension
S-2–S-4	Perineum & sphincters	Bladder & lower bowel function
S-4–S-5	Rectal muscles	

There may be some variation among references regarding actual nerve roots and innervated muscles (Burke & Murray, 1975; Chusid, 1985; *Dorland's Medical Dictionary*, 1962; Hoppenfeld, 1977; Sharrard, 1964).

Figure 3. The Frankel grading system: Neurological extent of spinal cord injury.

Frankel A	Complete	No sensation or motor function.
Frankel B	Incomplete	Preserved sensation only. Preservation of any demonstrable sensation, excluding subject phantom sensations. Voluntary motor function is absent.
Frankel C	Incomplete	Preserved motor (nonfunctional). Sensation may or may not be preserved.
Frankel D	Incomplete	Preserved motor (functional).
Frankel E	Complete recovery	Complete return of all motor and sensory function; abnormal reflexes may persist.

From *Spinal Cord Injury: The Facts and Figures* (p. 27) by S.L. Stover and P.R. Fine, 1986, Birmingham: The University of Alabama Press. Copyright © 1986 by The University of Alabama Press. Reprinted by permission.

Case Study 1.

For a high-level spinal cord–injured person (C-1 through C-3), a mouthstick serves as a substitute for the hand. Traditional mouthstick training enables the person with this level of injury to achieve some independence and control in his or her life.

K.T. was an active high school senior when he dove into a shallow pool and hit his head on the bottom, resulting in a C-3 spinal cord injury. He received comprehensive rehabilitation, including strengthening of preserved neck musculature and mouthstick training. He learned to turn pages of a book, type, and write. Once discharged from the hospital, he decided to pursue a college degree in computer science. He was independently mobile with a chin-controlled power wheelchair and, therefore, was able to travel across the college campus without difficulty. However, he sometimes did find himself in buildings with elevators, and he had no way of depressing the elevator buttons. Frequently, passers-by would depress the buttons for him, but if no one was nearby he had to wait, which often made him late for class. Finally, he decided to call the occupational therapist who had worked with him originally and set up an outpatient appointment. After consultation and evaluation, the therapist devised a small, triangular-base-shaped mouthstick holder with suction cups on the bottom that was positioned on K.T.'s lapboard. It was strategically placed close to his body so that he could flex his head forward and bite the mouthstick to pick it up independently. He was instructed to drive his chin-controlled wheelchair close to the elevator buttons, positioning it so the side where the mouthstick holder was mounted was closest and parallel to the buttons. Then he could lift the mouthstick and call the elevator. Once inside the elevator, he repeated the process to select the floor he desired. Fortunately, the elevator buttons are accessible to him most of the time. However, he has found that he is unable to depress the buttons in all elevators, and at those times he politely asks for assistance. This relatively inexpensive mouthstick holder and a little creativity went a long way toward enhancing this young man's ability to pursue his education.

Case Study 2.

S.K. had sustained a spinal cord injury at the C-3 level. Prior to his injury, he had been an avid collector of small fish, which he kept in his aquarium at home. He had always enjoyed taking care of the aquarium; however, because he also enjoyed simply watching the fish, he was determined to find a way to care for them, even if it only involved feeding. He devised a plan to stabilize a small cup that held the fish food on a platform above the aquarium. He mounted a mouthstick holder at the level where he could drive his wheelchair up to it, access the mouthstick (which he had had adapted with a small spoon) and scoop the food up and into the aquarium. This task was not only fun for him, but it greatly increased his sense of accomplishment, self-esteem, and independence.

Eating and Meal Preparation

Eating

Head position and sitting angle may affect the individual's ability to chew and successfully swallow food or medications, especially if there is any involvement of the brain stem, the area of the brain that affects the swallow mechanism coordination. The individual with C-1 through C-4 quadriplegia can ensure safe swallowing of food if he or she can effectively communicate the body position that enhances this function. Every person has preferences for how to consume food, whether conscious of this or not. We all have our own eating rituals, such as which food item is eaten first, or how large a portion is eaten in one spoonful. An individual with a C-1 through C-4 injury will enjoy the meal more if able to direct another person verbally to feed him or her in the most accustomed manner.

Depending on the strength of the deltoid and biceps muscles, the individual with a lesion at C-4 may find a ball-bearing feeder orthosis (BBFO) or mobile arm support (MAS) useful for self-feeding and/or self-propulsion in a powered wheelchair (see Figure 4). With a Fair to Poor muscle grade in the anterior/posterior deltoid and biceps, a MAS with wrist support and an adapted utensil is a method of using the individual's maximum potential for self-care activities. An automated/automatic feeder is another option for self-feeding (see Figure 5).

Medication

Every person who is prescribed oral medications should understand what they are, be able to identify them visually, and know the dosage, purpose, and side effects. These specifications should be taught to those with C-1 through C-4 quadriplegia, so these individuals can be assured of receiving the appropriate medications. This also allows them to report verbally their medication regimes to any physician who may be involved in their care, but unfamiliar with the specific treatment protocol for persons with spinal cord injury.

Workbooks that are individually organized with the specific medications the person

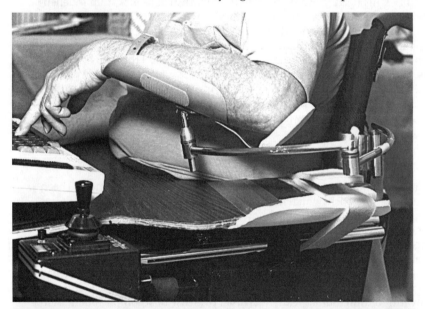

Figure 4. Mobile Arm Support (MAS).

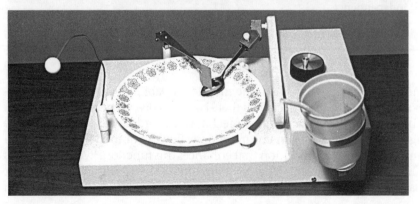

Figure 5. Electronic feeding device.

is currently taking can be provided to the family. It is not enough for this information to be given just to the caregiver; it must be committed to memory, and the person must be tested on the accuracy of the details. A mechanism to update medical information should be in place through the pharmacy so the workbook can be an accurate reference for the patient or caregiver.

Meal Preparation

The person with C-1 through C-4 quadriplegia uses verbal instruction to fulfill roles congruent with family life, such as instructing a child in preparing a simple meal, cooking, or using household appliances. The accuracy of the verbal direction will be critical to the child's successful and safe accomplishment of the tasks (Garber et al., 1988). While the patient is in the hospital, tasks can be planned in which the patient must give instruction, in order to provide practice and feedback on its accuracy. For example, he or she may initially direct another person to prepare a sandwich, then advance to giving direction in the use of a microwave.

The therapist is responsible for giving direct feedback to the patient about the effectiveness of the verbal instruction. The key word is "direct," because sometimes a person can verbally direct with an aggressive or negative tone, which will decrease others' willingness to listen and assist. The intonation of voice, and volume and word choice are just as important as accuracy of direction. To enhance learning and provide a satisfying experience for therapist and patient alike, the therapist should actually perform the task exactly as the patient gives the verbal direction.

Hygiene and Grooming

Dental Care

Brushing teeth, rinsing the mouth, and using mouthwash can be independently performed with the use of a commercially available dental device (see Figure 6). This specially mounted device can be set at the appropriate height from the floor so a person with C-1 through C-4 quadriplegia can drive the wheelchair to it and use its components

Figure 6.
Dental
hygiene device.

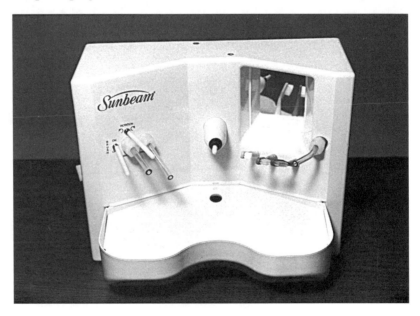

to complete dental hygiene tasks. Flossing of teeth must be performed by a caretaker. Since the individuals with C-1 through C-4 injury may use a mouthstick to accomplish certain tasks, dental hygiene is extremely important. The structure and health of teeth can affect a person's ability and comfort in using a mouthstick (see Figure 7). It is recommended that the individual be encouraged to have annual or more frequent dental evaluations to ensure healthy oral hygiene. A caretaker must clean dentures, due to the high level of dexterity necessary for this task.

For tasks such as washing and/or shaving the face, combing hair, and applying makeup, stable head support is important for safety and comfort. These tasks, as well as feminine hygiene and bowel/bladder care, must be performed by a caretaker. As with any task, the individual with quadriplegia has preferences for how they are to be performed. Accuracy in verbal direction is important to ensure that the tasks are completed in the manner that is familiar and pleasing. Repetition and practice in giving directions are essential to maximize effectiveness.

Bathing

Although the individual with C-1 through C-4 quadriplegia will be totally dependent in the task of bathing, there are different options available to allow it to be accomplished by a caregiver efficiently and effectively.

Many times, because an individual's bathroom is not accessible, or appropriate equipment is not available, bathing in the conventional location is not possible and must be done in bed. Some type of plastic covering can be used under the individual to protect the bedding from getting wet. A commercially available inflatable bathtub can be used on top of the bed to hold water. The inflatable bathtub is portable to allow bathing while traveling. A basin of water and all necessary items (i.e., soap, washcloth and towels, shampoo, razor) should be brought to the bedside before the bath begins to reduce the time the individual is exposed to the water and possible cool room air. An inflatable shampoo basin can be used to wash hair while the person is in bed.

If the bathroom is accessible, a tall back shower lift with head and neck support may

Figure 7. Mouthstick activity performed by an individual with high level quadriplegia.

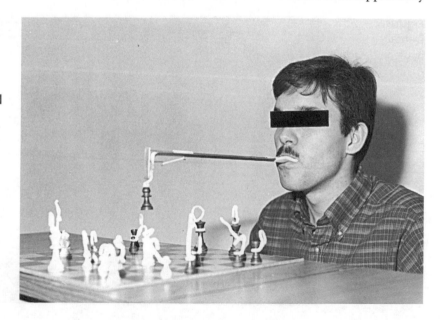

be used to support the body while the person sits in a shower chair, to assure safe transfer and body support under wet conditions. For those persons using a ventilator, protection to prevent water from entering the trachea must be assured.

Mobility

The individual with C-1 through C-4 quadriplegia will be dependent in transfers and manual wheelchair mobility.

Transfers

The most safe and effective type of transfer should be established with the patient and caregivers. This can range from a mechanical lift transfer, to a three-person lift, to a

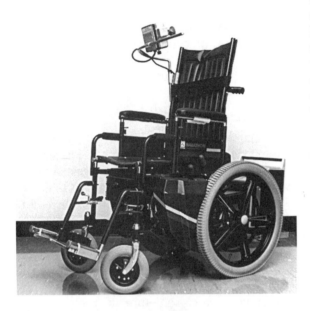

dependent slideboard transfer. Much depends on the size of the person being transferred, the abilities and strength of the caregiver performing the transfer, spasticity or other medical complications, and available equipment to be used. The individual with C-1 through C-4 quadriplegia must be able to direct each step of the transfer verbally with complete and accurate instructions.

Wheelchair Mobility

A manual wheelchair is generally used as a back-up means of mobility for a person with C-1 through C-4 quadriplegia. A person with this level of spinal cord injury generally uses a motorized wheelchair for mobility using a sip-and-puff, chin control, or head-control driving mechanism (Lathem, Gregorio, & Garber, 1985) (see Figures 8a & 8b).

Powered or motorized mobility can be achieved for the individual with a C-4 spinal cord injury in three different ways. One is to control the powered wheelchair by a small remote joystick mounted on a swing-away bar positioned near the person's chin. This allows the individual to

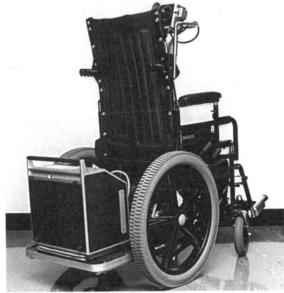

Figure 8a (top) and 8b (bottom). Powered mobility with chin control for the individual with high level quadriplegia.

access a proportional drive joystick. The individual may need to be transferred and positioned properly in the wheelchair, but once positioned has access to the community, home, or school.

The second way an individual can make use of powered mobility is to operate a sip-and-puff type pneumatic control switch. The individual puts a small tube in his or her mouth and sucks or blows air into it in order to activate a latching type switch. This is translated through the electronic module to activate the motors.

The third way is to use a MAS to access the regular joystick, which may need to be specially mounted or placed in an optimal place for the safest and most reliable control. It is helpful to have the on/off and high/low switches relocated on top of the joystick box so the individual can turn the wheelchair on or off when desired.

An automatic power reclining system on a motorized wheelchair will allow the individual to perform independent weight shifting to reduce the risk of pressure ulcers. If spasticity is a significant problem for a person, a power tilt control would be an alternative to allow for weight shifting, although it is less effective in totally shifting weight off of the buttocks, because it only tilts 45° to 60°, depending on the manufacturer of the system (Lathem et al., 1985).

Transportation

The person with C-1 through C-4 quadriplegia requires assistance with all community transportation. Information regarding adapted vans with power wheelchair lifts and tie-down systems must be discussed with the individual and caregiver. The wheelchair itself must have adequate positioning devices to support the person's body and to maintain stability while the van is in motion. This includes head supports, chestbelts, seatbelts, and lateral supports.

The clearance through the van door is a critical measurement, because the wheelchair back with head support tends to be higher than a conventional van doorway opening. People have different preferences for how they position their wheelchair once inside the van. The safest position for securing the wheelchair to the floor is facing forward. Visual restriction from the headliner of the van is sometimes a problem. Those individuals who are unable to afford a modified van for personal transportation should be educated in the use of public transportation systems. An actual community outing with supervision is the best preparation for a person with high-level quadriplegia to learn how to access public transportation.

Dressing/Undressing

An individual with C-1 through C-4 quadriplegia requires assistance with dressing and undressing. There are techniques, however, that can be employed by the caregiver to ease the task. It is important to give the individual choices in the selection of clothing. When purchasing clothing, consideration should be given to reducing the effort needed to dress and undress. Some suggestions are loose-fitting clothing, stretchable fabrics, touch-fastener closures, slip-on shoes, minimal zippers and buttons, and elastic sleeves and waistbands (Farmer, 1986).

Because individuals with injuries at these levels have impaired sensation, fabrics should be selected that do not irritate the skin. Clothing made of breathable materials, such as cotton, is best for air exchange between the atmosphere and the skin. Pants with double-welted seams and studs, or rivets, should be avoided because these can cause excessive pressure. Rear pockets of pants may be removed to reduce the risk of pressure from seams.

Watches, necklaces, rings, and bracelets should be carefully selected for size, taking tightness into consideration. If edema is a problem in the wrists or hands, tight jewelry could impede circulation and possibly need to be cut off.

Upper Extremity

Upper extremity dressing is accomplished by the caregiver through one of three methods: overhead, side-to-side, or around-the-back. The person with a C-1 through C-2 lesion needs assistance to extend the neck; the person with C-2 through C-4 lesion is able to assist in flexing the neck forward. Bras with front touch fasteners or hooks are easier to put on using the around-the-back method because of non-restrictive front access. Bras with back closures can be fastened first then slipped over the head. Clip-on ties or ties fastened midway are the easiest for a caregiver to put on a person with C-1 through C-4 quadriplegia.

Undressing the upper extremities requires the same techniques performed in reverse. If sitting in the wheelchair, the patient must be well-supported to maximize trunk balance.

Lower Extremity

Lower-extremity dressing presents additional concerns. Underwear may or may not be worn, based on personal preference. Sometimes brief-style underpants cause pressure over the ischial tuberosities, resulting in skin breakdown. In addition, if the person is rolled side-to-side for the garment to be pulled up over the hips, enough shearing and friction could be produced to damage the skin. Extreme caution must be taken to prevent this. Loosely fitting socks are much easier to pull over the foot than tight, elasticized socks. Slip-on or self-fastening closure shoes are also recommended.

Dressing or undressing the person with C-1 through C-4 quadriplegia provides a convenient opportunity for the caregiver to perform a complete skin inspection to identify pressure sores or other lesions.

Communication

Communication tasks may comprise the category of activities in which the person with C-1 through C-4 injury is the least restricted. In a comprehensive rehabilitation program much time is usually devoted to training in these skills, which could mean a return to independence in socializing with family and friends, as well as having a safety tool to call for help, if necessary. Many communication tasks can be translated into potential vocational pursuits. Descriptions of tasks such as turning pages, typing, writing, operating a tape recorder, using the phone, painting, and verbal instruction are presented thoroughly in the literature (Garber et al., 1988; Kovich & Presperin, 1986; Lathem et al., 1985).

It is noted that due to their limited head and neck control, persons with C-1 through C-2 quadriplegia are more successful in completing tasks such as turning pages, typing, and activating a tape recorder and telephone if they use electronic equipment. People with C-3 through C-4 quadriplegia use either electronic devices or a mouthstick to accomplish these tasks. Mouthsticks often are used to enable the person with a spinal cord injury at this level to participate in leisure and avocational activities, such as board games (see Figure 7). Other necessary associated equipment to be used in conjunction with communication skills are elevating tables, modified work stations, mouthstick holders, environmental control units, computers, electric typewriter keyguards, bookholders, electric page turners, voice amplifiers, speaker phones, phone flippers, and gooseneck supports, some of which are pictured in Figure 9.

Figure 9. Work station modified for the individual with high level quadriplegia.

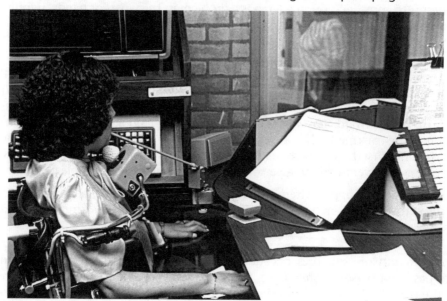

With the advent of voice-activated computer access, communication for persons with disabilities has greatly expanded. Environmental control systems and computer input devices now operate reliably with voice commands. Access to phone systems may require a combination of mouthstick skills, voice activation, and setup by another individual.

Bowel and Bladder Care

The individual with C-1 through C-4 quadriplegia requires assistance in all bowel and bladder management and feminine hygiene, except for emptying a legbag. This can be accomplished with the use of an electric legbag emptying device, which receives its power from the electric wheelchair battery. It is activated by a breath control or lever switch mounted in an accessible place. The emptying device is connected to the clamp that surrounds the legbag tubing. When not activated, the tube is held closed by pressure and does not allow urine to pass. When the electric switch is activated, the pressure is released from the tube, allowing the urine to leave the legbag. This device limits a person to emptying the legbag into a floor drain, basin, cat litter box, or outdoors. For those persons active in the community this can be a very liberating device, because they do not have to ask others to perform this personal task for them.

Another method of urine collection is to mount a sealed container onto the wheelchair. The legbag tubing extends to reach around the wheelchair and into the container. The container must be emptied daily by another person and cleaned regularly to avoid an odor. A sitting position during a bowel program can assist in bowel evacuation. A commode chair with a high back and head positioner is needed to give proper body support during this procedure.

Education on managing autonomic dysreflexia and the ability of an individual with C-1 through C-4 quadriplegia to instruct others verbally on how to manage him or her during this medical emergency is essential. Bladder or bowel distension, suppository insertion, skin irritation, clothing or legbag straps that are too tight, or pressure ulcers can lead to a dangerous increase in blood pressure. This increase in blood pressure can lead to cerebrovascular accident or death if not relieved.

Following spinal cord injury, ovulation and fertility usually are not altered in the female once spinal shock resolves. Special precautions for delivery may be required to lower the likelihood of autonomic dysreflexia. Women with C-1 through C-4 quadriplegia are dependent on a caregiver to manage menstrual needs and birth control. Respect should be given to the person's choice, as these activities are very intimate and personal.

Quadriplegia: Levels C-5 Through C-8

Persons with C-5 quadriplegia have functional biceps and, therefore, are able to feed themselves and perform simple grooming tasks with the aid of adapted equipment. At level C-6 wrist function occurs, enabling the person to require only minimal to moderate assistance in grooming, bathing, and meal preparation. At the C-7 through C-8 levels, many of these individuals can live alone or without assistance with home modification (Stover & Fine, 1986).

Eating and Meal Preparation

Eating

Meal preparation and eating are challenges for individuals with a spinal cord injury at levels C-5 through C-8. Eating is generally accomplished using a variety of adapted devices. The universal cuff (an elastic or self-fastening strap attached to a leather pocket) is easily donned and simply used with a regular utensil inserted into the palmar pocket.

Case Study 3.

> S.M. is a 21-year-old male who sustained a C-4 through C-5 level spinal cord injury following a motor vehicle accident. He underwent spinal stabilization and was placed in a halo brace postoperatively. He was transferred to The Institute for Rehabilitation and Research for comprehensive rehabilitation. During the first 4 weeks of hospitalization, S.M.'s occupational therapy program focused on progressive wheelchair sitting (to enable him to achieve the 90° sitting angle), strengthening and range of motion to the upper extremities, and the initiation of independent living skills training. At week 5, he was fitted with a ball bearing feeder orthosis (BBFO) to facilitate such activities as feeding, turning pages, and typing. He particularly practiced the skill of typing because this encouraged fine placement control. S.M. gradually improved his ability to move the BBFO in the directions he desired. After 2 weeks of practice, it was time to mount the BBFO onto a powered wheelchair so he could develop skill in accessing and moving the joystick control. Initially, he found this to be a very difficult task because the momentum of the wheelchair interfered with the movement control of his arm in the BBFO. With continued practice, encouragement, and motivation, he improved both his skills and his self-esteem. His occupational therapist reports that she will never forget the excitement or the look on his face when, for the first time, he independently drove the wheelchair in a straight direction for approximately 10 feet. This independence in mobility boosted S.M.'s spirits and gave him the needed motivation to work even harder to achieve the goals he had set for himself.

> Although S.M. quickly learned to drive the wheelchair forward and to the right, driving in reverse and turning left were more difficult. An orthotist was consulted and, together with the occupational therapist and the patient, devised a spring assist to add to the proximal arm of the BBFO. This spring served as an active resist to retract the shoulder to the point that these difficult directions (reverse and left) of the drive path were also accomplished with relative ease. Except for the placement of his arm in the BBFO trough, the patient became totally independent in driving the wheelchair in approximately 4 weeks.

Most people prefer to use this if possible because it is less noticeable in public, quickly put into a pocket, and easily carried when eating out.

The person with a spinal cord injury at levels C-5 through C-6 is able to pick up a modified cup or glass using a wrist stabilizing device. A cup or glass can be given a modified handle so the hand can passively lift it to the mouth. Some prefer using a long straw so they do not need to lift the cup or glass from the table. Usually a straw holder is used to keep the straw pointed toward the face for ease of reach.

If the person is using a ratchet-type orthosis or an electric prehension orthosis, the orthosis itself can be positioned around the cup or glass for lifting. Usually after all equipment is procured and in position, the person will be able to drink independently. A nonbreakable, lightweight cup or glass is safer and gives less stress to arm musculature.

Eating with utensils can be accomplished with a variety of adaptations. The wrist must remain stabilized in a neutral position. The plate-to-mouth pattern is accomplished through a combination of shoulder flexion, horizontal shoulder adduction, external rotation, and elbow flexion. If these motions are too weak, a BBFO or monosuspension feeder can assist in overcoming the effects of gravity and the weight of the utensils. A hand orthosis with a utensil pocket, a long opponens orthosis, or a wrist stabilizing splint with the ability to attach a spoon or fork can be used.

If the person has a difficult time keeping the food on the utensil due to a lack of forearm rotation, swivel utensils may be used. However, in some cases the swivel mechanism makes the scooping motion more difficult. Plateguards may be useful as a border for food to be scooped against, so as not to fall off of the plate. Initially, a person may be unable to self-feed an entire meal. The therapist may have the person practice feeding him- or herself one serving only; then, as strength and endurance increase, more food can be added to the plate. A ratchet-type or electric prehension orthosis can be used to hold utensils in the conventional way. After this equipment is prepositioned the person can scoop and bring food to his or her mouth independently.

Cutting food takes much practice, and the person with quadriplegia at levels C-5 through C-6, usually requires minimum to moderate assistance and adapted equipment. Again, the wrist must be stabilized in a neutral position. A rocker knife can be used if the individual has good shoulder internal rotation. A knife with a serrated edge can be used if a sawing motion is used to cut. Commercially available modified serrated knives with a quad cuff can be purchased. Care must be taken to assure that the thumb is out of the way of the blade while cutting food. Some individuals with C-5 lesions choose to have others who prepare the food cut it for them because it is safer and neater. This should be a respected choice of the person.

Individuals with lesions at levels C-7 through C-8 can live without personal assistance using only a minimum number of assistive devices. They may intertwine the utensil between their fingers for stability. However, cutting devices require the use of both hands or some adaptation, such as a cuff, to secure the knife. These individuals should be able to drink from a cup or glass utilizing a tenodesis grasp or using both hands but may need assistance opening milk cartons or canned drinks.

Medication

Medications can be placed in an easy-to-open container or open cup. A person with C-5 quadriplegia may use an electric prehension orthosis to pick up and place the medication in his or her mouth independently. If the medication is placed in a small shallow cup, a person with stabilized wrists will be able to raise the cup between two hands brought together to the mouth. Safety issues must be considered with this method, such as the consequences of dropped medications or of open containers, which could be handled by small children if they are in the home.

The individual should experiment with different types of containers and request that the pharmacist provide the type most easily manipulated. These often have flip-top or regular screw-off lids. The push and turn, or "child-proof," type are the most difficult but should be attempted during rehabilitation training so the individual knows the consequences of selecting medications in this type of container.

Meal Preparation

Meal preparation can be a very difficult and time consuming task for persons with C-5 quadriplegia, and individuals with lesions at the C-6 level may require moderate assistance. Each person determines which parts of meal preparation are safe and reasonable to perform. By using an electric prehension orthosis or ratchet type orthosis, the individual will be able to accomplish more meal preparation tasks than someone using a passive wrist stabilizing orthosis.

There are many labor saving devices and small appliances that facilitate chopping or grating. The major challenge is safely lifting pans into and out of the oven. A microwave or toaster oven may eliminate the problem and be adequate if preparing meals for just one or two people. Cooking on top of the stove is accomplished with over-the-stove mirrors, long-handled utensils, large-handled pots, shallow fry pans, and long oven mitts to prevent burns. A suction stabilizer that holds the pans stable increases safety when preparing hot food items. Using adapted utensils or a palm-to-palm method to grasp utensils, the individual can accomplish many mealtime tasks.

When transporting food from one place to another, it is easiest to slide the item along the counter or to use a laptray. Commercially available one-handed can openers with adjustable stands to support the can are difficult for an individual with C-5 quadriplegia to use but with practice may be mastered. A blender or mixer can conserve the individual's energy. Controls should be levers or push buttons.

Cutting can be done using an adapted knife and a cutting board with a stainless or aluminum nail through it to stabilize the food. Suction cups on the bottom provide stability on the countertop. This allows a two-handed method to be used, either palm-to-palm or allowing one hand to be the antagonist or stabilizer. A table or lower counter is helpful because the objects are then close and the elbows are supported. Due to a lack of triceps and trunk balance, the individual is most successful when working close to the body. Jars can be opened by holding them between both hands and pushing against serrated edges while turning. The jar lids should be kept loosely engaged for ease of opening.

Ovens can be difficult to handle, because of the weight or spring action of the door. Lifting pans into and out of the oven can be very unsafe. Usually a toaster oven or a broiler used on a low table top is a safer way to bake. Lever action is used to open the door and depress buttons. Microwave ovens are also safer than conventional ovens if placed on a table at an accessible height. The door is often controlled by a button or lever. Loops can be added to the door handle to aid in opening.

The refrigerator door can be made easier to open by adding loops to the door handle. Frequently used items should be placed on the shelves of the refrigerator that are eye-level or lower. Food storage containers should be lightweight plastic, in case they are dropped or slip from the person's grasp.

Cleanup is easier if the sink is accessible. This is accomplished by removing lower cabinets, insulating the pipes, and lowering the counter. A scrubber with soap in the handle is a useful step saver. Brushes with large open handles that the hand can fit through provide a better grasp. A rubber pad on the bottom of the sink will decrease the likelihood of breakage. An adapted scrub brush and a liquid soap dispenser, a bottle brush, a wash mitt, and levers on sink controls can help during dish washing. The dishes can be dried either in the sink or in a sink rack. A dishwasher can be used, but this is difficult due to the weight of the door. A loop can be added to assist in opening it.

Lightweight, nonbreakable dishes are economical and safer to use than china, especially as the person adjusts to the spinal cord injury. Prepared foods and microwave dishes may be relatively expensive, but they save time and energy and reduce frustration. Conventional meal preparation presents challenges that may include: getting the food out of the pantry, refrigerator, or freezer; reaching the pots and pans; opening plastic, frozen, or metal containers; operating manual and small electric kitchen appliances; setting the table; and using large kitchen appliances.

The kitchen area should have room for wheelchair maneuvering in order to open drawers and doors. The cabinets should be easy to open, with glides and handles to facilitate operation for those with limited strength and hand function. Items need to be placed within reach at wheelchair level, and one may choose to eliminate doors on the cabinets altogether. These individuals will utilize a reacher to access those items that are above the head. The best refrigerator is a side-by-side, because both the freezer and the refrigerator compartments are accessible.

Small manual kitchen appliances need to be on a work surface at desk height in order to be operated with little or no adaptation, but they require more energy to operate and often are not as effective as electric ones. There are several electric appliances now available to perform those same tasks: electric can openers, electric peelers, food processors, and mixers are a few. Small electric appliances, like electric can openers, may require a supporting base and lever switches or special push buttons for efficient and safe operation.

The person with an injury at this level needs to be careful around sharp surfaces and extreme temperatures, due to sensory deficits. Operating the range or oven requires the switches to be at eye level and within reach, eliminating the need to reach over hot burners.

It takes creativity to adapt the kitchen environment appliances and utensils to meet the needs of an individual with C-5 through C-8 quadriplegia. Preplanning can help save time and increase efficiency in meal preparation.

Hygiene and Grooming: Levels C-5 Through C-6

Dental Care

The first prerequisite to brushing teeth is to develop a functional hand-to-mouth pattern. Several different types of orthoses or assistive devices can be used by someone with C-5 quadriplegia. If the individual is unable to lift his or her arm against gravity, a MAS can be used for this task. A person using a MAS must be set up with the toothbrush in a utensil holder and toothpaste on the brush. The person then brushes one side of the mouth, turns the toothbrush around, and brushes the other side to completion. The toothbrush can be turned within the utensil holder by holding the brush between the teeth and rotating the head, or grasping the brush between the teeth, removing it from the holder, then reinserting it into the holder. A cup of water with a straw, previously set up by another person, can be used to rinse the mouth.

If a person has adequate muscle strength to move his or her arm against gravity, other orthotic devices, such as a Universal cuff, a long opponens splint, or an electric or reciprocal orthosis, can substitute for lack of wrist extension to stabilize the hand (see Figure 10). Other assistive devices, such as a Wanchik writer, dorsal wrist cock-up splint, or elastic wrist brace, may be used for this activity as well. These devices are usually less costly than the previously mentioned orthoses. Most individuals find it easiest to clasp the toothpaste tube with both hands to bring it to the mouth to obtain the toothpaste. In this case, a flip-top cap is preferred so it can be easily opened A pump tube can be mounted onto a fabricated stand to stabilize it while dispensing toothpaste.

Combing Hair

Without triceps, brushing and styling the hair require maximum assistance. An individual with C-5 quadriplegia who uses a MAS is unable to perform this task without assistance. Long-handled brushes are useful, as are the small octopus type scrubbers with the ring handles, found in drugstores. Using a curling iron requires maximum assistance. An adaptation may be for the person to get a permanent or a low-maintenance hair style.

Someone with this level of injury who can move his or her arm against gravity needs to use an orthosis to stabilize the wrist. A comb with an extended handle stabilized in the previously mentioned orthoses or assistive devices is best. A phone holder or Universal cuff can also be used in conjunction with these devices.

Figure 10. Universal cuff with toothbrush.

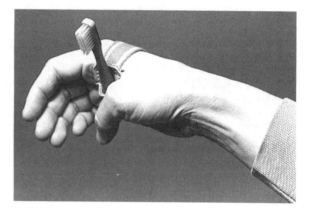

Shaving

Shaving the face can be performed with either an electric or safety razor depending on personal preference. Many individuals change to electric razors to avoid the cuts and nicks experienced with blades. Not being able to keep the razor from falling is a major problem but can be overcome with a two-handed technique. The therapist should be sensitive to this fact and work to achieve safety and independence in the selected method. A person using a MAS needs assistance setting up the razor and shaving cream. In some cases, assistance is needed to shave difficult-to-reach contours of the face and neck.

An electric razor can be held by using a reciprocal orthosis, an electric prehension orthosis, or a specially adapted cuff (see Figure 11). The razor's weight is a major consideration, because it may give more resistance than the limb can support. Safety razors can be adapted with a variety of low-temperature plastics for ease of handling. If the person can move his or her arm against gravity, a utensil holder can be used to stabilize the razor. Commercially available razor holders can be purchased but must be used in conjunction with a wrist-stabilizing brace. Commercially available shaving cream dispensers that have a long lever handle can assist with this aspect of the activity.

Most women with C-5 quadriplegia require assistance in shaving their underarms and legs due to the necessary trunk stabilization during forward leaning and for maintaining upright balance while using both upper extremities for the task.

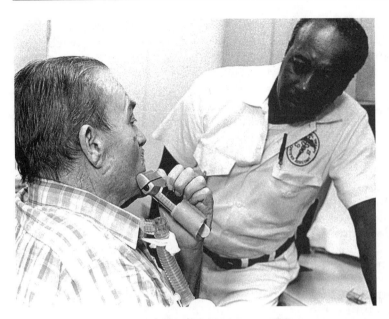

Figure 11. Shaving with an adapted electric razor (C-5 through C-6 quadriplegia).

Washing Face and Hands

In order to perform this task independently, the person must be able to maneuver the wheelchair up to a sink. The water faucet controls must have a lever so the person can turn them. A wash mitt with a D-ring strap must be placed on the person's hand. Some people may want to use a stabilizing wrist device under the mitt. Soap can be secured to the sink by a suction pad. If a MAS is employed, the person uses a combination of head, neck, and upper extremity movements to reach all areas. Excess water is squeezed out of the wash mitt by pushing it against the side of the sink. After the face and hands are cleaned, the mitt is removed. A towel can be clasped between both hands and brought to the face for drying.

Makeup Application

The female with an injury at level C-6 can use a reciprocal orthosis to grasp makeup brushes, pencils, or wands. Sanding or slightly filing the clasps on blush and eye shadow compacts makes them easier to open. Small tubes, such as those containing mascara, can be held in the mouth, enabling the individual to achieve greater independence.

Bathing

An individual with C-5 quadriplegia requires maximum assistance from another person for the greatest effectiveness and safety during bathing. If the individual has an accessible shower, a shower commode chair is used for transporting and positioning him or her for bathing.

A D-ring wash mitt may be used by the individual to perform a small part of the bathing task, allowing washing of the face, neck, anterior chest, and upper legs. Long-handled brushes help to get those hard-to-reach places, like the feet and in between the toes. A hand-held shower head may be useful, but the occupational therapist may need to add an adapted handle to it. Skin protection, postural support, and adapted handles make bathing a more independent, more private activity. Bed baths are an alternative way of cleaning the body should home modification and/or equipment procurement preclude using a roll-in shower for the task.

Washing and Drying Hair

Washing hair is most easily performed in conjunction with showering or bathing. Since the ability to stabilize the trunk while leaning forward over a sink is necessary, assistance is required; therefore, most choose to have someone else wash their hair. A commercially available shampoo basin can be used when bathing in bed. This basin holds the water and has a drain tube leading from it that can be placed in a bucket to collect the excess water.

Due to the difficulty of holding up a hair dryer against gravity, drying hair is most easily achieved by using a blow dryer mounted onto a gooseneck stand. The person then moves his or her head toward the direction of the blowing air.

Hygiene and Grooming: Levels C-7 Through C-8

Persons with a C-7 through C-8 injury can perform sink hygiene and grooming without assistance and with few or no adaptive devices. The important issue concerns accessibility of the sink and faucets. If the person is unable to approach the sink facing front, then he or she may be able to approach it from the side; however, this may affect balance. Lever controls are easiest for the person to utilize, although he or she also may be able to utilize some twisting controls. Towels should be placed close to the sink and at a low level for ease of accessibility.

Dental Care

Individuals may position the toothbrush in between their fingers to secure it or use a built-up handle to increase their grip. Some individuals may choose to utilize an electric toothbrush. Getting the toothpaste onto the brush may require using the countertop to get enough pressure to push the paste out, or the paste may be put in the person's mouth before the brush. A small, prethreaded dental flossing tool is also helpful.

Washing Face and Hands, Combing Hair, Shaving, and Makeup Application

Persons with C-7 through C-8 quadriplegia are able to use a wash cloth for face and hand washing without difficulty. They may use liquid soap but also should be able to use bar soap. Hair grooming can be done with a regular brush and comb but may require an adapted handle if the hair is very thick. Men with injuries at this level may decide to use an electric razor to shave. This allows reaching facial hair with maximum safety, but the weaker hand may need a strap to secure the heavier razors. A safety razor can be used, but may not be as secure in the hand and may require frequent repositioning. Women should be able to put on most makeup, except fine eye applications, without difficulty. Applicators for eye liner, eye shadow, and mascara may need to be built up, and containers may need to be adapted for easier opening.

Bathing and Hair Washing

Persons with this level of injury need assistance with bathing to prevent falls and to assure cleansing each area well. They either use a roll-in shower with a shower chair, or transfer to a bath bench with a back into the tub. They may use a hand-held shower and long-handled bath brushes to reach areas they cannot bend to reach. They probably will not be able to reach their buttocks well due to poor balance, and will also need assistance washing their feet. They should be able to shampoo their hair if well-supported on the bath bench or in the shower chair. Rinsing the soap out will be best done with a hand-held shower. Towels should be placed where they can stay dry but are still within the person's reach. Transfers are more complicated when one is wet, so drying off well is very important.

Mobility

Transfers

For the person with C-5 through C-6 quadriplegia, transferring or moving the body from one surface to another can require a tremendous amount of effort. Many persons at this level choose to rely on others to perform the total task for them due to the energy expenditure necessary for completion. In most cases, moderate assistance from another is needed for transferring to and from level surfaces. In transfers between positions of different heights, maximal to total assistance is required. A transfer board provides a smooth surface to slide across, which decreases resistance during the task.

Individuals with a level C-7 through C-8 injury can use a sliding board to transfer to and from the wheelchair. Eventually they may be able to transfer without the use of a transfer board. Removable armrests and footrests are essential for safe transferring for both the person and the assistant.

Manual Wheelchair

An individual with C-5 quadriplegia can be independent in wheelchair mobility over both level and uneven surfaces with a manual wheelchair. The wheelchair must be specifically measured to accommodate the body for proper support and function (see Figure 12). The wheelchair's back must be high enough to support the trunk, so arm function can be maximized. "Quad" rim projections are necessary to be able to push the wheelchair forward and in reverse. The scapular stabilizing musculature must be sufficiently strengthened so as not to over-stretch supporting shoulder structures. Some type of wrist stabilizing splints are usually used to enhance hand placement between the rim projections.

A grade aid (or hill climber), a secondary braking device, is recommended for propelling the wheelchair up an incline or ramp. The grade aid is mounted under the wheelchair brakes and is engaged by pushing the lever handle downward. The device lies on the surface of the tire, allowing the tire to be pushed forward. When the push stroke is completed the grade aid clutches the tire, preventing it from rolling in reverse, thereby maintaining the ground gained. When the incline or ramp has been climbed, the lever is pushed upward to disengage.

Brake extensions are also useful for providing a greater lever advantage to operate the wheelchair brakes. On lightweight model wheelchairs anti-tip bars are a safety option to consider should the person tend to be back heavy in the wheelchair. These bars prevent the wheelchair from tipping backwards on an uneven surface.

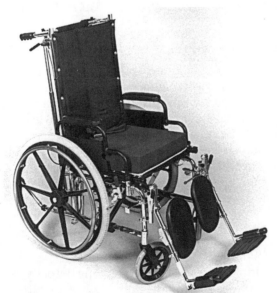

For some individuals with spinal cord injury, propelling the weight of a manual wheelchair takes too much effort, and endurance is compromised. Sometimes the slowness of the propulsion precludes functional mobility in the community or long-distance trips. Rough terrain, long distances, and/or shoulder pain challenge the person's

Figure 12. High-back reclining manual wheelchair for individuals with quadriplegia.

abilities and may necessitate a powered wheelchair. This may conserve energy and allow the individual greater mobility, as well as expand the opportunities for school or work. A manual wheelchair is usually purchased to serve as a back-up should mechanical failure of the powered wheelchair occur or transportation of the powered wheelchair not be achievable.

The individual with an injury at level C-7 through C-8 can be independent in mobility using a manual wheelchair. The wheelchair may have friction-coated hand rims to assist in propulsion. This person will still have difficulty pushing up steep inclines or over rough terrain but may begin to participate in wheelchair sports.

Motorized Wheelchair

A motorized wheelchair with a hand control is usually the mode of mobility for spinal cord–injured persons at the C-5 through C-6 level. The ease of powered mobility allows for the conservation of energy and the time efficiency needed for community accessibility. A person who uses a MAS needs extensive supervised practice initially to master driving a hand-controlled motorized wheelchair, due to the effects of the arm positioned in the orthosis while in motion. It is important to look for the position of the MAS that provides the greatest mechanical advantage.

The hand control must be adapted with an extended joystick to move the wheelchair effectively and safely. The wrist is stabilized with an orthosis or assistive device. A powered recliner interface may be a consideration for weight shifting, should the person be unable to lean side-to-side independently to relieve pressure.

Individuals with injuries at level C-7 through C-8 will be independent with powered mobility using a joystick for power control. Powered mobility conserves energy and allows the individuals to perform other independent living skills, such as dressing and vocational activities.

Community Transportation

New technology in adapted driving, including modified vans with low- or zero-effort steering and electric lifts, enables some persons with injuries at the C-7 through C-8 level to be independently mobile (see Figure 13). Some assistance is necessary for transfers, as the person usually drives from a motorized wheelchair that is stabilized to the floor with a 4-point electric tie-down system. Evaluation and supervised driver's training are critical to ensure safety. Those individuals unable to achieve this level of independence must rely on another person to drive. The individual with C-5 quadriplegia either can be transferred into the passenger seat of a van or have the wheelchair tied to the floor for transport safety. Whenever the van is in motion, the wheelchair seat belt, as well as the van safety restraint, should be fastened.

If the person does not own a van, he or she must be transferred into a car with assistance. The wheelchair is then loaded, either in the back flooring or in the trunk of the car by the caregiver. If a person uses a motorized wheelchair, loading is a very difficult and time consuming task due to the necessary dismantling and handling of the batteries. A manual wheelchair is usually used in this case, which may mean less function for the person once at the destination.

In some cities, van or bus service with modified lifts is available. If trunk balance is a problem, the use of a chest strap worn during public transportation assures upright sitting to counter the force of the motion. Wheelchair lifts on buses, para-transit, or agreements with cab companies will be more widely available due to the passage of the Americans with Disabilities Act. In one major city, the bus system recently converted an entire route, adding buses with lifts.

Figure 13. Driving controls in an adapted van.

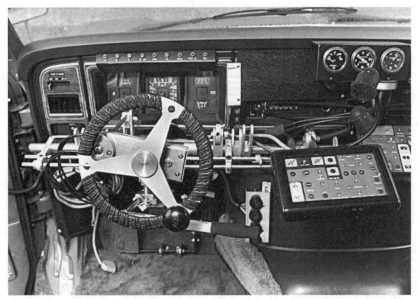

Persons with a C-7 through C-8 injury should be able to drive personal vehicles adapted with appropriate controls. Most should be able to transfer independently into a passenger car but will need assistance with wheelchair loading, car top loaders, or special lifts. Some of these individuals may choose to drive from their wheelchairs in a modified van. This will save energy but is more expensive. Regardless of the vehicle they drive, these individuals need adaptive steering devices, hand controls, and adaptations for secondary controls (such as turn signals and windshield wipers). Regardless of the position from which they drive, it is important that special attention be given to the appropriate securing system.

Dressing/Undressing

Upper Extremities

The individual with a C-5 spinal cord injury needs moderate assistance to dress upper extremities with pullover garments due to the inability to raise the arms functionally overhead and the lack of trunk stability. The person is able to assist in donning shirts and jackets by placing the arms through the sleeves in preparation. The garment must then be lifted overhead by a caregiver and pulled down over the trunk.

A person with C-5 spinal cord injury can use the around-the-back method of donning a front-fastening shirt or jacket with moderate assistance if he or she is sitting in a wheelchair or on an electric bed. Easy-to-reach enclosures, such as buttons or zippers, may be fastened by the individual with the use of a buttonhook-zipper pull device. Bras that either close in the front or use self-fastening closures can be donned by putting the thumb through sewn-in loops added to the garment. Many men will choose either to use a clip-on tie or to have the caregiver fasten a conventional tie. Most persons with spinal cord injury prefer to put on a shirt, tie, and jacket once seated in the wheelchair.

Lower Extremity

Due to the lack of bed mobility skills at the C-5 level, the person requires assistance in lower extremity dressing. Slacks and skirts cut slightly larger in the hips and with longer length are easier to put on and fit a person sitting in a wheelchair with flexed knees more precisely. Modified clothing is commercially available through catalogs (such as Avenues), and modified sewing patterns are available (through Simplicity) to assure a more functional fit for a person with a physical disability.

An exceptionally motivated individual with C-6 through C-8 quadriplegia may learn to complete both upper- and lower-extremity dressing without assistance. The rolling side-to-side method of dressing in bed is quite energy consuming, and many decide to save their efforts in favor of vocational or educational goals. Donning and doffing footwear will most likely require assistance, but may be achieved independently using specially adapted shoes.

Communication

Communication, whether it be written or oral, is critical for any person. It helps one stay in contact with others and complete home management educational or vocational tasks. Many adaptations can help to achieve these important activities.

Writing

Initially, devices to assist in writing, such as a MAS in conjunction with an electric prehension, reciprocal, or long opponens orthosis may be indicated. Most individuals gradually reduce the use of a MAS but continue to need a wrist stabilizing orthosis with an adaptation to hold a pen or pencil.

The first trials of writing will be very difficult, so it is advisable to have the person draw lines or circles. To ask the person to form letters or numbers at this time can lead to disappointment or frustration because of the unrefined arm movement. Assistive devices, such as a Wanchik writer (see Figure 14), a flexor hinge orthosis (see Figure 15), or a dorsal wrist cock-up splint with cuff can help to hold the wrist in a neutral position, as well as position the writing utensil. A Dycem pad is useful for holding the paper in place while writing. As arm control improves, letters and numbers may be attempted. At first the writing will be large and slow. Practice is the key to improving this skill.

Typing may be the choice of written communication for someone with this level of spinal cord injury due to its visual presentation. As in writing, initial attempts at typing may be frustrating if too much skill is called for before arm control is developed. The most efficient typing is achieved using either an electric typewriter or a computer. The wrists must be stabilized and a typing implement must be attached in order to depress the keys for typing. An automatic paper feeder on an electric typewriter is desired to assist in loading the paper. A continuous roll of computer paper is generally recommended for advancing from page to page. In most cases, another person must remove the typed text from the typewriter or computer printer to decrease the likelihood of tearing.

Typing can be used as an exercise for a MAS due to the fine control of the arm necessary to select exact keys to depress. Usually the person is asked to type each row of keys individually from right to left, left to right, then up and down, before actually typing words. Once control of arm placement is achieved, the individual can type words.

Telephone Use

Accessing a telephone is very important for continuing interaction with others in the community, emergency contacts, and managing life tasks. Several methods can be employed to achieve telephone access. Some choose to use a gooseneck stand to hold the telephone receiver to ear height while using a phone flipper (an extended lever) to depress

Figure 14. Wanchik device for daily living activities.

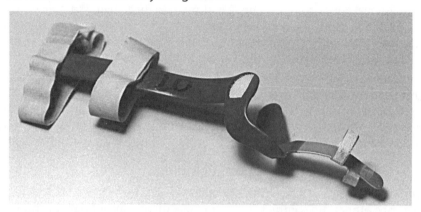

Figure 15. Flexor hinge/reciprocal orthosis.

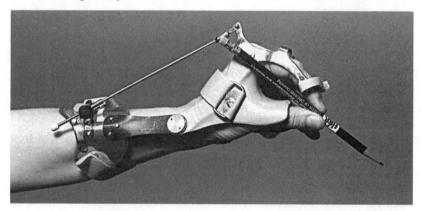

the switch hook connector on the phone base. This lever is lifted to obtain a dial tone or to receive a call when the phone rings. Most people using mobile arm supports employ this method, due to their inability to hold the receiver to the ear.

For those who have adequate arm strength to hold the receiver to the ear, a phone holder is added to the receiver to allow for handling. Depending on the skill of the individual, either a push button or rotary style phone may be used. Telephones that have the functions of automatic dialing, memory, or redial often increase efficiency. A speaker phone also decreases necessary hand function, although this interferes with privacy. A telephone with the dialing buttons on the receiver is usually not recommended, due to the increased hand function necessary to manipulate it.

For persons with a spinal cord injury at level C-6 through C-8, using the phone can be made easier with an adapted handset, universal cuff, or reciprocal used to press the buttons. In a vocational setting, ear phones or a headset can streamline the requirements of simultaneous note writing and phone use. Writing and typing are skills essential to independent living and handling one's own affairs, and many aids are available on the market. Most individuals with this level of spinal cord injury do not require wrist support and can don and doff a simple device without help. The same device selected to dial a phone can be utilized to type or use the computer. The wrist-driven orthosis gives dynamic grasp, which is useful for loading paper and computer disks, and for picking up and moving objects. Using a reciprocal may decrease the need for many other pieces of adapted equipment.

Bowel and Bladder Management

Persons with a spinal cord injury at level C-5 require assistance in bowel and bladder care due to the lack of hand function and body positioning necessary for completion. The person with C-5 quadriplegia should verbally be able to direct bowel and bladder care, particularly if subject to dysreflexia. Accurate and timely direction and instruction reduce the risk of a potentially life-threatening event.

An individual with C-5 quadriplegia may be able to empty his or her legbag with the use of either a manual pneumatic legbag clamp or an electric legbag emptier. The emptying clamp is released by a switch that the person can access easily. The legbag may be emptied into a floor basin or cat litter box, or onto grass. The automatic legbag emptier must be mounted onto the wheelchair. Gravity assists in draining urine from the tubing.

Proper food intake regulate waste elimination. Foods with a proper balance of fiber, nutrients, and liquids aid bladder and bowel regulation.

For the person with C-6 through C-7 quadriplegia, self-catheterization may be facilitated with bilateral reciprocal orthoses. However, the need to manage clothes and transfer may not make this activity functional on an every-4-hour basis. The individual who must rely on him- or herself is usually more motivated to develop the fine motor skills necessary to manage bowel and bladder care. Practicing fine motor skills such as sewing, lacing, and writing facilitate the problem-solving necessary to successfully complete a clean, safe, self-catheterization.

Persons with spinal cord injuries at levels C-7 through C-8 need assistance managing a regular bowel program due to difficulty with body positioning. However they should understand the bowel program thoroughly and be able to give the caregiver specific directions. Two examples of devices for bowel management are illustrated in Figure 16. The individual may be able to manage an intermittent catheterization program if he or she can self-position appropriately, either in the wheelchair or in bed. He or she should be able to empty the legbag with minimal adaptations. A woman with this level of injury should be able to position a sanitary napkin appropriately when dressing, but will have difficulty inserting a tampon.

Self-care is a tedious and demanding regimen for an individual with a spinal cord injury, involving tasks that are often difficult and frustrating to master. Support, humor, praise, and practice are the therapists' tools to encourage the patient to reach his or her maximum potential of independent living.

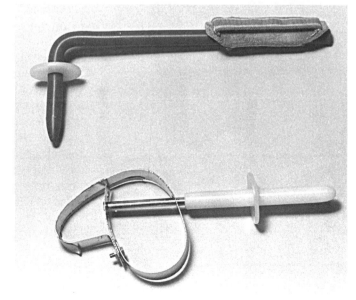

Figure 16. Bowel management devices.

Paraplegia: Levels T-1 Through T-6

The muscles of the trunk and thorax have their roots from T-1 to L-4. They include the intercostals (T-1 through T-10), serratus posterior superior (T-1 through T-4), rectus abdominis and external oblique abdominis (T-5 through T-12), transverse abdominis (T-7 through L-1), internal oblique abdominis (T-8 through L-1), serratus posterior inferior (T-9 through T-12), and quadratus lumborum (T-12 through L-4). In general, they are responsible for elevation and depression of the ribs during respiration, contraction of the abdomen, and anterolateral flexion of the trunk.

Individuals with a spinal cord injury at the T-1 through T-6 level have full use of their upper extremities and should be able to live independently in a wheelchair-accessible environment. Although breathing improves at this level, trunk balance is still compromised and therefore appropriate safety precautions should be implemented. The wheelchair is the primary mode for mobility, although ambulation may be encouraged for exercise purposes (Hoppenfeld, 1977).

Eating and Meal Preparation

Persons with a T-1 through T-6 spinal cord injury can eat and prepare meals without assistance. They have full function of the upper extremities, but have impairments in trunk control and, therefore, balance. Mealtime skills including cutting, drinking, and hand-to-mouth eating can be performed without assistance as long as there is a supportive surface from which to eat (see Figure 17). This person has no difficulty taking medications independently, as long as the medications are stored at a height that is within reach from a wheelchair.

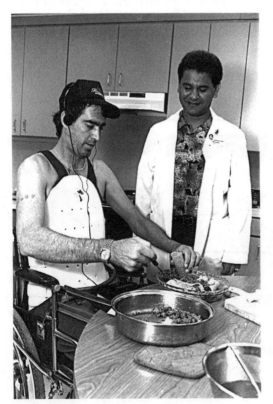

Meal preparation may require some adaptive devices or modifications due to poor trunk balance. The area for food preparation, whether the kitchen or another area set up with accessible appliances, needs to be wheelchair accessible. Lowered counter tops or work surfaces are essential to provide support for the person while preparing the meal without putting him- or herself at risk by compromising balance. A mirror over a standard range is helpful for seeing inside of the pans and avoiding touching hot areas that are not visible from the wheelchair level. It is important to consider the accessibility of the oven and the refrigerator from the wheelchair. Usually a side approach is best for securing items from each, as well as for maintaining balance. Dishes, glasses, and cooking pans

Figure 17. Meal preparation by the individual with paraplegia: Level T-6.

are most accessible if located at a level no higher than the shoulders. These few adjustments to the kitchen allow the person with this level of injury to function without assistance in meal preparation and eating skills.

Sink Hygiene and Grooming

Persons with a T-1 through T-6 level injury are able to perform sink hygiene if the sink and the faucets are within reach from the wheelchair. Items for brushing teeth, brushing or combing hair, and shaving or applying makeup need to be stored at an accessible level. The mirror may need to be repositioned to be fully visualized. The rack for the towels and wash cloths may need to be lowered to make these things accessible.

Bathing

The person with this level of injury needs some adaptations to accomplish bathing. Utilization of a shower commode chair in a roll-in shower probably provides the optimum level of independent functioning for bathing. The person could use a bathtub bench seat with a back, if able to transfer into the tub independently. Assistance may be needed for transfers when the person is wet. A hand-held shower allows for greatest independence in showering. There may be some difficulty reaching the buttocks and lower back for cleansing; however, long-handled sponges or brushes should allow access as long as the person can anchor him- or herself to maintain balance. Hair washing is best done when the person is supported in the shower or tub. He or she will be able to wash, rinse, and style hair appropriately, but may tire due to the excessive use of the arms above the head and the struggle to keep balanced.

Mobility

Persons with this level of paraplegia have the arm strength to transfer independently; however, transfer independence is complicated by body weight and height, transfer surfaces, position of the wheelchair, and general endurance level. Extremes in weight and height, in combination with the poor trunk control, may complicate independent transfer enough for these persons to choose to obtain assistance with this task. Transfers into and out of the car may be the activity for which assistance is frequently requested. Spasticity and muscle tone can be helpful in some instances or compromise transfer safety in others.

Mobility is usually independent from a manual wheelchair. The wheelchair should be lightweight and its back height should be just below the scapula. Armrests and footrests should be removable to allow for maximal independence (see Figures 18a & 18b). Some persons with T-1 through T-4 injuries eventually may choose to use a powered wheelchair to save energy and time.

Persons with this level of injury are able to drive using hand controls, a steering knob, and an emergency brake extension in either a car or a van (see Figure 19). The decision about the type of vehicle will be determined by the person's transfer skill and overall endurance. Transferring independently into a car is possible, but it requires additional energy to load the wheelchair. Some may chose to use a wheelchair loading device or to drive a van. If the person decides to drive a van, he or she should transfer from the wheelchair to the captain's chair to drive safely.

Dressing

Individuals with a T-1 through T-6 injury can dress without personal assistance. Dressing loops and larger-sized clothing enhance lower extremity dressing independence. These

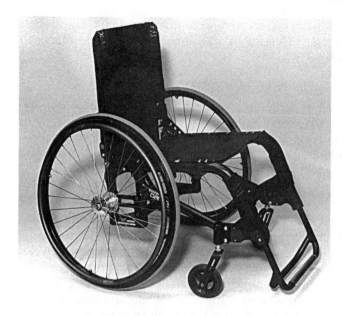

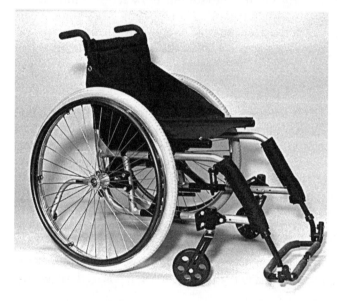

Figures 18a and 18b. Manual wheelchairs for individuals with paraplegia.

individuals do not require assistance in upper extremity dressing but may have to use the support of the bed or wheelchair to maintain balance. Shoes and socks can be put on independently if there is good hip range of motion and little interference from spasms.

Communication

These individuals are able to use telephones that are at a wheelchair-accessible height. They are also independent in all other communication skills, such as typing and writing. Computers can be easily accessed by these individuals, utilizing either a standard keyboard or mouse options.

Bowel and Bladder

Men are able to apply an external catheter and, if utilizing an intermittent catheterization program, can do it independently. Women with a T-1 through T-6 injury can catheterize, but need special positioning for the legs, and, possibly, adaptive equipment. Bowel program management is accomplished independently by utilizing suppositories. Again, positioning may be the one area requiring assistance. Women can place sanitary napkins independently, but may need a mirror and an adaptive device to help position their legs when inserting a tampon.

Paraplegia: Levels T-7 Through S-5

For the individual with paraplegia affecting levels T-7 through S-5, upper extremity and thoracic function are intact, enhancing trunk stability, wheelchair sitting balance, and transfers. Functional ambulation with long leg braces and crutches is possible below level T-8. The paraplegic person with a spinal cord injury at level L-4 through S-2 can ambulate with short leg braces and forearm crutches.

Figure 19. Adapted vehicle with hand controls.

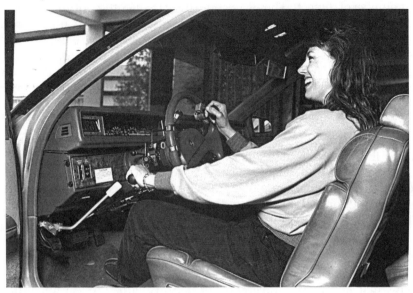

Functionally, these individuals are independent in self-care, although they may use some adapted equipment for energy conservation, efficiency, and maximum control. One of the primary concerns, however, is preventing secondary complications of the spinal cord injury. These include urinary tract infections and pressure ulcers (Pearman, 1985; Turner, 1985). Although management of these potentially serious problems is usually addressed during the initial rehabilitation, once the person returns to the community, family, employment, or school, secondary complications are often ignored or neglected until the situation reaches a crisis level. Persons who return to outpatient clinics at facilities where they originally were rehabilitated are reeducated about effective infection-free bladder management and skin care. Often, equipment such as new wheelchair cushions or wheelchairs is recommended.

Equipment: From Tradition to High Technology

The appropriate prescription of upper-extremity assistive devices is a major focus during the rehabilitation of persons with spinal cord injury. Until recently, little was reported in the literature about the use of the many devices prescribed during rehabilitation once the patient returned to family, community, and employment. In 1990, Garber and Gregorio reported the results of their study that identified the utilization of, and satisfaction with, devices prescribed to persons with quadriplegia secondary to spinal cord injury during initial rehabilitation. The first part of the study focused on categorizing devices and describing the frequency with which they had been prescribed to a population of 56 persons with spinal cord injury and resultant quadriplegia. The device categories included feeding (71%), splints and slings (79%), dressing (29%), hygiene/grooming (23%), communication (41%), and miscellaneous (23%) (Garber & Gregorio, 1990). They found that 54% of the devices prescribed were still in use 1 year after discharge from the rehabilitation hospital, representing a significant decline in use ($p = .001$). Furthermore, by the end of the second year following discharge, only 35% of all prescribed devices were still in use ($p = .01$).

Feeding devices and the splints and slings categories were prescribed most often for the largest number of subjects. These categories most frequently continued to be used, and include the more expensive devices (Garber & Gregorio, 1990). In contrast, dressing and hygiene devices were prescribed for the fewest number of subjects and, in combination with the miscellaneous device category, represented the greatest decline in use. The investigators concluded that although the most frequently discarded items were low-cost, therapists must identify ways to prescribe only the most necessary equipment. One approach would be to provide devices to patients during their rehabilitation hospitalization but wean them from those devices prior to discharge.

Advances in technology pervade every aspect of daily life and have a major impact on the quality of life for persons with spinal cord injury. From the automatic teller machines in banks to voice-activated telephone systems, technology often provides unique and dynamic solutions to otherwise insoluble problems. For the person with a spinal cord injury, technology expands opportunities for independence and productivity.

In the early 1970s, the U.S. government demonstrated its commitment to improving the vocational and self-care goals of persons with severe physical impairments through the establishment of rehabilitation engineering centers. These centers combined the efforts of medicine, engineering, and related sciences to identify practical solutions to problems that limited the integration of persons with physical impairments into productive community life (Traub & LeClair, 1975).

In 1988, with the passage of the Technology-Related Assistance for Individuals With Disabilities Act (Public Law 100-407), the U.S. government further demonstrated its support for the development and utilization of technological systems and devices that would enhance the outcome of rehabilitation of persons with severe physical disabilities. Assistive technology, then, has become the byword of the 1990s for consumers and health care providers alike. Assistive technology is defined as "any item, piece of equipment or product system, off-the-shelf, modified, or customized that is used to increase, maintain or improve function" (Public Law 100-407). It consists of both high and low technology that includes, but is not limited to, environmental control units, computer access systems, augmentative communication devices, and mobility and seating systems.

Occupational therapists have a prominent role in the assistive technology clinics that operate in many rehabilitation facilities or are established in the private sector. Occupational therapists evaluate each person with spinal cord injury and other neuromuscular and musculoskeletal dysfunction for the potential to use technology to enhance and expand the skills needed to be more independent in self-care, return to school, or become involved. The occupational therapist, as part of the assistive technology team, makes recommendations and trains these individuals to use technology to achieve maximum potential (Mann & Lane, 1991).

Technology changes at an extraordinarily rapid rate. Occupational therapists keep pace through their attendance at training courses, conferences, and special academic programs in rehabilitation technology. As an area of specialization, assistive technology is still in its infancy. Yet it provides occupational therapists with the opportunity to utilize their training and experience in evaluating and recommending devices that maximize ability in the patients they serve.

A number of robotic devices have been developed and evaluated at rehabilitation centers in the United States, Canada, and England (Glass & Hall, 1987). Their primary purpose is to help persons with very limited upper-extremity function perform daily living and vocational activities. This technology has the potential to reduce dependency on full-time attendant care and provide the person with severe physical impairment with a mechanism of control.

Most of the robotic systems are voice-activated and microprocessor-based. They are usually mounted either on a work station or on the wheelchair. Therapists and patients reported favorable experiences with robotic systems, and several systems are being modified to render them more functional. However, financing the purchase of robotic systems still presents a major impediment to acquisition.

In the future, acceptance and use of robotic systems will depend on several factors. Because a robotic system can cost in excess of $25,000, cost-benefit analyses must be done. The systems' reliability and durability must be determined to assess how many hours the physically disabled person could depend on it and not on attendant care. Another factor is its acceptance by the health care professional, who must learn the system and transmit the crucial information to the consumer. It has been estimated that the care of a person with quadriplegia, including attendant care, approaches $50,000 per year (Hammel et al., 1989). Advances in robotic technology can provide opportunities for new levels of self-care, independence, and employment. More importantly, robotic technology can return a measure of personal autonomy that until recently was only imagined.

Summary

Few fields in medicine are changing more rapidly than occupational therapy. The impact of high technology has not yet been fully realized, but it must be anticipated. It is apparent that systems and devices that maximize functional potential will continue to be a major concern in the rehabilitation of individuals with spinal cord injuries. With the explosive expansion of electronic technology, microprocessor-controlled preprogrammed "smart" devices are forthcoming in the areas of wheelchair mobility, environmental control, adapted driving, and vocational training (Seplowitz, 1984; Youdin, Dickey, Sell, & Stratford, 1980). The area of technological innovation presents new challenges to occupational therapists on the rehabilitation team because their specialty remains one of flexible adaptation to patient needs.

References

Burke, D.C., & Murray, D. D. (1975). *Handbook of spinal cord medicine*. London: MacMillan.

Chusid, J.G. (1985). *Correlative neuroanatomy and functional neurology* (18th ed.) (pp. 134–161, 200–221). Los Altos, CA: Lange.

Clifton, G.L., Donovan, W.H., & Frankowski, R.F. (1985). Patterns of care for the patient with spinal cord injury. *Current Concepts in Rehabilitation Medicine, 2*, 14–17.

Diasio, K. (1971). Occupational therapy—A historic perspective: The modern era—1960–1970. *American Journal of Occupational Therapy, 25*, 237–242.

Dorland's medical dictionary. (1962). (20th ed.). Philadelphia: W.B. Saunders.

Farmer, A.R. (1986). Dressing. In J.P. Hill (Ed.), *Spinal cord injury—A guide to functional outcomes in occupational therapy* (pp. 125–143). Rockville, MD: Aspen Publishers.

Fine, P.R., Kuhlemeier, K.V., & Stover, S.L. (1979). Spinal cord injury: An epidemiology perspective. *Paraplegia, 17*, 237.

Garber, S.L. (1985). New perspectives for the occupational therapist in the treatment of spinal cord–injured individuals. *American Journal of Occupational Therapy, 39*, 703–704.

Garber, S.L., & Gregorio, T.L. (1990). Upper extremity assistive devices: Assessment of use by spinal cord–injured patients with quadriplegia. *American Journal of Occupational Therapy, 44*, 126–131.

Garber, S.L., Lathem, P., & Gregorio, T.L. (1988). *Specialized occupational therapy for persons with high level quadriplegia*. Monograph funded in part by Grant No. G009300044 from the National Institute on Disability and Rehabilitation Research, (NIDRR), U. S. Department of Education, awarded to the Research and Training Center for the Rehabilitation of Persons with Spinal Cord Dysfunction at Baylor College of Medicine and The Institute for Rehabilitation and Research (TIRR).

Glass, K., & Hall, K. (1987). Occupational therapists' views about the use of robotic aids for people with disabilities. *American Journal of Occupational Therapy, 41*, 745–747.

Guttman, L. (1976). *Spinal cord injuries: Comprehensive management and research* (2nd ed.). Boston, MA: Blackwell Scientific.

Hammel, J., Hall, K., Lees, D., Leifer, L., Van der Loos, M., Perkash, I., & Crigler, R. (1989). Clinical evaluation of a desktop robotic assistant. *Journal of Rehabilitation Research & Development, 26*, 1–6.

Hoppenfeld, S. (1977). *Orthopaedic neurology—A diagnostic guide to neurological levels*. Philadelphia: Lippincott.

Kovich, K., & Presperin, J. (1986). Communication. In J.P. Hill (Ed.), *Spinal cord injury—A guide to functional outcomes in occupational therapy* (pp. 95–108). Rockville, MD: Aspen Publishers.

Kraus, J.F., Franti, C.E., Riggins, R.S., Richards, D., & Borhani, N.O. (1975). Incidence of traumatic spinal cord lesions. *Journal of Chronic Disease, 28*, 471–492.

Lathem, P., Gregorio, T.L., & Garber, S.L. (1985). High-level quadriplegia: An occupational therapy challenge. *American Journal of Occupational Therapy, 39*, 705–714.

Lindberg, A. (1976). Occupational therapy. In W.M. Jenkens, R.M. Anderson, & W.L. Dietrich (Eds.), *Rehabilitation of the severely disabled* (pp. 191–194). Dubuque, IA: Kendall/Hunt.

Mann, W.C., & Lane, J.P. (1991). *Assistive technology for persons with disabilities: The role of occupational therapy*. Rockville, MD: American Occupational Therapy Association.

Monroe, D. (1943). Cervical cord injuries: Study of 101 cases. *New England Journal of Medicine, 229*, 919–033.

Mosey, A.C. (1971). Occupational therapy—A historic perspective: Involvement in the rehabilitation movement—1942–1966. *American Journal of Occupational Therapy, 25*, 234–236.

Pearman, J.W. (1985). Prevention and management of infection—The urinary tract. In G.M. Bedbrook (Ed.), *Lifetime care of the paraplegic patient* (pp. 54–65). Edinburgh: Churchill Livingstone.

Reilly, M. (1971). Occupational therapy—A historic perspective. The modernization of occupational therapy. *American Journal of Occupational Therapy, 25*, 243–246.

Scott, S.J. (1984). The medicare prospective payment system. *American Journal of Occupational Therapy, 38*, 330–334.

Seplowitz, C. (1984). Technology and occupational therapy in the rehabilitation of the bedridden quadriplegic. *American Journal of Occupational Therapy, 38*, 743–747.

Sharrard, W.J.W. (1964). The segmental innervation of the lower limb muscles in man. *Annals of the Royal College of Surgeons of England, 35*, 106–122.

Spackman, C.S. (1968). A history of the practice of occupational therapy for restoration of physical function: 1917–1967. *American Journal of Occupational Therapy, 22,* 67–71.

Stover, S.L., & Fine, P.R. (1986). *Spinal cord injury: The facts and figures.* Birmingham, AL: The University of Alabama at Birmingham.

Traub, J.E., & LeClair, R.R. (1975). The rehabilitation engineering program. *American Rehabilitation, 1*(2), 3–7.

Trombly, C.A. (1989). Spinal cord injury. In C.A. Trombly (Ed.), *Occupational therapy for physical dysfunction* (3rd ed.) (pp. 555–570). Baltimore: Williams & Wilkins.

Turner, A.N. (1985). Prevention of tertiary complications and management—Decubiti. In G.M. Bedbrook (Ed.), *Lifetime care of the paraplegic patient* (pp. 54–65). Edinburgh: Churchill Livingstone.

Youdin, M., Dickey, R.E., Sell, G.H., & Stratford, C.D. (1980). Instrumentation for the severely disabled: An update. *Model Systems Spinal Cord Injury Digest, 2,* 16–24.

Young, J.S., Burns, P.E., Bowen, A.M., & McCutchen, R. (1982). *Spinal cord injury statistics.* Phoenix: Good Samaritan Medical Center.

8

Self-Care Strategies Following Stroke

Kathleen Okkema

Kathleen Okkema, MBA, OTR/L, practices in Harvard, IL.

Chapter 8 Outline

Medical and Functional Problems Associated With Stroke

Prognosis

Precautions

Age-Related Changes

> Predictors of Successful Outcome

Case Descriptions

Assessment of Self-Care Skills of the Stroke Patient

Psychosocial Factors

Specialized Evaluations

> Assessment of Dysphagia

> Driving Assessment

> Work Assessment

Treatment Approaches

Compensation Techniques and Contextual Training

Case Descriptions of Treatment

> Rose

> Carmen

Remediation Techniques

Discharge Planning

References

Occupational therapy treatment for stroke survivors is a challenge. Not only does each individual have unique interests, roles, coping skills, and prestroke capabilities, but the deficits resulting from the stroke vary tremendously from one person to another. The therapist must use sophisticated problem-solving abilities to help the patient set meaningful, role-appropriate, and achievable goals, given the many changes in motor, cognitive, and perceptual status that may occur. This chapter emphasizes treatment principles to enhance independence in self-care for stroke survivors exhibiting a variety of interests, physical abilities, and cognitive/perpetual skills. Two case studies illustrate the described principles.

This chapter presents definitions of major medical and functional sequelae of stroke, and descriptions of the pros and cons of various treatment procedures, including contextual training, restorative approaches, and compensation. Specific techniques that may be helpful in ADL training are also presented. Using the problem-solving approach to treatment of the stroke survivor is emphasized.

Medical and Functional Problems Associated With Stroke

Approximately 400,000 people have a cerebral vascular accident (CVA) each year (Roth, 1988). A stroke results from a disruption of the blood supply to the brain. In approximately 75% of strokes the interruption of blood supply is caused by thrombosis, or narrowing of an artery (Roth). Embolism, the blockage of an artery due to a traveling mass, and hemorrhage, the rupture of a blood vessel, also commonly cause strokes. High blood pressure, high cholesterol levels leading to atherosclerosis, cigarette smoking, and diabetes increase the risk of a cerebral vascular accident (Garrison, Rolak, Dodaro, & O'Callaghan, 1988).

Both cerebral hemorrhages and subarachnoid hemorrhages result when a blood vessel in the brain ruptures. Like an embolism or thrombosis, a hemorrhage disrupts blood supply. In addition, blood flows into the surrounding brain tissue and eventually clots. The pressure the clot exerts can compress nearby blood vessels, leading to further cell death. While occlusion of a blood vessel results in localized symptoms, a hemorrhage produces more diffuse brain damage.

Knowledge of common symptoms associated with various lesion sites can help the therapist anticipate possible problems. Although individual variations in the extent and location of the lesion, as well as neuroanatomical differences between each person, will result in a unique presentation, the therapist's evaluation can be tailored to detect the most common symptoms associated with the location of brain injury. A summary of symptoms that correlate with damage to the major arteries of the brain follows.

Middle Cerebral Artery: Approximately 85% of strokes are due to thrombotic or embolic occlusion of this vessel (Roth, 1988). Symptoms include contralateral hemiplegia, with the upper extremity more involved than the lower extremity; hemisensory loss; and hemianopsia.

Dominant Hemisphere Lesion: Expressive and/or receptive aphasia, apraxia, and astereognosis are found (Chusid, 1973).

Nondominant Hemisphere Lesion: Damage results in visual spatial deficits, impaired body awareness, and visual construction deficits (Easton, 1981).

Internal Carotid Artery: The patient exhibits a combination of the problems associated with anterior, middle, and, at times, posterior cerebral artery occlusion, including hemiplegia, unilateral sensory loss, and aphasia if the dominant hemisphere is affected (Chusid, 1973).

Anterior Cerebral Artery: Frontal lobe functions, such as behavioral control, arousal, and attention, may be diminished. Contralateral hemiplegia with the lower extremity more involved than the upper extremity, mild contralateral sensory loss predominantly in the lower extremity, urinary incontinence, gait apraxia, and akinetic mutism may also be noted (Easton, 1981).

Posterior Cerebral Artery: Contralateral hemiplegia, hemianesthesia, and homonymous hemianopsia may result.

Dominant Hemisphere Lesion: Aphasia occurs.

Nondominant Hemisphere Lesion: Visual spatial deficits are found (Chusid, 1973).

Bilateral Hemispheric Involvement: Results in bilateral hemianopsia, cortical blindness with denial of visual disturbance, and amnesia (Easton, 1981).

Brainstem Involvement: The patient demonstrates contralateral hemiplegia, contralateral ataxia, and a contralateral increase in the pain and temperature threshold. When pain and temperature stimuli are strong enough to be detected, the sensation is unpleasant (Easton, 1981).

Vertebrobasilar Artery: Cranial nerve palsy; unilateral or bilateral motor, sensory, or cerebellar signs; nystagmus; and/or coma may result (Easton, 1981).

Lacunar Infarct: Some strokes are not the result of occlusion of an entire branch of an artery, but rather are due to lesions in small vessels near the end of the arterial course. These are called *lacunar strokes* and affect a relatively small segment of the brain. Nineteen percent of cerebral infarctions can be characterized as lacunar strokes (Miller, 1983). In contrast to the multitude of symptoms that may result from large vessel occlusion, one or two striking features are evident. These features have been used to classify four lacunar syndromes. A pure motor stroke results in hemiplegia, a pure sensory stroke leads to paresthesia, while ataxic hemiparesis leads to hemiparesis and ipsilateral ataxia. The fourth syndrome, dysarthria and clumsy hand syndrome, are self-descriptive (Miller) in that they result in difficulty with speech and fine motor incoordination of the upper extremity. Because lacunar syndromes result in motor and sensory changes without cognitive deficits, patients are capable of participating fully in their therapy and can be expected to reach a high level of independence.

Prognosis

Patients frequently show spontaneous recovery during the first 2 months following stroke, due to the reabsorption of edema. However, many patients continue to show functional gains for several years (Bach-y-Rita, 1980). Therapeutic treatment can influence the recovery process. As the therapist provides encouragement and helps the patient choose activities based on the patient's interests, skill develops. Neuronal sprouting and unmasking are two mechanisms that may contribute to recovery following a CVA. Central nervous system neurons sprout new dendrites in response to functional demands, and previously suppressed neural pathways may become "unmasked," taking over some of the jobs previously performed by the damaged areas (Bach-y-Rita, 1981). Women and left-handed people often have more generalized neural pathways and may be better able to find a substitute way to accomplish an activity following a stroke. Motivation, age, sex, handedness, lesion location, intelligence, and participation in structured treatment influence these neural changes (Moore, 1990).

Precautions

The therapist must be conscious of precautions pertinent to each patient. Cardiac problems including hypertension, coronary artery disease, and congestive heart failure, often are associated with stroke (Roth, 1988). It is important that the therapist review the patient's chart, understand emergency procedures, and discuss any concerns with the physician prior to engaging the client in strenuous activity. Physicians can routinely provide parameters for heart rate and blood pressure for at-risk patients. These patients then must be monitored prior to, during, and after activity to determine whether the activity is too stressful. It should be realized that isometric, heavily resistive, and overhead activities increase cardiac stress and should be carefully monitored or avoided, depending on the patient's cardiac status. In addition, community activities in extremely cold or hot weather should be postponed.

Dysphagia often accompanies stroke and may affect as many as one-third of the patients (Roth, 1988). If the patient has swallowing difficulties, the therapist must follow dietary guidelines. These may range from no food or liquid by mouth, to restrictions in texture or liquidity. Confused patients who are not able to manage thin liquids must be carefully supervised so they don't accidently ingest water during oral facial hygiene. The use of commercially available thickening agents is recommended for appropriate patients.

When a patient uses specialized medical equipment, the therapist must be familiar with the equipment's operation and precautions. A patient using intravenous (IV) fluids or a gastrostomy tube must be monitored to ensure that the tubing is not disrupted during activity. The therapist should know when gastrostomy feedings are given, since the patient must be maintained in an upright position (at least 45°) generally for 1 hour following meals. This prevents back flow of the feeding, which can lead to aspiration pneumonia.

Patients with respiratory problems should not be exposed to noxious fumes, excessive dust, or pollutants. Therefore, caution should be exercised to ensure that the work and recreational environments used during therapy do not put the patient at unnecessary risk.

Clients with balance deficits must not be left alone in a potentially unsafe position. Safety belts should be used in wheelchairs and on the toilet if sitting balance or judgment is impaired. A gait belt may be useful when transferring, standing, or walking with a patient. Brakes on the wheelchair, bed, or other unstable items should be locked prior to a transfer.

Elderly patients frequently have some degree of joint damage. Those who have had hip replacements should avoid adduction and internal rotation of the hip. Proper alignment of all joints must be maintained during self-care and passive range of motion to avoid impingement and injury to internal tissues. The affected shoulder is particularly vulnerable to injury following stroke. Optimally, the patient should be taught to position the affected arm correctly during all tasks. When the patient is unable to position the arm safely, the therapist can assist the patient by placing the arm on a stable surface, or by providing manual guidance to help incorporate the limb during activity. As a last resort, static support may be provided by using a sling during stressful activities if injury may otherwise result. The use of a Harris hemisling, an arm trough, or a lapboard can be effective in correcting subluxation (Brooke, deLateur, Diana-Rigby, & Questad, 1991). However, care in fitting by an experienced therapist is an important factor in the use of these devices. All caregivers must be careful to avoid pulling on the affected arm and should mobilize the scapula before attempting overhead movement of a spastic arm. The therapist should be alert for signs of shoulder-hand syndrome, or reflex sympathetic dystrophy, which include: (a) swelling of the hand; (b) trophic changes, including altered skin color, nail appearance, sweating or hair growth; and (c) pain at rest or upon motion, especially during metacarpal phalangeal (MP) and shoulder flexion, abduction, and/or external rotation (Eto, Yoshikawa, Ueda, & Hirai, 1980).

Patients with cognitive and perceptual problems involved in activities that pose potential danger require careful supervision. Confused patients or those with motor planning deficits may try to drink shaving lotion, shave their eyebrows, eat lipstick, or reach beyond their balance point. Visual perceptual disturbances may result in a finger that is dangerously close to a knife. Patients with unilateral or left-sided neglect offer particular challenges and must be trained to compensate for their visual field loss. Butter and Kirsch (1992) have reported that the use of monocular eye patching (wearing an opaque patch over the right eye) combined with lateralized visual stimulation is effective and may be more beneficial than the use of trained scanning techniques for generalizing to daily living skills. Those with impaired attention may stand when it is unsafe to do so, fail to survey the street adequately prior to crossing, or be unaware of obstacles and hazards, such as a hot burner. Although the therapist gradually challenges the patient and reduces structure in the therapy setting, he or she must first ensure the patient's safety.

Age-Related Changes

Age-related changes combine with the effects of the stroke and make rehabilitation efforts more complex. Visual acuity may decline due to cataracts or glaucoma, color discrimination may decrease as changes in the lens cast a yellow hue on all that is seen, and sensitivity to glare may occur (Christenson, 1990). Decreased auditory discrimination can make noisy environments very distracting and can reduce the ability to hear high-frequency sounds, such as a high-pitched voice (Christenson). Balance and strength also decrease with age, making falls in the elderly a common problem. Coupled with osteoporosis, falls can result in fractures of weakened bones.

Predictors of Successful Outcome

Recent studies (Granger, Hamilton, & Gresham, 1988; Granger, Hamilton, Gresham, & Kramer, 1989) have attempted to determine the factors associated with favorable outcome following stroke. These studies have shown that 80% of stroke survivors will be able to attain independence in mobility, while 67% will attain independence in activities of daily living (ADL). Independence in bowel control, eating, grooming, and bladder control have a cumulative influence on predicting the ability of a survivor to live independently in the community following discharge. Davidoff, Keren, Ring, and Solzi (1991) found that patients receiving inpatient rehabilitation services were able to maintain the gains in functional independence a year following discharge, and that outpatient therapy services permitted further gains, particularly in patients with unilateral neglect, impaired joint position sense, urinary incontinence, or complete upper or lower extremity hemiplegia.

Bernspång, Viitanen, and Eriksson (1988) found that even several years after a stroke, visual and visuo-perceptual deficits were more significant than motor impairment in determining the extent to which survivors could manage self-care requirements. The authors speculate that it may be easier for individuals to compensate for motor impairment than for perceptual limitations.

Social factors are also important to satisfactory outcome. Evans, Bishop, and Haselkorn (1991) found that patients at risk for less-than-optimal home care had caregivers who were more likely to be depressed, had a below-average knowledge of stroke care principles, and had a greater incidence of family dysfunction.

Case Descriptions

The following case histories present a variety of concepts important to care of individuals undergoing treatment for a stroke. Different evaluation approaches, goals, and treatment techniques are used, based on the individual's background, coping style, and the unique challenges imposed by the stroke. Two stroke survivors are described on the following pages. Throughout the remainder of the chapter, evaluation and treatment principles are illustrated based on these case descriptions.

Case Study 1.

Rose is a 68-year-old woman who, prior to her stroke, lived with her daughter in a bi-level home in the city. She helped with meal preparation, cooking, and light cleaning. She took pride in her appearance and enjoyed talking with her family, attending church services, and playing with her great-grandchildren. Most of her leisure time was spent watching television, although occasionally she knit small gifts for her family. She had not completed high school and throughout her life had viewed herself primarily as a mother and a homemaker.

Two weeks prior to admission to the rehabilitation hospital, Rose had a right fronto-parietal CVA, with resulting left hemiplegia and 7th cranial nerve paralysis. Computerized tomography (CT) scans showed a right parietal image consistent with multiple infarcts. She had additional medical problems of obesity, severe dysphagia, hypertension, and insulin dependent diabetes mellitus (IDDM).

Although their relationship had not always been smooth, Rose's daughter felt strongly about caring for her mother at home. She stated her willingness to learn all that was necessary and requested the assistance of a personal care assistant upon her mother's discharge. Her main concerns centered on home accessibility, learning how to perform basic care, and positioning her mother safely and comfortably.

Rose's initial occupational therapy evaluation revealed severe limitations in all self-care activities and in cognitive, perceptual, and motor component skills. She was dependent in all basic self-care except washing her face, which required moderate assistance. She had deficits in arousal, attention, orientation, memory, safety awareness, error recognition, frustration tolerance, initiation, and the ability to follow simple commands. She was unable to attend to visual or tactile information left of midline. Consequently, body scheme was impaired, and she could locate her left arm only with constant verbal cues and physical assistance. Rose was unable to participate in formal visual perceptual testing; however, severe deficits in visual spatial organization were seen in simple daily living tasks.

Her right upper extremity (RUE) was functional; however, no active movement was seen in the left upper extremity (LUE), and a moderate amount of spasticity was present in a flexor synergy pattern. Due to obesity, lack of left-side motor function, and poor body awareness, she was unable to move in bed effectively and required a Hoyer lift and the assistance of two people for transfers. She could not sit unsupported, and when in a wheelchair, she used her right arm to push herself toward the left side, quickly losing midline orientation. Her head was oriented to the right, and tightness in the neck muscles was noted.

Case Study 2.

Carmen is a 24-year-old bilingual mother of a 3-year-old child. She had formerly worked in a factory, packing and folding items for shipment. She lived with her mother, her sister, and her son in a second-floor walk-up apartment. She had been very involved in her church and enjoyed making decorations for religious celebrations. She also liked to shop, watch TV, and visit with friends. Her family is very supportive and they willingly assist with child care and homemaking tasks. Prior to her stroke, Carmen was responsible for cooking several meals a week, making her bed, cleaning the apartment with other family members, and caring for her son.

Carmen had an Arterial Venous Malformation (AVM) resulting in a left parietal CVA with right hemiplegia and aphasia. She had numerous medical complications following her stroke and remained in the acute care hospital for approximately 1 month. Toward the end of her acute care stay she was able to engage in an active therapy program and had focused on feeding techniques, oral facial hygiene, bed mobility, and transfers.

When admitted to the rehabilitation hospital, she was stable and did not experience further medical problems. Her self-care status at admission is shown in Figure 1.

During the initial occupational therapy evaluation, Carmen showed some difficulty with safety, and her ability to follow commands was reduced, due to language deficits. She had poor awareness of her affected extremity and needed consistent cues to position it properly. Visual-perceptual skills were sufficient to perform basic self-care; however, she showed difficulty integrating changing visual information in the community. Testing revealed that she had problems separating foreground from background information and attending to relevant visual details. Motor planning deficits, especially sequencing problems, were evident when learning new activities, such as wheelchair propulsion, or when attempting to copy unfamiliar motor patterns. She was able to use objects appropriately and used some familiar gestures for communicating her needs.

Left upper extremity motor function was within normal limits (WNL); however, the RUE showed severe sensory deficits. Beginning active motion at the shoulder and elbow in a flexor synergy pattern was present, and she was able to achieve minimal isolated forearm, wrist, and metacarpal phalangeal motion. A moderate anterior subluxation with pain at the glenohumeral joint and intermittent minimal edema of the right hand was present.

Carmen was able to roll and move from supine to sitting with minimal cues to incorporate her RUE. She could maintain dynamic sitting balance while reaching in moderate ranges without support. She could stand with minimal assistance, using one arm for support. When engaged in dynamic activities, however, she required moderate assistance.

The speech pathologist reported that Carmen showed a moderately severe Broca's aphasia with no functional speech other than the ability to say "si" and "no" inconsistently. She could understand simple conversation related to familiar topics; however, the speakers often needed to repeat themselves. She was unable to write, but used gestures to communicate basic needs.

Carmen was able to walk several steps with moderate assistance and unequal weight bearing. She had difficulty with wheelchair propulsion and sequencing the use of a quad cane during ambulation. She was able to ascend and descend three steps with moderate assistance and a hand rail.

Assessment of Self-Care Skills of the Stroke Patient

Assessment is an ongoing process in which the therapist provides activity, evaluates

Figure 1. Initial ADL status: Carmen

	ADL Skill	Initial Status
Feeding	Help needed to cut meat, spread butter, and open containers.	Modified I
UE Dressing	Shirt	Moderate Assistance
	Bra	Maximum Assistance
LE Dressing	Shoes/socks	Moderate Assistance
	Pants—help to put over feet and pull over hips	Moderate Assistance
Toileting		Minimum Assistance
Bathing	Sponge—help for affected arm and feet	Minimum Assistance
	Tub/shower	Moderate Assistance
Hygiene	Set up to open containers, put paste on toothbrush, and obtain supplies from cabinet	Modified I
	Nail care	Dependent
Meal preparation	Two-dish, hot meal—Help needed to reach items, cut food, open packages, transport items, and manage hot dishes	Moderate Assistance
	Shopping: grocery and clothing	Moderate Assistance
Transportation	Public bus/train	Maximum Assistance
Child care	3-year-old son	Dependent
Light homemaking	Vacuum, dust, wash dishes, change and make bed	Maximum Assistance
Work	Factory work—folding and packing sheets	Dependent
Leisure	Hand crafts, TV, visiting with friends, movies, shopping	Moderate Assistance

responses, and modifies the task to match the patient's needs. During the initial days of patient contact, a wide range of information is collected in order to understand the patient's strengths and weaknesses and to guide treatment. Carefully performed initial assessments can save time and prevent patient frustration by helping the therapist choose tasks and techniques that match the patient's hopes, skills, limitations, and interests. Evaluation continues as the therapist works with the patient. Based on new information, changes in the patient's status, or new goals, the therapist updates the assessment data and treatment plan. As many leaders in occupational therapy have acknowledged, the ongoing process of getting to know a patient and refining treatment goals is important to successful outcome (Fleming, 1991; Mattingly, 1991; Rogers & Holm, 1991).

Although the most skillful and experienced therapists can detect many aspects of the stroke survivor's cognitive, perceptual, and motor performance through observation of ADL, the pattern of strengths and deficits is often complex. Therefore, comprehensive and holistic treatment planning frequently requires specific evaluation of certain skills. Slater and Cohn (1991) identify five levels of professional accomplishment in occupational therapy, ranging from novice to expert. Structured observation appears to aid problem identification and subsequent treatment planning for therapists who are at Level 1 ("novice") through Level 4 ("proficient"). While "experts" (Level 5), seem to function at a more intuitive level based on years of experience, they also use systematic problem solving techniques when they encounter obstacles or new situations. It is therefore recommended that after the initial observation of relevant basic self-care and instrumental ADL activities, the therapist further evaluate components that seem to limit function, with thoughtfully chosen assessment devices. Many approaches are available to measure motor, cognitive, and perceptual function. The final result should be a performance baseline relevant to the patient's and the family's goals, as well as a description of specific factors that limit independence.

Both of the patients described in the case studies benefited from early evaluation of pertinent self-care skills. The therapist observed those activities that were goals for the patient. During the functional evaluation, the influence of component skill deficits was noted. Then further assessment was directed toward the areas that appeared to be limiting performance. During her evaluation of Rose, the occupational therapist found severe deficits related to arousal, attention, body awareness, and visual-spatial skills. As expected, these deficits significantly limited Rose's ability to participate in self-care activities. Based on her review of the chart, the therapist had anticipated severe deficits and was prepared to engage the patient in simple self-care tasks during the initial treatment session.

Carmen was able to perform the full range of basic self-care tasks during the initial evaluation period. In addition, standardized motor, cognitive, and perceptual tests were used to help quantify the problems that were evident during basic self-care and to help detect more subtle deficits. Because her goals included activities like work and child care, it was important to test a wide range of skills that would affect future performance. While Rose's evaluation focused on basic self-care and the appropriate prerequisite skills, Carmen's assessment was much more extensive because she had set high-level goals.

Psychosocial Factors

Psychosocial and cultural factors can influence the evaluation and treatment process. The person who has had a stroke may feel helpless, hopeless, fearful, anxious, angry, or apathetic. Cognitive, language, and perceptual deficits may cloud the expression of these feelings; however, their impact on the evaluation and treatment process should be recognized. Estimates of depression among stroke survivors range from 25% to 60% (Roth, 1988). Although the site of the lesion may provide an organic basis for depression, reduced self-care ability, with poor self-esteem and feelings of helplessness also contribute (Ross & Rush, 1981; Roth). Throughout the evaluation and treatment process the occupational therapist must provide support, anticipate and verbalize feelings that the aphasic patient is unable to express, encourage discussion of feelings when the patient is able, and provide opportunities to experience success in relevant tasks. Furthermore, the occupational therapist should be aware that emotional distress may be interfering with performance.

In addition to considering emotional factors, an effective evaluation must use age-appropriate, culturally relevant activities. Activities are best selected in consultation with the patient. However, the family or friends can also provide valuable information if the patient is unable or unwilling to express interests. Barney (1991) states that ethnic identification is often an important part of the elderly patient's self-concept. Despite good intentions, gaps frequently exist in therapist's knowledge of other cultures. The therapists treating Rose and Carmen willingly listened to them and their families in order to understand better each patient's values and life-style. This openness enhanced collaboration and led to effectively individualized treatment.

Forcing all patients to perform a defined set of activities may be useful for departmental consistency, but it provokes anger in patients who do not see these tasks as relevant to their interests, goals, or life-styles. For example, evaluating tub bathing was unnecessary for Rose, who was returning to a home with an inaccessible bathroom, who had insufficient finances for remodeling, and whose size made tub bathing impractical. If the therapist had decided that tub bathing should be a goal, she was likely to alienate Rose and her family. Careful selection of pertinent tasks is much more likely to elicit cooperation and investment in the evaluation process.

Because interests, emotions, and cultural differences were considered, the tone and content of each patient's evaluation was unique. Rose was upset by the unfamiliar hospital regime. Her cognitive and perceptual limitations made it difficult for her to adjust to an unfamiliar environment. She benefited from a very slow, indirect approach to evaluation. During the initial evaluation, the occupational therapist assisted Rose with washing her face, combing her hair, and applying hand lotion. Through handling the affected arm, the therapist gathered information about tone and ROM. She and Rose discussed previous roles and interests, and the therapist provided reassurance and praise for small accomplishments. Although she did not use structured evaluations initially, the therapist gathered information through observation of motor, visual perceptual, self-care, and cognitive skills, without upsetting the patient. Over the course of several days, the therapist performed pertinent formal evaluations but returned to familiar activities whenever Rose began to seem frustrated. Rose's daughter was included in the initial evaluation and helped to encourage and reassure her mother. She also provided some relevant orientation topics that were discussed in a conversational manner. Evaluation results were shared in a simplified manner with Rose and discussed more extensively in a private session with Rose's daughter.

Carmen was initially reluctant to take an active role in treatment planning and felt more secure when the therapist provided direction and structure. Her therapist, therefore, took a more directive approach during the initial sessions, but was sensitive to nonverbal responses and spent time suggesting various activities and goals, allowing Carmen to indicate which of them seemed relevant. Because some of the self-care evaluation procedures, especially toilet use and putting on a bra, made Carmen frustrated and embarrassed, the therapist initially focused on activities that were less threatening, then readdressed the more sensitive issues when rapport was established. Carmen was able to participate in formal evaluations of motor, cognitive, and perceptual status, and seemed very interested in her performance. As Carmen improved, she selected more advanced self-care skills, which were then evaluated.

Specialized Evaluations

Although occupational therapists are well trained to observe and evaluate most daily living skills, several specialized evaluations call for advanced training, due to their inherent safety risks. These specialized evaluations include dysphagia evaluation, driving evaluation, work evaluation, and independent living evaluation. A patient who is incorrectly evaluated may be cleared for an activity that could present a serious threat to health or safety. On the other hand, a person who is improperly excluded from an activity may be denied basic rights and important opportunities. Clearly, the therapist who is involved in making such important recommendations must be well trained through advanced clinical courses or practice under the supervision of an expert therapist.

Assessment of Dysphagia

Dysphagia evaluations may be performed by an occupational therapist or a speech and language pathologist. Territorial issues should be laid aside, allowing the professionals who are best trained to perform the evaluation. Often speech and language pathologists have received more extensive academic preparation than occupational therapists in the evaluation and treatment of swallowing dysfunction. When both disciplines have important skills to contribute, they can share evaluation data and provide cotreatment. The patient benefits from the expertise and collaboration of two professionals.

The dysphagia evaluation should include observation of the following phases of swallowing: (a) anticipatory phase—note the patient's ability to decide what and how much to eat; (b) oral phase—note lip closure, the ability to chew, and the tongue's ability to manipulate food in order to form a bolus; (c) pharyngeal phase—note laryngeal elevation signaling closure of the airway, and signs of coughing or choking; and (d) esophageal phase—reflux may indicate improper cricopharyngeal closure (Glickstein, Olson, Cherney, & Pollard, 1989). The duration of each phase should also be noted, because an abnormally long transit time indicates swallowing difficulty. In many cases, a video-fluoroscopic examination is the best tool for detecting deficits in oral control and swallowing. Food and liquid of various consistencies are mixed with a substance that is visible on the video monitor and is given in small quantities to the patient. The movement of the food is observed in the mouth, through the pharynx, and into the esophagus. Any abnormality that suggests risk of aspiration can readily be detected, and specific recommendations about the types of food that are safe can be made. Clinical observations or repeat video-fluoroscopy can be used to upgrade the diet if it seems appropriate. Specific treatment techniques are applied based on the type of deficit that is found. These may include thermal stimulation, oral exercises, special breathing techniques, conscious throat clearing, cues to monitor the rate of eating, checking the mouth for pocketing, and/or positioning the head and neck to optimize control.

In Rose's case, the dysphagia evaluation and video-fluoroscopy showed poor oral manipulation of solids, decreased oral initiation, delayed pharyngeal swallow, and coughing on a ½ teaspoon of thick liquid. In addition, her reduced attention caused her to "forget" food in her mouth and subsequently cough. Rose did not tolerate attempts at thermal stimulation, becoming agitated. It was recommended that gastrostomy tube feedings be continued since Rose was unable to understand the abstract techniques required to improve swallowing, and significant functional improvements were not expected.

Driving Assessment

When driving is a realistic consideration, the evaluation should include a thorough assessment of higher-level cognitive and perceptual skills, specialized testing of visual fields, visual acuity, and depth perception (Quigley & DeLisa, 1983), appraisal of reaction time, and evaluation of general driving knowledge. Access to a driving simulator is helpful, particularly for younger patients, to screen for problems prior to a road test. Clinic screening tests, simulator tests, and driving in a parking lot are important to detect potential problem areas, to counsel the patient about skills that require improvement, and to eliminate unsafe drivers from the road test. However, these tests cannot be used exclusively to predict driving performance (Galski, Ehle, & Bruno, 1990). The actual driving evaluation should therefore occur in a variety of settings that replicate those the patient will encounter once discharged. To ensure adequate treatment, the therapist must be knowledgeable about the applicable requirements and procedures for driver's training, as determined by the local laws.

Work Assessment

A work evaluation generally has several phases. When a possible job has been identified, the occupational therapist and/or vocational specialist can define requirements for strength, dexterity, speed, mobility, endurance, decision making, verbal skills, writing abilities, interpersonal interaction, or other pertinent job skills. This may be done by consulting with the employer or by visiting the workplace and observing the job. The patient's capacity to meet these requirements is tested through activities that imitate the demands of the job. Specific treatment then can be aimed at improving the component skills necessary for returning to work. When job skills seem sufficient, the therapist may accompany the client to the work site for evaluation in the work environment. Recommendations may include further training, modifying the job, returning to work independently or with a coach, or working a reduced schedule. The therapist should be familiar with equal employment and workers' compensation laws, and should understand the insurance system in order to best advocate for his or her clients.

When a patient is hoping to live alone, the occupational therapist, in conjunction with the rehabilitation team, must help determine whether he or she will be safe. This decision is complex. When a patient demonstrates subtle cognitive and perceptual problems, it may be difficult to ascertain whether the limitations are severe enough to interfere with routine decision making. If possible, the optimal evaluation takes place in the patient's own home for a period of 4 to 6 hours and includes observation of self-care, home care, cooking, shopping, financial management, and child care, if indicated. When a home visit is not possible, reliable friends or family may report performance during a home pass, and the therapist can provide simulated tasks in the clinic. In all but the mildest cases of stroke, a caregiver or a structured community support system is required to ensure safety. Given time and an opportunity to develop increased independence in a supportive environment, some patients may reach a sufficient level of adaptation to live independently. This ability is generally not present upon inpatient discharge. While Rose was clearly unable to be left alone, Carmen had sufficient cognitive skills and self-care independence to remain alone for short periods of time. Eventually she was able to care for herself completely; however, she appreciated the assistance of her family with complex financial matters and with demanding physical chores.

Treatment Approaches

Compensation Techniques and Contextual Training

Once the therapist completes the initial evaluation, treatment begins. A variety of treatment approaches can be used and are generally combined to maximize both the level and the quality of independence.

Contextual training can improve basic self-care skills. This type of training emphasizes practice of the desired activity in a standard way in a specific environment until it becomes habitual. This repetition of specific task sequences has been found to be effective for improving independence in the brain-injured population (Soderback, 1988). In addition to the benefit of practicing familiar functional activity, contextual training requires the patient to integrate various motor, cognitive, and perceptual skills. The therapist can structure the activity to provide an appropriate level of challenge and can incorporate component skill retraining techniques.

Instrumental ADL, such as home care, child care, community living skills, and work, provide a wide assortment of cognitive, perceptual, and motor challenges. When involvement in these activities is feasible, a whole range of high-level functional goals and corresponding component skill goals can be set. These activities are best performed in the actual environment where they will take place. Since this often is not possible for the hospital-based therapist, he or she should attempt to simulate the discharge situation as closely as possible. With guidance, patients who participate in high-level tasks are frequently able to apply principles learned in simulated settings to their own situation. For example, the therapist was not able to go to Carmen's neighborhood store, but compensated by accompanying Carmen on several trips to a store near the hospital in order to identify problem areas and improve performance.

Home visits are time consuming, but are one of the most useful services an occupational therapist can provide to a stroke survivor and his or her family. The visit helps to plan treatment, as well as to prepare for discharge. It provides an opportunity to evaluate the accessibility of all rooms, home safety, furniture arrangement, and organization of storage spaces. In addition, specific tasks can be evaluated in a familiar environment. For example, Carmen was asked to prepare a cup of tea in her kitchen, obtain items from the bedroom closet, use the bathroom, and get on and off the couch. Her interaction with her son and other family members was observed, as was her response to greetings from neighbors. Since patients who have difficulty in the clinic may be able to perform better in a familiar environment, home evaluation helps ensure that treatment addresses real difficulties and allows the therapist to solve problems within the environment. The visit provides clues about the prestroke life-style that are often not learned through discussion with the patient or family and, as an added benefit, it provides a relaxed setting for family training.

As an adjunct to practice in real environments, adapted methods, specialized equipment, and environmental modifications can promote function, despite deficit areas. Selection of an adaptive technique must be based on careful thought. Some adaptations, such as bathroom modifications or environmental changes, are very helpful if the patient is willing and able to change his or her home. Successful integration of other techniques, like learning new methods or using adaptive equipment, requires that the patient be highly motivated for independence, that the equipment or techniques truly simplify the task, and that the patient has sufficient cognitive/perceptual skills. The therapist must present a variety of options to the patient, but then must listen and observe performance carefully to determine which suggestions are practical.

Some patients become very frustrated during ADL training. This may be because their limitations make the tasks seem overwhelming. Even after the therapist breaks the task into small components, the patient sometimes remains upset because of the inability to perform as he or she did prior to the stroke. Other patients may be frustrated when they feel capable of independent problem solving and resent the therapist's well-intentioned presence during ADL. The occupational therapist must remain sensitive to the emotional, physical, and cognitive/perceptual aspects of the task and make modifications, give more freedom, or provide encouragement as needed. At times it may be necessary to delay involvement in a self-care skill until prerequisite abilities improve.

Many clever devices and methods have been developed to help a person accomplish tasks single-handedly. Therapy-supply catalogs offer a variety of equipment, and written resources are available to provide specific information in this area (see Chapter 14). The ADL training process and techniques that helped Rose and Carmen are discussed in the following section to provide examples of methods useful in addressing the self-care needs of persons in which CVA is the primary diagnosis.

Case Descriptions of Treatment

Rose

Contextual training was helpful for Rose, who was unable to understand the purpose of abstract clinic tasks. She was most invested when performing simple morning self-care routines. Activities that improved her appearance and were accompanied by socialization were the most enjoyable. Consequently, hygiene and grooming tasks were a major goal for therapy. At the sink, a washcloth was prepared, and Rose was given verbal cues and physical assistance as needed to wash the left side of her face. Brushing her hair required similar cues. Applying lip gloss was performed more independently, due to the midline position of the task. Application of lotion to the left hand, positioned in midline, required numerous cues. When practical, the left hand was manually guided by the therapist during functional tasks. For example, when a container needed to be stabilized, the therapist placed her hand over the patient's in order to allow Rose to "hold" the object. This provided additional sensory input and movement to the affected arm. These activities, although slow and somewhat tedious to perform, provided numerous opportunities for sensory motor input in the context of a familiar, enjoyable, and relevant task.

Due to her extremely poor sitting balance and large size, the hospital bed was used to facilitate dressing. While seated in bed, Rose's pants were pulled to her mid-calf, and she was then able to pull them to her thighs. The bed was lowered, and rolling was facilitated using Proprioceptive Neuromuscular Facilitation (PNF) techniques. Rose could help pull the pants up on the right side, but was unable to assist on the left. When the pants were on, the therapist put Rose's socks and shoes on her and facilitated sitting from a side-lying position using Bobath techniques. Because Rose pushed strongly to the left and was very large, a sliding board and the assistance of another person were required to complete the transfer.

Once in her wheelchair, Rose helped to put on her shirt. Positioning her affected LUE in the sleeve provided tactile input and a simple visual perceptual challenge. The therapist gave encouragement and assistance when needed, in order to avoid undue frustration. Due to her severe cognitive and perceptual deficits, coupled with motor limitations, Rose easily became frustrated during even simple activities. When overly challenged, she "shut down" and refused to cooperate. The therapist learned to be sensitive to signs of overload and modified the task or the environment accordingly.

Finding appropriate leisure activities was difficult. Because Rose had limited interests before the stroke, there was not a wide range of activities upon which to draw. Perceptual and cognitive deficits prohibited playing cards or checkers, and motor deficits interfered with knitting. Rose showed poor memory for new learning, did not follow directions well, and demonstrated severe visual perceptual problems, making adaptive equipment impractical. A rug punch was attempted. Although Rose enjoyed the activity, and her performance was fair, carryover at home was doubtful due to the need for special stretching frames, clamps, and constant supervision. Rose's favorite activity continued to be socializing with friends and family. This was encouraged because it promoted eye contact with another person and helped provide orientation information and cognitive challenge. It was suggested that only one or two people visit with Rose at a time and that they sit at her midline, gradually moving to the left as her left awareness improved. She was encouraged to look at picture books with her great grandchildren. Finally, since TV was a former interest, Rose practiced using a remote control in order to change channels and turn the TV on and off independently. This proved to be a perceptual motor challenge that she worked diligently to meet. It was also suggested that Rose be given simple tasks to help with home care roles that she formerly enjoyed. For example, she could pat lettuce dry then put it in a bowl, sprinkle nuts on a cake, or use a feather duster.

A home visit was important to ensure a smooth transition from the hospital. The physical therapist and the occupational therapist accompanied Rose to her home. Access was possible either through the front or a side door, and no ramps were required. Although the bathroom was upstairs, Rose and her daughter were content with sponge bathing, and using a commode and bedpan for toileting. A bedroom was arranged on the first floor, which allowed access to the kitchen and living room. The family was advised to remove scatter rugs and to clear a pathway so that Rose could be moved easily from room to room. A hospital bed was ordered to facilitate self-care and caregiver tasks. Because the daughter did not work outside the home, and a personal care attendant was scheduled to work 20 hours a week, an emergency call system was not considered necessary.

The therapist gave Rose's daughter suggestions for improving her mother's function despite the cognitive, perceptual, and motor deficits that remained. An easily read calendar and clock were recommended to help maintain orientation. It was suggested that distractions be reduced by keeping clutter to a minimum where possible, turning off the TV when conversing, and limiting the number of visitors. Using objects that contrasted with the background (i.e., a dark washcloth on a white counter) and presenting only one or two objects at a time, helped decrease the effects of Rose's visual perceptual problems. In addition to the compensatory techniques, remedial approaches were also recommended. Left awareness was to be encouraged by providing verbal, visual and tactile cues. Items were first presented at midline and, as improvements were made, gradually moved left.

Because Rose had poor body awareness and control, proper positioning in the wheelchair was crucial to improve function and comfort. In addition, this decreased the amount of time the caregiver needed to spend repositioning Rose. An extra-wide wheelchair with a solid seat and back, a firm foam cushion, an angled lap belt, elevating leg rests, and desk arms was ordered. The seat height allowed Rose's feet to reach the floor to assist with propulsion. A custom arm rest supported the LUE in a functional position and prevented injury. The rotational capability of this arm rest allowed it to be positioned partially within the patient's visual field. A lap board was ineffective because Rose pushed against it with her right arm, further displacing her body to the left. The therapists considered lateral supports, but they felt Rose might develop pressure areas and sustain skin damage, due to her tendency to push to the left. A splint was constructed for periodic use to maintain optimum hand position.

Rose was not expected to gain a significant level of independence in self-care. She remained dependent in bathing and toileting, and required maximal assistance with most ADL tasks other than oral and facial hygiene. She and her daughter acknowledged that she would always require assistance, but the achievements she did make lessened the burden of care for her daughter, gave her a small measure of independence (especially in oral and facial hygiene), and provided movement and perceptual challenges in a functional, nonthreatening way. Facilitating maximal involvement from Rose in transfers and bed mobility was therapeutic because it provided vestibular and sensory input and practice in following simple functional commands, and helped her actively improve midline orientation. Despite significant gains, she continued to require maximal assistance for transfers, and a Hoyer lift was recommended for home use to avoid injury. Extensive family teaching was necessary because there were many activities Rose was incapable of performing, and most of those that were possible required special set up and cuing.

Carmen

Carmen generally responded well to ADL training. She realized the importance of practice so that she could meet her goal of independence. In addition, she was embarrassed to ask for help, and thus was motivated to improve. Despite her motivation, she sometimes resisted the therapists' efforts to engage her in self-care tasks because she dreaded the long struggle with her limitations that each ADL session required. When her resistance was especially strong, she complained of fatigue and feeling sick. On these occasions, or when Carmen's patience was strained, the therapist negotiated a compromise and agreed to assist with difficult and frustrating portions of the task. Little by little Carmen's frustration decreased, and she performed more of the activity without requesting assistance or showing resistance.

Due to mild motor planning problems and language deficits, all ADL techniques required initial demonstration by the therapist and subsequent hand-over-hand assistance or tactile cues to guide Carmen through the correct movement. Short verbal cues to help sequence the activity were also provided. It is believed that people carry out a dialog within their mind when learning a new task. This dialog is used to give oneself cues about the next step in a sequence. Since Carmen lacked this internal language, due to aphasia, short verbal, visual, or contextual cues helped her move from one step to the next. Although unfamiliar equipment and methods should generally be avoided when working with a patient who demonstrates motor planning deficits, Carmen's motor planning deficits related more to sequencing an activity. She was able to use familiar objects and gestures correctly. She was therefore able to learn new methods and to use equipment when necessary.

Carmen received feedback to encourage her in her progress. The therapist praised slight improvements in the time it took to complete a self-care activity or in the amount performed without assistance. Positive reinforcement seemed to make Carmen more accepting of herself and willing to try again. For each new technique, the therapist explained how it would be helpful and assisted Carmen in her initial attempts to use it. By working with Carmen, rather than just giving instructions, the task became collaborative. Together they decided whether a technique was working and, if unsuccessful, tried to determine the source of the difficulty. They could then modify their approach or work on component skills to improve performance. This collaborative problem solving provided many opportunities for Carmen to express opinions and occasionally identify a new solution. In contrast, techniques imposed in the hospital that do not match the person's goals or are not practical for his or her environment are soon discarded. Rather than teaching a set of techniques, teaching the ability to generate solutions is crucial for independence. A capable patient, like Carmen, can be given a framework for making

independent decisions. Modeling problem solving techniques, providing encouragement to try new alternatives, and working in collaboration helped Carmen gradually
learn to tackle new problems alone.

Although aphasia and the fact that English was a second language limited the verbal
interchange that could take place, the therapist was sensitive to Carmen's facial expressions, level of enthusiasm, and gestures. The therapist also provided many opportunities
for Carmen to express herself by asking questions that required "yes" or "no" responses.
When possible, a family member aided translation. Because the therapist had developed
a supportive relationship and encouraged differing opinions, Carmen felt comfortable
expressing herself even when she knew that her feelings did not match the therapist's.

Performance of self-care skills improved rapidly. Initially Carmen used Dycem to
stabilize her plate and a rocker knife to cut meat. As control of her right arm improved,
these were discontinued. She was eventually able to stabilize her meat using the fork in
her right hand while cutting with the left. During outpatient treatment, Carmen's goal
of using her right hand to eat finger foods was attained after much practice and focus on
refining control of the RUE.

As her balance improved, Carmen was able to cross her legs independently while
sitting on the edge of the bed in order to place her foot in her pants leg, and put on socks
and shoes. She then stood with minimal assistance to pull up her pants. Since she was very
sensitive, the therapist was careful to maintain Carmen's sense of privacy by allowing her
to wear her gown until her pants were on. Touch-fastener shoe closures were discussed;
however, RUE motor function improved enough for Carmen to use her right hand to
stabilize the laces when tying. A step-in shoe horn was issued to help her slide her right
foot into the shoe.

Carmen learned the overhead method of putting on a shirt, and although the new
method of performance was somewhat difficult at first, it caused less RUE pain by allowing
better control of her arm position. With the collar close to her stomach and the front of
the shirt facing up, she dropped the sleeve between her legs, and, using the minimal active
motion she retained, positioned her RUE in the sleeve. She then placed her LUE in the
sleeve and brought the shirt overhead. She learned to put on her bra by fastening it in
front, then sliding it around her back. Carmen tried touch-fastener bra closures, closing
the bra first and then putting it on overhead. She also tried using a clip to stabilize the bra
on the waistband of her pants while fastening the hooks; however, she found that she
preferred using her right thumb hooked through a strap to stabilize the garment while
fastening with her left hand.

During grooming, Carmen learned to stabilize an object with her right hand while
opening it with her left. Initially she applied roll-on deodorant with her LUE. She was able
to reach her left armpit with her left hand, although it was a bit awkward. As she improved,
she used her right hand to apply deodorant to her left armpit. Early in her hospitalization,
items such as a toothbrush stabilizer, a makeup basket holding small containers in place
so she could open the lids easily, a soap stabilizer, and a suction nail brush were
considered. As her right-hand function improved, it became clear that these items would
not be necessary.

Because Carmen was accustomed to well-groomed nails, the therapist recommended using a one-handed clipper with a clamp-on emery board or taping a file to a table
edge. Carmen also tried polishing her nails using a device that holds the nail polish brush.
When the brush was positioned in the holder, Carmen was able to polish the nails on her

unaffected hand. She was not satisfied with the quality of the job, however, and decided to obtain assistance from family or friends. While the therapist would have liked her to practice more diligently, she recognized that Carmen was more interested in the quality of her appearance than in performing independently. The therapist felt that Carmen's family and friends would gladly assist with this task and that it would be an opportunity for socialization.

Carmen was able to bathe using a tub bench, a grab bar, nonskid mats inside and outside the tub, and a shower hose. The therapist suggested mounting a dispenser for liquid soap and shampoo near the tub bench to make the task easier. A hand-held hair dryer with a built-in brush helped Carmen style her hair.

Requiring assistance for toileting and feminine hygiene was an undignified experience for Carmen. As a result, she was motivated to gain independence as quickly as possible. Early in her stay she was routinely encouraged by the nursing staff to request assistance; however, she frequently attempted to perform on her own. She fell on one occasion, without serious consequences. She was labeled impulsive. Yet in reality, using the bathroom on her own was a conscious decision. Her decreased ability to express her needs; the busy schedule of the staff, which often led to waiting for bathroom assistance; the neurological changes that made bowel and bladder control more difficult; and her embarrassment at needing assistance for such a private task gave her the impetus to attempt using the bathroom alone. The therapist spent time during morning ADL and clinic sessions helping Carmen learn to safely perform the task independently. Standing to pull her pants up or down for toileting was difficult. The therapist suggested that the pants be pulled up much as possible while sitting. Carmen stood with her right side near a wall so she could brace against it if her balance was momentarily offset. With practice, she was able to manage feminine hygiene products independently with one hand.

Carmen continued to be interested in leisure and craft activities. She used a card holder to play games with her sister. Although making tissue flowers was initially difficult and frustrating, as her RUE function improved she was able to fold the paper while a friend wired the stems. She also found that she was able to use a latch hook to make a rug. She decided to make this rug for her mother and sister in thanks for their help. She also tried an embroidery hoop mounted on a gooseneck, but found the activity too tedious. Socializing with her family remained enjoyable, although her aphasia limited conversation and made her reluctant to visit with friends. As time went on and language, especially Spanish, improved, she became more active with her friends and resumed church and social activities.

Carmen had been responsible for cooking several meals each week at home and hoped to continue this activity. She was able to prepare a simple, familiar, two-dish, hot meal with assistance opening containers, transporting items, stabilizing objects, reaching low and high shelves, handling hot items, and cutting. Her difficulties were primarily due to motor limitations, although she also had mild problems in sequencing, problem solving, and attention. The therapist felt that as the task became more familiar and less difficult, these cognitive/perceptual problems would not interfere with performance.

Various options for opening containers were considered, including using special adapted box openers, opening packages with a knife or scissors, using a one-handed electric can opener, and using a wall-mounted jar opener or rubber pads to improve grasp. Carmen felt that using scissors was most effective for opening boxes, and the therapist issued a pair of loop scissors. Since hand function was returning, Carmen did not want to invest in a hand-held electric can opener. After some practice, she was able to use a manual can opener. She felt there were enough people at home to help with tight jars on occasion, but was able to wedge the jar in a drawer and use Dycem to improve her grasp if necessary. She also practiced using a piece of Dycem under the jar to help stabilize it when opening the lid.

Transporting items presented a bigger problem. Carmen's kitchen was tiny, and a wheeled cart would take up too much room. Counter space was limited and did not provide continuous surfaces on which to slide items. She required her cane for balance when walking, thus did not have a free hand. She was able to stand at the refrigerator and place items on the kitchen table. A full-length chef's apron with a large pocket was used to carry items that were not too bulky or fragile. Hot items could be cooled slightly on the stove with the burners off. The food was then removed to a plate using an appropriate utensil. She needed assistance from her family to move a hot, bulky, or fragile item across the room. She was able to prepare a simple meal for herself or her child independently, but needed assistance when cooking a full meal for her family.

Stabilizing items on the table or counter was accomplished through the use of Dycem. The therapist demonstrated a pot-handle stabilizer on the stove, but Carmen preferred to brace the handle against a tea kettle partially filled with water. As RUE function improved, she was able to use her right hand to stabilize a pot while stirring with the left.

The therapist issued long oven mitts for checking food in the oven. A wooden tool to pull out the oven rack was discussed; however, Carmen did not feel she wanted the extra equipment. She was advised not to put items into, or remove them from, the oven, due to compromised balance and limited right upper extremity function. Baking was to be done only when a family member could help.

Carmen was able to cut simple items for her son, such as a sandwich or fruit, using an adapted cutting board. Other options for cutting were discussed. She felt that using the blender she owned, buying pre-cut foods, or asking her family to help would be acceptable.

Carmen could wash dishes using her right hand to stabilize and her left to scrub. The therapist suggested using a rubber mat in the sink to cushion the dishes in case they slipped, and demonstrated a suction bottle brush for washing glasses; however, Carmen was confident of her ability to do an adequate job without the equipment. Although this task was slow, Carmen felt that she was making an important family contribution by helping with the dishes. Due to her difficulty transporting the dishes, they were left to air dry, and another family member put them away.

Carmen was reluctant to resume caring for her 3-year-old son. During her hospitalization Carmen's mother had cared for him and was continuing this role now that Carmen was home. Carmen felt incompetent and had difficulty physically or verbally guiding his activities. He seemed to want her attention, yet frequently challenged her authority and seemed uncomfortable with the changes brought about by the CVA. Because she did not want to distance herself further, Carmen agreed to choose several tasks that she could perform to increase her involvement in her son's care gradually. She chose to fix his breakfast and to purchase loose fitting clothes and touch-fastener strapped shoes so she could help him dress. Finally, she felt that she could play with him using blocks, crayons, simple picture books, cars, and stuffed toys. Although she could not pick him up, she encouraged him to sit in her lap to look at a book, color, do a puzzle, or receive a hug. This level of involvement seemed appropriate, given the many changes to which Carmen was adjusting in her own life. Independent care of a young child required physical abilities, language skills, and problem-solving capabilities that Carmen was still developing. Carmen's mother and sister continued to assist with discipline and other daily care responsibilities.

Community trips were planned and carried out to meet goals of independent grocery shopping and use of the bus to visit friends for social outings. Cues and assistance were initially required for monitoring hazards in the environment, establishing topographical orientation, efficiently organizing her shopping trip, locating items in the store, maintaining balance on uneven surfaces, negotiating bus steps, moving through narrow bus aisles, handling money, and transporting items. Little by little, the therapist reduced her intervention and provided assistance only when a danger existed. Topographical orientation was enhanced by discussing a route prior to a trip, pointing out landmarks, and writing the destination on a card. When Carmen first attempted to ride the bus, she selected a simple route. Later she practiced going from the hospital to a friend's apartment. The therapist advised her to practice any new route several times with a friend or family member prior to going alone.

When shopping, Carmen was able to push the grocery cart and maintain good balance. She could obtain most items but occasionally needed to ask for help reaching high shelves. She did not want the inconvenience or stigma of carrying a reacher. She was able to carry a small number of items home using a backpack or large canvas shoulder bag that was placed diagonally across her chest. Extensive purchases were delivered or were made only when her sister or mother accompanied her.

Returning to work had been a primary goal when Carmen was first admitted to the rehabilitation hospital. As she realized the changes that her stroke imposed on her life, she became more interested in meeting her own self-care needs and those of her family. She did not think that she would be able to handle the pace of her former factory job. She was referred to vocational counseling, where she completed interest and aptitude tests. Her options were limited because she was unable to speak fluently due to aphasia, and because her motor performance was slowed by the hemiplegia. It was possible that she could be retrained to handle a light duty job that required skilled use of only one hand; however, Carmen decided to wait to begin such retraining.

Carmen's ADL training followed the normal progression, from addressing basic self-care to working on home care, community, and child-care tasks. Although she was not completely independent in all areas, the progress she did make gave her a sense of satisfaction. She knew that she was ultimately in control of her progress. Goals were adjusted according to her expressed desires and based on the way she participated in treatment. When she showed little enthusiasm for a goal that had previously been set, she and the therapist discussed it. At times the goal was modified—at other times she was challenged to work harder toward its accomplishment—but she was always held responsible for the direction of treatment.

Remediation Techniques

Remediation techniques are often used to improve the cognitive, perceptual, and motor skills needed for optimal function. This approach is often the most acceptable to the patient and his or her family, at least in the initial phases of disability. Patients are eager to regain lost function, and concentrating on a specific aspect of performance is sometimes less threatening than facing formerly simple tasks that have become very difficult. When remediation techniques are effective, they may enable the patient to perform tasks "like I did before," using automatic and familiar methods. This is especially helpful when cognitive or perceptual deficits make learning new, adapted methods very difficult. Finally, remediation techniques can enhance the quality of performance by making the task easier and more spontaneous. Although Carmen was able to learn to perform many tasks with one hand, they were accomplished more quickly and efficiently when she was able to incorporate her affected extremity. Balance and mobility training helped both Rose and Carmen during all self-care. Rose became more aware of her left side and could gradually see objects at midline. She could also locate her affected arm, using verbal cues, in order to position it for safety and to apply lotion. Skilled use of remediation techniques can be the most efficient way to promote positive changes that ultimately enhance ADL performance.

Used alone or in combination, techniques employed by proprioceptive neuromuscular facilitation (PNF) theorists, Bobath theorists, and motor learning theorists, can be effective for retraining motor function. All techniques rely on careful observation of patient performance and ongoing modification of treatment techniques to enhance movement. Bobath methods for the adult hemiplegic stress treatment of the whole body, provision of normal sensory input, inhibition of abnormal tone, facilitation of movement through sensitive handling, and use of key points of control (Bobath, 1972). PNF relies on facilitating diagonal patterns of movement through multisensory input and repetition, using manual contacts to provide sensory cues for motion, providing stretch to facilitate motion, and applying just the right amount of manual resistance to require effort without decreasing control (Voss, Ionta, & Myers, 1985). Motor learning theory, as described by Carr and Shepherd (1987), uses a sequential clinical reasoning process. A functional performance problem is identified; the limiting motor components are analyzed; the defective components are practiced in isolation through visual, verbal, and manual guidance; and, finally, the motion is practiced in the context of the functional task with the intent of integrating the components.

These motor facilitation and retraining techniques are useful to improve UE function, trunk control, and balance necessary for optimal performance of self-care skills. They can be used in the clinic to build prerequisite skills needed for ADL. For example, specific techniques can enhance functional mobility while rolling, sitting, standing, or kneeling. Working on various surfaces, such as a table mat, bench, chair without arms, bed, ball, or rocker board can provide graded challenges to balance. Reaching activities and eye-hand coordination games can introduce speed and control. Carmen initially worked on gross motor activities, such as picking up items from the floor and placing them overhead in diagonal patterns. Later she was able to stand on a rocker board while performing gross RUE control tasks. The therapist facilitated symmetrical weight bearing in sitting and standing during functional activities like dressing and oral and facial hygiene. The therapist encouraged trunk rotation during reaching and functional mobility and used manual contact and facilitation through key points of control to enhance the quality of motion. Carmen then used improved balance and mobility skills in functional activities, such as a community shopping trip, riding the bus, or playing with her son.

Upper extremity use can be facilitated to improve bilateral function. The therapist can influence improvement by properly positioning the patient to enhance distal motor control and encouraging concentration on the desired movement patterns, and can demonstrate skillful use of inhibition and facilitation techniques. In addition to neurorehabilitation approaches, functional electrical stimulation (FES) and biofeedback training are being successfully used to improve upper extremity motor control and functional abilities.

When working on remediation of component skills, the therapist must be sure that the patient views the activities used as meaningful. Rather than creating artificial activities, such as stacking cones, the therapist can often gain the same results through a more straightforward approach. For example, Carmen wanted to be able to use her RUE to eat finger foods. Portions of many treatment sessions were exercise-oriented, with a focus on refining RUE control and enhancing movement. Activities were not consistently used during the exercise phase of treatment, because carefully guided training allowed better isolation of the desired motion. During these "exercise" treatments, the goal of picking up and eating finger foods remained clear. Following the isolated movement practice, Carmen used the motions in a portion of the functional task. If the therapist had chosen just to practice eating finger foods, it is doubtful that the careful analysis of movement and focus on retraining specific motions would have occurred. The quality of movement would have suffered and Carmen may have become frustrated by her lack of control. By using specific motor remediation techniques, Carmen realized her functional goal more quickly.

Carmen's treatment sessions initially emphasized controlled use of the RUE in bilateral tasks. As improvements were seen the focus changed to use of the RUE as the dominant hand for reaching needed items, using utensils, and operating fasteners. She used inhibition techniques prior to functional reach-and-grasp activities, and she used facilitation techniques to promote improved overhead reach and multiple joint control. By remaining conscious of normal movement, the therapist facilitated and corrected abnormal patterns as they occurred and ultimately taught Carmen how to monitor and correct movement independently. Carmen learned how and when to use inhibition techniques to improve function. She was also encouraged to observe and feel desired movements with her non-affected extremity, then to duplicate them with her right arm.

The therapist addressed tactile awareness by asking Carmen to consciously attend to various temperatures, textures, and sensations encountered during self-care tasks. As awareness of primary sensory modalities improved, the therapist addressed simultaneous tactile sensation by asking Carmen to concentrate on two different sensations in each hand. For example, when holding the toothbrush in one hand and the toothpaste in the other, Carmen was asked to stop, look at each object, close her eyes, attend to the sensations, then open her eyes again. Initially, she was unable to perform bilateral manipulative tasks because sensory input on the left overrode sensory input on the right. She was unable to maintain control unless she visually guided right hand movement. With improved tactile attention, however, she could perform gross tactile manipulations without visual guidance, and coordinated movements with visual assistance.

Cognitive and perceptual remediation can be incorporated into many activities. For instance, planning a meal, setting time guidelines for an activity, solving problems encountered in ADL, focusing on a new movement pattern, learning a new exercise sequence, following a pattern for a latch hook rug, carrying over exercises at home, attending to the environment during a community excursion, finding her way in a store, asking for help, or discussing her feelings, provided cognitive challenges for Carmen. Paper and pencil activities were not appropriate, due to Carmen's language limitations and a prestroke life style that did not rely heavily on reading and writing. Similarly, puzzles and other tabletop perceptual activities were used only when they corresponded to a desired functional task. For example, Carmen occasionally practiced a child's game, such as a simple puzzle, so she would have the confidence to play with the toy with her son.

For Rose, the therapist provided clinic treatment in a quiet corner or an individual therapy room to minimize confusion. The session often began with simple orientation information, carried out in a conversational tone. Throughout all clinic activities, the therapist used simple commands and graded the length of attention required to build these skills gradually. The therapist incorporated left awareness into almost all tasks, and used verbal, tactile, and visual cues. The treatment focused on midline orientation, but due to Rose's large size and her tendency to push to the left, it was difficult for one person to facilitate normal movement patterns. Cotreatment with the physical therapist was arranged 2 days per week so that midline orientation and motor skills could be jointly addressed. Cotreatment also ensured that the therapists taught consistent methods and recommendations to the daughter.

While remediation of deficits is very beneficial, it can be a long process. The occupational therapist must be careful to maintain a functional perspective and combine ADL training and compensatory techniques with remediation efforts. In this way the stroke survivor can maximize independence within the limits of his or her disability. Then, as improvements are made, equipment and special techniques may be abandoned in favor of more conventional methods.

Discharge Planning

When goals have been met or changes in functional ability no longer occur, it is time for formal therapy to end. Discharge planning, however, should begin at the onset of treatment to ensure that the patient and family will feel ready for the return home. Although they may hope for further gains, they should feel prepared to deal with current abilities and limitations. Throughout the course of treatment, the therapist should direct therapy sessions, self-care instruction, home visit recommendations, equipment provision, and patient/family teaching toward the discharge goals and environment.

When a patient is able to follow a home program independently, the activities should be selected in collaboration. The therapeutic benefits inherent in various daily activities should be explained and, when possible, should serve as the basis of the home program. The therapist can make suggestions for stretching muscles, facilitating a particular response, or practicing a movement prior to activity. Some people find exercise satisfying and enjoyable. For them, specific home exercises can also be a meaningful activity. All tasks should be practiced and revised routinely in the clinic long before discharge to ensure that they are performed correctly and remain appropriate. Home programs may use written instructions, diagrams, or photographs, based on the patient's language and visual perceptual skills. Experience suggests that Polaroid photos of the patient performing the activity often serve as better cues than drawings. Personalized videos or audiotapes that provide cues for activities or exercises have also been useful.

A caregiver should be trained when the patient is unable to carry over his or her home plan. It may be very difficult for one person to be responsible for all aspects of the patient's care at home, especially if he or she is also caring for other family members. As Hasselkus (1991) discusses, caregivers often experience ethical dilemmas when faced with conflicts between taking good care of the patient and meeting other family and personal responsibilities. The therapist must be sensitive to the demands on the caregiver and should collaborate with him or her to develop a home program that meets the client's needs and is realistic for the caregiver. While some family members are anxious to provide therapeutic intervention during the day and are willing to carry out a comprehensive home program, others are overwhelmed by their responsibilities and feel guilty when unable to do all that has been suggested. When a hired caregiver will be helping the patient, it can be tempting to expect more extensive follow-through with home activities.

Experience suggests, however, that many personal care assistants may have language, training, or educational barriers that prevent optimal follow-through. Prior to discharge, the home program should be demonstrated and plenty of opportunity given for practice. Picture diagrams or photographs of each activity may be helpful. All caregivers appreciate suggestions and techniques to make their job easier and should be encouraged to help streamline their responsibilities. Chapter 16 covers caregiver instruction in depth.

Prior to discharge Rose's daughter attended therapy, although not as frequently as originally planned. She learned the basic techniques and home program suggestions. She seemed capable, but a bit overwhelmed and somewhat quick to intervene when her mother encountered difficulty. The therapist stressed the importance of giving Rose time to perform portions of a task, while acknowledging the time constraints inherent in caring for Rose and running a home. Together they decided that the extra time needed to help Rose with dressing and grooming should be scheduled when the personal care attendant was working. Suggestions were given about how to set up tasks for Rose, such as face washing, hair brushing, and applying lip gloss, as well as how to put on her clothes most easily, the types of clothing that might be easier to use, and how to wash her hair. Because of the safety implications and the potential for the daughter to injure herself, the physical therapist spent a good deal of time teaching her how to use a Hoyer lift for transfers to and from the bed and commode, as well as methods of rolling. Before discharge, the daughter demonstrated the ability to perform the necessary skills. She took her mother first on a day pass, then on an overnight pass, both of which were successful. The personal care attendant also came to therapy one day to learn ADL techniques and home exercises.

At the time of discharge, Rose had met her functional goals. Equipment was in place and she was able to return home with her family. This had been her primary goal during rehabilitation, and though she was cognitively unable to participate fully or make major gains in self-care status, she did improve enough to make care at home reasonable for her daughter.

The occupational therapist's role in treating Rose consisted of facilitating optimal performance through setting realistic goals; encouraging participation; minimizing frustration and overload; selecting appropriate, meaningful activities; providing necessary equipment in conjunction with physical therapy; teaching the daughter how best to manage self-care activities and therapeutic techniques; and ensuring that the home was accessible. Although patients like Rose often do not make tremendous gains, occupational therapy enhanced her quality of life by helping her perform several small, but meaningful, tasks. In addition, the caregivers' quality of life was enhanced by helping them prioritize activities and by teaching methods to care more easily for a severely disabled person.

Carmen made progress in many areas; however, the gap between her prestroke capabilities and her current status remained very apparent. Following an extensive period of outpatient treatment, Carmen reached the goals that had been set and, even with prodding from the therapist, was unable to identify new functional goals. Initially the therapist had imagined further progress in work, home care, and child care, but it was evident that Carmen was not taking the necessary responsibility for developing these areas at home. While the therapist had hoped to inspire a greater desire to perform these tasks, Carmen was not interested in expanding her roles unless her motor and language skills improved. Carmen enjoyed therapy and was willing to attend occupational therapy for RUE control and balance activities. Using the conditional reasoning process described by Fleming (1991) and considering the importance of relating occupational therapy treatment to meaningful occupation as described by Mailloux, Mack, and Cooper (1983), the therapist decided that in the absence of concrete functional goals, further occupational therapy was not warranted. Carmen had made significant improvements in motor function and ADL skill. She was independent in basic self-care, contributed to some of the home maintenance and child care activities, was involved in several leisure activities, and was interacting satisfactorily with her family (see Figure 2).

Figure 2. ADL changes: Carmen.

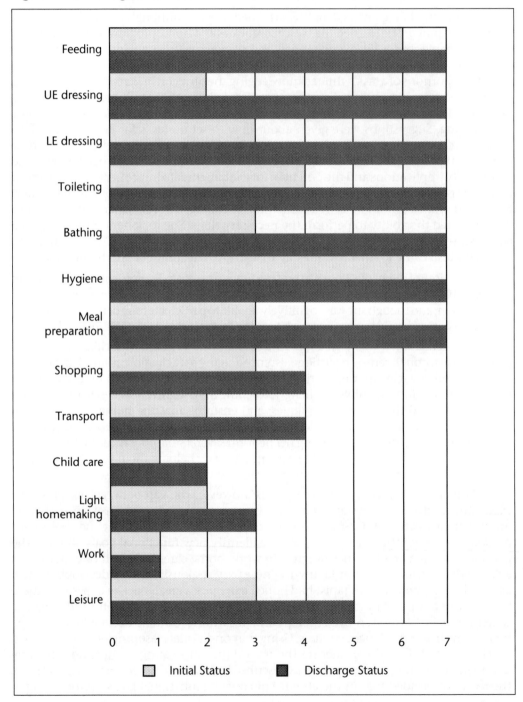

Carmen was given a comprehensive home program, which she demonstrated independently prior to discharge. Her sister, who often accompanied her to treatment, had observed the problem-solving methods used in therapy and was able to facilitate this approach when she met obstacles. Carmen was to return for an occupational therapy checkup 1 month after discharge to monitor adjustments at home and changes in ADL status or goals. She was aware that therapy could be resumed if specific functional goals were identified and diligently pursued. Carmen accepted this plan and acknowledged that a new phase of treatment was beginning in which she would need to decide her direction and goals independently. She had received guidance and training in important functional tasks and now needed to meet new challenges using the techniques she had learned. ◆

References

Bach-y-Rita, P. (Ed.). (1980). *Recovery of function: Theoretical considerations for brain injury rehabilitation*. Baltimore: University Park Press.

Bach-y-Rita, P. (1981). Brain plasticity as a basis of the development of rehabilitation procedures for hemiplegia. *Scandinavian Journal of Rehabilitation Medicine, 13*, 73–83.

Barney, K. (1991). From Ellis Island to assisted living: Meeting the needs of older adults from diverse cultures. *American Journal of Occupational Therapy, 45*, 586–593.

Bernspång, B., Viitanen, M., & Eriksson, S. (1989). Impairments of perceptual and motor functions: Their influence on self-care ability 4–6 years after a stroke. *Occupational Therapy Journal of Research, 9*(1), 38–52.

Bobath, B. (1972). *Adult hemiplegia: Evaluation and treatment*. London: William Heinemann Medical Books.

Brooke, M.M., deLateur, B.J., Diana-Rigby, G.C., & Questad, K.A. (1991). Shoulder subluxation in hemiplegia: Effects of three different supports. *Archives of Physical Medicine and Rehabilitation, 72*, 582–586.

Butter, C.M., & Kirsch, N. (1992). Combined and separate effects of eye patching and visual stimulation on unilateral neglect following stroke. *Archives of Physical Medicine and Rehabilitation, 73*, 1133–1139.

Carr, J.H., & Shepherd, R.B. (1987). *A motor relearning programme for stroke* (2nd ed.). Rockville, MD: Aspen Publishers.

Christenson, M.A. (1990). Adaptations of the physical environment to compensate for sensory changes. *Physical & Occupational Therapy in Geriatrics, 8*(3/4), 3–30.

Chusid, J.G. (1973). *Correlative neuroanatomy and functional neurology*. Los Altos, CA: Lange Medical Publications.

Davidoff, G.N., Keren, O., Ring, H., & Solzi, P. (1991). Acute stroke patients: Long term effects of rehabilitation and maintenance of gains. *Archives of Physical Medicine and Rehabilitation, 72*, 869–873.

Easton, J.D. (1981). *TIA, progressing stroke, and stroke: Recognition and response*. (Telecourse No. 374). New York: The Network for Continuing Medical Education.

Eto, F., Yoshikawa, M., Ueda, S., & Hirai, S. (1980). Posthemiplegic shoulder-hand syndrome, with special reference to related cerebral localization. *Journal of the American Geriatrics Society, 28*(1), 13–17.

Evans, R.L., Bishop, D.S., & Haselkorn, J.K. (1991). Factors predicting satisfactory home care after stroke. *Archives of Physical Medicine and Rehabilitation, 72*, 144–147.

Fleming, M.H. (1991). The therapist with the three-track mind. *American Journal of Occupational Therapy, 45*, 1007–1014.

Galski, T., Ehle, H., Bruno, R., (1990). An assessment of measures to predict the outcome of driving evaluations in patients with cerebral damage. *American Journal of Occupational Therapy, 44*, 709–719.

Garrison, S.J., Rolak, L.A., Dodaro, R.R., & O'Callaghan, A.J. (1988). Rehabilitation of the stroke patient. In J. DeLisa, D. Currie, B. Gans, P. Gatens, J. Leonard, & M. McPhee (Eds.), *Rehabilitation medicine: Principles and practice* (pp. 565–584). Philadelphia: Lippincott.

Glickstein, J.K., Olson, D.A., Cherney, L.R., & Pollard, E. (1989). Feeding and swallowing problems in the elderly: An interdisciplinary approach. *Focus on Geriatric Care & Rehabilitation, 2*(7), 1–8.

Granger, C.V., Hamilton, B.B., & Gresham, G.E. (1988). The stroke rehabilitation outcome study: Part I. General description. *Archives of Physical Medicine and Rehabilitation, 69*, 506–509.

Granger, C.V., Hamilton, B.B., Gresham, G.E., & Kramer, A.A. (1989). The stroke rehabilitation outcome study: Part II. Relative merits of the Total Barthel Index Score and a four item subscore in predicting patient outcomes. *Archives of Physical Medicine and Rehabilitation, 70*, 100–103.

Hasselkus, B. (1991). Ethical dilemmas in family caregiving for the elderly: Implications for occupational therapy. *American Journal of Occupational Therapy, 45*, 206–212.

Mailloux, Z., Mack, W., & Cooper, C. (1983). Knowing what to do: The organization of knowledge for clinical practice. In G. Kielhofner (Ed.), *Health through occupation*. Philadelphia: F.A. Davis.

Mattingly, C. (1991). What is clinical reasoning? *American Journal of Occupational Therapy, 45*, 979–986.

Miller, V.T. (1983). Lacunar stroke: A reassessment. *Archives of Neurology, 40*, 129–134.

Moore, J. (1990, October). *Sensory learning: Application of a sensory integration treatment approach to adult stroke and head injury*. Workshop presented at the Rehabilitation Institute of Chicago, Chicago, IL.

Quigley, F., & DeLisa, J. (1983). Assessing the driving potential of cerebral vascular accident patients. *American Journal of Occupational Therapy, 37*, 474–478.

Rogers, J.C., & Holm, M.B. (1991). Occupational therapy diagnostic reasoning: A component of clinical reasoning. *American Journal of Occupational Therapy, 45*, 1045–1053.

Ross, E., & Rush, J. (1981). Diagnosis and neuroanatomical correlates of depression in brain-damaged patients. *Archives of General Psychiatry, 38*, 1344–1354.

Roth, E.J. (1988). The elderly stroke patient: Principles and practices of rehabilitation management. *Topics in Geriatric Rehabilitation, 3*(4), 27–61.

Slater, D.Y., & Cohn, E.S. (1991). Staff development through analysis of practice. *American Journal of Occupational Therapy, 45*, 1038–1044.

Soderback, I. (1988). The effectiveness of training intellectual functions in adults with acquired brain damage. *Scandinavian Journal of Rehabilitative Medicine, 20*, 47–56.

Voss, E.W., Ionta, M., & Myers, B. (1985). *Proprioceptive neuromuscular facilitation* (3rd ed.). New York: Harper & Row.

9

Self-Care Management for Adults With Movement Disorders

Margaret McCuaig

Margaret McCuaig, MA, OT(C), is a Senior Instructor, Division of Occupational Therapy, School of Rehabilitation Sciences, at the University of British Columbia, Vancouver, BC.

The author expresses her sincere thanks to the clients and colleagues—in particular Donna Brown, occupational therapist at George Pearson Centre, Vancouver—whose contributions and reflections helped shape the ideas in this chapter.

Chapter 9 Outline

Individuals With Movement Disorders

Framework for Identifying Problems in Self-Care

Occupational Therapy and Adults With Movement Disorders

Choice of Adaptive Strategy

Adaptive Strategies Using Equipment and Techniques

Meal Management

Mobility

Communication

Adaptive Strategies Using Routines and Social Supports

Communication

Homemaking

Meal Management

Facilitating the Development of Routines
and Social Supports

Summary

References

Suggestions for Further Reading

Science works with concepts of averages which are far too general to do justice to the
subjective variety of individual lives. (Jung, 1961, p. 3)

This chapter presents anecdotal accounts of how adults with movement disorders view and manage their self-care. Principles for problem solving from the perspectives of the client and the occupational therapist are drawn from case examples. Emphasis is given to the individual's perspective and experience of self, within the context of his or her social and physical environments, as they relate to the management of self-care requirements. The occupational therapist's role in assisting the individual to develop adaptive strategies is also described. A framework is used that considers techniques, equipment, routines, and social supports as categories of adaptive strategies that help individuals with movement disorders compensate for the paucity or excess of movement with which they must contend.

Individuals With Movement Disorders

Individuals with movement disorders face the challenge of living with too much or too little movement, associated with some degree of paralysis or weakness. For people with these disorders, actions are frequently difficult to initiate, terminate, or control. Many conditions carry with them a progressive component, often rapid, and some create a disturbance in cognitive functioning. Memory, concentration, and an ability to organize and sequence events may be affected. Sensation, including proprioception, may be impaired. Problems with functional abilities are often exacerbated by stress as well as the aging process, even if the medical condition itself is stable (Lohr & Wisniewski, 1987). Many individuals with movement disorders experience pain, and have constant fatigue and low energy; poor balance; and difficulties with most areas of self-care, including communication, mobility, eating, dressing, toileting, bathing, and grooming.

The scope of this chapter includes people with movement disorders, including amyotrophic lateral sclerosis, cerebral palsy, dystonia, Huntington's chorea, multiple sclerosis, muscular dystrophy, Parkinson's disease, tardive dyskinesia, and Tourette's syndrome. This nonexhaustive list provides examples of conditions of both hyper- and hypokinetic movement disorders (Jain & Kirshblum, 1993). A list of supplementary readings at the conclusion of the chapter provides sources for detailed descriptions of the medical conditions under discussion. Figure 1 provides common definitions of frequently used terms, and Figure 2 describes features and problems of selected movement disorders.

Framework for Identifying Problems in Self-Care

The Independent Living Movement, a consumer-driven style of life, calls for a redefinition of disability as originating in the social and physical environment, rather than within the person, and for laws and policies that eliminate barriers to full participation in society (DeJong & Lifchez, 1983). This movement embraces the principle that less-handicapping environments result in less-disabled individuals (Browne, Connors, & Stern, 1985). A person's environment has a profound influence on supporting or inhibiting independence. Social supports, cultural beliefs and values, environmental designs and furnishings, and the availability of structures and tools are all salient factors in an individual's ability to perform tasks of daily living. For this reason, when addressing problems of self-care, it is important to assess and to intervene within the context of the individual's social, cultural, and physical environments (Christiansen, 1991).

Figure 1. Terms describing movement disorders, with examples of associated conditions.

Ataxia: Movement, usually of the extremities, that is reduced in speed and distorted in terms of timing and direction (multiple sclerosis; Charcot-Marie-Tooth).

Athetosis: Slow sinuous movement with fluctuations in tone, and most commonly found in the distal extremities; more rhythmic and slower than choreiform movements; exacerbated by anxiety and attempted voluntary movements (cerebral palsy; tardive dyskinesia).

Bradykinesia: Slowness of movement resulting in a person "freezing"; often misinterpreted as depression and withdrawal; presents as a loss of spontaneity (Parkinson's disease).

Chorea: Usually describes a random pattern of rapid, irregular, unpredictable, and involuntary contractions of a group of muscles; resulting clinical picture may be one of a "dancing" or "clownish" gait, with the distal extremities more involved than the proximal ones; movements attenuated during sleep, exacerbated with stress and attempts at action (Huntington's chorea, tardive dyskinesia).

Dystonia: Although often found as a clinical descriptor, is in fact used to describe a neurological syndrome in which there is an abnormality of tone; affects muscle groups in the trunk, neck, face, and proximal limbs; presents with slow, sustained, involuntary twisting movement patterns that may be generalized, segmental, or focal; confused with athetosis when slow, and chorea when rapid.

Hyperkinesia and **hypokinesia**: An excess and a paucity of movement respectively; difficulty with initiation and enacting of a normal speed of movement (all movement disorders, with exception of amyotrophic lateral sclerosis).

Spasticity: Extreme or excessive muscle tone; presents as resistance to passive movement; a constant cocontraction of muscle groups inhibiting relaxation pulls the body into abnormal patterns, rendering it vulnerable to deformities; exacerbated by effort (cerebral palsy; multiple sclerosis).

Rigidity: Resistance of proximal and axial muscles to passive movement; frequently experienced as stiffness and associated with pain (Parkinson's disease).

Tremor: Simple, involuntary, rhythmical movement, frequently starting in the hands; difficult to differentiate from a generalized shivering or shaking; frequently found at rest, but disappears in sleep; most pronounced under stress (Parkinson's disease; multiple sclerosis).

Problems related to self-care are often addressed through adaptive strategies within the domains of techniques and equipment, routines, and social supports. In this chapter, case studies describe specific occupations of self-care within these adaptive domains. The emphasis of this approach differs from the traditional presentation of problems according to disability, and solutions in terms of physical performance.

Traditionally, medical rehabilitation focused on the assessment and elimination of the impairment (Christiansen, 1991). Consistent with the themes expressed elsewhere in this book, this chapter focuses on the process of adaptation of the individual to the physical and social environments. Its objective is to show that self-care needs can be met despite the presence of movement disorders and without emphasizing remediation of physical dysfunction. The importance of an individual's social and physical contexts is highlighted as a critical consideration in the assessment and intervention of self-care problems (Corbin & Strauss, 1988).

Figure 2. Summary data of major motor control disorders: Manifestations and presenting problems.

Condition	Features	Movement Problems
Amyotrophic lateral sclerosis	Motor neuron disease of rapid onset; more prevalent in men over 30; affects central and peripheral motor neurons.	Progressive muscle weakness and atrophy distally, then proximally; fatigue.
Cerebral palsy	Motor disorder resulting from a nonprogressive lesion in the developing brain, resulting in abnormal and fluctuating muscle tone and reflexes.	Ataxia; athetosis; flaccidity; spasticity; or mixed pattern of movement affecting the limbs, trunk, head, and neck.
Charcot-Marie-Tooth	Inherited, progressive, sensorimotor disorder of nervous system; includes mild loss of sensation.	Progressive muscle weakness starting in extremities resulting in loss of balance, and tripping.
Duchenne muscular dystrophy	Hereditary and progressive disease of the muscles; onset in males ages 2–6; marked wasting of proximal muscle groups; moves distally.	Rapidly progressive muscle weakness; initially pelvic and pectoral groups; fatigue.
Huntington's chorea	Hereditary, progressive disorder of the basal ganglia; characterized by abnormal, involuntary choreiform movements; amplified by progressive cognitive impairment.	Abrupt, involuntary choreiform movements exacerbated by stress and effort.
Multiple sclerosis	Lesions in the central nervous system; demyelination results in a series of exacerbations and remissions; progressive weakness; sensory disturbances; cognitive damage.	Progressive muscle weakness and spasticity; tremors; ataxia; and fatigue.
Parkinson's disease	Degeneration of the basal ganglia; progressive; found most frequently in men and women over 50; results in muscle rigidity, postural changes, dementia, loss of autonomic reflexes.	Slowness in motor planning; difficulty initiating movement; tremors at rest and with intention; shuffling gait; slurred speech; symptoms exacerbated by fatigue and stress.
Tourette's syndrome	Involuntary movement disorder; onset ages 2–5, primarily males; includes sensory disturbances, impulsivity, compulsive and ritualistic behaviors, with possible attention deficits.	Recurrent involuntary, repetitive, rapid movements; hyperactivity; symptoms increase with stress.

Occupational Therapy and Adults With Movement Disorders

Self-care for adults with movement disorders calls for a new framework of self-direction, rather than a focus on task-oriented behaviors such as brushing teeth or combing hair (Cole, 1983). The occupational therapist's role is to be knowledgeable about the context of an individual's life, and to be committed to supporting the perspective of the consumer, using nontraditional approaches reflecting the principles of independent living. This framework requires occupational therapists to support an individual's acquisition of skills and capabilities for self-direction and to acknowledge the person's ability to be a manager who can communicate effectively, identify and use resources, make choices and decisions, set priorities, and make sound judgments (Burke, Miyake, Kielhofner, & Barris, 1982). Such a framework encompasses a belief that one learns when the teacher organizes information according to the hierarchy of importance perceived by the learner (Carpenter, 1991). In this hierarchy, timing assumes critical importance. The occupational therapist's primary challenge in working with adults with movement disorders is to consider the person as a unit consisting of personality, movements, and thoughts engaged in activity within a social and physical context. In meeting this challenge, the therapist must note what elements contribute to a successful outcome for that individual, and how learning takes place.

Teaching strategies that minimize fatigue, enhance safety, and foster adequate stability (particularly postural) are essential for managing self-care for people with movement disorders (Gauthier, Dalziel, & Gauthier, 1987). Organization, pacing, timing, and energy conservation are critical components of teaching techniques and strategies in self-care. The use of auditory and visual cues may be necessary to facilitate initiation and speed of movement in individuals with movement disorders. In particular, occupational therapists should consider equipping individuals with an array of adaptive strategies from which they can choose for managing their self-care. A person who fatigues easily through the course of the day may need to have at least three strategies for getting to the toilet: one using bars on the wall, one using a sliding transfer board, and one requiring the presence of another person for physical support. The choice of strategy will depend on the individual's energy level, resources available, urgency, and timing.

Choice of Adaptive Strategy

This chapter is organized according to adaptive strategies in the domains of techniques and equipment, and routines and social supports. Strategies consist of actions an individual employs to accomplish certain tasks, which in turn make up a larger system of a way of organizing a life. Within these domains of adaptive strategies, examples of self-care activities such as eating, communicating, mobility, homemaking, grooming, and dressing are described, and strategies for occupational therapy intervention are discussed.

An individual's choice of a specific adaptive strategy is not based on function alone (McCuaig & Frank, 1991). Deciding how to accomplish a task is a complex process, and highly dependent on values that determine the importance and order of potential actions. The decision to choose one piece of equipment, technique, or routine rather than another is also based on the context, possibilities, and requirements of the situation. Occupational therapy literature on self-care for adults with movement disorders would be enriched by descriptions from the perspective of the individual with the disability— a view from "the other."

All too often, the clinical focus in occupational therapy intervention has been to enhance function without due consideration of the context in which it is performed. Adaptation to living with a movement disorder involves more than learning a repertoire of techniques in a clinical setting or choosing a particular piece of equipment. Rather, it is a complex process related to the meaning of actions to the individual. Physical and social supports and limitations, as well as individual constraints and beliefs, strongly influence adaptation. Behavior is organized by values and beliefs that individuals hold about themselves and those around them, and affects functional choices in a particular context. An individual's choice of action or adaptive strategy will be shaped by temporal factors, personal values, and beliefs about the activity, self, and environment (Fleming, 1991).

Meghan, a woman with cerebral palsy, has personal criteria for choosing her adaptive strategies in self-care activities. These choices are influenced by her need to present herself as capable (McCuaig & Frank, 1991). For Meghan, important criteria thus include being viewed as mentally competent, physically able, and socially acceptable. To carry out her activities, she chooses from a variety and combination of strategies that include techniques and equipment, routines, and social resources. As might be expected, Meghan's choice of strategy is frequently based not on functional efficiency, but on self-presentation. The techniques, pieces of equipment, routines, or people supporting her appearance as a competent, and socially and physically able individual are given preference as adaptive strategies.

Meghan's athetosis, physical deformities, and inability to speak, affect her ability to function. Therefore, if she makes tea for her sister, whom she believes views her as incompetent and dependent, it is critical that she complete every step herself, from boiling the water to pouring the cream in the cups and serving the food. When she is with those whom she feels acknowledge her as a competent individual, her desire to present a social self and to communicate takes precedence over demonstrating her physical abilities. Under these circumstances, she will ask her guest to fix and serve the tea. This leaves her free to use her hands for pointing to her communication system to "chat" with her visitors. During these situations, Meghan directs the activity, indicating which dishes to use, and noting where the items are located and where tea will be served. Thus, Meghan has a repertoire of strategies for "making tea" and chooses one based on the context of the event. Who is present and how she is perceived are more important considerations that simply accomplishing the task of getting the tea from the kettle into the cups.

Adaptive Strategies Using Equipment and Techniques

Adaptive strategies to address self-care management for people with movement disorders often include methods or techniques involving either specialized or commonplace equipment. See Figure 3 for factors to consider when making recommendations.

Highly specialized equipment used by people with movement disorders might include powered wheelchairs for those unable to walk. Features such as a custom joystick

Figure 3. Factors to consider when recommending adaptive strategies.

- What is important to the individual about the task?
- Is the strategy viewed as compatible with the particular social context?
- Does the strategy enhance the individual's sense of personal control?
- Does the strategy minimize effort?
- Does the strategy interfere with social opportunities or diminish the presentation of self?
- Is the recommended strategy temporally realistic given the context?
- Does the strategy provide for safety?

add flexibility and control of the chair. This is important, particularly if the individual's movements lack stability. Joysticks can be adjusted to compensate for excess or diminished movement. The effects of excess movement can be absorbed by the controls, and the driving of the chair is not affected. Alternatively, the sensitivity to movement can be increased so that a minimum amount of movement from the individual produces a maximum degree of movement of the wheelchair.

Another example of highly specialized equipment is an environmental control unit. Using this equipment, stereo sound systems, telephones, apartment intercoms, lights, fans, and televisions can be accessed through a wide variety of switching devices. Individuals lacking the dexterity, coordination, or strength to turn knobs or push buttons directly have easy access to many functions within their living environments through the use of environmental controls. Dickey and Shealey (1987) have provided a useful overview of these devices, in which they identify the assessment information necessary to determine the type of transducer or activator device appropriate for a given client. These include (a) muscle strength and range of motion, (b) endurance, (c) sensation, (d) visual and auditory perceptual status, and (e) gross and fine motor coordination.

By contrast, equipment may be transparent (not readily identifiable as an adaptive device). Included in this category are conventional items widely available commercially, yet considered adaptive because of specific characteristics and application. There are several important advantages to such equipment, including cost, availability, and service and maintenance warranties that frequently accompany major items. Useful equipment can be found in shopping malls and local hardware stores or through consumer catalogues. Often, commercially available items have easily replaced parts, minimizing the "down time" for malfunctioning equipment. Manufacturers should be contacted before making modifications, to ensure that such adaptations will not jeopardize the item's warranty (Gordon & Kozole, 1984).

Examples of "transparent" adaptive equipment include a typewriter with widely spaced keys as a useful communication device for someone lacking the coordination and dexterity to write; felt-tipped pens enabling an individual too weak to exert pressure to mark a page; and front-opening, lightweight clothing providing independence in dressing for someone with excess movement. A lightweight kettle with a plug attachment at its base may compensate for a person's lack of muscle strength in homemaking tasks (see Figure 4). Wall bars are becoming common in many apartment dwellings, and provide stability for someone transferring to the toilet. Commercially available nonskid mats and stripping for tubs are used by many individuals with movement disorders.

Assessment, prescription, and adaptation of equipment are familiar activities for occupational therapists. Batavia and Hammer (1990) have noted the general absence of consumer-based criteria for the evaluation of equipment. Criteria formulated by consumers could benefit designers, manufacturers, funding agencies, occupational therapists, and ultimately the consumers themselves in the process of choosing appropriate equipment. Batavia and Hammer cite research showing that in addition to identifying the need for the equipment, important criteria from the consumers' perspectives included effectiveness, affordability, operability, and dependability. It is also interesting to note that criteria ranking changed according to the equipment function. Acceptability (the esthetics, or psychological "fit") were a high priority for something as personal as a powered wheelchair, but of little consequence in an environmental control unit to operate the stereo.

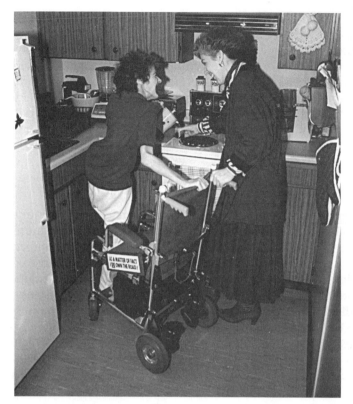

Figure 4. Meghan stabilizing herself on a kitchen counter and wheelchair, using a lightweight kettle to make tea.

Criteria for equipment specifically to be used by people with a movement disorder include an ability to undergo unusual physical force or stress, which includes falling and inadvertent, uncoordinated hitting. Equipment often needs to be both lightweight to compensate for weakness, and durable to withstand being dropped or struck through excess movement. If an individual has involuntary movement, safety factors such as stability, absence of sharp edges, and flexibility must be considered. Equipment may need extra padding, bolts may need to be covered, and raw edges may need to be smoothed or sanded. If the individual has difficulty initiating and sustaining movement, then sensitivity to touch and the use of lightweight material are important features of equipment. If the individual's condition is deteriorating, it is critical that the equipment be flexible and able to be adapted easily and with as little expense as possible to meet changing requirements.

An important aspect of equipment is its appropriate and effective use. Techniques refer to the methods an individual has developed or been taught in order to accomplish a task, and often include equipment. Adults frequently use methods that have evolved over the years, often by trial and error, through family intervention, persistence, and experimentation. Often techniques that appear to be awkward, uncoordinated, and precarious are in fact finely honed and efficacious elements of a highly integrated system.

Witty Ticcy Ray, a man with Tourette's syndrome (Sacks, 1970) developed a unique set of techniques to adapt to his excess movement. Sacks writes, "When I first saw Ray he was 24 years old, and almost incapacitated by multiple tics of extreme violence coming in volleys every few seconds" (p. 97). Ray had so incorporated his surfeit of movement into his everyday life and activities that when he was under the influence of Haldol, a medication to rid him of his tics, he was virtually unable to function. Without the tics his sense of timing, and his reflexive actions, balance, and poise, which he had incorporated into his "techniques" enabling him to be a jazz drummer (with astounding improvisations arising from the tics) and a contestant to be reckoned with in games such as ping-pong, were all askew and his life was catastrophic. He had so adapted to the presence of tics in his life that without them he banged into things, was literally off-balance, fell, and had a strong feeling that a part of him was missing.

The occupational therapist's role in teaching adaptive techniques to people with movement disorders is to observe closely and assess the individual in context, to give attention to the larger and potentially fragile system of movement. Techniques designed for individuals with movement disorders require observation of timing and an understanding of peoples' adaptive use of their physical abilities and limitations. Body postures that decrease excessive movements and provide trunk support and proximal stability need to be taught and developed. For those with a poverty of movement, finding the body part that provides consistent, voluntarily controlled movement and does not fatigue easily is important. Rhythmic counting may assist someone who has difficulty initiating movements.

Meal Management

Occupational therapists have paid considerable attention to the development of equipment and specialized techniques for meal management. They make recommendations for built-up handles to compensate for weakness, and for weighted utensils to dampen extraneous movements. Very sophisticated feeding apparatuses, such as the Winsford feeder (Einset, Deitz, Billingsley, & Harris, 1989) move food from the plate to the mouth by means of a spoon set in motion with an electronic switch, for adults with cerebral palsy. In other instances, highly individualized devices are fabricated, such as a feeding harness developed for a man with amyotrophic lateral sclerosis, reported by Takai (1986). Stability for people with movement disorders is often enhanced by the use of nonskid mats, plate guards, and utensil holders, such as the universal cuff (Pedretti & Zoltan, 1990). Commonplace equipment, such as straws and heavy mugs, may be used by people with poor coordination.

Dysphagia, or difficulty swallowing, frequently occurs in individuals with movement disorders, particularly those with amyotrophic lateral sclerosis, cerebral palsy, multiple sclerosis, or Parkinson's disease. This condition, which is potentially life threatening because of the possibility of aspiration and inadequate nutrition, results from a disturbance to the swallowing mechanism. Dysphagia may result in food retention in the mouth and throat, while delayed swallowing and poor lip closure may result in drooling. There may also be weakness of the tongue and palate, leading to difficulty maneuvering food in the mouth, and a hyperactive gag reflex, resulting in choking. Often, correct assessment and diagnosis, coupled with simple intervention, helps to normalize oral food intake. Occupational therapy intervention for individuals with dysphagia has been well-documented (Asher, 1986; Fearing, 1989; Pedretti & Zoltan, 1990).

We return to the example of Meghan, a woman with athetoid cerebral palsy, for nontraditional examples of how techniques and equipment can be part of an adaptive strategy for meal management. Meghan, who has deformities in her trunk and limbs and an inability to communicate verbally, has developed many adaptive techniques that use her body as a tool to compensate for the fluctuations in tone that make her movements difficult to predict and control (McCuaig & Frank, 1991). She holds a fork woven unconventionally in and out of the fingers of her right hand. She is unable to grasp the handle adequately, and prefers the stability this position gives the utensil. She spears the food with her fork, and, balancing on her forearm and elbow, brings the food to her mouth. Her chin rests on her chest with her neck rotated so that her left ear is almost touching her shoulder. This seemingly contorted body position provides the balance she lacks when sitting erect, and minimizes the effects of the extraneous movements in her arms when her elbow is not stabilized. A colorful, plastic-coated mat provides the stability for her dishes, countering the excess movement in her hands. Meghan is not set apart as different from her mealtime partners by her use of "adapted" equipment. She uses ordinary utensils in extraordinary ways.

Equipment and techniques address only the functional aspect of moving food from the plate to the mouth. Of equal or greater importance for Meghan is the social context of meal management and eating. Although Meghan often invites people for tea or lunch, she rarely eats at these functions. The physical stress of eating, the ensuing fatigue, and the fact that when she is eating she cannot use her hands to access her communication systems, have led to her decision not to eat with others. She explains her decision in the following comment: "The reason I very often don't eat with people is I feel I can eat after they go, but I won't be able to talk [after they are gone]." Like most of us, Meghan uses the occasion of tea or a meal for social purposes. This social aspect has sometimes been overlooked by therapists who emphasize the functional and nutritional aspects of mealtime management.

Thus, important considerations for occupational therapists in recommending equipment and techniques may be the extent to which they permit social interaction and whether independence in meal management is important to the individual. Is eating viewed as a social occasion? Is eating "independently" with equipment more important than the length of time or the physical effort it takes to finish a meal? Are esthetics important, and, if so, are the utensils attractive and pleasant to hold to the tongue and lips? Does the plate guard blend with the plate? Does the color of the nonskid mat clash with that of the table? Do the techniques, such as sliding rather than lifting, minimize effort? Does the independent use of the equipment detract from the potential social opportunities available when a person is fed by another (Einset et al., 1989)? What are the temporal considerations and the fatigue factors? Would several smaller meals a day be more manageable than the traditional three main meals? These are some of the questions that may be important to determine appropriate adaptive strategies for mealtimes. Further suggestions for adaptive strategies for meal management are described in the section, "Adaptive Strategies Using Routines and Social Supports."

Mobility

Another factor identified as central for adults with movement disorders is independent mobility, both within and outside the individual's dwelling (DeJong, 1979; Neuman, Schatzlein, & Sparks, 1987). The physical control a person has over the environment and the ease and freedom with which he or she can navigate within it, influence feelings of autonomy and competence. The ability to move at will and as efficiently as possible in terms of speed and conservation of energy adds to a person's sense of independence, grace, and dignity.

Equipment recommended for mobility must be considered from perspectives other than function. A person's apparent unwillingness to use a piece of equipment may have nothing to do with the equipment's potential functional opportunities. Stronger than the desire to be mobile may be the need to maintain a view of an able self, which may not include using a wheelchair.

A woman in her 50s with muscular dystrophy describes why she would not accept a wheelchair as an alternative to stumbling and falling:

> I wanted a cure for my wobbly legs. I wanted to maintain my denial of what was happening to me . I disconnected from my old way of life before being committed to the new. I had to mourn the loss of using my legs before I could put energy into using a wheelchair instead. (Wagner, 1985, p. 58)

Meghan uses a conventional powered wheelchair with a joystick, with the footrests removed. This chair, in combination with ramped sidewalks, paved roads, and an accessible apartment, gives her the independence she requires to get about in her home environment, go to her appointments, do her shopping, and visit friends who are within commuting distance. After opening a levered-handled door with her right hand, Meghan hyperextends her knee to hold the door open with her foot (acting like a hand), while she uses her hand to operate the joystick on her powered chair (acting as her legs) to move herself out of doors. Her feet often act as "hands" as she pushes items out of the way, backed by the power of the wheelchair. She controls her direction with the joystick, and her speed by separate switches on the control box.

Meghan's ability to extend her body image to include the wheelchair appears to be an important adaptation in her mastery of techniques and the use of equipment. A straight cloth sack made by a friend hangs over the wheelchair handles, enabling Meghan to carry items in the same manner in which a person might use a backpack or a tote bag over a shoulder. Meghan hangs her purse, which holds, among other things, her Canon Communicator (a portable printing device and word board) on the right side of the chair. She has personalized the chair with a sticker saying, "Writers have the last word." When looking at Meghan, one has the sense not of a person sitting in a wheelchair, but of a unit, a "goodness of fit." In her chair, Meghan has access to all aspects of her apartment, the building, and the environs. The use of a powered chair provides Meghan with independence she did not have in her initial manual wheelchair. She can approach and leave clerks, friends, store displays, and buildings with the same timing and grace as the general public. She can cross busy streets during the prescribed "walk" interval. The powered chair allows Meghan to move with dignity, ease, and at a speed comparable to the average walking pace of her peers.

Particular concerns for occupational therapists in addressing powered mobility for people with movement disorders are physical and cognitive control, flexibility, and safety. Positioning for maximum stability is critical. This may require special seating, with trunk and head supports, as well as adaptations to provide proximal control for the extremities. Proximal joints and limbs must be stabilized, and extraneous movements controlled to enhance distal control. In general, individuals with severe movement disorders involving abnormal or fluctuating muscle tone require customized seating systems involving carefully fabricated seating surfaces. Taylor (1987) has provided a useful overview of the issues of seating and positioning for clients with varying levels of need.

Sophisticated technology has much to offer people with movement disorders. Once the most reliable, consistent, voluntarily controlled body movement and location have been determined, the powered wheelchair's control mechanism (usually a joystick) can be adapted to compensate for almost any degree of excess or lack of movement. Latching, or "cruise control," is an option for individuals who fatigue easily. Tremor dampening can be adjusted to almost any degree of excess movement. The speed at which the braking system engages can be adjusted for someone with a startle reflex.

For individuals with cognitive impairment, occupational therapists may consider including the provision of safe environments for practice, extended time to experiment with moving in the powered wheelchair, obstacle courses, and simulation exercises. They may need to emphasize demonstration and doing, rather than verbal instruction.

Individuals with movement disorders may experience substantial fluctuations in ability and endurance over time, even during the course of a day. Accordingly, they may require highly flexible mobility systems. For example, a person with multiple sclerosis may wish to use a manual wheelchair as a way to exercise in the morning, and a powered chair for transportation as the day and ensuing fatigue progress. When choosing a control mechanism for a powered wheelchair, it may be important to consider a remote joystick, which can be mounted easily in various places on the chair—on the right, the left, centrally, under the chin, or at the back or side of the head.

Particular safety points for powered mobility systems include replacing square-headed bolts with round ones, padding sharp edges, removing heel loops if necessary, and using safety belts and antitipping devices.

Communication

Communication, whether graphic, verbal, or physical, is central to human interaction. In order for communication to take place there must be an idea or a feeling, a sender and a receiver of the message, and a vehicle for its transmission. An idea or feeling is most commonly transmitted via words representing language, in the form of human speech accompanied by body language, and is received by the ears and eyes of the listener. When any element of this process is damaged, alternative techniques and equipment may need to be introduced (Vanderheiden, 1983).

Individuals engage in different modes of communication. Conversation, commonly a brief, temporal, and often spontaneous verbal exchange, is usually thought of as the most common. According to Vanderheiden (1983), conversation using the voice as a tool usually takes place at a rate of 120 to 180 words per minute and is augmented by facial expressions, gestures, and body language. These verbal exchanges include changes in intonation and timing. Conversation takes place in face-to-face situations, over the telephone, or simultaneously with an activity. Messaging, another mode of communication, is the delayed presentation of previously prepared information. Common tools for messaging include pens or pencils, typewriters, FAX machines, telephone answering devices, and computers. When an individual is unable to use the conventional modes and tools of communication for conversation or sending messages, the dynamics and quality of the interaction are affected.

Augmentative communication includes any personal or technical system that enhances a person's present communication abilities. These devices may produce speech, a visual display, or a written message. They are accessed directly or indirectly by body parts, such as a hand, the head, or eyes.

Communication aids may take many forms. A man unable to move from the neck down uses a pointer held in his teeth to dial his telephone. He has learned to use his mouth as his hand to manipulate the pointer, and uses the pointer as his finger to dial the numbers (Zola, 1982).

Meghan has a wide variety of universal or commonplace communication devices, including felt-tipped pens, an electric typewriter with widely spaced keys, a computer, and a telephone. She also uses specialized equipment, including an 8" x 11" Letter Board indicating the letters of the alphabet, to which she points to spell her message; a Canon Communicator, a small, portable, battery operated device with keys that she presses to produce a ticker tape–printed message; and a Vocaid, a device producing synthesized sounds in the form of letters, attached to her telephone that enables her to spell messages to her caller. Meghan also uses her voice, facial expressions, and gestures to convey a message. She has a repertoire of equipment and techniques from which to choose, based on the context of the communication taking place.

Meghan's decision regarding which piece of equipment to use is based not only on the criteria of wanting to present an able self, but on her perceptions of the demands of the situation and on her expectations of the exchange. If Meghan is having an intimate conversation with a friend, she likes to sit close to that person with the Letter Board on her lap, point to the letters as she spells out her message, and have her friend repeat the letters and say the resulting words. Although this method is slow (approximately 12 words per minute) it has elements that Meghan highly values. Using her Letter Board allows Meghan to make frequent eye contact and to stay engaged with her partner. She can use her other hand to gesture, and she can use her face and body to express feelings. The "voice" is personal and not synthesized. Meghan can augment the spelling with vocalizations and with nodding and shaking her head. The result is a personal and intimate conversation (see Figure 5).

When Meghan is in a place like the drug store, a situation that has very different requirements and for which Meghan has fewer personal communication expectations, she uses her electronic Canon Communicator. This device resembles a small pocket calculator, looks attractive, produces a written message that is easy to see, and is understood by all who can read. Meghan has tried to use her Letter Board in public, but says, "People just think I'm retarded pointing to this dumb piece of paper, and ignore me." She finds that people are interested in her Canon Communicator, and that it can be an ice breaker for people who are not familiar with her methods. Meghan does not need to express her feelings or to communicate intimately with a store clerk. She needs only to deliver a message that will not be ignored, and that will get her the items she requires. Meghan's desire to present a sophisticated and capable image is supported by her use of this device in public.

In assessment and intervention for communication needs, occupational therapists should work closely with speech and language pathologists to determine access to the equipment and the requirements of the social and physical environment. For people with movement disorders, specific recommendations for addressing communication needs

Figure 5. Meghan communicating through her letter board.

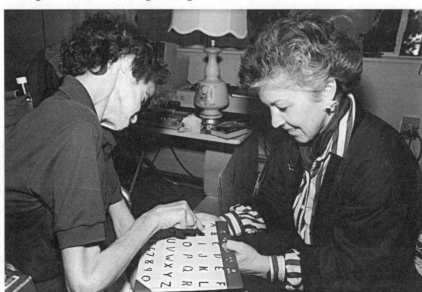

include the use of enlarged pencils, writing aids that hold a pen or pencil, and felt-tipped pens. For people capable of using typewriters or computers (or electronic communicators), key guards that prevent more than one key from being pressed at the same time can help those with poor coordination. Enlarged keyboards for computers are useful for people who lack the fine motor skills to access a standard-size keyboard. Mini keyboards are available for people who lack range and muscle strength in their upper extremities.

Often a person has sufficient control of the head and neck to permit the use of mouthsticks or head wands for operating augmentative communication devices. Mouthsticks made of lightweight doweling with rubber tubing on the end may be useful for people with adequate neck and jaw control and movement. Smith (1989) has noted that inadequate attention has been given to the potential problems of improperly fitted mouthsticks. In addition to oral problems, fatigue, gagging, and temporal mandibular joint dysfunction are known consequences of improperly fitting mouthpiece components. Therapists are urged to consider the standards developed by Blaine and Nelson (1973) when prescribing mouthsticks. Head pointers offer another option for using augmentative communication devices, and these can be custom made or obtained commercially.

Other important considerations when determining appropriate equipment and techniques for communication are rate of transmission, portability of the system, reliability, flexibility, spontaneity, and the system's potential for expressing the fullness of the message. An augmentative system should require as little expenditure of energy as possible, for both for the sender and receiver of the message. It must enhance an individual's personal abilities and, wherever possible, encourage physical gestures and expressions of sound. The equipment must also meet the requirements of the physical and social environment.

Adaptive Strategies Using Routines and Social Supports

Behaviors that are repeated over time and organized into patterns and habits form routines that can be viewed as part of a person's adaptive strategies for increasing independence in self-care (Cohen & Lazarus, 1983). Often these behavioral routines are unconscious, while at other times they are planned and deliberate. The development and establishment of routines frequently involve attention to temporal considerations, including the ability to plan ahead, efficiency in organization, and the capacity to remember past experiences. Routines and the use of social supports can be considered adaptive for people with movement disorders, because they compensate for the inability to perform certain activities, the extended length of time and energy required to accomplish a task, and limited coordination and strength. Frequently an individual's strategy for accomplishing a task employs a unique combination of equipment, techniques, routines, and social supports. These social supports may take the form of family and friends, casual acquaintances, formal and informal organizations, or health care workers within and without institutions.

The use of adaptive strategies employing routines and social supports is often dependent on specific factors. The individual needs to know that a certain activity or interaction is going to take place and what the requirements of the situation will be. The individual must also have adequate time for planning, have a well-developed ability to organize personal and environmental resources, have the perception of how long an activity will take, understand what the specific steps will involve, and know how much energy will be needed. Routines generally have a sense of predictability and familiarity, in that they have usually been used successfully in the past under similar, if not exact, conditions. Social supports need to be initiated, nurtured, and developed.

Adaptive routines and social supports are not necessarily developed in a systematic and consciously planned manner. Often, it is a process of trying to establish a "goodness of fit" between resources and demands (King, 1978). Routines are frequently developed through repeated action over time. When Meghan was asked how she had developed certain routines she replied:

> I have never thought of that, I just keep trying until I figure it out. I mostly learn by trial and error. I have a real flare for making mistakes, blunders, and everything else, but I'm too stubborn to quit. . . . I am a terrifically stubborn person, which has been a great assistance to me in my condition. But I also think I know when I have reached a point that enough is enough.

Meghan, now in her 50s, credits her mother and others in her family for having the determination to let her try things on her own—to think and do for herself since she was very little. The following examples illustrate adaptive strategies using routines and social supports for self-care activities, including communication, homemaking, and meal management.

Communication

Emma, a woman who has amyotrophic lateral sclerosis and lives in a long-term-care unit, uses a variety of techniques and pieces of equipment for communication to adapt to her inability to speak and her paucity of movement in her limbs. She has a letter/word board to which she can point with hand movements that are slow and laborious. She also has a computerized message system, which she operates with a microswitch in her palm; and a system of eye-blinking, which she uses in conjunction with the communication partner's verbal spelling. In addition, Emma has established routines for communication that are considered adaptive because of their premeditated, compensatory nature.

Emma, like Meghan, determines which strategy to use after considering outcome, context, and values. She decides in advance the purpose of the communication, the intended recipient of the message, what she expects from the exchange, and what is important for her to achieve. Emma decides ahead of time whether it is more important to save the other person time by having information ready, or whether the conversation process and the elements of the interaction are of greater significance than the message itself. One of Emma's routines for communicating is to provide her communication partner with a bulk of information in the format of a printout from her computer. Depending on her partner, this may include news of her family, humorous anecdotes of her day, specific information needs in the form of questions, or follow-up responses to a previous conversation.

This routine necessitates Emma's foreknowledge of the visit, adequate time for Emma to compose her thoughts and messages at the computer, and the ability of her communication partner to read. Emma often chooses this routine, out of consideration of the time and energy constraints of her partner. She is very aware of the importance of her social support system and consciously works at sustaining these networks. It requires much more of Emma's time, but significantly less of her partner's, if she puts her thoughts on paper before the interaction. It also provides the partner with something to read, and on which to focus. Emma can work at her own pace at her computer when she has the energy, and can take rest periods, which in conversation would be awkward and possibly stressful for the partner.

Many people with movement disorders that include loss of speech struggle with "spread," or the assumption of one disability based on the presence of another (Wright, 1983). An inability to speak is frequently equated with an inability to think. The strategy

Emma has developed for communicating with people through a prepared note helps to dispel any misconceptions the partner might have of her cognitive abilities. The notes contain witticisms, inquiries about the partner's well-being, social comments about the news or weather, descriptions of her sons' activities, and her feelings about events on the ward. Emma presents herself as a socially competent woman, full of ideas and feelings, and actively engaged in life.

The words of one of Emma's more recent friends reflects the impact of her writing. "The notes helped me to see who Emma was; they really touched me, and made me feel as if I knew her, and gave me insights I hadn't had before." Comments from a health care worker confirm this view. "The use Emma makes of humor and her expressions of appreciation help to build a bridge between us. I find that it has enhanced my receptivity to her desire to communicate, which is very time consuming and exhausting."

Homemaking

The following incident demonstrates the use of routines and social supports as an adaptive strategy for homemaking activities. Lee is a woman who has Parkinson's disease with resulting intention tremor in her upper extremities, head, and neck; a slow and shuffling gait; rigidity in her trunk; and slurred speech. She lives with her elderly husband in their own home. Having friends in for tea once a week is an important social event for Lee. When her guests arrive, the cups and saucers are out on a tea trolley, along with the cream, sugar, and napkins. Lee directs one of the woman to open the oven door and remove the cake made at the local bakery. She often stores baked items in the stove—it is a large space that she can easily reach from her scooter, and it keeps items fresh. She asks another of her guests to pour from the thermos and to serve the tea. Lee is the conductor of the orchestra. She directs the play and the players.

The dimensions of this seemingly simple event that render it an adaptive strategy are time, effort, and forethought. In order for Lee to execute this very ordinary but important occasion she must invest considerable planning time and effort. She needs to travel in her scooter to the local mall to buy the cake and other grocery items, and transport them safely home. She has to have her cups clean and arranged on the tray ahead of time. Her problems with strength, balance, dexterity, and coordination make an apparently easy task one that requires considerable orchestration. During the tea Lee plays the host, directing the event. She manages everything, deciding when to hold the tea, what to serve, and who will pour. She has a keen sense of timing, is extremely gracious and social in her requests, is well-organized, and gives clear directions.

Meal Management

For many individuals with movement disorders, eating can be an exhausting and undignified experience, whether managing food independently or being fed. The physical and emotional strain of getting the food on the utensil, safely negotiating it to the lips, keeping it in the mouth, chewing adequately, swallowing smoothly, and maintaining a comfortable posture can be excessive. Weighted handles, nonskid mats, plate guards, and even automatic feeding devices are often not adequate to support a person's nutritional, social, and personal needs related to eating. As with other self-care activities, function alone is not sufficient for a satisfying experience at meal time. While being fed brings its own set of problems, it is often the strategy of choice for people unable to manage a meal in a reasonable amount of time and with a minimum of effort.

Catherine, a young woman with cerebral palsy living in an extended-care facility, prefers to be fed, rather than to feed herself. She has spent countless hours practicing, trying different pieces of equipment and physical positions. The combination of her severe athetoid movements, poor head control, and general weakness makes eating independently an unpleasant chore. She now prefers to spend her energy writing at her computer, visiting with friends, and going to school. Catherine has done several things to make her mealtime pleasant. She has asked to be fed in her room, and to invite one other person who also needs to be fed to join her and the aide who is feeding her. When she orders her meal she includes an extra tea and biscuit for the aide. This is a treat for the aide, and adds to the feeling of the meal being more of a shared and social experience. Catherine also has the television turned on to her favorite soap opera at noon, and to the news in the evening. This too is a treat for the aide, and gives them something on which to focus and to discuss. The conversation, the tea, and the company promote a relaxed atmosphere and help to minimize the potential tedium, and therefore the stress of the aide.

When occupational therapists plan mealtime interventions, they should always consider how to create an environment that promotes eating as an enjoyable social event rather than simply a nutritional exercise. At its best, eating is an intimate affair; at its worst, it is traumatic. Wherever possible, the physical environment should promote relaxation and comfort. Attention should be given to room temperature, noise level, and visual stimulation, particularly if the individual has a sensitive startle reaction. A quiet room may suit one person, whereas another person might prefer company. Individuals who require feeding can be taught how to engage the interest and attention of the person feeding them. They can be encouraged to take control of choices, determining what food to eat and when, and how quickly items are presented and in what order. They can also help to identify what elements of the mealtime event are stressful, and collaborate with the therapists in addressing them.

Facilitating the Development of Routines and Social Supports

Research in multiple sclerosis (Brooks & Matson, 1982) has suggested that social psychological variables are the most salient explanatory models of adjustment to the disease. In particular, integrating the realities of the disease into the life-style, and depending on strong social support networks, have each been identified as important variables for persons with this progressive, episodic, and debilitating neuromotor condition. Thus, the development of adaptive routines and social supports has empirical support in the literature as an effective therapeutic strategy.

Therapists can help individuals with all types of movement disorders to develop strategies that use routines and social supports by facilitating a person's repeated action beyond basic problem solving until a routine is established and acceptable to the individual and those in his or her environment. During this process, therapists should help develop routines that minimize stress and conserve energy. Routines require planning and organization to allow people to do the most important activities when they have the most energy, maximizing both safety and enjoyment.

Therapy sessions can be planned to support a person's shift from focusing on the physical to the cognitive domain. A person who is no longer able to execute an activity physically may need to learn to organize and plan in order to direct care. Overvaluing the concept of independence may lead to goals that seek to achieve levels of function that are too costly in terms of expended energy. Assistance with personal care may be preferable to independence in activities of daily living if the physical and mental costs of attaining independence interfere with social interaction or life satisfaction (Gillette, 1991). Social supports must be sought out, developed, nurtured, and maintained. Attention must be given to ways in which the distress, enormous effort, and tedium of living with and of supporting someone with a physical disability can be managed so that important social supports can be maintained as integral components of a person's adaptive strategies.

Summary

Strategies that minimize fatigue, enhance safety, and reduce stress are essential. Attention to organization, pacing, timing, and energy conservation are also important for managing self-care by people with movement disorders. A philosophy of independent living that emphasizes the importance of an individual's acquisition of skills and capabilities for self-direction in managing physical and social resources has been embraced. However, this philosophy also acknowledges that a person can exhibit an independent spirit while accepting assistance from others, and that all adaptive strategies must be considered in terms of their contribution to overall well-being and life satisfaction. In working with individuals with movement disorders, the role of the therapist is to identify, in conjunction with clients, an array of adaptive strategies that can be used comfortably within the context of the client's daily life. ◆

References

Asher, I.E. (1986). Dysphagia in the adult population: The role of occupational therapy. *Occupational Therapy in Health Care, 3*, 5–21.

Batavia, A.I., & Hammer, G.S. (1990). Toward the development of consumer-based criteria for the evaluation of assistive devices. *Journal of Rehabilitation Research, 27*, 425–436.

Blaine, H.L., & Nelson, E.P. (1973). A mouthstick for quadriplegic patients. *Journal of Prosthetic Dentistry, 29*, 317–322.

Brooks, N., & Matson, R.R. (1982). Social psychological adjustment to multiple sclerosis. A longitudinal study. *Social Science and Medicine, 16*, 2129–2135.

Browne, S.E., Connors, D., & Stern, N. (Eds.). (1985). *With the power of each breath: A disabled women's anthology*. San Francisco: Cleis Press.

Burke, J., Miyake, S., Kielhofner, G., & Barris, R. (1982). The demystification of health care and demise of the sick role: Implications for occupational therapy. In G. Kielhofner (Ed.), *Health through occupation: Theory and practice in occupational therapy* (pp. 197–210). Philadelphia: F.A. Davis.

Carpenter, C. (1991). *Spinal cord injury and adult learning*. Unpublished master's thesis. The University of British Columbia, Vancouver, BC.

Christiansen, C. (1991) Occupational performance assessment. In C. Christiansen & C. Baum (Eds.), *Occupational therapy: Overcoming human performance deficits* (pp. 376–424). Thorofare, NJ: Slack.

Cohen, F., & Lazarus, R. (1983). Coping and adaptation in health and illness. In D. Mechanic (Ed.), *Handbook of health, health care, and the health professions* (pp. 608–635). New York: Free Press.

Cole, J.A. (1983). Skills training. In N.M. Crewe & I.K. Zola (Eds.), *Independent living for physically disabled people* (pp. 187–204). San Francisco: Jossey-Bass.

Corbin, J.M., & Strauss, A. (1988). *Unending work and care: Managing chronic illness at home*. San Francisco: Jossey-Bass.

DeJong, G. (1979). Defining and implementing the independent living concept. In N.M. Crewe & I.K. Zola (Eds.), *Independent living for physically disabled people* (pp. 4–27). San Francisco: Jossey-Bass.

DeJong, G., & Lifchez, R. (1983). Physical disability and public policy. *Scientific American, 248*, 40–49.

Dickey, R., & Shealey, S.H. (1987). Using technology to control the environment. *American Journal of Occupational Therapy, 41*, 717–721.

Einset, K., Deitz, J., Billingsley, F., & Harris, S.R. (1989). The electric feeder: An efficacy study. *Occupational Therapy Journal of Research, 9*, 38–52.

Fearing, G. (1989). *Eating dysfunction: Program guidelines for occupational therapists.* Unpublished manuscript, University Hospital (UBC), Department of Rehabilitation Services, Vancouver.

Fleming, M. (1991). The therapist with the three-track mind. *American Journal of Occupational Therapy, 45*, 1007–1014.

Gauthier, L., Dalziel, S., & Gauthier, S. (1987). The benefits of group occupational therapy for patients with Parkinson's disease. *American Journal of Occupational Therapy, 41*, 360–365.

Gillette, N. (1991). The challenge of research in occupational therapy. *American Journal of Occupational Therapy, 45*, 660–662.

Gordon, R.E., & Kozole, K.P. (1984). Occupational therapy and rehabilitation engineering: Team approach to helping persons with severe physical disability to upgrade functional independence. *Occupational Therapy and Health Care, 1*(4), 117–129.

Jung, C.G. (1961). *Memories, dreams, reflections.* New York: Vintage Books.

King, L.J. (1978). Eleanor Clark Slagle Lectureship: Toward a science of adaptive responses. *American Journal of Occupational Therapy, 32*, 429–437.

Lohr, J.B., & Wisniewski, A.A. (1987). *Movement disorders: A neuropsychiatric approach.* New York: Guilford.

McCuaig, M., & Frank, G. (1991). The able self: Adaptive patterns and choices in independent living for a person with cerebral palsy. *American Journal of Occupational Therapy, 45*, 224–243.

Neuman, S.S., Schatzlein, J.E., & Sparks, R. (1987). Technology. In N.M. Crewe & I.K. Zola (Eds.), *Independent living for physically disabled people* (pp. 245–270). San Francisco: Jossey-Bass.

Pedretti, L., & Zoltan, B. (1990). *Occupational therapy: Practical skills for physical dysfunction* (3rd ed.). St. Louis: Mosby.

Sacks, O. (1970). *The man who mistook his wife for a hat and other clinical tales.* New York: Harper & Row.

Jain, S.S., & Kirshblum, S.C. (1993). Movement disorders, including tremors. In J. DeLisa & B. Gans (Eds.), *Rehabilitation medicine: Principles and practice* (2nd ed.)(pp. 700–715). Philadelphia: Lippincott.

Smith, R. (1989). Mouthstick design for the client with spinal cord injury. *American Journal of Occupational Therapy, 43*, 251–255.

Takai, V.L. (1986). Case report: The development of a feeding harness for an ALS patient. *American Journal of Occupational Therapy, 40*, 359–361.

Taylor, S. J. (1987). Evaluating the client with physical disabilities for seating. *American Journal of Occupational Therapy, 41*, 711–716.

Vanderheiden, G. (1983). Non-conversational communication technology needs of individuals with handicaps. *Rehabilitation World, 7*(2), 8–13.

Wagner, M. (1985). A four-wheeled journey. In S.E. Browne, D. Connors, & N. Stern (Eds.), *With the power of each breath: A disabled women's anthology* (pp. 57–62). San Francisco: Cleis.

Wright, B. (1983). *Physical disability: A psychosocial approach* (2nd ed.). New York: Harper & Row.

Zola, I.K. (1982). *Missing pieces: A chronicle of living with a disability.* Philadelphia: Temple University Press.

Suggestions for Further Reading

DeVeaugh-Geiss, J. (1982). Tardive dyskinesia: Phenomenology, pathophysiology and pharmacology. In J. DeVeaugh-Geiss (Ed.), *Tardive dyskinesia and related involuntary movement disorders* (pp. 1–18). Boston: John Wright PSG.

Hashimoto, S.A., & Paty, D.W. (1986). *Disease-a-month: Multiple sclerosis.* Chicago: Year Book Medical.

Jeste, P.V., & Wyatt, R.J. (1982). *Understanding and treating tardive dyskinesia.* New York: Guilford.

Marsden, C.D. (1990). Neurophysiology. In G. Stern (Ed.), *Parkinson's disease* (pp. 57–98). Baltimore: Johns Hopkins University Press.

McGill, F. (1980). *Go not gently: Letters from a patient with amyotrophic lateral sclerosis.* New York: Arno.

Montgomery, M.A. (1984). Resources of adaptation for daily living: A classification with therapeutic implications for occupational therapy. *Occupational Therapy in Health Care, 1*(4), 9–24.

Rose, F.C. (Ed.). (1990). *Amyotrophic lateral sclerosis.* New York: Demos.

Scott, S.G. (1988). Movement disorders, including tremors. In J. DeLisa, D. Currie, G. Gans et al. (Eds.), *Rehabilitation medicine: Principles and practice* (pp. 463–475). Philadelphia: Lippincott.

Selby, G. (1990). Clinical features. In G. Stern (Ed.), *Parkinson's disease* (pp. 333–388). Baltimore: Johns Hopkins University Press.

Trombly, C.A. (1989). *Occupational therapy for physical dysfunction* (3rd ed.). Baltimore: Williams & Wilkins.

10

Managing Self-Care in Adults With Upper Extremity Amputations

Diane J. Atkins

Diane J. Atkins, OTR, FISPO, is Coordinator of the Amputee Center at The Institute for Rehabilitation and Research (TIRR) and an Assistant Professor in the Department of Physical Medicine and Rehabilitation, Baylor College of Medicine, Houston, TX.

Chapter 10 Outline

The Preprosthetic Therapy Program

Common Functional Issues

    Hook Versus Myoelectric Hand

    Unilateral Amputation

    Bilateral Amputation

    Traumatic Amputation

    Unilateral Partial Hand Amputation

    Unilateral Wrist Disarticulation and Below Elbow Amputation

    Unilateral Above Elbow Amputation

    Unilateral Shoulder Disarticulation Amputation

    Bilateral Partial Hand Amputation

    Bilateral Wrist Disarticulation and Below Elbow Amputation

    Bilateral Above Elbow Amputation

        Prosthetic Options Available

    Bilateral Shoulder Disarticulation Amputation

Summary

References

In 1990 there were more than 1 million people in the United States who had experienced the loss of one or more limbs (U.S. Department of Health and Human Services, 1991). Limb loss can be acquired or congenital. The majority of upper extremity amputations in adults are the result of traumatic causes and occur most often to men ranging from age 15 to 45. Other amputations are necessitated by disease and tumors.

Regardless of the cause, rehabilitation of the amputee can be one of the most challenging and rewarding opportunities a therapist can experience. In 12 years of working exclusively with children and adults with upper limb amputation, the author has never encountered the same type of patient twice. Each is as individual as the unique characteristics of his or her residual limb and the circumstances that necessitated the amputation.

The occupational therapist is a key player in assisting the person with upper extremity amputation to become self-reliant. The individual with a unilateral upper extremity amputation is often grateful for even seemingly small accomplishments introduced to him or her, such as tying a bow, using a knife and fork, or hammering a nail. When this individual chooses to wear a prosthesis, the occupational therapist is typically the designated professional to orient him or her to one-handed activities.

The individual with bilateral upper extremity amputation presents an entirely different set of functional needs and desires. In the majority of cases, this person requires assistance with all aspects of self-care and daily living until the prosthesis is fabricated. The occupational therapist literally becomes a "lifeline" for this patient. This is where the real challenge of understanding the human emotions of frustration, anger, and anxiety come into the total picture of the treatment process. However, the joys of helping individuals to eat for the first time, brush their teeth, or write their name are beyond measure.

Prior to beginning any treatment program, it is important to remember that the patient is usually quite uncomfortable and self-conscious when he or she first begins to wear a prosthesis. Often patients enter the clinic on the first day of therapy with the prosthesis in a bag or cloth sack. Although they may have tried the "new arm" at the prosthetist's several times during the fitting process, many individuals are very self-conscious about wearing it publicly.

It is recommended that a person with a recent amputation be taken to a quiet room, without distraction, where the therapist can begin to familiarize him or her with the new prosthesis. The training progression includes learning prosthetic terminology, donning and doffing the prosthesis, and orienting the person to body movements to operate it. This is followed by simple grasp and release activities. As the treatment program progresses and the patient becomes more comfortable with a new body image, the therapist should involve him or her in the clinic treatment area. The therapist may introduce the patient and try to encourage socialization with others. If possible, it is useful to include another person with a similar level of limb loss in the same treatment time.

Within this chapter, several case studies describe some very special individuals who have been instrumental in teaching the author more than she could have learned in any text. The descriptions of these patients also reveal situations in which the occupational therapist has become a vital and essential link in the individual's total rehabilitation process.

The Preprosthetic Therapy Program

From the time the sutures are removed to the time that the prosthetic prescription is being discussed, there are many goals that the occupational therapist, who is often the primary person managing and monitoring the prosthetic training program, needs to address. The objectives of the preprosthetic program are to

1. promote residual limb shrinkage and shaping,
2. promote residual limb desensitization,
3. maintain normal joint range of motion,
4. increase muscle strength,
5. provide instruction in the proper hygiene of the limb,
6. maximize self-reliance in the performance of tasks required for daily living,
7. determine the electrical potential provided by various muscles (this is known as Myoelectric site testing, and is necessary if myoelectric prosthetic components are prescribed),
8. inform the patient about prosthetic options, and
9. explore the patient's goals regarding the future (Atkins, 1989a).

The postoperative and preprosthetic phase generally begins 2 to 3 weeks after surgery. Healing has essentially occurred by the 21st postoperative day (Meier, 1984) and should allow for a vigorous program of prosthetic preparation. Malone et al. (1984) have suggested that the 1st month after upper extremity amputation is the "golden period" during which prosthetic fitting should occur in order to maximize the level of acceptance and use of the prosthesis.

Common Functional Issues

There are various functional issues that are primary considerations in managing the training programs for individuals with different types of limb loss. These functional issues change depending on the number of limbs affected, whether the amputation is acquired or congenital, and whether a myoelectric or conventional prosthesis is prescribed. The following sections describe some of these considerations.

Hook Versus Myoelectric Hand

One of the first decisions to be made is whether to fit a patient with a myoelectric hand or more conventional hook-type terminal device. Some of the advantages of a hook-type terminal device include improved function in many activities, lighter weight, greater ease in seeing the object being manipulated, less expense, greater durability, and improved sensory feedback.

Several advantages of the myoelectric hand include improved appearance, less harnessing, an improved ability to use the device overhead and in all planes of movement, better grip strength, the ability to grasp larger objects, stronger prehension force, and minimal body movement and effort necessary for control.

The most effective method of determining the appropriate terminal device follows a thorough evaluation of the patient by the entire team. The individual's needs and goals should always be forefront in the decision-making process. If finances permit, a prosthetic prescription that includes both a hand and a hook is desirable. Training proceeds with both devices, and the choice to use either component is determined by the patient.

Before initiating a program of upper extremity prosthetic training, the therapist must realistically orient the patient to what the prosthesis can and cannot do (Atkins, 1989b). If the individual has an unrealistic expectation of the usefulness of the prosthesis as a replacement arm, he or she may be dissatisfied with its ultimate functioning and may reject it altogether. Alternatively, if the patient's expectations are realistic at the beginning of training, then ultimate acceptance will be based on the ability of the prosthesis to improve performance. It is imperative that the therapist be honest and positive about the function of the prosthesis. If the individual believes in and understands the functional potential of the prosthesis, success can be more realistically achieved.

Unilateral Amputation

Depending on the level of amputation, the individual may integrate the "arm," "hand," or "hook" into all of the daily functional tasks or may totally reject the prosthesis if it is not found to be useful. It is important for the therapist to know as much as possible about the patient. Here, narrative reasoning, as described by Mattingly (1991) is an important part of clinical decision making. Narrative reasoning involves understanding the patient's "story," which enables the therapist to learn the patient's interpretation of the amputation in the context of his or her current circumstances and life history. This narrative reasoning process helps the therapist to plan learning experiences that will be relevant to the patient's specific situation, which in turn will engage the patient and foster a high level of motivation for training.

Narrative reasoning individualizes therapy and avoids inappropriate goal setting. To cite an obvious example, a man injured on his farm in a corn-picking machine would not be taught the finer points of meal preparation if he had never cooked a meal in his life, had no desire to learn, and for 30 years had depended on his wife to do it. Through careful listening and thoughtful interaction, a milieu can be created where the patient feels comfortable expressing needs and becomes open to the therapist's explanations about the rationale for a certain activity. The success of therapy, reflected in the patient's willingness and motivation to use a prosthesis, depends greatly on the rapport that develops between the therapist and the person with the amputation. Within this milieu, useful, interesting, and successful therapeutic activities are more readily planned.

Fisher (1989) recommends that throughout use training the therapist involve the individual in the activity analysis process. This enables the individual to determine how to use the prosthesis in new activities learned after discharge. A prosthesis can make a difference in various daily living tasks such as cutting meat, tying a bow, buttoning a shirt, or managing a snap or zipper. A simple checklist has been designed by Northwestern University that identifies and rates performance on personal needs, eating procedures, desk procedures, general tasks such as opening locks and windows, various housekeeping procedures, use of tools, and driving and maintaining vehicles. This checklist can be used as a guide and reviewed with the individual when planning treatment goals.

Early learning experiences for patients should be selected with success in mind. This will reduce anxiety and frustration. It is important to practice activities of daily living (ADL) that are useful and purposeful. Thus, cutting food, using scissors, dressing, opening jars and bottles, washing dishes, using household tools (such as a hammer), and driving are all functionally important activities that can be practiced during treatment. Atkins (1989b) has stressed the importance of prepositioning prior to approaching functional tasks, because most difficulties are related to improper positioning. The person should be instructed to orient the components of the prosthesis in space to a position that resembles that of a normal limb engaged in the same task.

A few techniques can be mentioned here. The prosthesis always functions as the nonpreferred extremity did—as a stabilizer of objects. When cutting meat, the fork is placed between the hook fingers and behind the prosthetic thumb. The knife is held in the unaffected extremity. Principles of dressing are the same as for the stroke patient: The prosthesis is dressed first and undressed last.

Those who successfully master the prothesis wear it daily, incorporate the new arm in the majority of bilateral activities, and essentially see this "tool" as an important extension of the body. A revised body image should incorporate this new look and appearance. The level of a unilateral amputation is a significant factor in whether the prosthesis is both used and accepted.

Bilateral Amputation

The person with bilateral amputation presents an entirely different set of functional and emotional needs. When an individual loses both hands, he or she temporarily loses the ability to complete important daily tasks without assistance. The person's world is suddenly focused on someone else to help accomplish the most basic of human requirements—feeding, dressing, and toileting, to name but a few. The reality of this experience is often enough either to plunge a person into depression or enable him or her to discover an inner resource to beat the odds, conquer the challenge, and make the two prosthetic body "extensions" work.

Training procedures for both limbs are the same as for someone with a unilateral amputation, except separation of controls must be accomplished. When using body-powered prostheses, this involves keeping one terminal device closed to maintain the grasp of an object while simultaneously opening the other terminal device.

Loss of self-reliance is a difficult idea for any individual to accept. The occupational therapist's challenge is to listen to each patient; attempt to understand that person's emotional status, family dynamics, and level of frustration; and help him or her to identify short- and long-term needs and goals. What is possible and practical to achieve is primarily dependent on the level of the amputation. Motivation, family support, a job to return to, and a strong desire to overcome adversity are also critical factors in determining success.

Traumatic Amputation

The individual who has lost a limb or limbs secondary to trauma constitutes the type of amputation that is most frequently seen by the occupational therapist. A single moment in time literally changes the course of these individuals' lives.

The anger experienced by the patient can be significant if the accident was the fault of someone else. The emotional adjustment of someone who loses a limb secondary to trauma is generally much more of a challenge to address than the emotional well-being of someone who has a congenital amputation. The congenital, limb-deficient child and adult generally adapt extremely well to limb loss.

On-the-job accidents account for a large number of traumatic injuries. If the injured worker is insured through workers' compensation, financing for rehabilitation care is generally comprehensive. Money may be available for the most advanced type of prostheses.

Unilateral Partial Hand Amputation

The individual with partial hand amputation presents one of the most challenging situations for the physician, clinical team, and prosthetist. When sensation is present, the surgeon attempts to save any functional part of the hand in lieu of a wrist disarticulation (Wilson, 1989). The clinical picture can include the loss of a single digit or part of a digit, as well as numerous combinations of digits and part of the palm.

Amputations through the carpals or metacarpals are individual problems requiring specialized fitting. Using prostheses only for cosmetic purposes sacrifices function and often covers the valuable tactile areas of the fingers and palm. Ensuring that a prosthesis provides functional improvement requires special evaluation and prescription. Often standard components can often be modified for adaptation to the partial-hand case, but many times custom-made devices are indicated. For the hand that has a thumb amputation, deepening of the first web space is a viable option that increases mobility and allows better pinch and grasp.

The functional types of prostheses that are generally prescribed include

1. an opposition post, where fingers are present and thumb opposition is required; this is good because sensation is preserved;

2. an opposition pad, prescribed for transmetacarpal amputations to provide a broad opposition surface; sensation is preserved; and

3. a handi-hook, prescribed when a holding or handle device is necessary; this is generally fitted in the palm of the hand and requires a cable control system.

Cosmetic options include "life-like" replacements for digits, the thumb, or the entire hand. Depending on the skill of the artist or prosthetist (often the same person), these cosmetic replacements may look very real and often are not discernible as being artificial. As with the glove of a myoelectric hand, these gloves are also prone to staining, tears, and discoloration. Water and hot and cold extremes should be avoided. Unless the amputation is at the carpal-metacarpal joint, myoelectric options are difficult and often impossible for the person with a partial hand amputation.

In general, there are no standard components or procedures for obtaining optimal function for a partial hand amputation. The prosthetist must devise a solution for each individual case. For further explanation of several of these prosthetic options, refer to Muilenburg and LeBlanc (1989).

Very little, if any, device training is required for individuals with unilateral partial hand amputations. An orientation to the partial hand device's application and potential is helpful. If a cosmetic glove is prescribed, a review of glove care and maintenance is recommended.

Typically, the individual with a partial hand amputation uses the sound arm and hand to perform the majority of ADL and does not require assistance. The partial hand is a very good functional assist, with or without a prosthetic appliance. Eventually, the majority of these patients reject any prosthetic device, custom-made tool, or holding appliance. They find ways of doing their activities without "gadgets" and generally prefer this simpler mode of operation. The following case study describes the management of a man with a unilateral partial hand amputation.

Case Study 1.

J.J. is a 44-year-old male who sustained an amputation of the right hand at the distal interphalangeal (DIP) joint of the right thumb and a transmetacarpal amputation of the remaining digits, on May 30, 1989. This occurred at a rubber manufacturing plant where his hand was caught in a paddle-wheel portion of a machine.

J.J. required several plastic surgical procedures, including pedicle grafting and the eventual deepening of his web space and removal of the residual metacarpal bone of the index finger (see Figure 1).

Two prosthetic prescriptions were generated: one for work purposes and one for cosmetic use only. Excellent cosmetic results were achieved (see Figure 2).

The residual thumb is covered; however, the remaining movement at the MP joint allows a mug handle to be grasped. Note the short zipper installed in the palmar aspect of the glove in order to allow greater ease in donning and doffing (see Figure 3).

J.J. has returned to work full time as a mail clerk. He rarely wears his work appliance and wears his cosmetic hand an average of 2 hours each day for social reasons. He does not require either device for his ADL or his various job activities.

Unilateral Wrist Disarticulation and Below Elbow Amputation

Following the loss of a hand, a wrist disarticulation or a long below elbow amputation is desirable because supination and pronation are preserved. It is important to remember that as much as 50% of pronation and supination can be transferred to the prosthesis if 50% or more of the length of the forearm is preserved. Therefore, preservation of this movement is critical. This range of motion is frequently lost if exercise is not performed in early therapy. Pronation and supination are not possible in amputations of the proximal one-half of the forearm. Flexion and extension at the elbow are critical, and as little as 1.5 inches of the residual limb are preferable to an amputation through the elbow (Louis, 1982).

One of the problems in fitting the wrist-disarticulation stump is keeping the overall length of the prosthesis consistent with the normal arm. The development of very short wrist units, especially for wrist disarticulation cases, has materially reduced this problem.

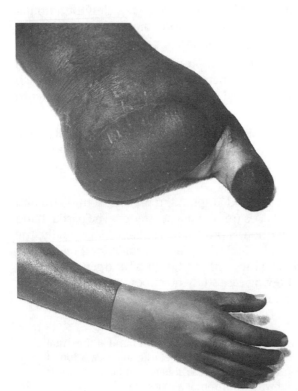

However, these units are available in only the screw or thread type. They cannot be obtained in the bayonet type, which lends itself to quick interchange of terminal device.

The socket for the wrist-disarticulation patient need not extend the full length of the forearm. It is fitted somewhat loosely at the proximal end to permit the wrist to rotate. A simple figure-eight harness and Bowden cable are used to operate the terminal device.

The socket for a below elbow prosthesis is similar to that described above. The figure-eight ring-type

Figure 1 (top). A partial hand amputation with remaining thumb (to IP joint).

Figure 2 (bottom). Cosmetic glove for this partial hand amputation.

Figure 3. Grasping a mug with a partial hand and cosmetic glove.

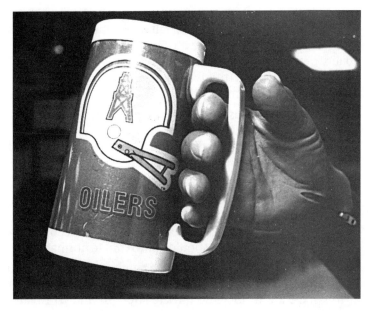

harness is generally used, but a chest strap harness may be required when the amputee expects to engage in heavy work. Where possible, flexible hinges and an open cuff are used. When more stability between socket and stump is needed, rigid metal hinges and a closed cuff can be used.

A distinctly different option exists for the individual with a below elbow amputation: the myoelectric arm which did not achieve widespread commercial availability until the 1960s. The concept of myoelectric control is very simple. One uses an electric signal from a muscle to control the flow of energy from a battery to a motor. In a myoelectric prosthesis, the control signal comes from a muscle remnant (the wrist flexor and wrist extensor in a below elbow amputation), which still has normal innervation and thus is subject to voluntary control. The motor actuates a prosthetic hand, wrist, or elbow (in above elbow amputees). Scott (1989) provides an excellent reference for more information about myoelectric protheses.

During the first and second training visits of a person with an amputation, the following goals should be addressed: orientation to prosthetic component terminology, independence in donning and doffing the prosthesis, orientation to a wearing schedule, and care of the residual limb and prosthesis.

Prior to actually applying the prothesis, several motions need to be reviewed.

a. *Scapular abduction.* This provides tension on the figure-eight harness in order to open the terminal device.

b. *Humeral flexion.* This motion also applies pressure on the cable and allows the terminal device to open. Scapular abduction and humeral flexion are the basic motions to review with someone with a below elbow amputation.

c. *Elbow flexion/extension.* It is extremely important to teach the person with a below elbow amputation how to maintain full elbow range of motion. This range enables the person to reach many areas of the body without undue strain or special modifications in the prosthetic design.

d. *Forearm pronation/supination.* This motion is very important for someone with a long below elbow amputation to maintain. It enables the person to position the terminal device where he or she chooses, without prepositioning the wrist unit.

Before beginning functional training, it is important that the prosthesis fits comfortably and that the components function well. The therapist is encouraged to communicate openly and frequently with the prosthetist— not only initially, but also when fit or operation concerns arise.

Functional use training is the most challenging and prolonged stage of the prosthetic training process. The success or failure of the individual's acceptance and use of the prosthesis depends on: (a) the motivation of the patient; (b) the comprehensiveness and quality of the tasks and activities practiced; and (c) the experience and enthusiasm of the occupational therapist (this is critical). The functional training experience is most effective if the same therapist remains with the patient throughout the entire process (Atkins, 1989b).

The decision to use a myoelectrically controlled prosthesis must be evaluated by the entire team, and, particularly, by the individual who will be using it. As yet there is no definitive standard by which to determine the ideal candidate for myoelectric use. The prescription process is dynamic and may change as the evaluation progresses.

If the evaluation determines that a myoelectric prosthesis is indicated, muscle sites need to be tested to determine their potential to activate a prosthesis. Location of appropriate muscle sites, and training these sites in proper control, are by far the most important aspects of successful operation of a myoelectric prosthesis. Muscles that control the prosthetic movements should approximate normal movements as much as possible.

Initially, the individual must be taught to understand the feedback modalities used on the myotester (like biofeedback) and to use this feedback to train the muscles. The goals at this stage are to increase muscle strength and to isolate muscle contractions. The importance of good training at this point cannot be emphasized enough. Control of these signals is the basis for successful prosthetic use. As with a body-powered prosthesis, the training process for a myoelectric prosthesis includes orientation, control training, use training, and training in ADL.

During orientation, the individual is provided with the information needed for care and use of the myoelectric prosthesis. Along with proper terminology, he or she is taught how to charge the battery and various other techniques. For example, the arm must be stored with the batteries removed, and a myoelectric hand should be fully opened for storage in order to keep the thumb well-stretched.

Hygiene of the residual limb and cleaning of the prosthesis, are also part of the orientation. The prosthesis can be cleaned with soap by using an almost dry cloth. It should not be immersed, and exposure to water should be avoided. Cosmetic gloves stain easily from ink, newsprint, mustard, grease, and dirt, and a special cream is available from the prosthetist for cleaning. The glove should be replaced if torn, but will normally be replaced every 6 months.

Control training teaches proficiency in the actual operation of the myoelectric prosthesis. The control sites should have good contact with the electrodes. Good use and control of the basic mechanical operations of the prosthesis help develop the strong base of automatic control needed for higher level functional skills. Less cognitive energy used for mechanical operation of the prosthesis leaves more stamina to focus on actual tasks.

As prosthetic skills increase, training should progress from gross motor activities to fine motor and manipulative functions. When an individual has achieved approximately an 80% accuracy rate for control, activities can be initiated to increase skill and dexterity. Training is complete when the person can use the prosthesis while his or her attention is focused elsewhere (Spiegel, 1989).

The individual with a unilateral wrist disarticulation and below elbow amputation should be expected to achieve complete independence. The majority of any bilateral task will be accomplished by the sound arm and hand, with the prosthesis providing a good functional assist. Certain activities, such as buttoning, tying shoes, and cutting meat, may initially require special adaptive equipment. Eventually, however, it has been observed that many individuals with unilateral wrist disarticulation and below elbow amputations reject adaptive devices and learn their own techniques for accomplishing virtually all of their activities. The following case study provides an example of the management of this type of patient.

Case Study 2.

> F.A. is a 20-year-old male from Lima, Peru. He was a professional soccer player who had finished practice one afternoon and found what turned out to be a grenade on the soccer field. He did not know what this was at the time. He was holding the grenade in his right hand, turned to give it to his friend, and the grenade exploded. F.A. lost his right arm below the elbow. His friend was killed.
>
> Within 3 weeks, F.A. was flown to Houston and was involved in an active preprosthetic program. Following wound healing, his program consisted of Ace wrapping the residual limb, range of motion and muscle strengthening exercises, desensitization techniques, and change of dominance activities.
>
> F.A. lived in Peru with his parents and four brothers. He was studying to be a lawyer while playing soccer for his father's professional soccer team. Appearance was extremely important to this patient and his family. He understood the reasons for a hook-type, body-powered prosthesis, but he was very focused on the myoelectric arm.
>
> The family was wealthy, and they were prepared to pay for a body-powered, as well as a myoelectric, arm without hesitation. They understood the importance of occupational therapy in learning how to use the prosthesis. In fact, they were eager to stay as long as necessary.
>
> F.A. did exceptionally well in occupational therapy and completed his training with both prostheses in 2 weeks. An orientation to many two-handed activities was included in his therapy program. Because he was fitted so early, F.A. still thought of himself as having two hands and, therefore, problem solved in a two-handed manner; he had not become unilaterally independent. Although functional with his left hand, he preferred to use his right myoelectric prosthesis in many one- and-two-handed activities (see Figures 4 and 5).
>
> F.A. is now actively involved in school and will return for follow-up during the next semester break.

Unilateral Above Elbow Amputation

With the loss of the elbow joint, prosthetic planning demands additional time, componentry, and problem-solving on the part of the prosthetist. The elbow is an extremely valuable joint in the biomechanics of arm movement. At best, the above elbow prosthesis provides a good functional assist in most bilateral activities. The ability to use an above elbow prosthesis takes additional commitment and strong motivation on the part of the individual.

At this level of amputation, a prosthetic "internal locking" elbow is sometimes used. If the amputation is at the level of the elbow, "outside locking" hinges are used. Because the individual must control both the terminal device and the elbow lock, he or she must use a dual-control type of shoulder harness. When the elbow unit is unlocked, a pull on the main control cable flexes the elbow. When the elbow unit is locked, a pull on the main control operates the terminal device. Humeral rotation is passively controlled by prepositioning the turntable in the proximal prosthetic elbow unit. The wrist unit and terminal device type are chosen based on the patient's preference or need.

There are a number of electric elbows also available for this individual. The main

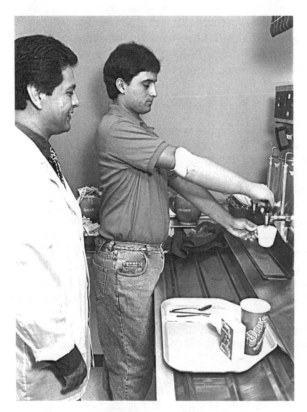

Figure 4 (top). Operating a spigot to pour coffee necessitates the use of a myoelectric hand as an assist.

Figure 5 (below). Tying bows is an excellent bilateral activity to practice with a myoelectric hand.

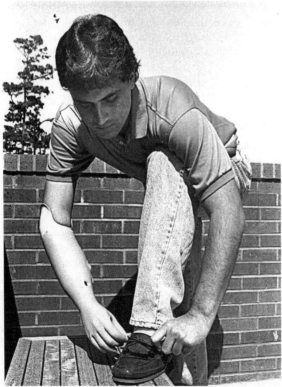

ones include the Utah elbow, Boston elbow, and Hosmer elbow. Each has its own unique characteristic and incorporates myoelectric or switch control. A comprehensive overview of these elbows is given in Prout (1989); Sears, Andrew, and Jacobsen (1989); and Williams (1989).

If myoelectric operation of the above elbow unit is selected, control with remnant biceps and triceps muscle contractions is usually possible. In cases where the independence of these two muscle contractions is lacking, or both do not remain, a biceps/posterior deltoid control pair, or biceps/infraspinators, as well as a pectoralis/posterior deltoid can be used. The anterior deltoid is avoided because it also contracts when the humerus is flexed.

Typically, an intimate-fitting, total contact socket is used for the person with an above elbow amputation. This provides a good feeling of control of the prosthesis via the residual limb. A very low trim line is often utilized in order to allow full shoulder range of motion. Suspension is usually provided by a modified figure-eight harness because of simplicity. A suction type socket, with or without auxiliary harnessing, might also be used. However, this socket requires precisely fitted dimensions. Small changes in body weight (5 to 10 pounds) can easily affect the suction fit.

The patient, other team members, and prosthetist have many options when choosing an above elbow prosthetic prescription. Various combinations of body-powered and electric elbows, used in conjunction with myoelectric hands and body-powered hooks, can be utilized in a hybrid prosthesis. Some hybrid prostheses allow an interchangeable hook with a myoelectric hand in the same prosthesis. This is an excellent alternative for individuals who value function and appearance (see Figure 6).

Financial sponsorship is a significant factor to consider when determining an above elbow prostheses. A total myoelectric prosthesis, such as the Utah arm, can be very costly. Insurance carriers often require lengthy documentation to determine why a $35,000 to $45,000 arm is indicated. Hybrid type prostheses may offer an affordable alternative if financial coverage becomes an issue.

The reader is referred to Prout (1989), Sears et al. (1989), and Williams (1989) for an in-depth discussion of the operation, advantages, disadvantages, and application of several of these prosthetic options.

Many of the principles of training an individual with an above elbow amputation are identical to those for below elbow amputee training. In addition to scapular abduction and humeral flexion to open the terminal device, the following motions need to be reviewed for this individual:

a. *Chest expansion.* This motion should be practiced by deeply inhaling, expanding the chest as much as possible, then relaxing slowly. Harnessing this motion with a cross-chest strap is determined by the prosthetic design. In some instances of extensive axillary scarring, a cross-chest strap may be used in lieu of the figure-eight harness.

b. *Shoulder depression, extension, and abduction.* This is the combined movement necessary to operate the body-powered, internal locking elbow. It is advisable to have the patient practice this motion by cupping one's hand under the residual limb and instructing him or her to press down into the palm. This simulates the motion required to lock and unlock the elbow unit.

As described previously, the functional use training segment of the occupational therapist's program is the longest and most challenging. It is es-

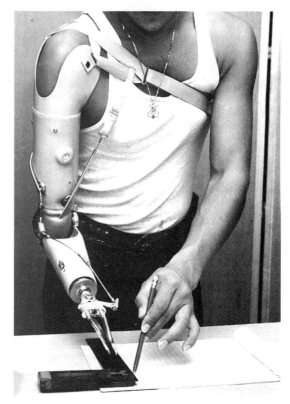

Figure 6. A hybrid prothesis allows a myoelectric hand to be interchanged with a body-powered hook (note electrode over biceps).

pecially important to review thoroughly the operation of the prosthesis in grasp and release exercises with fine and gross objects. When bilateral activities are attempted, the patient must be given simple and positive learning experiences. Initially it can be frustrating for the person with an above elbow amputation, particularly when he or she is required to work at different heights, incorporating the mechanical elbow. More advanced bilateral activities, such as building a woodworking project and using various tools, can be attempted later.

The primary aspects of training an individual with an above elbow myoelectric prosthesis differ little from those for an individual with a below elbow myoelectric prosthesis. When training an individual with a complex myoelectric arm, providing positive learning experiences is essential for success. An electric arm is perhaps the most frustrating prosthesis one can operate. Total concentration is required to train the muscles to contract as the myoelectric arm demands. Fatigue of the muscles used for electrode sites is not unusual, and should be expected. One may mistake a tired muscle for a problem in the prosthesis. Reinforcing the importance of practicing isometric exercises with the myoelectric sites is crucial. The weight of the myoelectric arm may also be a detriment. Short wearing periods, to build up tolerance, are strongly suggested.

All individuals with above elbow amputation should be able to achieve a level of modified or complete independence in functional tasks required for daily living. Minimal assistance may be required in complex bilateral activities; however, with time and practice the individual will eventually develop his or her own techniques, which will require little or no assistance. It is important to note that an individual who chooses not to wear a prosthesis becomes equally adept at the ability to function independently with one arm. Case study 3 provides a description of the management of a patient with an above elbow amputation.

Case Study 3.

S.B. is a 30-year-old female with a history of synovial sarcoma in her right elbow. This necessitated an above elbow amputation. She had a long history of pathology with her right arm, including a shoulder fracture. This resulted in limited range of motion demonstrated by the lack of 50° of extension and 30° of flexion. She remained right dominant, however, and her arm was fully functional in spite of her range-of-motion limitations.

Following her amputation surgery to the above elbow level, S.B. was involved with therapy at another hospital. This included figure-eight wrapping and a home program of range-of-motion exercise. Pain was a significant problem for S.B. She had not been exposed to any occupational therapy to help desensitize it. Additionally, she had not received any training to achieve independence in ADL with her nondominant left hand.

When therapy began at a new rehabilitation setting, S.B.'s program included change of dominance activities, teaching techniques of figure-eight wrapping to shrink the residual limb, and desensitization exercises. During therapy, S.B.'s pain gradually lessened with medication and desensitization techniques. Her therapy also included a comprehensive orientation to prosthetic componentry. This orientation is a very important element in the preprosthetic program; the individual needs to know, see, and understand the available options.

After reviewing the various alternatives, S.B. felt that the "state of the art" Utah arm was her prosthesis of choice. Appearance was important, as was her ability to function independently at work as a data entry clerk, and at home. The doctor and team agreed with S.B.'s choice and recommended the Utah Arm.

S.B. made many attempts to receive sponsorship from her insurance company and the state-funded insurance agency, but was repeatedly denied. She resorted to approaching her friends and family and to using personal savings for money to pay for the Utah arm. Finally, following months of personal fund raising, she was able to purchase this sophisticated prosthesis.

Her therapy included an orientation to many two-handed activities. She has done extremely well, and is seen in the clinic on a regular basis with the amputee team and her prosthetist. She prefers her myoelectric hand over her hook and has had very few problems that require maintenance for the elbow or hand. S.B. is very pleased with her Utah arm and feels it was an excellent choice for her.

Unilateral Shoulder Disarticulation Amputation

Any amputations proximal to the axillary fold are treated as shoulder disarticulations, since abduction and adduction are lost. If the deltoid is preserved in a shoulder disarticulation, some shoulder contour is maintained. The loss of a shoulder joint may significantly restrict an individual's activities. Although prosthetic shoulder joints exist, they have limited range. Additionally, they must be prepositioned by the individual. This proximal level of limb loss provides an even greater challenge in fitting for the prosthetist. Motivation, attitude, and perseverance are the determining factors of success.

At this level of amputation, the shoulder unit that is most frequently prescribed is the Shoulder Flexion-Abduction unit that allows flexion/extension and abduction/adduction. It is passively controlled, or prepositioned, by the sound hand. Unfortunately, at this high level of loss the person has more joints to control and less body with which to do it. A triple control system, which controls the elbow unit, terminal device, and a forearm flexion assist may be used. There are no electric shoulder units available at this time—the weight and cost increases are obviously not desirable.

The philosophy, training progression, and functional goals for the person with a unilateral shoulder disarticulation are generally the same as for other conditions. The positioning of the shoulder joint in abduction and flexion is usually accomplished by the sound arm. Adduction, however, is often accomplished by leaning the arm against a hard surface, such as a wall or the arm of a chair.

Locking and unlocking the elbow joint is generally controlled by a nudge control button mounted on the right side of the thoracic shell. The chin depresses this control button to operate the prosthetic elbow. Training someone with a shoulder disarticulation amputee takes approximately 8 to 10 hours, with additional verbal cuing from the therapist.

The techniques for training an individual with a shoulder disarticulation amputation fitted with electric prosthetic componentry are very similar to those for the individual with an above elbow amputation. The primary difference, however, is that the individual with shoulder disarticulation amputation must use proximal muscle sites in the shoulder, upper chest, and upper back regions. Careful and deliberate muscle site testing must be done prior to fabrication of the prosthesis. This determines the strength of the muscle contractions and, most importantly, the ability of these two muscles (anterior and posterior) to separate their control. Equally important when training an individual with the Utah arm is the ability of these two muscle sites to cocontract in order to unlock the myoelectric elbow.

In some instances the individual with a shoulder disarticulation amputation may choose to wear the arm only for certain occasions or not at all. The conscious effort, energy, and concentration of utilizing this type of prosthesis are significant. The weight of a shoulder disarticulation prosthesis may be an additional drawback. There are, however, many individuals who choose to wear the prosthesis on a regular basis. They feel they are more balanced, symmetrical, and "complete" with two arms.

Whatever the choice of the person—to wear or not to wear a prosthesis—he or she should be expected to achieve a level of complete independence with the remaining arm and hand. The shoulder disarticulation prosthesis will serve as a gross functional assist. Occasional assistance might initially be necessary, but eventually the individual finds his or her own way of doing things independently that have personal importance.

Case Study 4.

> D.B. is a 26-year-old male from Missouri, who was injured in a "power take off" (PTO) shaft of a tractor while working on his parents' farm. He sustained a left traumatic shoulder disarticulation on February 15, 1982. D.B. was initially fitted with a body-powered prosthesis, but he had no training, developed some skin breakdown, and eventually rejected it.
>
> D.B. was living by himself when he was seen for evaluation 4 years following the accident. He was unilaterally independent, worked at a service station, had "little social life," and expressed being "embarrassed in public."
>
> D.B. was of average intelligence and had a strong desire to attend a local college. He was noted to be achievement oriented, willing to take risks, and opposed to giving up without a strong effort.
>
> At the suggestion of his attorney and others, D.B. explored various prosthetic alternatives and decided he would like to be fitted with the Utah myoelectric arm. He felt that although he was unilaterally independent, another arm would help him in many two-handed activities that now took him extra time and effort to complete.
>
> Funding for a Utah myoelectric arm became available in a legal settlement. Fabrication proceeded, and training with the prosthesis followed. D.B. was exceptionally well-coordinated and motivated to learn to use the Utah arm. He perfected the operation of this complex prosthesis in less than 1 week.
>
> At last contact, D.B. was attending college, finding his prosthesis helpful when carrying a briefcase on campus, and accomplishing several cooking activities in his kitchen at home. Because of the weight and heat of the arm, as well as the effort to use it, D.B. decided that his prosthesis was helpful for a total of 2 to 3 hours a day.

Bilateral Partial Hand Amputation

Each individual with bilateral amputation presents a new and different challenge to the health care team. For almost every individual, function is primary over appearance. The reason is obvious, yet sometimes overlooked. The ability to be self-reliant is often critical in one's life, and many cosmetic alternatives do not provide this.

As discussed in the section on unilateral partial hand amputations, the thumb and tactile sensation are perhaps the most important components to "save" in the partial hand. Therefore, in lieu of prosthetic alternatives, hand surgery is often the treatment of choice. A toe transfer, index pollicization, or deepening of the web space are viable options for the individual with a bilateral partial hand amputation. Sensation is preserved and adequate function is achieved.

Prosthetic options for a person with a partial hand amputation are discussed in the section, "Unilateral Partial Hand Amputation." If the level of the hand amputation extends beyond the carpal-metacarpal joint, a myoelectric prosthesis is not an option, as the electric components and battery are simply too large. However several research centers are pursuing componentry miniaturization.

If the patient is fitted with a functional post, handi-hook, or cosmetic hand, little, if any, training is required. The person should receive an orientation to the device's use, as well as an overview of its general care and maintenance.

If myoelectric hands are fitted on an individual with intact carpals, the arm will be a bit longer in order to accommodate the carpal bones. Training is accomplished in the same manner as described for the individual with a below elbow amputation. However, essential ADL are emphasized first (eating, writing, and brushing teeth) so the person can experience short-term success and independence. Complex bilateral tasks should be attempted only when simple bilateral activities are successfully and efficiently completed.

The level of independence achieved depends on what remains functional following surgery or prosthetic intervention. The ability to grasp both large and small objects is essential. The thumb, or opposition post, is therefore critical to successful independence. With little grasping ability, independence in bilateral activities creates a greater challenge, and adaptive devices may be required. However, many times individuals will find "their own way," and succeed in achieving the level of independence important to them.

Case Study 5.

L.L. has a congenital bilateral partial hand amputation. At first glance, one could guess that she had a bilateral wrist disarticulation amputation. However, a row of carpals, or part of her carpal bones, were present when she was born.

As a child, L.L. had been fitted with bilateral body-powered wrist disarticulation prostheses. She eventually rejected these prostheses at age 13 and realized she could accomplish many activities with her residual limbs.

She was evaluated in the Amputee Clinic at age 19, at which time she requested bilateral myoelectric prostheses. During her clinic evaluation, L.L. stated that she was totally independent in eating, dressing, and combing her hair (see Figure 7), and was even able to tie her shoes using her teeth. Her teeth become an important "clamp" when she needs the ability to hold. (This is true for everyone with an amputation.) L.L. was also independent in driving a standard transmission automobile, was a full time

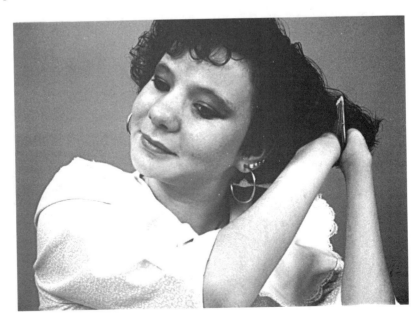

Figure 7.
Holding a comb is possible with congenital partial hand amputations.

student in college, and worked 4 hours a day as a data entry clerk. Her career goal was to become a certified public accountant.

L.L.'s desire for myoelectric arms came at a time in her life when her appearance became more important, particularly as she planned to deal with the public as an accountant. Also, because L.L. never had the opportunity to try myoelectric arms, she thought it might be a valuable experience and that her level of independence would improve. The increased grip and grasping ability the myoelectric hands provide was an additional incentive for her.

All these reasons were valid and convincing. Unfortunately, as a student L.L. had no insurance and had to seek financial help. Thanks to a generous gift presented by a local service organization, L.L. was fitted with bilateral myoelectric arms.

She was delighted with the outcome. A skillful prosthetist was able to incorporate the battery in the forearms without an unsightly "bulge" in the socket, and the length was kept to a minimum. L.L. enjoyed painting her "nails" on the glove and wearing rings (see Figure 8).

Although L.L. liked the appearance of the myoelectric hands and found them helpful in school and on the job, she discovered that she greatly missed the valued ability to feel. She noted improvements in her ability to grasp and hold objects, but she had to "attend" every activity visually to make certain the grip was not too secure, or was secure enough, to accomplish the task adequately. Additionally, L.L. found that her myoelectric hands did not enable her to be as quick, responsive, or reliable in many school and work tasks as she was without them.

L.L. does not use the myoelectric hands on a regular basis, but she is glad she has them.

Bilateral Wrist Disarticulation and Below Elbow Amputation

The loss of both hands is traumatic indeed. For persons with this circumstance, the prostheses become an integral and essential tool in the ability to achieve independence in school and work activities. Without the prostheses, an individual is dependent in the majority of his or her daily activities.

While the principles described for the unilateral below elbow prosthesis apply here,

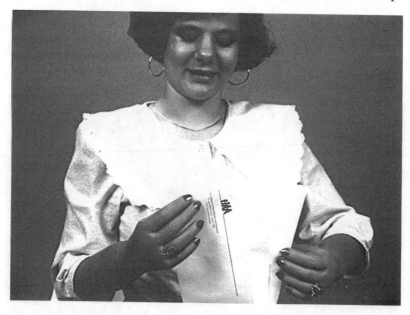

Figure 8. Often the fingernails are painted and rings are worn on a myoelectric hand.

an additional component is considered valuable, if not essential. Because of the many mid-line activities we do each day, a wrist flexion unit is a necessary consideration. Several types are available, but the typical Sierra "dome-type," constant friction, wrist unit allows three settings of the terminal device in relation to the wrist. Many individuals choose this wrist unit on one side only and prefer a locking wrist unit on the other side.

The design and development of a spring-loaded forearm rotator unit is also immensely beneficial for these individuals. With a quick movement of the arm to the side of the body, this mechanism positions the forearm at the desired angle for a better bio-mechanical position of the terminal device. This replaces the sometimes awkward movement required to position the terminal device in a conventional wrist unit.

Body-powered terminal devices are often the prescription of choice because of the valuable proprioceptive and kinesthetic feedback an amputee has with a cable-controlled prosthesis. The individual can "feel" when the terminal device is open, closed, or open halfway without looking. This is important feedback when tactile sensation of the hand is missing. A myoelectric hand does not provide this as effectively as a body-powered terminal device. Additionally, the ability to see "through" the hook when doing various tasks is an advantage over the "bulkiness" of the myoelectric hand, and the myoelectric hand is considerably heavier than a conventional hook.

Because of their limitations, bilateral myoelectric prostheses are not often pre-scribed. Function is of utmost importance for individuals with bilateral amputation, and many feel that the body-powered terminal devices offer them greater independence. On occasion, an individual may choose to wear one body-powered and one myoelectric prosthesis. The decision for this, or any other prosthetic terminal device, should be discussed fully with the patient at the time of the initial evaluation. If sponsorship is available for both types of prostheses, it is the ideal solution for these individuals.

Prosthetic training for this bilateral level of limb loss should proceed as in other examples, whether for body controlled or myoelectric prostheses. Simple, positive learning experiences should be provided, with a gradual increase in the level of difficulty. It is essential to begin with six important activities of daily living: Writing, eating, brushing teeth, toileting, bathing, and dressing. These activities reestablish a sense of control and self-esteem. Following mastery of self-care tasks, vocational, avocational, and recreational activities can be explored and attempted. The recommended duration of prosthetic training is approximately 3 weeks.

The individual with a bilateral below elbow amputation using prostheses can almost always achieve a level of considerable self-reliance with very few, if any, adaptive devices. Individuals with this condition prove to be the most consistent wearers and users of prostheses. With few exceptions, the prostheses tend to become an essential part of life and body image.

Case Study 6.

S.D. is a 35-year-old male who, while working as a lineman for an electric company, sustained an injury through electrocution, which entered his right arm and exited his left. This resulted in bilateral below elbow amputations on February 17, 1989. He required ongoing surgical treatment for approximately 1 year and was eventually fitted with a pair of body-powered prostheses. He was never comprehensively trained in the use of these prostheses and therefore required assistance in many of his ADL. It was thought that myoelectric prostheses might be the answer, so bilateral myoelectric below elbow prostheses were also prescribed.

S.D. was referred to another rehabilitation facility in order to evaluate his prostheses, assess his independence, and increase this level of independence. His goals were to return to an independent life-style at home and at work.

S.D. was independent in feeding but required assistance in set-up. He needed minimal to moderate assistance with dressing, toileting, and showering. His goal was to be completely independent in all ADL, including driving. He also expressed a desire to meet other bilateral below elbow amputees. This proved to be a valuable learning experience for him.

At the time of his evaluation, S.D. stated that he preferred his myoelectric arms but did not feel adequately trained in the use of either prostheses. He remained a total of 3 weeks, during which time all aspects of ADL were explored using both hooks and hands (see Figure 9). He completed a woodworking project and a meal, and perfected all aspects of bathing, showering, and dressing. S.D. also completed driver's training. It was recommended that he use a driving ring on his steering wheel.

It was also recommended that S.D. be considered for spring-loaded forearm rotator units in the future. These automatically position the forearm in one quick and easy maneuver. Additionally, a backup set of body-powered prostheses was strongly recommended in the event that his prostheses required repairs. This is a recommendation routinely prescribed for all bilateral upper extremity amputees who depend on their prostheses on a daily basis.

At the time of discharge, S.D. felt equally independent using either set of prostheses and could make the choice of which to use according to the specific activity.

Bilateral Above Elbow Amputation

This individual is at a distinct disadvantage compared to the individual with bilateral

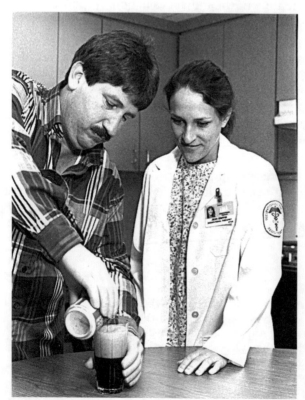

below elbow amputations. The value of the human elbow joint and its function cannot be over emphasized. When both elbows are lost, the prosthesis must provide all motions at the elbow, wrist and terminal device. Although a great deal of energy and effort have gone into perfecting an above elbow prosthesis, the challenge of achieving independence with it is great.

Prosthetic Options Available

The body-powered prosthetic options have been addressed. The addition of bilateral spring-loaded forearm rotator units, and unilateral or bilateral wrist flexion units, is an important consideration.

Figure 9. Demonstration of control and coordination in this two-handed activity.

For reasons already stated, bilateral hook-type terminal devices are often preferred over mechanical or myoelectric hands. A hook-type terminal device weighs less than a myoelectric hand. As with unilateral above elbow amputations, a number of hybrid combinations can be explored with the elbow, forearm, and terminal device.

The myoelectric choices are essentially the same as for the individual with unilateral above elbow amputation. Hybrid prosthetic alternatives are often considered. Powering one side with myoelectric or switch controls and one side with body-powered controls is gaining favor. If mechanical problems occur with the electric arm, the body-powered prosthesis can be utilized to avoid being totally dependent.

The process for training an individual with bilateral above elbow prostheses is similar to what has been presented regarding the individual with bilateral below elbow amputation. There is one important consideration, however, at the outset of training. Realistic expectations *must* be discussed in order to avoid setting the person up for failure.

Goals that include unilateral functions such as writing, eating, and brushing teeth are realistic. Toileting, dressing, and bathing are possible, but require a great deal of time, energy, and perseverance. Complex bilateral activities, such as preparing a meal or building a woodworking project, are unrealistic at the outset of training. Complex bilateral activities may be expected to be accomplished after months of practice and a sincere desire to be as proficient and skilled as possible with the above elbow prosthesis.

During the initial phase, prosthetic training can take from 4 to 6 weeks. Following several months of practice, a second admission may be necessary to refine and improve many activities. More complex tasks may be attempted during this second admission if the therapist feels the individual is able to experience some degree of success.

Training for the myoelectric prosthesis proceeds in the same manner as mentioned above. Realistic expectations should be discussed prior to receiving the prostheses. When the training process begins, success, no matter how small, should be praised and reinforced. A tremendous amount of frustration is often experienced when first learning to operate bilateral above elbow myoelectric prostheses. Simple unilateral activities should be attempted before trying anything in a bilateral manner. The fact that only time and lots of practice will enable the individual to feel any degree of success or functional independence must be reinforced. Myoelectric hands for this level of amputation tend to be replaced with body-powered terminal devices.

Goals should be set according to the interest, motivation, and coordination of the individual. Motor coordination is perhaps the most important component in this process. The therapist should be prepared to encounter people, who, no matter what the activity, are unable to coordinate their movements (or muscles) to operate the prosthesis. This should not be considered a failure. I would suggest discharging the patient and allowing him or her to practice at home, with follow-up visits at a later date.

The first 6 months to a year are the most difficult for an individual with bilateral above elbow limb loss. Generally only limited success in functional independence is seen. If, however, the individual perseveres and has a strong desire to be independent, it is sometimes possible to become completely independent in all activities of daily living.

Case Study 7.

E.N. is a 39-year-old male who was injured in a high voltage electrical burn injury in Wyoming on December 14, 1983. He sustained bilateral above elbow amputations and

Figure 10. An adapted bath towel can be used by the individual after a bath or shower.

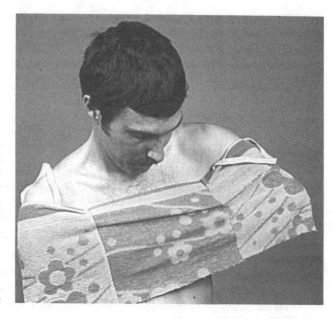

was treated locally until both residual limbs had healed. E.N. was fitted with bilateral Utah myoelectric arms that included myoelectric hands and hook-type terminal devices. He was also fitted with body-powered prostheses at that time; however, they did not fit properly, caused skin breakdown, and were eventually rejected.

E.N. was never comprehensively trained in the use of his myoelectric arms. Consequently, although he wore the arms daily, he did not use them in a functional manner. He was referred to another rehabilitation facility 9 months following his injury. The purpose of this hospitalization was to evaluate and upgrade his level of function with and without prostheses.

E.N. was essentially dependent when first admitted to rehabilitation. He was, however, able to write his name, pick up various objects, and feed himself certain foods. His primary goals were to be independent in eating, brushing teeth, shaving, showering, toileting, and dressing. Morning ADL activities had not been comprehensively explored with his residual limbs.

E.N. owned an electrical contracting company in Wyoming. His financial coverage was provided through insurance and workers' compensation. He had a strong desire to return to his electrical contracting company in whatever capacity was possible.

E.N. was hospitalized for rehabilitation as an inpatient for nearly 4 weeks. Rehabilitation goals included evaluating his present status and upgrading all areas of "essential" ADL (feeding, toileting, bathing, etc.). Several of these activities were attempted with and without his prostheses. Because his residual limbs were of sufficient length to meet his mid-line, there were many activities that could be accomplished with adapted clothing, devices, and custom-made equipment (see Figure 10). A "dressing tree" proved to be helpful (see Figure 11).

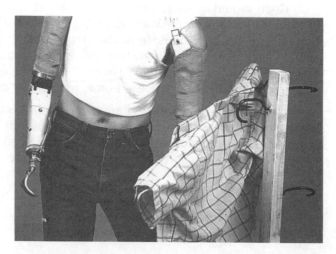

Figure 11. A "dressing tree" can be designed in various ways to provide optimal assistance.

Figure 12. Using a fork to eat requires control and coordination of the biceps and triceps in order to operate the elbow.

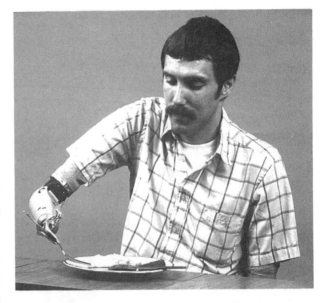

At the conclusion of his hospitalization, the majority of E.N.'s rehabilitation goals were met. These activities were accomplished with and without his prostheses. When E.N. used his prostheses (with Utah electric elbow), he preferred to use his body-powered hooks in lieu of his myoelectric hands. He felt he had better control and feedback with these terminal devices (see Figure 12).

Additional practice was the key to E.N.'s eventual functional independence. He was extremely motivated, coordinated, and committed to becoming independent. Today, E.N. is independent (with some environmental adaptations) in all ADL, and he has remarried and relocated. He started college and wants a degree in counseling. He has decided that he prefers body-powered internal locking elbows over his Utah myoelectric elbows as he feels they are more reliable and dependable, and are lighter and essentially easier to operate than his myoelectric units.

The Bilateral Shoulder Disarticulation Amputee

The loss of both arms at the shoulder presents, without question, the most difficult challenge for the prosthetist. Needless to say, for the patient this is the most serious and extensive of all upper limb amputations. Even under optimal circumstances, this individual will require maximum assistance for the majority of his or her activities of daily living. The utilization of one's feet is an alternative for many congenital upper limb amputees; however, adults encounter a great deal of difficulty due to their lack of hip range of motion and toe dexterity.

Unfortunately, there are no total body-powered prosthetic systems that address the many needs of an individual with bilateral shoulder disarticulation amputation. No system is available that can control the elbow, forearm, and terminal device with the few body motions that remain for this individual. Hybrid or complete electric prosthetic systems are the only answer.

The myoelectric prosthetic options should include an electric elbow, electric forearm rotators (if possible), and electric hands or body-powered hook-terminal devices. As stated previously, these individuals show a strong preference for body-powered terminal devices rather than myoelectric hands. Reasons stated include better proprioceptive feedback, fewer repairs, and increased fine motor dexterity skills with a hook versus a myoelectric hand.

A complete body-powered prosthetic system is not available. Training with a hybrid type of prosthesis should proceed as previously discussed. It is important to focus on simple ADL tasks such as writing, feeding, and brushing teeth. Providing positive learning experiences is crucial to success. This individual will need maximum assistance with dressing and bathing. The use of a bidet is strongly recommended in order to allow independence in toileting.

Training an individual in how to use myoelectric or switch-controlled prostheses is the most complex and time-consuming process a therapist will experience. Anxiety, frustration, anger, and depression are frequently experienced by individuals with this type of disability.

The skills and experience of the occupational therapist are critical. It is essential that the therapist thoroughly understands how the prostheses operate, the appropriate progression of prosthetic training, and, most importantly, what is realistic for the individual. A great deal of patience and understanding are necessary in order to achieve any degree of success with this complex problem.

It is appropriate to be cautious in estimating the individual's ability to be self-reliant in day-to-day activities. Some environmental modifications will be required, such as special sponges or brushes on the shower wall; special equipment, such as a dressing tree; and many clothes and towel adaptations. The process of prosthetic training and learning techniques to adapt to one's environment is a lengthy one. Staged admissions may be indicated in an attempt to avoid an overly discouraging situation when training is first initiated.

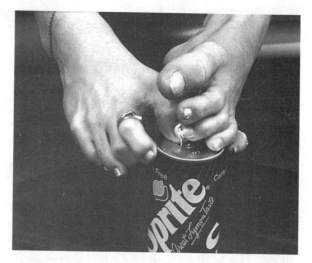

Some individuals will achieve independence in writing and eating. Aspects of dressing, bathing, brushing teeth, washing the face, and toileting can be attempted using foot skills, the prostheses, and/or environmental modifications. Manipulation of certain objects is also possible, but generally with only one prosthesis. Bilateral activities are extremely difficult.

Driving is also a possibility through the use of additional specialized equipment. If foot skills are perfected, it is possible to drive a car

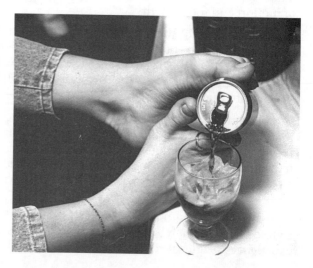

Figures 13 (top) and 14 (bottom). Opening a flip-top can and pouring it with one's feet demonstrates amazing dexterity in the person with congenital amelia (note rings on toes).

without adaptation, with the seat reclined, one foot operating the accelerator and brake, and one foot manipulating all elements of the dashboard and steering wheel.

An individual born without arms develops exceedingly fine motor manipulation skills with the feet and toes. It is not uncommon for these individuals to live independently, drive, pursue a career, and raise a family. To them, their feet have essentially become their "hands" (see Figures 13 and 14). An individual who loses his or her arms as an adult may acquire many of these skills through training. Case study 7 describes an experience involving a young male with bilateral shoulder disarticulation.

Case Study 7.

R.S. is a 34-year-old male who sustained bilateral shoulder disarticulation amputations at work. While working in a cherrypicker, he lost his balance and came in contact with 7,600 volts of electricity. He was hospitalized at a major burn center and had multiple surgical procedures in an attempt to preserve remaining viable tissue. Necrosis of the limbs was so severe, however, that bilateral shoulder disarticulation amputations were ultimately necessary.

R.S. was oriented in several areas of ADL during his original hospitalization, many of which included his feet. He was referred to a major rehabilitation hospital 1 month following the onset of injury for prosthetic fitting and training in order to increase his level of functional independence.

At the time of discharge from the burn center, R.S. was feeding himself with adapted equipment for his right foot. He was able to brush his teeth using an adaptive brush holder and used both feet to squeeze the toothpaste onto the brush. Using an adaptive cuff on his foot, he was able to shave independently. He remained dependent in dressing and toileting at the time of discharge from his initial hospitalization.

His primary goals included being as independent as possible with his bilateral Utah arms. His specific priorities included eating, toileting, and dressing. Although R.S. had attempted several ADL activities with his feet, his preference was to become adept with the upper extremity prostheses.

R.S. had been employed as a lineman for a major gas and power company. He was interested to returning to work for the same employer in a job requiring computer skills. While hospitalized, he was fitted and trained with bilateral Utah arms. R.S. underwent revision surgery for a large amount of redundant soft tissue over both shoulders. He was initially fitted with bilateral shoulder caps to establish a wearing tolerance.

Occupational therapy initiated many areas of ADL training; however, midway through his hospital course he and his wife needed to return home while she delivered their third child. Although he continued prosthetic training closer to home, he achieved little functional success. At one point he rejected his left prosthesis and found it easier to use the right arm only (see Figure 15). Ultimately, however, he found this "awkward and of limited use." Essentially, he felt his arms caused him "too much of a struggle for too little function."

Several home modifications were attempted. Some were successful (shower board, bidet, door knob extensions, and reading stand) and some were not (dressing tree and dental adaptation).

Following a recent conversation with R.S., the therapist discovered that he had just completed a specialized computer course recommended by the rehabilitation facility close to home. After being trained in the "Liaison" system, R.S. was able to control a chin-operated joystick to design electrical substations for his company. He was returning to work full-time and was extremely proud of his new abilities (see Figure 16).

R.S. had been highlighted on a morning talk show the week we spoke. That week, the Americans With Disabilities Act (ADA) had gone into effect. R.S. was featured as an individual who overcame disability and worked well with his employer in order to adapt his work environment. R.S. has been evaluated to learn to drive independently using a foot-operated system. This appears to be a viable alternative for him.

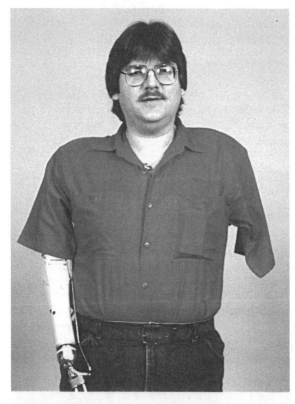

Figure 15 (top). At times, one shoulder disarticulation prosthesis is preferred over wearing both protheses.

Figure 16 (bottom). Workstation design by Carol Wheatley, OTR/L, and Judy Rein. Photograph copyright © by Carol Wheatley. Used with permission.

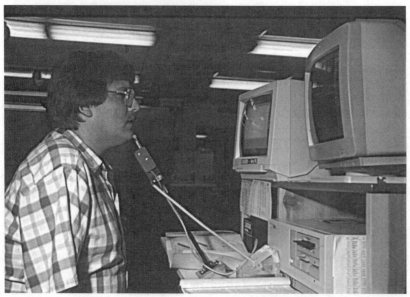

Summary

The complete rehabilitation process for an individual with adult amputations can be short, as with unilateral below elbow amputations, or long and ongoing, as with bilateral shoulder disarticulation amputations. Early fitting is crucial to achieve a successful, functional outcome for individuals with upper extremity amputations.

The amputee's potential is limitless. Adjustment to limb loss depends on many factors, including the quality of the prosthesis; medical considerations; the patient's history; and the ability of the therapist to devise a training program, in conjunction with the patient, that is tailored to meet the patient's needs. Motivation and the individual's desire to be self-reliant are perhaps the most important characteristics to cultivate and reinforce.

The patience, attitude, and experience of the occupational therapist are critical to the success of the patient. It is essential that the therapist believes in and understands the functional potential of the prosthesis. Success can then be more realistically achieved. The choice to use a prosthesis is one that only the individual can make. It should not be considered a "failure" if a person makes the choice not to wear a prosthesis. It is important, however, that he or she has had an opportunity to try. ◆

References

Atkins, D.J. (1989a). Postoperative and preprosthetic therapy programs. In D.J. Atkins & R.H. Meier (Eds.), *Comprehensive management of the upper limb amputee* (pp. 11–15). New York: Springer-Verlag.

Atkins, D.J. (1989b). Adult upper limb prosthetic training. In D.J. Atkins & R.H. Meier (Eds.), *Comprehensive management of the upper limb amputee* (pp. 39–59). New York: Springer-Verlag.

Fisher, A.G. (1989). Amputation and prosthetics. In C.A. Trombly. *Occupational therapy for physical dysfunction* (3rd ed.) (pp. 604–624). Baltimore: Williams & Wilkins.

Louis, D.S. (1982). Amputations. In D.P. Green (Ed.), *Operative hand surgery* (Vol. 1) (pp. 55–111). New York: Churchill Livingstone.

Malone, J.M., Fleming, L.L., Roberson, J.J., Whitesides, T.E., Leal, J.M., Poole, J.U., & Grodin, R.S. (1984). Immediate, early and late post-surgical management of upper limb amputation: Conventional electric and myoelectric prostheses. *Journal of Rehabilitation Research and Development, 21*(1), 33–41.

Mattingly, C. (1991). The narrative nature of clinical reasoning. *American Journal of Occupational Therapy, 45*, 998–1006.

Meier, R. (1984). Amputations and prosthetic fitting. In S. Fisher (Ed.), *Comprehensive rehabilitation of burns* (pp. 267–310). Baltimore: Williams & Wilkins.

Muilenburg, A.L., & LeBlanc, M.A. (1989). Body-powered upper-limb components. In D.J. Atkins & R.H. Meier (Eds.), *Comprehensive management of the upper limb amputee* (pp. 39–59). New York: Springer-Verlag.

Prout, W. (1989). The New York electric elbow, the New York prehension actuator, and the NU-VA synergetic prehensor. In D.J. Atkins & R.H. Meier (Eds.), *Comprehensive management of the upper limb amputee* (pp. 221–226). New York: Springer-Verlag.

Scott, R.N. (1989). Biomedical engineering in upper-limb prosthetics. In D.J. Atkins & R.H. Meier (Eds.), *Comprehensive management of the upper limb amputee* (pp. 173–189). New York: Springer-Verlag.

Sears, H.H., Andrew, J.T., & Jacobsen, S.C. (1989). Experience with the Utah arm, hand and terminal device. In D.J. Atkins & R.H. Meier (Eds.), *Comprehensive management of the upper limb amputee* (pp. 194–210). New York: Springer-Verlag.

Spiegel, S.R. (1989). Adult myoelectric upper-limb prosthetic training. In D.J. Atkins & R.H. Meier (Eds.), *Comprehensive management of the upper limb amputee* (pp. 60–71). New York: Springer-Verlag.

U.S. Department of Health and Human Services. (1991). *Vital health statistics: Current estimates from the National Health Interview Survey, 1990.* (Series 10, 181). Washington, DC: Government Printing Office.

Williams, T.W. (1989). Use of the Boston elbow for high-level amputees. In D.J. Atkins & R.H. Meier (Eds.), *Comprehensive management of the upper limb amputee* (pp. 211–220). New York: Springer-Verlag.

Wilson, A.B. (1989). *Limb prosthetics* (6th ed.). New York: Demos Publications.

11

Self-Care Strategies Following Severe Burns

Cheryl Leman Jordan

Rebekah Allely

Joanne Gallagher

Cheryl Leman Jordan, MA, OTR/L, is a Burn Rehabilitation Therapist and a Consultant at the Burn Center at the Washington Hospital Center, Washington, DC.
Rebekah Allely, OTR/L, is a Burn Rehabilitation Therapist at the Washington Hospital Center, Washington, DC.
Joanne Gallagher, MSc, OTR/L, is Chief Burn Rehabilitation Therapist at the Washington Hospital Center, Washington, DC.

Chapter 11 Outline

Introduction

Phases of Recovery

Burn Injuries
 Burn Depth
 Mechanism of Injury
 Percent Total Body Surface Area Involved
 Severity of Injury
 Wound Care
 Scar Formation
   Occupational Therapy
 Assessment
   Acute Care Phase
   In- and Outpatient Phases
 Acute Care Phase
 Rehabilitation Phase
 Outpatient Phase
 Facial Scars
 Burn Reconstruction
 Case Examples
   Case One
     Acute and Inpatient Rehabilitation
     Outpatient Rehabilitation
   Case Two
     Acute and Inpatient Rehabilitation
     Outpatient Rehabilitation
   Discussion

Summary

References

Acoordinated team approach is necessary to manage effectively the medical, functional, and psychosocial problems encountered during burn recovery. Functional independence is possible following a severe burn, but pain, discomfort, scar contracture, cosmetic disfigurement, and adverse psychological reactions to the burn injury can limit the patient's independence.

Throughout burn recovery, the rehabilitation treatment emphasizes patients returning to their preinjury ways of life. The occupational therapist uses splints and positioning, exercise and activity, functional skills performance, compression garments, skin and scar treatments, and patient and family education to prevent dysfunction and to support independence. Frequent assessment of the person's physical function, social needs, and emotional status is necessary for effective treatment programming. The patient's compliance and motivation are also essential for a successful outcome.

Introduction

A multidisciplinary team approach is a key component of functional recovery for people with severe burns. This team approach should start the day a patient is admitted to the hospital and continue through the wound-maturation phase. Only through continual interactions with the patient and each other can the burn team work efficiently. Today's burn team usually consists of a physician, nurses, occupational and physical therapists, social worker, and nutritionist. Many times, respiratory therapists, a chaplain, and a psychiatrist are additional members of the burn team. This continuum of comprehensive care is necessary to manage all the medical, functional, and psychosocial problems associated with burn injury recovery.

Medical advancements have improved burn survival and morbidity for the past several decades. For example, at one burn center, mortality was approximately 50% in the early 1970s, 13% by the 1980s, and 5.6% in 1990 (M. Jordan & M. Lewis, personal communication, November 14, 1991). Progressive surgical management and wound care; critical care monitoring; the use of pharmacokinetics for antibiotic dosing; nutritional support; and early, comprehensive rehabilitation are just a few of the advances that have improved burn injury outcomes.

When a patient is described as having a severe burn injury, it infers that an extended period of rehabilitation will be needed for recovery. The burn depth and extent, and the quality of wound healing, are primary determinants of potential outcomes. A patient's motivation, compliance with treatment, preinjury personality and emotional stability, psychosocial reactions, general health, and family support are other factors that affect burn injury outcomes.

Traditionally, a burn patient's recovery was a success if he or she survived the injury, returned home, and was able to perform basic self-care (either independently or with adaptation), including eating, dressing, grooming, toileting, and ambulating. Today, expanded burn care objectives include the quality of life following a burn injury. Severe burn injuries can cause functional, psychological, and cosmetic impairment; therefore, functional recovery for a severely burned patient now includes assuming responsibility for him- or herself and the role(s) in the home, returning to work or school, and resuming social and recreational activities.

Phases of Recovery

Burn rehabilitation treatments are usually discussed as they relate to stages of burn recovery. There are essentially four phases: acute care, inpatient rehabilitation, outpatient rehabilitation, and outpatient follow-up.

During acute care, the focus is on survival. Medical and surgical management are the principal goals of the burn treatment plan. As soon as the patient is medically stable, self-care is emphasized. When a patient's medical status limits basic self-care, other rehabilitation treatments (i.e., splinting, positioning, range of motion [ROM], etc.) are continued to prevent dysfunction. Patient and family education are integral components of acute care and all stages of recovery. The acute care phase continues until extensive wound care needs are minimal.

When a burn patient is transferred from the intensive care unit to an intermediate care unit in the hospital, he or she usually enters the inpatient rehabilitation phase of recovery. Independent function and prevention of disability become the central themes of treatment. Wound care continues, but patient participation in self-care and wound-care activities increases. In addition to independent eating, dressing, and grooming skills, there is an emphasis on general conditioning (including strength, flexibility, and endurance), independent skin and scar care, and socialization. The inpatient rehabilitation phase can extend 6 to 8 months postinjury for burn injuries involving major body surface areas (more than 60% to 70% of the body surface), although the average length of stay for a major burn injury is 3 to 4 months after the initial injury.

The emphasis of care during the outpatient rehabilitation phase is to: minimize scar contracture formation; improve flexibility, strength, and endurance; assure proper skin and scar care techniques; and promote independence in normal daily activities, including social and recreational pursuits. It is an extension of the rehabilitation phase, but patients live at home and attend therapy during the day. Community reintegration and socialization issues become more apparent, making the patient's adaptation to the injury a primary objective.

Most burn patients are discharged from intensive outpatient rehabilitation when they achieve the skills needed to function at home independently and can return to school or work full time. They can reach this phase before wound maturation is complete. The total time required before returning to work has been found to be related to the site and severity of the burn, age of the patient, the patient's occupation, and the location where the thermal injury occurred (Bowden, Thomson, & Prasad, 1989; Helm, Walker, & Peyton, 1986). To prevent unforeseen problems, a schedule of follow-up visits to a burn clinic is established to monitor wound maturation (Petro & Salisbury, 1986).

Burn Injuries

The burn team considers numerous factors while developing treatment plans and goals for specific patients. Potential functional outcomes can also be predicted from an analysis of these factors. Primary considerations are the depth of the burn, the mechanism of injury, the percent of total body surface area (%TBSA) burned, specific body areas burned, and associated problems (i.e., an inhalation injury or other trauma). The patient's age, past medical history, and preinjury health also affect medical and rehabilitation care plans.

Burn Depth

The depth of the burn is estimated from clinical observation of its appearance, sensitivity,

Figure 1. Burn wound characteristics.

Burn Depth	Tissue Depth	Clinical Findings	Healing Time
Superficial	Superficial epidermis	Erythema, blisters; painful	3–7 days
Partial thickness; superficial	Epidermis	Red, weeping, large blisters; painful	2 weeks or < 21 days
Partial thickness; deep	Epidermis and varying depths of dermis	Hemorrhaghic, waxy, white, ± pain	> 21 days
Full thickness	Epidermis, dermis; may involve subcutaneous tissues, tendons, or muscles	Tan, dry, leathery, thrombosed vessels; insensate	Surgery required

and pliability. Burns were traditionally classified as first-, second-, and third-degree; however, they are now described as superficial, partial, or full-thickness (see Figure 1).

Functional problems encountered during burn recovery can be predicted from an assessment of the burn depth. Partial-thickness burns can heal without surgical intervention. Once healed, they tend to be dry and itchy, and are frequently prone to shear forces (e.g., rubbing or scratching), which can cause blisters and altered skin integrity. Deep partial-thickness and full-thickness burns can result in scarring and cause hypo- or hyperpigmentation of the area once it heals. Full-thickness wounds usually require surgical wound closure and have a greater potential for contracture formation than do partial-thickness wounds.

Mechanism of Injury

The annual incidence of burn-related injuries in the United States is estimated at 2.5 million, more than 70,000 of which require hospitalization (Feller & Jones, 1984). Predominated etiologies of burn injuries, as identified in a 1988 national survey by the American Burn Association's Committee on Organization and Delivery of Burn Care, are flame or flash exposure (55%). Hot liquids and immersion scalds account for 35% of all the injuries. Electrical contact and chemical burns each account for approximately 5% of all admissions (M. Lewis, personal communication, October 19, 1991).

The severity of a burn injury depends on the area exposed and the duration and intensity of thermal exposure. Superficial partial-thickness burns typically occur after a brief contact with hot liquids, surfaces, or flames. Deep partial-thickness burns are caused by longer exposure to intense heat, such as with hot water immersion scalds, or skin contact with flaming materials or hot surfaces. In the home, superficial or deep partial-thickness burns frequently occur when cooking or bathing. Full-thickness burns result from prolonged immersion scalds, electrical contact, longer exposure to flames, contact with hot grease or tar, or contact with chemical agents.

Percent Total Body Surface Area Involved

Two methods for estimating %TBSA are the rule of nines, and the Lund and Browder chart (Solem, 1984). The rule of nines is simple and quick, but relatively inaccurate. It divides the body surface into areas comprising 9%, or multiples of 9%, with the perineum making up the final 1%. The head/neck is 9%, each upper extremity is 9%, each leg is 18%, and the front and back of the trunk are each 18%.

The Lund and Browder chart provides a more accurate estimate of the total body surface area (Lund & Browder, 1944) and is used in most burn centers. This chart assigns a percent of surface area to body segments. For example, the arm is divided into the upper arm, forearm, and hand. As a rough estimate, a patient's palm print, excluding the fingers, is approximately 1% of the total body surface area. (Due to the chart's detail, readers are referred to the reference.)

Severity of Injury

The %TBSA and depth of burn are frequently used to determine the severity of injury. A deep-partial or full-thickness burn to more than 20% of the body is often the determining factor for admission to a burn intensive care unit. Depending on the patient's age and preinjury health, small partial- or full-thickness burn wounds (less than 20% TBSA) can be considered severe burn injuries. For an average adult, a deep-partial and full-thickness burn of greater than 40% TBSA is severe. The time involved to achieve wound closure may be protracted, and functional recovery requires intensive rehabilitation.

Burn involvement of certain body areas also is used to classify injury severity, although the %TBSA burn is limited. For example, deep-partial or full-thickness burns of the hands, face, or perineum are usually considered severe (Wachtel, 1985). Burns of the face, eyes, and neck may cause respiratory compromise and difficulties in seeing and eating, and can result in long-term functional and cosmetic impairment. Bilateral hand burns may initially limit the individual's self-care ability and can also result in long-term functional disability if not properly managed.

Wound Care

Various topical agents are available to treat burn wounds. Their purpose is to delay colonization and reduce bacterial counts on or in the wounds (Hartford, 1984). When a topical agent is used, the dressing must be changed at least twice daily. Although all burn wounds are usually treated with a topical antibacterial agent, the extent and depth of the burn wound determines the need for surgical treatment. When a wound will take more than 2 weeks to heal, surgery can usually decrease morbidity.

Surgical treatment for burn wounds consists of excision (removal) of the burned tissue (eschar) and placement of skin grafts. Transplanting the person's own skin from one body area to another is an autograft. Following surgical excision and autografting, the area treated is immobilized for a minimum of 3 days.

Biologic dressings are used as a temporary wound covering when adequate autograft is not available or when burn depth limits graft adherence. Examples of biologic dressings are homografts, which are processed cadaver skin; xenografts, which are processed pig skin; and synthetic products or artificial skin substitutes.

Scar Formation

The most common burn injury sequela limiting function is the development of scar and contracture during wound maturation. The quality of burn-wound maturation is affected by numerous factors, some of which can occur during the early phases of care (Helm & Fisher, 1988). A significant determinant of scar development is the time needed for wound closure. Bacterial infections in a wound increase the inflammatory response and delay healing. The spontaneous healing of full-thickness burns can be lengthy and contributes to collagen overgrowth. Race, age, anatomical location, and depth of the burn wound also influence scar formation.

Hypertrophic scars develop after wound closure, and are initially thick, rigid, and hyperemic in surface appearance. Histologically, immature hypertrophic scars have increased vascularity, fibroblasts, myofibroblasts, and whorls or nodules of collagen (Abston, 1987). Their functional or cosmetic significance depends on their anatomical location. Joint motion is limited when the scar complex crossing a joint surface contracts. Scars on the face distort facial features and can also limit function.

Regardless of the wound-care method used and the time taken for wound closure, scar maturation differs with each patient. Nonhypertrophic scars can mature in 5 to 8 weeks, whereas hypertrophic scars can take up to 1 or 2 years to mature. Although it is sometimes possible to predict outcomes from the initial appearance of the wound, many factors can affect the end results.

Occupational Therapy

The role of the occupational therapist in the treatment of severe burns is multifaceted and changes as healing progresses and the patient moves through the phases of recovery. It is necessary to maintain or increase range of motion, strength, and endurance so that the patient may be functional to perform activities of daily living (ADL) (Trombly, 1983). These goals are essential to prevent contractures and deformities (Parent, 1983). Modalities used may include splints, ADL, and exercise programs.

A view of human occupation developed by Kielhofner (1980, 1985) and others (Kielhofner & Burke, 1985) serves as a useful model to consider the impact of a serious burn injury on the life of a patient, assists the therapist in understanding relationships between various aspects of treatment, and provides a method for problem identification. This model suggests that restrictions in the ability to move and perform tasks reduce the patient's ability to accomplish necessary roles, which in turn influences his or her views of self as a competent being. Over time, this can affect interests and values and reduce motivation.

When patients sustain severe burn injuries, they are unable to complete activities of daily living due to the depth and extent of the wounds, medicated dressings, and pain. Their restricted function and isolation result in a dramatic change in their ordinary daily routines, and their roles are temporarily or permanently altered. For example, the hospital routine does not allow a patient to sleep uninterrupted because policy frequently dictates that vital signs be taken on certain predetermined schedules during the nurses' shifts. The new role of patient replaces the roles of worker, parent, and/or spouse (Reilly, 1962).

Psychological affects are a significant concern (Fleet, 1992). Changes in motivation may occur at the time of injury and could continue for many years after discharge. Values can change, and self-esteem and confidence may be impaired due to body-image issues. Social and personal interests may be affected, particularly if the injury occurred during a specific activity or event. A patient who was injured at a friend's outdoor barbecue may become anxious at the mention of social gatherings and often refuse to participate.

Cheng and Rogers (1989) studied men who had completed rehabilitation for severe burn injuries to determine how their role performance changed in the areas of self-care, leisure, home management, and work. They found that some patients experienced minimal role reduction, while others managed their self-care requirements but were experiencing role disruption in their leisure, work, and home management. A third pattern seemed to be substantial disruption of all roles. In this study, role loss was commonly associated with reduced endurance, the presence of impaired grip strength and upper extremity skill, and difficulty walking and standing. While most of the individuals studied had achieved independence in self-care within a year after discharge, this did not coincide with role resumption in home management, work, and leisure areas. The authors suggest that further study is needed to examine how residual burn impairment affects performance and achievement in occupational roles.

By viewing the patient within a dynamic conceptual framework of occupation such as that proposed by Kielhofner, rehabilitation focuses on the relationship between the injury and the patient as a social being. Within this context, the need to address the emotional, as well as the physical, dimensions of the injury becomes more apparent, and both assessment and intervention strategies should be planned accordingly.

Assessment

Acute Care Phase

Whenever possible, a patient should be evaluated by an occupational therapist within 24 hours of admission to the hospital. An initial review of the medical record helps to determine the mechanism of injury, %TBSA affected, depth of burn, and the patient's age, sex, and past medical history. This information can also be obtained or confirmed by assessment, observation, and communication with the patient. (When a patient is intubated for a thermal injury to the airway, the therapist should consult with other burn team members to obtain this information.) A visual assessment of the patient prior to applying dressings provides a more accurate understanding of the %TBSA and burn depth. Attention should be directed to joint surface areas involved and any circumferential burns, in order to prioritize patient treatment needs.

Once the patient is stabilized and nursing care is completed, a comprehensive occupational therapy assessment can be started. If the patient is able to communicate, information pertaining to hand dominance, home environment and responsibilities, work skills, and any past medical or musculoskeletal problems affecting function, family, and social support systems should be discussed. Developing an understanding of the patient's premorbid level of function is important to support effective communication and program planning. The functional component of an acute care assessment should include range of motion evaluation, general strength, and functional abilities.

To evaluate range of motion during acute care, verbal instructions should be given and the motion should be demonstrated for clarification. A goniometer should be used to assure accuracy when recording motions for both involved and uninvolved joints. If the patient demonstrates motion limitation, it is important to determine and document the cause. Frequently a patient resists motion because of apprehension, pain, or confusion. Other reasons include edema and bulky dressings. An assessment of active range of motion is preferred; however, if the patient is unresponsive or not willing, the therapist should evaluate active-assistive and, in some cases, passive range of motion (see Figure 2).

Initial assessment of gross strength is easily performed by a manual test of major muscle groups. Because muscle strength is not initially affected by the burn, this test can help identify any associated injuries or preexisting conditions that were not reported.

Actual performance of ADL skills should be continually assessed during acute care. Observation of eating and grooming skills is important to determine if normal or

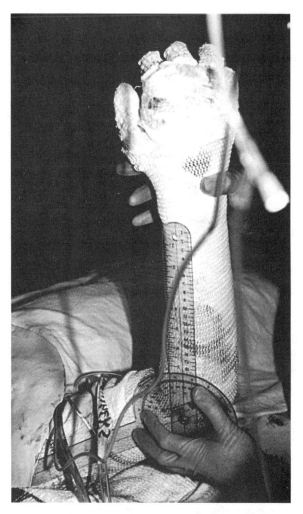

Figure 2. After identifying the joint axis through observation of active or passive motion, goniometer measurements can be taken over burn dressings by controlling the position of the longitudinal axis during the motion.

compensatory motions are being used. Often adaptive methods are used, due to interference from dressings or edema, and are associated with positional changes.

In- and Outpatient Phases

Assessments during both in- and outpatient rehabilitation include evaluating range of motion, strength, endurance, self-care activities, work skills, skin and scar condition, and social and emotional adaptation.

Goniometric measurements of range of motion should be done weekly, biweekly, or as needed, depending on the frequency of treatment. Strength can be evaluated by the patient's performance of various activities or use of different treatment modalities. When the patient has hand burns, dynamometer recordings of grip strength and pinch gauge measures of pinch strength should also be frequently documented.

Progressive scar formation usually causes discomfort when the patient stretches to achieve full range of motion. It is important to evaluate a scar visually, tactually, and in terms of its effect on range of motion or combined joint motions. Scar contracture, causing banding of the skin over a joint surface, requires close supervision because it may affect the patient's ability to maintain adequate range of motion. Early observation, documentation, and therapeutic intervention can help prevent the need for future surgical release of a scar contracture.

Continual assessment of a burn patient's functional skills is a primary objective. Visual observation of self-care activities is necessary to instruct and encourage the patient in normal movement patterns. For example, a patient with upper-body burns involving the trunk and extremities may feel unable to perform any upper-body dressing activities. When attempting the task, the patient will struggle and use abnormal posturing and motions. Therapy intervention should include instruction and demonstration of normal movement patterns. The patient's ability to integrate correct motions for the activity should be closely monitored.

Awareness of the patient's emotional status is important throughout recovery. Due to pain, frustration, fatigue, and other difficulties encountered with rehabilitation activities, patients commonly demonstrate emotional turmoil. To assess coping skills, the therapist should carefully inquire how a patient is dealing with the many issues encountered during burn recovery. When appropriate, the patient should be encouraged to discuss problems with the burn center's social worker.

Acute Care Phase

During acute care, pain is a principal concern of patients. Patients with a severe burn injury often respond to pain by being noncompliant with treatment and resistive to motion. When this occurs, the therapist should gently talk to the patient, explaining what is being done and why. Counting out loud or describing the motion frequently helps patients attend to what is occurring. It is not uncommon for intensive care patients to be disoriented or unresponsive to verbal cuing, however. With these cases it is important to continue verbal communication during passive exercise. Full range of motion should be achieved during every treatment session (see Figure 3).

Patients with smaller burn injuries often complain of pain by describing dressing tightness and other sensations. To achieve treatment objectives, patient education at this early stage is critical. The patient should be assured that the tightness of the dressings will not harm the skin, and that the discomfort is real, but must be tolerated to regain normal function. Deep breathing techniques or other relaxation exercises can help the patient deal with pain during various activities.

Controlling edema is another acute care objective. This is frequently achieved through positioning techniques that prevent dependent posturing. Many of the positions used initially are continued throughout recovery. When a patient has hand burns, the hands should be elevated above heart level. This can easily be achieved by using pillows. Volar hand splints also assist in edema control. Patients should be encouraged to use their

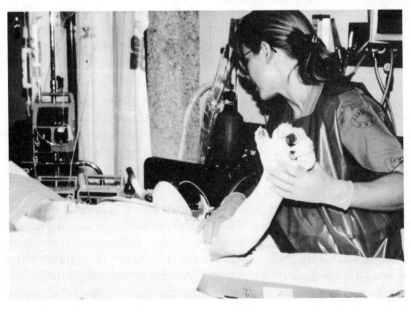

Figure 3. During passive or active-assistive range of motion, the therapist should continually talk to the patient and describe what is being done.

Figure 4. Proper positioning for burn injuries.

Body Area Burned	Antideformity Position	Modalities/Techniques
Neck	Extension	No pillow
Shoulder	90° abduction	Arm boards, traction
Elbow	Extension	Arm boards, elbow extension splint
Dorsal hand	Wrist extension, MCP* flexion, PIP+ and DIP‖ extension	Volar splint, arm elevated above heart
Volar hand	Full digit and palmar extension	Volar extension splints
Hip	Extension	Hospital bed flat
Knee	Extension	Knee extension splint
Ankle	Dorsiflexion	Dorsiflexion splint

*metacarpophalangeal; + proximal interphalangeal; ‖ distal interphalangeal

hands for eating, grooming, and other functional activities as much as possible. As adequate nutrition is very important for wound healing, feedback on calorie and protein intake can be useful in fostering patient involvement during mealtimes (Mahon & Neufeld, 1984). The combination of exercise, performance of self-care activities using normal motions, elevation, and splints applied with elastic bandages for night positioning not only helps control or decrease hand edema, but also promotes normal recovery (see Figure 4).

Patients are often so overwhelmed by the trauma of being burned that they do not hear what the therapist is telling them. Some patients perceive their injury in a paralyzing manner. Regardless of the education provided, they frequently experience decreased self-confidence and believe they are dependent on staff and family. When asked to perform a task, they will say they are unable to do it. In these situations, therapy should focus on accomplishing simple skills, such as holding a spoon with a normal pinch. Although a considerable amount of time can be involved in completing simple tasks, improved patient confidence for trying complex tasks can be achieved. A social worker also helps by providing supportive counseling.

Prior to surgery, patients should be informed that a period of immobilization may follow the procedure, but under supervision certain rehabilitation activities will continue. For example, if a patient's hands and forearm burns are surgically excised and autografted, the therapist may still provide shoulder activities at the patient's bedside during the postoperative immobilization period.

Postoperative immobilization can restrict functional independence. When a patient's hands are in postoperative dressings, self-feeding is only possible using adaptive equipment. If adaptations are used for postoperative function, the patient should understand that they are only temporary.

Deconditioning is frequently a result of prolonged bed rest, the hypermetabolic demands of a severe burn, and a generalized decrease in daily activity. To limit deconditioning, intensive care unit patients should be involved in exercise, activity, and ambulation throughout the day. Range-of-motion, stretching, and functional activities are a few techniques that can be used. A therapist should communicate daily with the burn team to determine when to increase or decrease activity. If the patient is on bed rest, grooming and eating tasks and bedside activities, such as pegboards or other upper extremity exercises performed while wearing cuff weights, can promote flexibility and strength.

When a patient is medically cleared to ambulate, the treatment program should be adjusted to include out-of-bed exercise and activity. Walking to a chair or standing to do exercises, standing at a sink for grooming tasks, and sitting in a chair for meals can help limit deconditioning. Patients often complain of fatigue during this phase of increased activity. Consistent support and encouragement for them to ambulate, perform stretching and range of motion activities independently, and increase self-care are necessary.

During the transition from dependency on staff to independent activity, patients frequently demonstrate alterations in posture and lethargy. Abnormal posturing is often a guarding response to avoid pain and discomfort. Splints may be necessary to emphasize normal posture. For example, a patient with an arm burn may hold the elbow flexed and resist extending the arm. This can cause difficulties with an activity such as dressing. If the problem is allowed to continue, the patient may be unable to don slacks, shoes, or socks, due to limited reach. As a prevention, use of an elbow extension splint when resting can help preserve elbow extension.

During acute care, a daily exercise and activity schedule may be needed to support appropriate patient behaviors and emphasize treatment objectives. The schedule should include morning and afternoon therapy; dressing changes and independent grooming, eating, and dressing tasks; visiting hours and rest periods; and frequent ambulation. The schedule should be developed with the patient, and the entire burn team should try to adhere to it.

The acute phase of a burn injury primarily affects the ability of the patient to move and act in the environment. Skills needed to complete tasks are impaired, constraining engagement in normal routines and contributing to the anxiety and frustration that comes from disrupted social roles. An acute burn injury does not inhibit the movement of joints and extremities, but it is painful. The dressings placed on the burn injury may limit motions that are necessary to finish a task in a timely and normal manner. An example is a patient with dressings on the dominant upper extremity. Self-feeding can (and should) be completed independently; however, manipulation of the utensil may be difficult due to edema and impaired sensation caused by the dressings and the burn injury.

Rehabilitation Phase

The patient's responsibility for self-care increases in the rehabilitation phase. Burn wounds continue to heal, reducing nursing care needs. The patient's role is to complete self-care activities (i.e., feeding, grooming, and dressing) as independently as possible. Continued patient education stresses the importance of resuming preinjury function and emphasizes daily routines and habits that will give the patient control over part of his or her care (see Figure 5).

Decreased range of motion, strength, and endurance may interfere with performance of daily living tasks. A patient can have difficulty donning an overhead shirt when there are limitations in shoulder motion, and donning socks when trunk mobility is limited. Poor strength may prevent the patient from performing repetitive activities, and decreased endurance prevents the task from being completed.

To increase range of motion and improve strength and endurance, various treatments and modalities can be used. A burn exercise program should include stretching exercises for all extremities, as well as strengthening activities. Flexibility exercises (i.e., jumping jacks, toe touches, etc.) should be performed at a full-length mirror so the patient can see his or her posture and progress. Endurance can be emphasized through paced ambulation activities in the hospital, in addition to riding a stationary bike. Equipment such as a BTE Work Simulator can simulate function motions to increase upper body ROM, strength, and endurance. It also provides written results to monitor patient performance. Other modalities, such as West II and Valpar Work Samples can be used to reproduce functional motions and to assess and simulate work skills (see Figure 6).

A positive rapport with patients is vital for their education on the importance of rehabilitation activities in preparing for return to work. Open communication is also instrumental in determining the skills needed for patients to eventually return to work.

Newly healed skin is extremely fragile and is prone to breakdown. Problems include blisters resulting from friction, and an increased sensitivity to touch. It is imperative that skin conditioning be initiated as soon as wound healing occurs. Skin-conditioning activities include using massage, using a moisturizing cream, and applying intermediate and custom-made pressure garments to desensitize the skin. Patients should be taught to

Figure 5 (top). Independent performance of self-care tasks is emphasized during the rehabilitation phase of care. **Figure 6 (bottom).** Work conditioning equipment can be used for ROM activities and general conditioning during burn recovery.

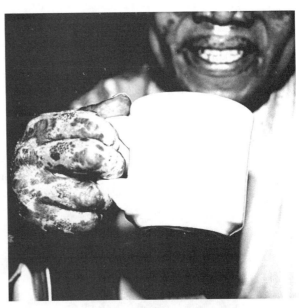

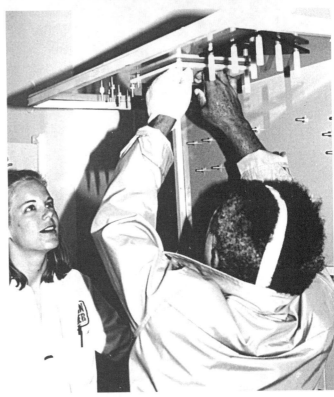

massage their skin whenever it feels tight and dry. Pressure garments should be used to provide continuous external vascular support. Garments are usually worn 23 hours a day and are only removed for 1 hour during bathing. Patients can perform most ADL tasks and participate in recreational activities and most work environments without interference from the garments. During hospitalization, patients should be taught the necessity of pressure garments and their responsibility in adhering to the wearing schedule.

Poor venous return in burned extremities is identified by increased edema in the limb; vascular pooling is apparent by the skin color. Edema is often the result of the extremity being dependent without garments for external support, the patient's altered movement patterns, and, sometimes, the patient's noncompliance with exercises. Gloves should be worn when there are hand burns, and vascular stockings or ace wraps should be applied to the legs when there are lower extremity burns, to increase venous return.

Hands that have been severely burned often become edematous due to decreased use and a lack of exercise. To reduce hand edema, compression wraps, using self-adherent elastic dressings (Coban), can be applied providing slight tension using a figure-eight wrap (see Figure 7). Care should be taken to avoid wrapping too tightly, which is evidenced by

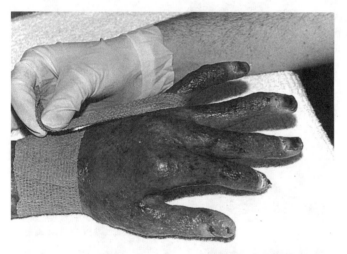

poor circulation and the patient reporting numbness or tingling. The self-adherent elastic wraps should include the thumb, all fingers, and web spaces, and the hand wrapping proximal to the wrist (see Figures 8 and 9). Exercises and ADL should be performed with the Coban wrap intact. To bathe, the Coban wrap can be protected by a rubber glove. Constant edema that does not respond to Coban wraps may be reduced by intermittent compression pump therapy.

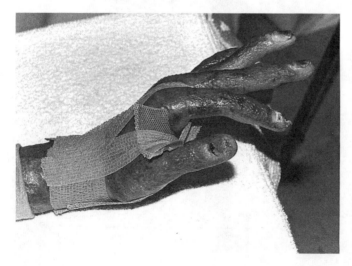

Figure 7 (top). To apply a compression wrap to the hand, inch-wide strips of Coban are first placed through the web spaces and attached at the wrist.

Figure 8 (bottom). Silicone gel can be used under Coban strips to apply added pressure to firm scars or to prevent the Coban wrap from pinching the skin.

Figure 9. Inch-wide Coban strips are then applied circumferentially working distal to proximal on the individual digits, then the hand. Hand motion is monitored to determine if the elastic wrap is too restrictive.

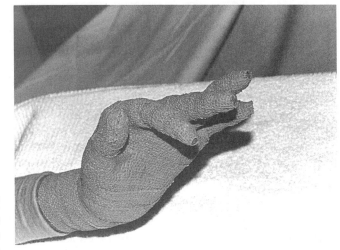

Performing activities of daily living is essential to the rehabilitative phase. Patients often prefer to be dependent on nurses and family because of pain, fear, or a lack of motivation. Dressings may inhibit full movement and prolong the time necessary to complete the task, but maximum independence should be emphasized. Performing ADL independently provides patients with some control during recovery. Wearing street clothes can help develop a feeling of approaching normalcy. To support independent self-care function, family members should be asked to bring the patient's clothes and grooming appliances from home early during hospitalization (see Figure 10).

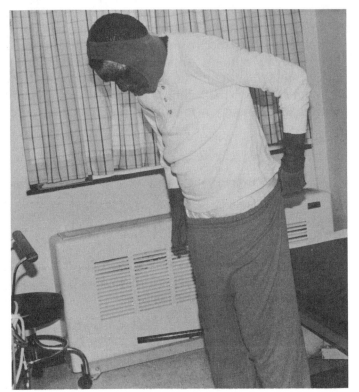

Patients who were injured while cooking or bathing may be hesitant or refuse to perform related tasks. It is crucial that these fears be identified and addressed. Treatment activities should include education in safety precautions and performance of the fear-provoking tasks with therapist supervision. A patient who was injured while cooking may be reluctant to return to the kitchen. One goal of therapy would be for the

Figure 10. Independent dressing using clothes from home can have a positive effect on a patient's outlook.

patient to use a stove for food preparation. Prior to the activity, safety precautions should be discussed so they can be practiced during the kitchen activity.

The rehabilitation phase of burn recovery primarily affects the habituation subsystem. Noncompliance with exercise programs often results in contractures that impair full range of motion. When this occurs, activities of daily living (habits) cannot be completed without adaptive equipment or compensatory techniques. Poor trunk mobility may inhibit a patient from donning socks and shoes without a sock aid or a long-handled shoe horn. Extended hospitalization or a daily outpatient treatment schedule can prevent a patient from resuming familiar roles of family member, student, or provider. It is imperative in this phase that patients see their progress and begin to assume roles on a part-time basis.

Outpatient Phase

Burn patients and their families must be educated about home care activities prior to discharge from the hospital. Throughout hospitalization, education about what can be expected following discharge can aid the process. Home care booklets, classes, and video tapes are some techniques that burn care facilities use to reinforce this information (Adriaenssens, 1988; Mason & Forshaw, 1986; Yurko & Fratianne, 1988). Discharge education and training cover a broad range of topics and activities, ranging from skin and wound care to home exercises (Kaplan, 1985). Appropriate home care can only be achieved when the patient and family have a thorough understanding of its procedures and activities (see Figure 11).

During the outpatient rehabilitation phase of recovery, burn patients may go through countless physical, functional, and emotional changes, despite continuous inpatient education. This is the time when they truly begin to experience the functional consequences of a burn injury. Psychological and social issues become more apparent and can have a significant affect on the patients' outlook. Although they leave the hospital eating and dressing independently, they may return unable to get a spoon to their mouths. Providing adaptive equipment is not the solution, because there are many reasons that may contribute to this change in function. Identifying the underlying causes

Figure 11. Home program content.

Topic	Points Covered
Wound care	When, method, precautions
Skin care	Frequency, method, supplies, blister care, sun protection
Exercises	Purpose, frequency, techniques
Self-care	Importance of independence, adaptive equipment use when appropriate
Recreation	Purpose, types, frequency
Pressure garments	Purpose, care, wearing schedule, insert use, precautions
Splint wear	Application, care, wearing schedule, precautions

is the first step toward developing an appropriate treatment plan. Although scar contracture is the most common cause, there are often physical factors and emotional reactions that contribute to the dysfunction. Some patients suffer from posttraumatic stress disorders (Perry & Difede, 1992), and others contend with emotional sequelae, sometimes related to premorbid psychological problems (Malt & Ugland, 1989; Tucker, 1986.) A review of the literature by Hill (1985) did not indicate a relationship between the severity or visibility of physical deformities and psychosocial adjustment following discharge.

Prior to discharge from the hospital, a patient's strength and endurance may be adequate for self-care independence. Once home, differences between the hospital and home environments may be so great that fatigue sets in before noon. This feeling of fatigue may be functional, but it may also be emotionally based. The normal reaction is to rest instead of participating in home activities and outpatient therapy. As a result, strength remains poor or decreases, while scars contract and cause decreased flexibility. The outpatient treatment plan should include a daily exercise program that emphasizes massage and stretch followed by flexibility and strengthening activities. The activities are similar to those used during inpatient rehabilitation, but their intensity and frequency increase. Although these activities should be done frequently throughout the day, scar massage and stretching prior to self-care activities can improve a patient's functional skills performance.

Scar contracture is the primary cause of functional deficits. Burn scars that cross joint surfaces limit range of motion and function because the skin shortens over the joint. If left untreated, muscle shortening and fibrous contracture of the joint capsule can occur (Abston, 1987). A scar treatment goal is to control maturation so that a minimal amount of scar tissue develops without adhering to underlying structures or limiting motion. Although pressure garments and flexible pressure inserts are used to minimize scar proliferation (see Figure 12), continuous activity is necessary to overcome the contractile forces of the scar. Splints, casts, stretching exercises, and activities accentuating flexibility also are effective scar treatments (Rivers, 1987). There are times when a scar contracture is so strong that preventing further loss of motion can be the only goal. This type of contracture eventually requires surgical reconstruction to restore functional mobility.

Because scar control and remodeling are possible during the early stages of wound maturation, limitations in self-care function can be temporary if appropriate treatments

Figure 12. Insert materials used under pressure garments.

Material	Areas Used
Aliplast	Thumb webs, shoe inserts
Plastazote	Finger webs, hand dorsum, axillary webs, any firm scar
Silastic elastomer, Otoform	Hands, face, chest
Prosthetic foam	Chest
Silicone gel	Hands, face, areas of limited friction
Aquaplast	Face contours, finger webs
Adhesive-backed, closed-cell foams	Concave areas

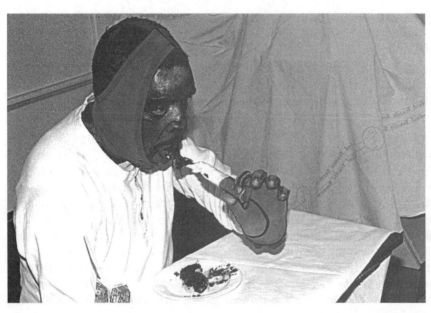

Figure 13. Extended handles on utensils should be gradually shortened to increase range of motion.

are implemented quickly and the patient actively participates. In addition to other outpatient burn treatment activities, performing basic self-care is an effective way to increase function. Despite the time it takes, patients should perform self-care without compensating or using substitute motions. With these patients, every effort should be made to avoid the use of adaptive equipment. If equipment is used, it should be frequently changed to increase motion. Built-up or extended handles on eating, dressing, and grooming aids can be continually adjusted to stimulate increased motion (see Figure 13).

There are cases where burn depth, extent, and involvement of underlying structures are so significant that adaptations are necessary for the patient to function. If the patient

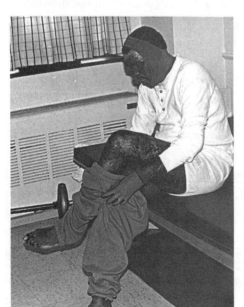

does not have additional physical problems affecting function, the adaptations should be simple and designed to utilize the range of motion available (see Figure 14). Until scar maturation is complete, functional skills can gradually improve. Tendon and joint adhesions may also eventually resolve if patients use the motion available and continue to stretch.

Depending on their personalities, some burn patients with permanent functional limitations develop their own adaptive methods to accomplish activities. These individuals fre-

Figure 14. Scar contractures of both shoulders, elbows, and hands made it necessary for this patient to develop compensatory techniques to accomplish lower-extremity dressing without adaptive equipment.

quently consider extensive adaptations to be an encumbrance. If they do use equipment, it usually must be small enough to fit in a pocket on their clothes, such as a button-aid. This type of attitude usually develops near the end of the wound maturation phase and is a sign that the patients are taking control of their own lives (see Figure 15).

During outpatient rehabilitation, patients may not participate with therapy or care for themselves due to the physical and emotional effects of the injury. Depression is common during recovery and is often demonstrated by noncompliance or apathy, which can affect function. Avoidance of pain is another common reaction that contributes to decreased function. Because burn patients tend to provide support for each other, attending a burn support group can help. These group discussions can facilitate understanding of where the patients have been and what they have to do.

Everyone has an individual perception of pain. Scar tightness and sensitivity that causes discomfort for one individual may cause severe pain for another. Skin conditioning techniques, massage, and the wearing of external vascular support garments are used to decrease hypersensitivity. Imagery techniques or redirecting the focus to functional activities, concentrating on the quality of performance, can sometimes distract a patient from the sensations being experienced. When a survivor of a burn injury concentrates only on scar sensations or on all of his or her problems, counseling should be recommended.

A patient's skin and scar status, functional skills, and return to work or school status are a few of the factors that should be periodically reevaluated. When return to work or school part-time may support skills recovery, the treatment schedule should be adjusted accordingly. A patient who achieves the skills needed to function at home independently and can return to school or work full-time should be discharged from the outpatient therapy program. Since burn scar maturation can take up to 18 months postinjury, a patient may still be wearing pressure garments and night splints after resuming normal activities.

The outpatient phase of burn recovery primarily affects psychosocial adjustment. The patient's prognosis and ability to resume preinjury function are assessed and should be fairly accurate. During this phase, personal interests and values are examined.

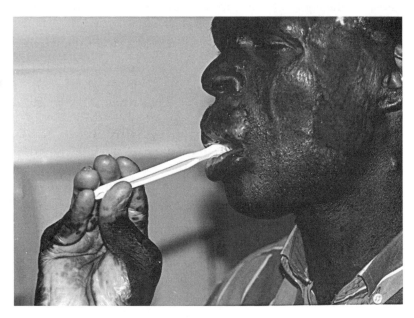

Figure 15. Many activities of daily living can be performed with restricted range of motion if the patient is motivated.

Acceptance of the inability to pursue further a favorite avocational activity, or the realization of the injury and its impact on one's life, helps the patient determine what values are important.

Facial Scars

Not all scars affect function by limiting range of motion. Scar contracture and hypertrophy can also cause devastating facial disfigurement. Facial structure is distorted by altered nasal contours, shortened eyelids that expose the conjunctivas, and malaligned lips and oral commissures. There are primarily two treatment choices for controlling facial scarring: a custom-made elastic face mask with inserts; or a rigid, total contact, transparent facial orthosis (Rivers, 1987).

An elastic face mask is custom-made and should be replaced every 6 to 8 weeks until the scar matures. It is often worn using silicone gel, elastomer, or thermoplastic inserts to distribute the pressure at and around facial contours. The mask should be worn continuously except during bathing, skin care, and meals. Skin care education should include lubrication and massage, with pressure applied during massage for scar desensitization. Instruction about facial exercises that stretch the skin when the mask is removed should also be provided.

Fabricating a transparent facial orthosis is an involved process, but more precise alterations and assessment of its fit are possible. The fabrication process consists of taking a negative impression of the patient's face, making a positive plaster cast of the impression, heating and stretching the plastic over the cast, finishing the edges, applying elastic straps, and fitting it to the patient (Rivers, 1984). The goal in fitting the orthosis is to see all the scars blanch once it is donned. Prior education is critical to prepare a patient for the fabrication process and fitting of a transparent facial orthosis.

A total contact, transparent facial orthosis should be worn all the time except when bathing, performing skin care, and eating. Skin care education and facial exercise instructions should be the same as for an elastic face mask. If a transparent facial orthosis will be worn exclusively, two orthoses should be made: one for day and one for night. The mold for the night orthosis should be made with the patient supine to include the soft tissue changes that occur with positional adjustments. Many patients prefer to wear an elastic mask at night and the transparent orthosis during the day. Individuals wearing either type of mask often report feelings of self-consciousness, awareness of people staring, and looking in the mirror and seeing someone else. All of these perceptions need to be acknowledged and addressed by those close to the patient. Many patients receive encouragement from speaking with someone who has previously worn a facial orthosis.

Burn Reconstruction

Throughout rehabilitation and follow-up visits to the burn clinic, the patient's functional skills and emotional adjustment to the injury should be continually reevaluated. When limitations in motion persist or the patient requests reconstruction, the burn team must assess the specific problems and make recommendations. These recommendations can range from increasing the frequency and intensity of rehabilitation to surgical reconstruction. A recommendation of surgical intervention depends upon several factors: (a) the amount of time since the injury, (b) the extent and strength of the scar contracture, (c) whether the patient is reliable and motivated, (d) the degree of disability and how it affects function, and (e) what effect surgery would have on immediate function (Salisbury, Petro, & Winski, 1987).

The appropriate time for reconstruction depends on the patient's needs. Early surgical reconstruction is usually indicated when a contracture deformity does not respond to scar treatment techniques and impedes rehabilitation and functional independence. If slow, gradual improvement occurs with therapy and the patient can function independently, the surgeon will attempt to delay reconstruction until scars are mature.

A patient's expectations of surgical reconstruction are frequently unrealistic. Many times functionally restrictive contractures develop because of the patient's noncompliance with home care and rehabilitation. These patients often believe that surgery will remove the problem. Since many reconstructive procedures to improve function require the same type of follow-up therapy as the acute injury, counseling is usually required before surgery will be scheduled. Whether it was a psychological or physical problem that caused the noncompliance, counseling is necessary to ensure that the patient will comply with postoperative instructions and rehabilitation. Developing a contract with the individual can also be used to try to ensure compliance.

There are various types of surgical procedures used in burn reconstruction. Most of them are for functional reconstruction; however, some are also used to improve appearance. Scar excision and grafting; advancement, rotation, pedicle, and myocutaneous flaps; steroid injections and dermabrasion; and Z-plasties are a few examples. To gain a better understanding of the procedures, their expected results, and their treatment implications, it is suggested that books dedicated to burn reconstruction (Achauer, 1991; Salisbury & Bevin, 1981) be reviewed.

Many face reconstructive procedures are done to improve both function and cosmesis, such as release of a lower eyelid ectropion or surgical opening of the oral commissures. When there is extensive facial distortion due to scarring, scar excision and autografting of aesthetic units can usually improve cosmesis once burn wound maturation is complete.

Normal skin cosmesis can never be achieved after a severe burn, but the illusion of normalcy is possible (Salisbury et al., 1987). Once the wounds are mature, the patient should be referred to a cosmetologist who has training in corrective makeup blending. Corrective makeups can be used on other body areas as well as on the face.

Burn reconstruction is usually the last option. Many burn rehabilitation techniques are designed to reduce the need for reconstruction. By providing early and continuous patient education and progressive rehabilitation, many reconstructive needs can be prevented. When reconstruction is inevitable, consideration must be given to appropriate timing for reconstruction, the type of procedure, and necessary follow-up treatment.

Case Examples

Case One

Mr. T., a 30-year-old maintenance worker living with his elderly parents, suffered an 89% TBSA burn and severe smoke inhalation injury during a house fire. His burn injury was deep partial and full thickness in depth. Face edema and the inhalation injury necessitated immediate intubation. Upper extremity burns were full thickness circumferentially and required escharotomies of both arms and hands upon admission to the hospital. Body areas not burned were the lower legs, the feet, and a small area on the back of the head and lower abdomen.

Initial wound care consisted of silver sulfadiazine dressings changed twice daily, with sulfamylon used later during hospitalization. The patient underwent multiple surgical procedures throughout the hospitalization to excise and cover the burn wound. Temporary biological dressings were initially used because of the lack of adequate donor sites for timely wound closure. Once all the dead tissue was removed and the wound bed was clean and free of bacteria, the patient was returned to the operating room for application of wide mesh (3:1) autografts. Because autograft was extremely limited, many areas healed by contraction of granulation tissue. When possible, these areas were later reexcised, releasing scar whorls, and wide mesh autografts were applied.

Acute and Inpatient Rehabilitation

Therapy activities, started the day after hospital admission, included active range of motion exercises and ambulation, positioning when resting, and the application of hand splints. Severe edema in the extremities, facial swelling occluding vision, inelastic eschar on the extremities, and an endotracheal tube prevented initial performance of any ADL. Once the endotracheal tube was removed and swelling in the eyelids had subsided, the patient began feeding himself. The handles of the utensils were temporarily enlarged, using gauze and adhesive tape. Since exposure could alter body temperature during bathing, the nursing staff performed most of the bathing activities during the acute phase. Initial grooming activities were limited to brushing teeth, since face dressings were extensive.

As the hospital course progressed, Mr. T.'s rehabilitation program expanded to include stretching and range of motion exercises, resistive exercises, flexibility activities, and positioning with the aid of splints when resting. For ADL, Mr. T. practiced donning and doffing hospital clothes, eating skills, and assisting with bathing and applying dressings.

Although the extent and depth of the burn injury were obvious limitations to functional recovery, persistent brawny edema and extensor tendon involvement in the hands complicated Mr. T.'s rehabilitation. Approximately 5 weeks into his hospitalization, he was taken to the operating room for placement of Steinmann pins in his hands. The pins were surgically inserted to hold the index, middle, ring, and little fingers' metacarpophalangeal joints (MCPs) in 70° of flexion with the interphalangeal joints extended, in an attempt to preserve tendon integrity. Unfortunately, infection limited wound healing and caused further tendon destruction. Edema persisted, necessitating therapy to apply Coban wraps over the hand dressings during the day, with intermittent compression pump therapy at night.

Despite the restrictions imposed by the pins and burn wound pain, Mr. T. continued to perform ADL, using universal cuffs to hold utensils and grooming aids. He was able to don and doff hospital clothes using an awkward, modified lateral pinch. Although burn depth and involvement of the upper extremities were significant enough to limit function, Mr. T. cooperated with his rehabilitation and went through the painful motions necessary to preserve as much motion as he could.

Due to finger tendon destruction and delayed wound closure, the Steinmann pins were left in place for approximately 4 weeks. When they were removed, the goal of rehabilitation was to help Mr. T. regain as much independence and function as possible. Therapist creativity and patient motivation and compliance were necessary to achieve this goal, because increasing digit mobility was not an option. To combat scar contracture, a progressive program of stretching and strengthening exercises was emphasized. Cuff weights were used for strengthening because of Mr. T.'s limited hand function. Stretching exercises were done for trunk and extremities' flexibility. Because the hands still required edema treatments, Coban wraps were used, progressing to intermediate compression gloves.

For additional scar control, intermediate compression garments were applied to the extremities as wound closure progressed. Extensive hand involvement and persistent edema restricted the use of custom fitted, external vascular support garments on the arms. When wound status allowed, Mr. T. was fitted with a custom elastic face mask with inserts for use at night, with a clear plastic facial orthosis used during the day. Although a microstomia prevention appliance (MPA) was initially used to limit contracture of the oral commissures, Mr. T.'s inability to manipulate the MPA caused the rehabilitation staff to discontinue its use when he was discharged from the hospital. Once discharged from the hospital, Mr. T. returned for therapy treatment 5 times per week for the 1st month. Since his parents were elderly and did not have a shower in their house, visiting nurses were arranged for home wound care.

Outpatient Rehabilitation

Mr. T.'s outpatient therapy program primarily consisted of the same goals initiated during the acute and rehabilitation phases, which were to increase ROM, strength, endurance, and ADL independence; and to monitor and provide instruction about scar control and skin care.

Due to the severity of Mr. T.'s hand injuries, his finger motion was extremely limited, although he had trace active motion at some joints. A lateral-type pinch, accompanied by forearm rotation, was his primary source of hand function. Modalities used to achieve optimal hand function included the BTE Work Simulator and Valpar Work Samples. All ADL skills and related activities were performed repetitively to achieve independence (see Figure 16).

Mr. T.'s limited mental and cognitive status made his home care difficult. As a result, his skin was dry and scaly, necessitating skin care by the therapist. Paraffin application, followed by massage with a moisturizing lotion, were performed daily. Improving Mr. T.'s understanding of proper skin care became a major objective.

Early in Mr. T.'s outpatient course, elbow flexion contractures developed. Serial dynamic casting was performed, and 25° of elbow extension was regained in less than a

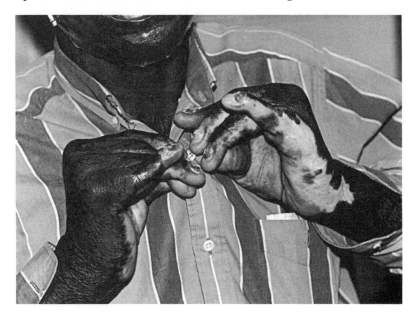

Figure 16. A lateral type pinch, along with wrist and forearm motion, were Mr. T.'s only source of hand function.

week. He resumed wearing his elastic compression garments. Regular adjustments and fractures of the transparent facial orthosis necessitated frequent new orthoses. An elastic face mask with thermoplastic inserts eventually became the primary treatment for the face.

After the first 3 months of outpatient rehabilitation, Mr. T. began to demonstrate a flat affect and started to miss or cancel appointments. He constantly stated that he was not feeling well or that he had too much pain in his face to attend. Due to low cognitive functioning, Mr. T. was continually confused about his facial scars and did not understand the sensations he was experiencing. As a result, he was referred to the hospital's outpatient crisis counseling center for assistance. Eventually, a referral to vocational rehabilitation followed.

Mr. T.'s hospital course was protracted because of the extent and depth of the burn, involvement of deeper structures, lack of unburned skin for donor sites, and infections limiting wound healing. Although his total length of stay for the acute admission was 3 $\frac{1}{2}$ months (104 days), his outpatient rehabilitation continued intensively for 6 months. Despite poor cognitive skills, Mr. T.'s perseverance and compliance with therapy goals helped him to achieve independence in ADL (see Figure 17).

Case Two

Mr. M., a 54-year-old health care administrator, suffered a 47% TBSA thermal burn while doing home repairs. Burn depth and extent were calculated as 36% TBSA partial thickness and 11% TBSA full thickness. Involved areas included the face, neck, right upper extremity, left forearm, posterior trunk, and lower left leg. There was no evidence of any inhalation injury. Past medical history was nonsignificant. Social history revealed he was married, and had children who were young adults.

Nursing care included hydrotherapy and twice-a-day dressing changes using silver sulfadiazine cream. He underwent a total of four surgical procedures acutely for burn wound excision and autografting.

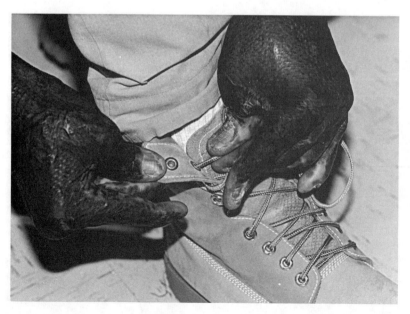

Figure 17. Mr. T. is independent in all self-care tasks, despite significant scar disfigurement and hand function limitations.

Acute and Inpatient Rehabilitation

The initial occupational therapy evaluation revealed right upper-extremity limitations in shoulder flexion and hand MCP and interphalangeal flexion. General muscle strength was good; grip strengths were less with the right hand. Mr. M. was independent in ambulation and feeding. Dressing and grooming were not evaluated initially due to his medical status. In order to maintain proper hand positioning, bilateral volar pan splints were fabricated and applied using elastic wraps. To prevent irreversible pressure damage to his burned ear, an ear protection device was also fabricated and applied.

Range of motion exercises to all extremities and patient education were initiated immediately following the initial evaluation. Patient education included the importance of maintaining independence in ADL and the need for frequent exercise.

Mr. M.'s pain tolerance was extremely low throughout all phases of care. He reacted to the anticipation of pain and did not perform any exercises without therapist supervision. Mr. M.'s wife constantly interfered with therapy treatment, stating that he needed to rest and would participate the following day. Mr. M.'s primary coping mechanism was denial. He appeared to believe that he would be fine because he would participate with rehabilitation at a later date.

Therapy consisted of range of motion, flexibility, strengthening, and endurance activities. Mr. M. was independent in feeding and grooming but used compensatory techniques when donning and doffing his shirt. His shoulder motion was functional (0-150° of flexion), but he could not tolerate stretch beyond that point. Range of motion of all other joints was normal.

As wound closure progressed, intermediate pressure garments were applied to begin skin conditioning and desensitization. Custom-made pressure garments were eventually fitted to control burn scar maturation. Mr. M. often complained that he could not tolerate the garments, specifically the body-brief. To improve his garment-wearing tolerance, a cotton undershirt was worn under his elastic body-brief.

Mr. M.'s length of hospital stay was 36 days. At hospital discharge, arrangements were made to begin outpatient therapy 3 times a week.

Outpatient Rehabilitation

Mr. M.'s outpatient rehabilitation program included scar massage and stretch followed by active, active-assistive, and passive range of motion exercises for the right shoulder and bilateral elbows. Strengthening of all extremities, flexibility exercises, and endurance training were additional treatment activities. A home program of independent exercises had been reviewed during his discharge training and during every outpatient treatment session. Because of his inability to follow through with his home exercises consistently, a continuous passive motion (CPM) device for the shoulder was prescribed for home use.

During the first 8 weeks of outpatient rehabilitation, active range of motion of the right shoulder and neck continually decreased, and Mr. M.'s posture regressed to right lateral trunk and neck flexion. Although a Watusi collar had been fabricated and fitted early during outpatient treatment, Mr. M. did not wear it. Surgical release of his neck scar contracture was performed 1 month after his hospital discharge. His postoperative care included fitting a triple component neck splint. This splint was designed to maintain the cervical angle while allowing some neck rotation and extension (Leman & Lowery, 1986).

Skin conditioning was a problem. Mr. M. frequently developed blisters as a result of friction from the compression garments. He used the blisters as a reason not to exercise.

At this time, he required assistance to don and doff his elastic bodysuit and oxford shirts. He also refused to perform his own skin care, stating his wife would do it.

He requested that he be returned to work part-time 2 weeks after his neck reconstructive surgery. This was approved primarily because of the limited physical demands of the job, his resistance to supportive counseling, his attitude regarding his health, and his reasons for noncompliance with home therapy. He was scheduled to continue with rehabilitation 3 times a week. Returning him to work was an attempt to help him realize what he needed to do to assume responsibility for his own care. Although his posture and range of motion of the right shoulder were poor, he was able to perform all skills necessary for his desk job. During the next 2 months, he frequently missed therapy appointments. When confronted with this behavior, he stated he was functional without rehabilitation because he was able to perform his job. If there were tasks he could not do, someone would help him.

Discussion

Current views of occupational therapy practice (e.g., Christiansen, 1991; Kielhofner & Burke, 1985; Mosey, 1981) recognize the individual as constantly changing within a dynamic set of environmental circumstances. Life satisfaction depends on a complex array of conditions, including motivation, experiences, social role expectations, and physical and cognitive capacities. Changes in any of these conditions affect the others.

In Case 1, Mr. T. was able to adapt to the requirements of his environment in several ways. He overcame his limitations in hand function by adapting various skills. He was able to perform ADL independently and enter vocational rehabilitation because he was motivated to do so. His attitudes and values allowed him to change and work within his limitations in a positive manner.

In Case 2, Mr. M. exemplified a different set of circumstances. Although he initially attended rehabilitation appointments, his motivation and compliance were poor. His main physical limitation was his right shoulder and neck area, which impaired his ability to perform the skills necessary to maintain independence in self-care, which in turn affected his interest in doing other things. Mr. M. now requires assistance in dressing and can no longer independently pursue his avocational interest of home restoration.

Summary

Functional independence is the primary goal of burn treatment; however, the depth and extent of the burn injury, scar contracture during wound maturation, and the patient's emotional reactions can limit recovery. A multidisciplinary team approach is necessary to treat the physical, psychosocial, and cosmetic problems associated with a severe burn injury effectively. To provide optimal rehabilitative care, it is necessary to consider the phase of recovery, the patient's functional problems identified by assessment, the level of patient compliance with treatment, the patient's emotional and psychological adjustment to the injury, and the personal goals of the patient. Dedication, patience, and knowledge of the potential problems encountered, and their treatments, are essential to help burn patients achieve functional independence. ◆

References

Abston, S. (1987). Scar reaction after thermal injury and prevention of scars and contractures. In J. Boswick (Ed.), *The art and science of burn care* (pp. 359–371). Gaithersburg, MD: Aspen Publishers.

Achauer, B. (1991). *Burn reconstruction*. New York: Thieme Medical Publishers.

Adriaenssens, P. (1988). The video invasion of rehabilitation. *Burns Including Thermal Injuries, 14,* 417–419.

Bowden, M.L., Thomson, P.D., & Prasad, J.K. (1989). Factors influencing return to employment after a burn injury. *Archives of Physical Medicine and Rehabilitation, 70,* 772–775.

Cheng, S., & Rogers, J.C. (1989). Changes in occupational role performance after a severe burn: A retrospective study. *American Journal of Occupational Therapy, 43,* 17–24.

Christiansen, C. (1991). Intervention for life performance. In C. Christiansen & C. Baum (Eds.), *Occupational therapy: Overcoming human performance deficits* (pp. 1–43). Thorofare, NJ: Slack.

Feller, I., & Jones, C. (1984). Introduction: Statement of the problem. In S. Fisher & P. Helm (Eds.). *Comprehensive rehabilitation of burns* (pp. 1–8). Baltimore: Williams & Wilkins.

Fleet, J. (1992). The psychological effects of burn injuries: A literature review. *British Journal of Occupational Therapy, 55,* 198–201.

Hartford, C. (1984). Surgical management. In S. Fisher & P. Helm (Eds.), *Comprehensive rehabilitation of burns* (pp. 28–63). Baltimore: Williams & Wilkins.

Hill, C. (1985). Psyochosocial adjustment of adult burns patients: Is it more difficult with people with visible scars? *British Journal of Occupational Therapy, 48,* 281–283.

Helm, P.A, & Fisher, S. (1988). Rehabilitation of the patient with burns. In J. Delisa, D. Currie, & B. Gans (Eds.), *Rehabilitation medicine principles and practice* (pp. 821–839). Philadelphia: J.B. Lippincott.

Helm, P.A., Walker, S.C., & Peyton, S.A. (1986). Return to work following hand burns. *Archives of Physical Medicine and Rehabilitation, 67,* 297–298.

Kaplan, S.H. (1985). Patient education techniques used at burn centers. *American Journal of Occupational Therapy, 39,* 655–658.

Kielhofner, G. (1980). A model of human occupation, part 3: Benign and vicious cycles. *American Journal of Occupational Therapy, 34,* 731–737.

Kielhofner, G. (1985). The human being as an open system. In G. Kielhofner (Ed.), *A model of human occupation* (pp. 2–11). Baltimore: Williams & Wilkins.

Kielhofner, G., & Burke, J.P. (1985). Components and determinants of human occupation. In G. Kielhofner (Ed.), *A model of human occupation* (pp. 12–36). Baltimore: Williams & Wilkins.

Leman, C., & Lowery, C. (1986). The triple-component neck splint. *Journal of Burn Care and Rehabilitation, 7,* 357–361.

Lund, C., & Browder, N. (1944). The estimation of area of burns. *Surgical Gynecology and Obstetrics, 79,* 352–355.

Mahon, L.M., & Neufeld, N. (1984). The effect of informational feedback on food intake of adult burn patients. *Journal of Applied Behavior Analysis, 17,* 391–396.

Malt, U.F., & Ugland, O.M. (1989). A long term psychosocial follow-up study of burned adults. *Acta Psychiatrica Scandinavia, 80* (Suppl. 355), 94–102.

Mason, S., & Forshaw, A. (1986). Burns after care: A booklet for parents—Your child at home after injury. *Burns Including Thermal Injuries, 12,* 343–350.

Mosey, A.C. (1981). *Occupational therapy: Configuration of a profession.* New York: Raven Press.

Parent, L.H. (1983). Burns. In C. Trombly (Ed.), *Occupational therapy for physical dysfunction* (2nd ed.) (pp. 399–408). Baltimore: Williams & Wilkins.

Perry, S., & Difede, J. (1992). Predictors of posttraumatic stress disorder after burn injury. *American Journal of Psychiatry, 149,* 931–935.

Petro, J., & Salisbury, R. (1986). Rehabilitation of the burn patient. *Clinics in Plastic Surgery, 3*(1), 145–149.

Reilly, M. (1962). Occupational therapy can be one of the great ideas of the 20th century. *American Journal of Occupational Therapy, 16,* 1–9.

Rivers, E. (1984). Management of hypertrophic scars. In S. Fisher & P. Helm (Eds.), *Comprehensive rehabilitation of burns* (pp. 177–217). Baltimore: Williams & Wilkins.

Rivers, E. (1987). Rehabilitation management of the burn patient. *Advances in Clinical Rehabilitation, 1,* 177–213.

Salisbury, R., & Bevin, A. (1981). *Atlas of reconstructive burn surgery.* Philadelphia: W.B. Saunders.

Salisbury, R., Petro, J., & Winski, F. (1987). Reconstruction of the burn patient. In J. Boswick (Ed.), *The art and science of burn care* (pp. 353–357). Gaithersburg, MD: Aspen Publishers.

Solem, L. (1984). Classification. In S. Fisher & P. Helm (Eds.), *Comprehensive rehabilitation of burns* (pp. 9–15). Baltimore: Williams & Wilkins.

Trombly, C.A. (1983). Biomechanical approach. In C.A. Trombly (Ed.), *Occupational therapy for physical dysfunction* (pp. 126–241). Baltimore: Williams & Wilkins.

Tucker, P. (1986). The burn victim: A review of psychosocial issues. *Australian and New Zealand Journal of Psychiatry, 20,* 413–420.

Wachtel, T. (1985). Epidemiology, classification, initial care, and administrative considerations for critically burned patients. In T. Wachtel (Ed.), *Critical care clinics* (pp. 3–26). Philadelphia: W.B. Saunders.

Yurko, L., & Fratianne, R. (1988). Evaluation of burn discharge teaching. *Journal of Burn Care and Rehabilitation, 9,* 643–644.

12

Self-Care Strategies for Persons With Cognitive Deficits

Mary Hall
Sherida Ryan
Estella Tse

Mary Hall, BSc, OT(C), is a Supervisor (Neuroscience, Musculoskeletal) at The Toronto Hospital, Western Division, Toronto, Ontario.

Sherida Ryan, BOT(C), is an Occupational Therapist at the Regional Geriatric Program, St. Michael's Hospital, Toronto, Ontario.

Estella Tse, BSc, OT(C), is an Occupational Therapist at the Regional Trauma Program, Sunnybrook Health Science Centre, Toronto, Ontario.

Chapter 12 Outline

Senile Dementia of the Alzheimer's Type

A Frame of Reference to Guide Intervention for SDAT

Level Six

Level Five

Mr. Morris

Level Four

Miss Olive

Level Three

Mr. Wills

Level Two

Level One

Traumatic Brain Injury (TBI)

Definition of Brain Injury

Medical Management

Severity

Factors Affecting Cognition

Frames of Reference

Self-Care Management Strategies

Cuing Program

Lewis

Summary

References

It is 8:30 a.m., and Joe has just finished his morning shower. He quickly dresses and goes downstairs for breakfast. Sarah, his wife, notices that his hair is dry, and asks Joe if he has washed it. Joe looks at her surprised and says, "Oh, I don't know, I can't remember." At this point Sarah realizes that while tidying earlier she had put the shampoo in the cupboard. Joe often forgets to wash his hair unless he sees the shampoo bottle in front of him.

People with cognitive dysfunction may have difficulty with even the simplest of self-care tasks that most of us take for granted. Cognitive disability cuts across a number of diagnostic categories and may be seen in conjunction with multiple sclerosis, congestive heart failure, AIDS-related dementia, Parkinson's disease, and other disorders. This chapter deals primarily with cognitive dysfunction as the result of Alzheimer's disease and acquired brain damage (traumatic brain injury). However, many of the intervention strategies described here may also be taken into consideration when assessing and developing treatment plans for persons with cognitive dysfunction as a result of other disorders.

Cognition refers to the process by which an individual uses information to understand and interact in a meaningful way with the environment. Cognitive function refers to processes such as attention, memory, language (communication), orientation, abstraction, goal setting, and problem solving. Self-monitoring or error recognition is necessary to ensure that the action or behavior is acceptable. A continuous feedback system exists to modify purposeful behavior.

The brain can be viewed as an information processing system, with perception of sensory information being the input, cognition being the throughput, and purposeful behavior being the output. Deficits can occur at each phase. For instance, impaired sensory information can interfere with input. Decreased attention can interfere with processing, and decreased physical status can interfere with performance of behavior. In many cases, more than one of these phases can present problems. Self-care requires the subtle integration of the senses, perception, cognition, emotion, motor skills, and the environment. Cognitive impairments, even when mild in nature, can affect the individual's ability to function independently.

When approaching the cognitively impaired client, the occupational therapist should employ a frame of reference to guide the problem-solving process. Frames of reference are "those portions of models that are methodological in focus" and are "mechanisms for linking theory to practice" (Christiansen & Baum, 1991, p. 12). Keeping in mind the complexities and individualistic nature of the cognitively impaired person, a core frame of reference may have to be augmented with methodologies borrowed from other models. An example is a brain-injured client who is depressed because of a weak right arm. When planning intervention, the occupational therapist may use methodologies from the psychodynamic model to address the depression, paired with neurodevelopmental techniques to facilitate upper extremity function using activities that would improve the client's attention span. Future treatment planning may also incorporate role acquisition theory in order to address return to the community. This problem-solving process is illustrated through case histories presented later in this chapter.

The first disorder presented is Alzheimer's disease. The frame of reference that has been chosen to link theory with practice is Levy's adaptation of Allen's cognitive disability model, where cognitive abilities are maximized through manipulation of the person/environment fit. An understanding of the Alzheimer's disease process and associated behaviors is necessary before this frame of reference can assist with self-care management.

Senile Dementia of the Alzheimer's Type

The dementias are a syndrome of neurological diseases characterized by progressive mental deterioration that impairs functional independence. It is important to recognize that dementia is a process that takes place over several years, culminating in a global impairment of all intellectual and functional abilities. It is estimated that 10% of the population over the age of 65 suffers from some form of dementing process, and the incidence of this condition rises rapidly with age (Evans et al., 1989; Mortimer, Schuman, & French, 1981). Given the increasing proportion of elders in our society, by the year 2010 the dementias will have a tremendous impact on our social and health care systems.

The two most common of these disorders are Senile Dementia of the Alzheimer's Type (SDAT), and multi-infarct dementia (MID). Approximately 50% of all dementias are of the Alzheimer's disease type (Glickstein, 1988). Alzheimer's disease can be distinguished from MID by the former's smooth progression, in contrast to the latter's step-wise progression. A definitive diagnosis of Alzheimer's disease can only be obtained through a combination of clinical findings and histopathological evidence obtained from a biopsy or an autopsy (McKhann et al., 1984).

Clinically, SDAT has an insidious onset, and its rate of progression and severity of symptomatology vary from individual to individual. The first signs of the disorder are short-term memory loss and word-finding difficulties. Abstraction, calculation, judgment, and visual-perceptual skills become impaired early in the disease (Edwards, Baum, & Duel, 1991; Liu, Gautier, & Gautier, 1991). Personality changes, depression, and persecutory delusions are common. The client becomes progressively disoriented and has increasing difficulty communicating. Throughout this process the person loses the ability to perform activities of daily living (ADL), and in the final stages impaired motor function leads to total dependence (Cummings & Benson, 1983). These features are only slightly changed from those found in Alois Alzheimer's original description of the disorder. Histopathologically, SDAT is confirmed by the presence of diffuse cortical atrophy, degeneration of specific nerve cells, neuritic plaques, and neurofibrillary tangles (Katzman, 1986).

In addition to the disease-related cognitive and behavioral changes (see Figure 1) the impact of normative age-related changes in vision and hearing is an important feature that determines the Alzheimer's patient's level of function. Although unrelated to the dementia itself, these sensory processes show an accelerating rate of decline after the age of 60 (Botwinick, 1973; Gilhome-Herbst & Humphry, 1980; Weale, 1963). This decline inevitably affects self-care skills.

Nolen (1988) studied patients with late-stage dementia and found that self-feeding was the best predictor of overall self-care functioning. However, less than 50% of the variation in self-care skills was explained by the Folstein Mini Mental State Examination (Folstein, Folstein, & McHugh, 1975). Overall, Nolen found that the loss of functional abilities in late-stage dementia seems to occur in reverse order of their development in childhood. During late-stage dementia, institutional care is often necessary.

It is important to remember that during early stages, the provision of care for people with SDAT is most likely to occur in the home, with caregiving provided by family members and friends (Select Committee on Aging, 1990). Often, the home caregivers are unaware of community resources for people with dementia, and the burden of care is a frequent cause of caregiver distress, elder abuse, and eventually the decision to institutionalize, as the strain of years of 24-hour-a-day caregiving takes its toll. A conceptual model can be very helpful for the caregiver's understanding of the disease and can provide guidance and structure in adapting self-care tasks.

Figure 1. Factors affecting cognition.

Category	Traumatic Brain Injury	Both	Alzheimer's Disease
Physical	Fractures, medical apparatus (i.e., fixators, lines)	Pain, tone, immobility, infection, nutritional status, previous brain injury, medications, environmental stimulation	Aging process
Perceptual		Impaired sensory systems, sensory deprivation	
Social		Substance abuse, family support, educational level, socioeconomic status, cultural background, involvement with legal system	
Emotional	Posttraumatic stress, accident-related loss	Psychiatric history, premorbid personality	Catastrophic reactions

A Frame of Reference to Guide Intervention for SDAT

Given the characteristics of dementia, the goal of occupational therapists working with demented elderly persons parallels that observed in any other clinical context—that is, to maximize functional independence, dignity, and quality of life. This is achieved by identifying an individual's strengths and recognizing that as cognitive impairment increases, it is necessary for the environment to be structured and to organize behavior (Lawton & Nahemow, 1973). The goal of occupational therapists working with persons with dementia and their caregivers is achieved, therefore, by maximizing person–environment fit or congruence (Kahana, 1979). Staging models of SDAT (i.e., Glickstein, 1988; Reisberg et al., 1989) have proven useful in achieving person-environment congruence. One of the more practical of these is Levy's adaptation of Allen's cognitive disability model (Allen, 1982, 1985; Levy, 1986, 1987, 1989). Levy's model provides the focus for the following discussion.

In Levy's adaptation of the cognitive disability model, three cognitive abilities are examined over six levels or stages: (a) attention, or the ability to focus on external cues without being distracted by irrelevant stimuli; (b) goal selection, or the ability to formulate and sustain intention; and (c) imitation, or the capacity to follow direction and, ultimately, to acquire new behavior. What follows is a description of SDAT at each level, the cognitive abilities present, and interventions that may enhance self-care management.

Level Six

Level Six is the highest level of performance in the cognitive disability model, representing normal cognitive function. An elderly person may suffer from normative age-related deficits but be able to sustain attention, employ goal selection, and acquire new behaviors using residual abilities to compensate for normative deficits.

Level Five

At Level Five, the earliest evidence of cognitive deficit and functional disability appears. Family members may observe that objects are more frequently misplaced, and word finding difficulties may emerge. The person may get lost when traveling to unfamiliar places, and coworkers may begin to notice a decline in occupational performance. Anxiety often emerges because the individual is aware of these difficulties and fears loss of control.

The person is capable of maintaining attention for four- or five-step processes while managing extraneous environmental stimuli, but begins to fail on purely symbolic tasks. Goal selection includes task completion and solving of emergent task-related problems. Imitation of concrete four- or five-step procedures is possible. In reasonably familiar environments no formal supervision is needed at Level Five.

The person at Level Five seldom comes to the attention of an occupational therapist. This may prove to be unfortunate if, as we suspect, early intervention has an impact that lasts throughout the course of the disease. Early intervention might include the consolidation of necessary routines and habits, and the adaptation or simplification of familiar tasks in order not to exceed the demands of attentional and goal-selection abilities. Perhaps adaptations in the home might best be introduced at this time, while the person is able to participate in decision making and to adjust to changes such as smoke alarms, emergency response systems, automatic shut-off kettles, and timed shut-off controls on the stove. At this stage, some reorganization of the home environment to cue and sustain particular instrumental or leisure tasks might be necessary. For example, bill paying routines would be assisted if a schedule of bill payments, and bills, writing supplies, and addresses were clustered in a specific area of the home. Ideally, it is at Level Five that the issue of safe driving should be addressed, with people with SDAT regularly referred to driver evaluation programs to monitor their ability to drive.

Long-range planning with the patient and caregiver, such as reviewing community resources (e.g., support groups, day programs, and respite programs) and clarification of legal issues (e.g., wills, power of attorney, and advance directives) may best be accomplished at this stage. These are still difficult tasks; however, sensitive counseling and providing the individual with information at his or her own level of acceptance can increase comfort and a sense of control while preventing longer-term difficulties when communication of wishes becomes impossible. The following case history illustrates occupational therapy intervention at this early level.

Mr. Morris

Background: Mr. Morris is 64 years old, married, and has two sons. He is a partner with one of his sons in a manufacturing firm that he started. During his annual physical, Mr. Morris complained of sleep difficulties that he attributed to his being worried about increasing forgetfulness and the feeling that he couldn't "pull all the strands of [his] life together like [he] could before." A screening of mental status revealed deficits in short-term memory, abstract reasoning, and word finding. Otherwise, Mr. Morris was in good general health, despite declining visual acuity. He was referred to a community occupational therapist for functional assessment and preretirement counseling.

Occupational Therapy Assessment: The evaluation supported previous test findings with functional examples of recent memory loss, such as misplaced invoices at work, forgotten social engagements, and declining bridge skills. Mr. Morris had no difficulties with self-care activities. His wife ran the household and managed the day-to-day expenses. He continued to drive his car but was having more difficulty at night because of glare. The couple had a strong relationship, with several joint leisure activities: travel, bird watching, music, gardening, and fishing. They had just sold their large, two-story house and were wondering what environment would most suit their needs as they got older. Mr. Morris had given some thought to retiring, as his son was a "dynamo" at the business, but he admitted that he would miss his business friends and associates.

Assets: Good health, supportive family, no financial worries, active in leisure pursuits, insight into aging process, outgoing, generally optimistic personality.

Deficits: Short-term memory loss, decreased abstract problem-solving ability, decreased vision, decreased ability to be involved in complex leisure activity (bridge), imminent relocation.

Intervention: Mr. and Mrs. Morris felt that their priority at this time was their relocation. In consultation with the occupational therapist, they decided to acquire a small, one-level house with a garden and with a layout and organization similar to their old one. An extra bedroom was recommended so that Mr. Morris could have an "office" at home and be able to work part-time. A schedule of activities and events was developed that reflected the couple's interests and responsibilities. They also decided to give their sons power of attorney.

Outcome: After 6 months, Mr. Morris was semi-retired but was still included in the decision-making activities of the firm. He and his wife were very involved in organizing their new home. Mr. Morris enjoyed his home office and spent many hours rearranging it. Mrs. Morris noted that her husband's forgetfulness had increased since the move and he frequently misplaced things.

Level Four

At Level Four, significant cognitive impairment is evident. The individual is unable to remember directions, may forget to shave or bathe, and has difficulty balancing a checkbook. New learning is not possible, and changes are made with great difficulty. Denial is a frequent form of coping, and anxiety and depression often lead to excess disability. Maximizing person/environment congruence at this stage can help to maintain functional independence and lessen the amount of supervision required.

In Levy's framework, a person's attention at this stage is limited to two- or three-step concrete processes. Goal selection is such that the individual continues to be able to form an intention, and imitation abilities allow him or her to follow two- or three-step directions to complete a concrete task. Level Four requires more detailed scheduling and organization by the caregiver. The impaired elder begins to respond more to concrete visual cues in the environment. Verbal instructions need to be supported by visual cues, and objects must be visually apparent to be utilized. The daily schedule should be displayed in the central part of the house (e.g., on the refrigerator). Crossing out activities and chores as they are accomplished may aid in temporal adaptation. Grooming supplies should be left out. Closets can be left open and illuminated. The person will need to be protected from "invisible" sources of danger (heat, electricity, chemicals). Labeling these areas, as well as labeling commonly used drawers and cupboards, becomes beneficial at this point. Figure–ground difficulties may become apparent at this stage (Powell & Courtice, 1983). Bright, intense colors on a contrasting background are optimal but may be offensive to the patient and caregiver. It is best to use pictures and symbols, as reading skills deteriorate with the progression of the disease.

The provision of adaptive devices and environmental supports should continue during this phase. Giving the person an electronic diary with an alarm connected to a daily calendar that records appointments and activities, such as taking pills, has been suggested. This is beneficial when introduced early, as it has a limited usefulness. In later stages the person will not remember the reason for the "beep" long enough to complete the task. Careful removal of hazards, such as scatter rugs, and the arrangement of furniture to provide clear spaces for mobility, should occur at this time to prevent accidents. Remote, motion-activated light switches are other inexpensive environmental manipulations. A private corner or room (see Mr. Morris) may be beneficial in allowing the impaired individual to organize and secure his or her possessions. This also provides the person with a contained area to control and fosters a sense of mastery over the environment.

Miss Olive's story illustrates how routine and environment can compensate for significant cognitive impairment.

Miss Olive

Background: Miss Olive is a 79-year-old retired bank personnel officer. She has never married, and her only close relative is a nephew, who acts as her power of attorney. He has been handling her finances for the past 3 years, as she has been experiencing short-term memory loss. She has lived alone in the same one-bedroom apartment for 19 years and is well-known in her apartment building and her neighborhood. Miss Olive has always been perceived as somewhat eccentric because of her obsessive habits and rituals.

Miss Olive was referred for psychogeriatric assessment because her nephew had become concerned about her ability to live alone. Her memory had significantly declined over the past 3 months, and she was getting lost going downtown. Her hearing had also become increasingly impaired. Community services had been involved for the past year, with a nurse visiting once a week for medication supervision and a homemaker providing service twice a week. Miss Olive would not always admit these community workers as she could not hear the doorbell, and would forget the appointment times because they were not consistent. The occupational therapist attached to the psychogeriatric clinic was asked to make a home visit to assess the client's ability to function in her own environment.

Occupational Therapy Assessment: Miss Olive appeared to be a pleasant but confused elderly lady whose social skills were very well-preserved. She proudly gave the therapist a tour of her apartment, pointing out exact places where she kept things that she used every day. She strongly believed in the maxim "a place for everything and everything in its place." Miss Olive gave a detailed (obsessive) description of her daily and weekly routine. She shopped for certain things on certain days and ate certain things on certain days. The timing of her daily schedule was dictated by her favorite TV and radio programs, which remained turned on (at moderate to moderate-high volume) during the assessment. She cooked her meals, never leaving the stove, at exact times between shows. She demonstrated this as she interrupted the assessment to make her lunch before the mid-day news. Miss Olive always shopped at the same stores and used the same bank clerk to help her with her bills. These people became concerned if they did not see her on schedule. Miss Olive had been considering a move to a more sheltered setting, but wanted to celebrate Christmas (a very special ritual) at her apartment.

Assets: Obsessive behavior, excellent social skills, well-known in neighborhood, regular community support visits, concerned nephew.

Deficits: Decreased hearing and memory, obsessive behavior, reliance on electronic media.

Intervention: Miss Olive had agreed to look at homes for the aged to find one she would be comfortable in, but not before Christmas (6 months away). Until this move was made, increased community services were arranged. These visits were timed to correspond with certain radio and TV shows. The doorbell was exchanged for a very loud buzzer. The TV and radio were serviced to make sure they were operating properly, and a portable radio was acquired. Miss Olive obtained a telephone with a flashing light and a permanent sound amplifier. A phone with memory capacity was tried, but Miss Olive could not adapt to this feature.

Outcome: Miss Olive moved into a private room at a home for the aged a month after Christmas and brought many of her personal possessions. Before this move her cherished routines had begun to break down, and she had become quite anxious. She was very suspicious of the people in her new setting but eventually settled in with structure and routine. Her functional capacities decreased to a lower level.

People with SDAT do not move from level to level in discrete steps. The boundaries often blur, and some behaviors normally found in a lower level appear in a higher level, and vice versa. For example dressing, which is a complicated activity, may change in Level Four. Most common is the inability to choose clothing appropriate to the weather. Disorientation to time and place can also slowly appear. These are early markers of the need for full-time assistance or supervision.

Level Three

Disorganized thinking is characteristic of Level Three. The person is no longer able to predict what consequences his or her behaviors will have, but is aware that the actions have some effect on the environment. The person is easily distracted and is not oriented to time or place—and sometimes not even to person. Wandering behavior may become a problem, and it is strongly recommended that the patient wear an identification bracelet and be registered with local police as a wandering risk. Tracking devices and alarm systems on doors may also prove useful. According to Levy's framework, at Level Three a person's attention is only oriented to his or her own actions, and goal selection is tied to the impact of these actions on the external environment. Imitation is limited to one-step, familiar, action-oriented commands.

The impaired person at Level Three is now very dependent on unambiguous visual cues and careful adaptation of the environment. All noxious liquids and sprays must be locked away. Conversely, all doors to important areas like the bathroom, bedroom, and clothes closet must be left open, and the toilet seat cover must remain up. Confusing or misguiding items, such as a waste basket next to a toilet, must be removed. Light and motion sensors may help the individual find his or her way around the house and help prevent falls or accidents in the dark. Perception is often quite impaired, so marking the edges of stairs with colored tape and putting decals on large plate glass doors and windows also increase safety.

Dressing and grooming become more difficult. Items of clothing for the day should be hung in plain view, and separate pieces may have to be handed to the person in sequence. This same procedure will eventually hold true for grooming and washing. The individual has difficulty entering and exiting the bathtub. Agitation increases when unexpected or novel stimuli are presented, and catastrophic reactions can occur. A safe, reliable routine is imperative at this stage. The impaired individual is calmed by repetitive action-oriented activity and can benefit from one-step maintenance tasks, such as drying dishes. Continued participation in routines such as religious services, Sunday drives, and daily walks structure time and convey a sense of normalcy. Mr. Wills is an example of a cognitively impaired elder moving from one level to another in the disease process.

Mr. Wills

Background: Mr. Wills is an 83-year-old retired musician whose closest relative is a distant cousin living in another city. He had been living in a subsidized bachelor apartment for 6 years. He was well-liked by his neighbors, who kept an eye on him as his memory deteriorated. They became increasingly concerned as Mr. Wills's cognitive decline accelerated over a 2-month period. Previously a very neat individual, Mr. Wills stopped shaving regularly and wore the same clothes for more than a week at a time. He would frequently have difficulty finding his apartment. His neighbors noticed he was losing weight and began to bring him food on a regular basis.

Mr. Wills was admitted to the hospital after a fall had made him bedridden for 2 days. He was delirious, with left lower lobe pneumonia. After the pneumonia was treated the delirium began to clear; however, significant cognitive impairment remained. Although still able to communicate, the patient was very confused and agitated, and tended to wander off the unit. He could no longer consistently recognize any of his neighbors. Mr. Wills could not function independently any longer, and he was waiting for placement. The patient was referred to the occupational therapy department by the nursing staff, who wanted assistance with a hospital care plan.

Occupational Therapy Assessment: Mr. Wills was only able to attend to stimuli for a few minutes and could not complete any task without prompting. An exception to this was when he played piano in the lounge. At those times he believed he was giving a performance and could play songs and classical pieces, although he would forget what he had just played and might repeat the same song. Mr. Wills required assistance with all self-care; however, he could feed himself if given one dish at a time. He was doubly incontinent, and the nurses had already instituted a bladder and bowel routine.

Assets: Mobile, able to play piano for periods of time, able to feed self.

Limitations: Agitated, wandering behavior, assistance required for self-care, no family supports.

Intervention: A schedule was devised for Mr. Wills that took advantage of his continued mobility and ability to play piano. Two periods were set aside each day when the patient was taken for a long walk and given the opportunity to play the piano. This activity was coordinated with his bladder routine and his meals.

Outcome: Mr. Wills became accustomed to this routine over a 3-week period. His agitation decreased, although he would repeatedly ask when he had to perform. His wandering behavior also decreased because he now watched for his "friends" to pick him up to walk to the show. He became increasingly content in his surroundings and visibly thrived on the praise he received for his musical abilities. Mr. Wills was admitted to a secure unit 6 months later. He was still able to walk; however, he could no longer play the piano. He continued to enjoy listening to piano music, and this was used to calm him when he became agitated in his new surroundings.

Level Two

Level Two represents a further deterioration in the behaviors encountered in Level Three. Behavior is highly disorganized and can seem bizarre and purposeless. Communication may be profoundly affected. Referring back to Levy (1986, 1987, 1989), attention can only be sustained for a few minutes by over-learned body movements (see Mr. Wills). Goal selection is related to the process of doing things, not to their outcome. The overall environment is largely ignored, as the person is only interested in the actions he or she is performing. Imitation holds only for one-step commands that have to be physically demonstrated. The impaired individual may engage in aimless pacing or repetitive tasks, such as moving objects from one end of the room to the other.

At this stage, assistance is required with all self-care activities. During dressing the person must be handed one article of clothing at a time and then given one-step directions (e.g., put your arm in the sleeve). Physical assistance is often needed to reinforce verbal cues. The client may become fearful and resistant during these activities, as he or she may not be able to understand the end product of the activity. Catastrophic reactions are common during bathing, often eliciting a high degree of uncooperative or agitated behavior. It is as if the tub is seen as a bottomless pit, and the person is afraid of being sucked under by the drain. Placing colored nonskid stickers on the bottom of the tub and using a plastic flower drain cover can be helpful (Butin, 1991).

Difficulties in self-feeding occur at this level. The impaired individual is distracted when a number of dishes are presented at the same time and is not able to handle various utensils. Foods should be presented one at a time on a contrasting background, and the use of spoons and nonslip, scoop-edged plates is recommended. The individual may also experience a decreased ability to perform the mechanics of toileting. Supervision and physical assistance are required to keep the person clean and to rearrange his or her clothing. "Clean-n-Dry" toilets that feature automatic flushers, warm water bidets, and hot-air dryers are available. These may be more frightening than useful to the impaired elder, however. Incontinence (urinary and, later, fecal) also occurs, making bowel and bladder routines essential. Often it is at this stage, when toileting becomes a problem, that institutionalization occurs.

Level One

Level One finds the individual globally impaired and most often institutionalized. Attention can only be sustained for a few seconds, and imitation is limited to one-word commands that may sometimes be followed. Motor abilities deteriorate significantly at this level. The person is often not ambulatory and may require seating intervention to prevent pressure sores and provide good positioning. Positioning is especially important during feeding to prevent aspiration. This is the terminal stage of SDAT, and interventions are aimed at providing comfort and a sense of security.

The maintenance of quality of life for individuals with Alzheimer's disease and their families is a major challenge. These cognitively impaired elders can retain some very important skills, despite their declining abilities. By using Levy's framework, an occupational therapist can provide the caregiver with practical suggestions to adapt the environment, matching abilities with the complexity of tasks, so that the person with SDAT can remain independent for as long as possible and retain some dignity and quality of life.

The remainder of the chapter focuses on individuals with traumatic brain injuries. Generally, these individuals improve over time. Strategies for self-care management are designed and graded to facilitate and maximize improvement. The Rancho Los Amigos Levels of Cognitive Functioning, as well as the Abreu and Toglia (1987) Cognitive Model, provide the discussion framework.

Traumatic Brain Injury (TBI)

Brain injury continues to be a major problem in North America and is one of the foremost killers and causes of disability in children and young adults. Citations of incidence have varied greatly in the literature (Kraus et al., 1984; Zahara & Cuvo, 1984). The Rehabilitation Research Training Center at the State University of New York at Buffalo (1992) recently estimated that in 1990 there were at least 316,285 individuals admitted to a hospital with a diagnosis of brain injury. Fifty percent of all TBIs are a result of motor vehicle accidents, and the remaining 50% are from falls, assaults, and sports injuries. Males between the ages of 15 and 24 have the highest rate of injury, and approximately 75,000 to 100,000 of these victims die. Some of the remaining survivors (70,000 to 90,000) often require lifelong assistance from social and/or governmental health care resources. These clients tend to be significant resource consumers of the health care system. The cost to care for a survivor of severe brain injury may exceed $4 million during a 5- to 10-year period (National Institute of Neurological Disorders and Stroke, 1989).

Definition of Brain Injury

Generally, the literature classifies traumatic brain injury as primary or secondary in nature. Primary injuries occur at the time of impact and include problems such as contusions, skull fractures, and lacerations. Secondary injuries are subsequent pathological processes, such as brain swelling, increased intracranial pressure, anoxia, and infection (Swan, 1988).

Each injury is unique because it is a result of the initial forces that are exerted on the brain tissue. Acceleration and deceleration of the brain against the cranium can result in focal (coup-contracoup) lesions as well as diffuse axonal shearing injury. Shearing forces are caused by the rotation of the brain within the cranial vault. These rotational forces often affect the brain stem, resulting in the clinical presentation of decreased level of consciousness (Ommaya & Gennarelli, 1974).

When diagnosing brain injury, physicians use both the clinical picture and radiological studies, such as computerized axial tomography (CAT) and magnetic resonance imaging (MRI). However, CAT scans often appear normal, even though there may be microscopic axonal injuries (Kay, 1986). In these cases, clients with normal CAT scans may demonstrate agitated and confused behavior. These clients, although medically cleared from organic brain injury, may demonstrate functional limitations and require treatment (Kay).

Medical Management

Initially, extensive pharmacological and/or surgical measures are taken to stabilize the acute problems and control or prevent secondary complications. Once this is completed, early intervention for rehabilitation is encouraged in order to maximize neurological recovery.

Severity

The severity of an injury depends on its nature, the location, the direction and magnitude of the impact's force, and the extent to which secondary factors interfere (Ommaya & Gennarelli, 1974). Initial severity is commonly measured by the Glascow Coma Scale (GCS) (Teasdale & Jennett, 1974). This 15-point scale examines a patient's level of response in the motor, visual, and verbal areas. It is commonly used in the acute phase of recovery. A GCS score greater than 13 is classified as mild head injury, between 9 and 12 as moderate head injury, and less than 8 as severe head injury. In addition to this initial medical scale, the duration of posttraumatic amnesia (PTA) has been correlated with future outcome.

PTA spans the time from the point of injury to a period when the client is able to demonstrate continuous and sequential memory, show orientation to place and time, and recount conversation or details of recent events. A PTA of less than 1 hour denotes a mild injury, a PTA of 1 to 24 hours a moderate injury, a PTA of 1 to 7 days a severe injury, and a PTA of greater than 7 days a very severe injury (Russell & Nathan, 1946).

Factors Affecting Cognition

The effects of brain injury can be compounded by the factors listed in Figure 1. In addition to the brain injury, these factors can produce a variety of either new behaviors or exacerbated premorbid behavior. It is important to realize that each client presents a unique neurobehavioral picture. Therefore, it is necessary to remain holistic when evaluating and meeting a client's needs. Although this chapter is concerned primarily with treatment strategies, appropriate and specific assessment techniques are necessary to identify a client's limitations and strengths (Abreu & Toglia, 1987; Arnardottir, 1990; Hartley & Griffith, 1989; Kovich & Bermann, 1988; Wang, 1990; Zencius, Lane, & Wesolowski, 1991).

TBI clients frequently exhibit multisystem involvement, primarily due to the mechanisms of injury. Clients who have sustained brain damage as a result of closed-head injury often have significant cognitive, as well as physical, deficits. There are commonly a number of cognitive, perceptual, and physical difficulties in severe-moderate injuries. For example, Jennifer had a moderate head injury with multiple fractures on the left side of her body. She was so focused on her physical changes (and her orthopedic devices) that she was unable to redirect her attention to any other tasks. The therapist working with Jennifer organized Jennifer's self-care activities to be done with her pelvic fixator covered up to produce the "out of sight out of mind" effect. Simple washing activities with moderate hand-over-hand and verbal step-by-step cuing were possible after this visual manipulation. In contrast, mild brain injuries can easily be masked by other, more pressing injuries or by their lack of appearance in empirical testing. However, the injuries can have just as devastating an effect on functional implications (Kay, 1986).

In the case of Bryan, he fell off his bike and sustained a small basal skull fracture and a fractured right arm. He recovered well in the hospital and was discharged home within 3 days. Bryan was able to carry out day-to-day self-care tasks at home; however, upon returning to work 2 weeks later, his colleagues noted that he was extremely moody and irritable, and that he demonstrated poor quality work. It was as if Bryan were a different person. In these situations it is best to monitor a client over a period of time in case difficulties occur in the various life roles.

Frames of Reference

This section concentrates on the Rancho Los Amigos Levels of Cognitive Functioning model (Malkmus, Booth, & Kodimer, 1980), and Abreu and Toglia's (1987) cognitive model as the primary framework in directing overall management of the client. Other optional frames of reference can be used to supplement treatment strategies. For example, a client with a great number of behavioral problems may require the creative use of behavioral modification, as well as appropriate cuing, based on his or her Rancho level.

It is important to recognize that a frame of reference may be changed to reflect a client's progress and unique clinical picture. Even though a therapist may use other frames of reference to supplement a treatment strategy, flexibility is necessary throughout a treatment program to provide the most appropriate intervention for a particular client at different levels of function (see Figure 2).

The Rancho scale is comprised generally of behavioral/cognitive descriptors that provide a way of compartmentalizing a client's progress (Malkmus, Booth, & Kodimer, 1980) (see Figure 3). Other scales can be used as a framework for managing a client (Allen, 1987; Kovich & Bermann, 1988).

In Abreu and Toglia's Evaluation Model, occupational behavior is achievable once a hierarchical series of subskills is in place. In this model there are five major steps or processes that have to be functioning prior to the ability to perform ADL independently (Abreu & Toglia, 1987). This process includes orientation (both to self and the environment) and the ability to attend and screen information (both internal, such as pain; and external, such as noise). It also includes an intact visual processing system; the ability to plan, select, and execute movements; and finally, the ability to use higher-level cognitive processes, such as memory, organization, and problem solving. Essentially, one cannot move to the next step without accomplishing the first.

Self-Care Management Strategies

The literature demonstrates numerous approaches and treatment strategies based on various combinations of frameworks (Arnardottir, 1990; Giles & Clark-Wilson, 1988; Giles & Shores, 1989; Hartley & Griffith, 1989; Kovich & Bermann, 1988; Poole, 1991; Smith & Wrinkler, 1990; Sohlberg, Sprunk, & Metzebar, 1988; Sudevan & Taylor, 1987; Szekeres, Ylvisaker, & Cohen, 1987; Tate, 1987a, 1987b; Zencius et al., 1991). However, none of these treatment methods have been proven to be effective in all cases. This may be a reflection of the challenge that therapists face when managing multidimensional TBI clients.

Central to any framework is the need for generalization from the therapy setting to the "real life environment" (Toglia, 1991). Generalization of learning requires knowledge of one's own ability to select, plan, and carry out strategies, and the subsequent evaluation of effectiveness (Toglia). Many clients with brain injuries demonstrate difficulties with this process, which is reflected in their daily functional tasks (Jacobs, 1988; Wehman et al., 1989). For example, a client with brain injuries may complete his or her morning

Figure 2. Case example: Client presents with a moderate closed head injury and a fractured left humerus and tibia.

Level	Problems	Frames of Reference
Rancho IV	• Inappropriate self-stimulation • Sexual aggressiveness • Violent outbursts	• Rancho (see manual) • Sensory integration • Neurodevelopmental • Spatial-temporal adaptation
Rancho VI	• Anxiety • Overwhelming fixation on pain in limbs, physical deformity, and abilities	• Occupational performance • Behavior modification • Rancho (see manual)
Rancho VIII	• Denial of cognitive deficits • Focused on return to work	• Rancho (see manual) • Role acquisition • Human occupation • Occupational behavior

Figure 3. Rancho Los Amigos Hospital scale of cognitive functioning.

Level	Behavioral Characteristics
I	**No Response** Patient is unreponsive to stimuli.
II	**Generalized Response** Patient reacts inconsistently and nonpurposefully to stimuli. Responses are limited and often delayed.
III	**Localized Response** Patient reacts specifically but inconsistently to stimuli. Responses are related to type of stimulus presented, such as focusing on an object visually or responding to sounds.
IV	**Confused, Agitated** Patient is extremely agitated and in a high state of confusion. Shows nonpurposeful and aggressive behavior. Unable to cooperate fully with treatments due to short attention span. Minimal assistance with self-care skills is needed.
V	**Confused, Inappropriate, Nonagitated** Patient is alert and can respond to simple commands on a more consistent basis. Highly distractible and needs constant cuing to attend to an activity. Memory is impaired, with confusion regarding past and present. The patient can perform self-care activities with assistance. May wander and needs to be watched carefully.
VI	**Confused, Appropriate** Patient shows goal-directed behavior, but still needs direction from staff. Follows simple tasks consistently and shows carryover for relearned tasks. The patient is more aware of his or her deficits and has increased awareness of self, family, and basic needs.
VII	**Automatic Appropriate** Patient appears oriented in home and hospital and goes through daily routine automatically. Shows carryover for new learning but still requires structure and supervision to ensure safety and good judgment. Able to initiate tasks in which he or she has an interest.
VIII	**Purposeful, Appropriate** Patient is totally alert and oriented, and shows good recall of past and recent events. Independent in the home and community. Shows a decreased ability in certain areas but has learned to compensate.

Used with permission of Adult Brain Injury Service, Rancho Los Amigos Medical Center, Downey, California.

hygiene routine and still appear unkempt. Therefore, an external feedback system is needed to facilitate task performance and to augment independence. This system is provided by the therapeutic staff and the family. The goal is for the client to develop an internal feedback system to replace the input of others.

The strategy of cuing focuses attention on a specific aspect of the task and provides information essential to performance of the task (Sudevan & Taylor, 1987). Larsson and

Ronnberg (1987) proposed that clients may be trained with material that is structured in advance or they may be taught to impose structure themselves. Diller et al. (1974) clarified this concept in their principle of "saturation cuing," which is the gradual and orderly delivery and removal of cues. This prepares the client to manage, through systematic training and over-learning, to assimilate and integrate cues, hence becoming capable of solving a problem free from structured cues. While occupational therapists often use cues, cues are at times presented in a random, unstructured context.

Cuing Program

In order to address basic self-care treatment strategies, the authors modified the process-oriented cuing system described by Abreu (1987). Instead of primarily using auditory cuing, cues were modified to be directed to all senses (see Figure 4).

The quality of cues depends on a number of factors. To be therapeutic, a cue must be easily identified and understood by the client. Ideally, cues should be single-step, positively reinforcing, and directed in a multisensory fashion. Examples include physical assistance, such as hand-over-hand guiding; verbal and nonverbal (gestures) cues; verbal cues only; or simply supervision. The therapist should be aware of the manner in which the cues are delivered (i.e., brief, repeated, and concrete words).

Occasionally, because of sensory deficits and other limitations, special approaches to cuing must be used, and can be successful. For example, Cook, Luschen, and Sikes (1991) described an approach to dressing training for an elderly woman with blindness and perceptual deficits that involved the successful use of audiotaped instructions. Their approach included the use of orienting prompts, stop cues, and a checking sequence, in addition to the requirement that clothes to be worn needed to be stacked at the foot of the bed each day in proper order by a family member. In cases such as this, task completion with the use of cuing mechanisms represents the highest level of functional skill that can be achieved.

As greater functional independence is achieved in patients who can progress, decreasing amounts and types of external feedback are needed. Quantitatively, therapists need to select and combine cues to optimize the situation, thus ensuring successful task performance.

Introduction of cues is based on three important criteria:

1. level of cognitive functioning, based on Rancho Los Amigos classification,
2. factors affecting cognition, and

Figure 4. Cuing system (Levels III–VI, Rancho Los Amigos Scale of Cognitive Functioning).

Cue Type	Description
Physical assist	Hand-over-hand through full movement; physical guide to initiate
Verbal and nonverbal	Gestures with step-by-step instructions
Verbal	Reminders, prompts
Supervision	Intermittent checking while supervisor is in the vicinity of the patient. Minimal or no visual or gestural cues.

3. detailed activity analysis (Llorens, 1986).

The following case study illustrates cue introduction using the eight levels of the Rancho Los Amigos Scale of Cognitive Functioning.

Lewis

Social History: Lewis is a 24-year-old man who comes from a large, rural family but is presently living with his girlfriend, Linda, in a rented house in Toronto. He is currently unemployed and thinking about upgrading his grade-9 education level.

Clinical Picture: Lewis fell 20 feet from his roof and sustained a skull fracture and dislocation of his right shoulder. His GCS upon admission was 7. The CAT scan revealed bifrontal contusions and a right frontal hematoma with shift to the left. He was taken immediately to surgery for a craniotomy and evacuation of the hematoma. Once his medical status was stabilized, occupational therapy became involved. Over the first 5 days, Lewis received a structured coma management program and progressed to level IV on the Rancho scale. At this stage, Lewis was agitated, restless, confused, and had decreased attention, which interfered with basic ADL. This was embarrassing for Linda and frustrating for the nursing staff. The therapist introduced a maximal cuing program, involving Linda as well as other caregivers. A full morning routine was considered unrealistic at this time. Certain basic tasks were selected from the perspective of number of steps, roteness of movement, and relevance to Lewis. These tasks were then analyzed, and clusters of cues were assigned to ensure successful performance. For example, in face washing Lewis required tactile, hand-over-hand, and verbal, step-by-step instruction, as well as visual demonstration (see Figure 5). To diminish the distracting effect of his painful right shoulder, this activity was scheduled around the administration of routine pain medication.

Within 2 weeks, Lewis was demonstrating behaviors from Rancho levels V and VI. He became more confused when tasks were complex and not structured. For instance, when asked by staff to get ready for therapy, certain ADL tasks were often omitted. At this point Lewis was ready to participate in a fully structured morning routine that involved a daily ADL checklist to assist with memory and organization. The level of cuing had

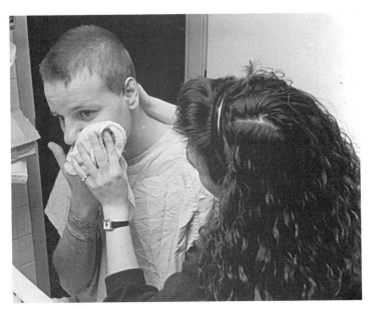

Figure 5. This client, recovering from traumatic brain injury, is provided with multisensory cuing to wash his face as part of a morning routine. The cues provided by the therapist include tactile physical assistance (hand-over-hand), and step-by-step verbal instructions with gestures to demonstrate the necessary actions.

decreased such that he required only verbal reminding and visual cuing from the checklist. Physical assistance was only necessary for tasks involving his right shoulder, such as donning a sweater (see Figure 6). Additional strategies that would be appropriate were also reviewed with Linda and the team. These included a daily diary to track Lewis's routine. Lewis and Linda completed the diary together twice a day. A large schedule was also placed on Lewis's door, indicating his appointments and daily activities.

At Rancho levels VII and VIII, the activities used in Lewis's treatment expanded to include instrumental ADL such as shopping, banking, and cooking. At this stage Lewis required primarily verbal cuing and supervision. In her treatment manual, Abreu (1987) describes a 6-point graded verbal cuing scale that would be most appropriate at this level. However, in unfamiliar and new learning tasks, the therapist would accompany verbal cuing with more supportive cues used in earlier stages.

Once he had attained Level VI, Lewis's program was not only directed at the overall reduction of externally provided cues, but also at introducing elements of change (i.e., a variety of staff and situations). This element required Lewis to begin solving problems, generating solutions, and evaluating his own behavior. This process helped to facilitate generalization (Toglia, 1991).

The case studies described in Figure 7 further illustrate the use of cues for specific

Figure 6. Activities of daily living checklist: Lewis.

Activity	Cuing Status	Mon.	Tues.	Wed.	Thurs.	Fri.	Sat.	Sun.
AM								
Toilet/bathroom	P + VC							
Eat breakfast	I + S							
Face & hands washed	VC							
Bed bath	N/A							
Bath/shower	VC + P							
Comb hair	I + VC							
Shave	I + VC							
Mouth & teeth cleaned	I							
Change clothes	VC + P							
Get up in chair	I							
Go for walk	I							
PM								
Eat lunch	I + S							
Toilet/bathroom	P + VC							
Eat supper	I + S							

Cuing Status: **D** = Dependent, **VC** = Verbal Cuing, **VD** = Visual/Demonstration, **P** = Physical Assistance, **S** = Supervision, **I** = Independent tasks at various Rancho levels. Note that the programs have taken into account the factors affecting cognition.

As shown in the case studies, different functional activities or goals are realistic in a range of stages. For instance, using the Rancho Los Amigos classification, it would be unreasonable to expect budgeting to occur before stage VI. General functional goals are illustrated in Figure 8. Therapists are encouraged to analyze each situation using an appropriate frame of reference to address identified deficits. In turn, a particular activity

Figure 7. Case studies: Traumatic brain injury.

	Carlos	Agnes
Clinical picture	Carlos is a 27-year-old man who, as a result of an MVA, sustained a closed head injury, fractures of the left tibia and fibula, left brachial plexus injury, and massive internal injuries.	Agnes is a 57-year-old woman who was a pedestrian struck by a speeding car. She sustained a Leforte III facial fracture, chest contusion, and fractures to her right humerus, right femur, and right acetabulum.
Glascow coma score	8 (on admission)	10 (on admission)
CAT scan findings	Generalized edema	Right frontal hematoma, no shift
Rancho Los Amigos level	Level VI within 8 weeks	Level V within 4 weeks
Factors affecting cognition	English not first language. Client had engaged in premorbid drug abuse and was unemployed. His education level was grade 11.	Client was self-conscious about her facial appearance. She had persistent double vision, a painful hip, and malaise due to immobility.
Problem	Carlos was unable to complete an entire morning care routine; however, he was able to do separate tasks.	Agnes was continually wiping and washing her face to "get rid of scars and bruises."
Cuing program	Carlos required visual cuing in the form of a Spanish activities of daily living checklist posted by his bed, and verbal reminding from the ward attendant. With this program in place, Carlos was able to complete his morning routine with less frustration and nursing supervision.	A grooming routine was set up where Agnes was assisted in hand-over-hand gentle face washing and supervised hair brushing. Mouth care was done by nursing, due to the facial reduction. A large visual checklist was provided where Agnes could check off completion of morning self-care tasks with supervision from the nurses. All caregivers were encouraged to explain to Agnes frequently why her face was scarred and bruised, and that face washing was already completed and checked off.
Environmental changes	Memory aids were used for all tasks, such as charts and lists. Anything written was translated into Spanish. Spanish-speaking staff were assigned where possible.	Environmental changes were made to limit the use of a mirror, provide contrasting materials for washing and grooming, and eliminating unnecessary clutter at the task site. An eye patch was provided to assist with decreasing double vision.
Frames of reference	Rancho, Toglia & Abreau, Occupational Performance	Rancho, Toglia & Abreau, Occupational Performance

can be analyzed and mapped out to meet each client's needs. This mapping process is demonstrated in Figure 9, and is comprised of cue ranges applied to a basic ADL routine. For instance, a client at level V may require different amounts and combinations of cues to complete a dressing routine, depending on the associated injuries and other contributing factors.

Figure 8. General functional goals.

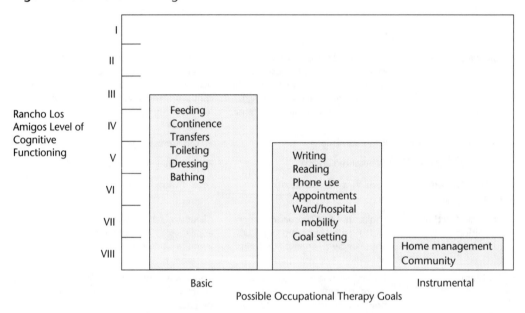

Figure 9. Level of cuing needed for basic ADL.

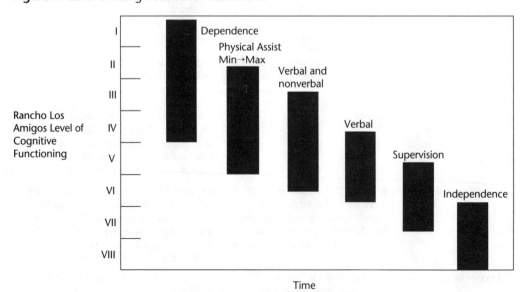

Summary

The performance of tasks, including self-care, involves a cognitive component. When cognition is impaired, the attention, memory, and behavioral control necessary for task performance may be inadequate. Moreover, after the loss of function following traumatic brain injury, the capacity for relearning skills may be compromised. As sensory processing is compromised, behavior may be erratic.

In their treatment of clients with cognitive deficits, occupational therapists must analyze, select, adjust, redirect, and modify their intervention strategies, using their knowledge of skill acquisition and activity. In clients with cognitive deficits, the necessary information for learning or performance is provided in the form of cues, which provide a means of compensating for attention and memory deficits. The demands of the environment must be matched with the capability of the client to manage them. Effective intervention requires therapists to understand the factors that affect cognition and the characteristics of different conditions so they can systematically apply appropriate cues to their client's changing needs.

In the individual with traumatic brain injury, the cuing program needs to diminish or become more subtle as the client improves. In contrast, the cuing program must expand for the client with Alzheimer's disease to support declining function. In all cases, careful cuing assists in optimizing performance of self-care tasks and adds to the quality of life for both clients and family caregivers.

References

Abreu, B. (1987). *Three frames of reference: Neurodevelopmental biomechanical cognitive rehabilitation.* (Available from Joseph P. Calnan, 3 Washington Square Village, New York, NY, 10012.)

Abreu, B., & Toglia, J. (1987). Cognitive rehabilitation: A model for occupational therapy. *American Journal of Occupational Therapy, 41,* 439–448.

Allen, C. (1982). Independence through activity: The practice of occupational therapy. *American Journal of Occupational Therapy, 36,* 731–739.

Allen, C. (1985). *Occupational therapy for psychiatric diseases: Measurement and management of cognitive disability.* Boston: Little, Brown.

Allen, C. (1987). Activity: Occupational therapy's treatment method. *American Journal of Occupational Therapy, 41,* 563–575.

Arnardottir, G. (1990). *The brain and behavior: Assessing cortical dysfunction through activities of daily living.* St. Louis: Mosby.

Botwinick, J. (1973). *Aging and behavior.* New York: Springer.

Butin, D.N. (1991). Helping those with dementia to live at home: An educational series for caregivers. *Physical and Occupational Therapy in Geriatrics, 9,* 69–82.

Christiansen, C., & Baum, B. (Eds.). (1991). *Occupational therapy: Overcoming human performance deficits.* Thorofare, NJ: Slack.

Cook, E.A., Luschen, L., & Sikes, S. (1991). Dressing training for an elderly woman with cognitive and perceptual impairments. *American Journal of Occupational Therapy, 45,* 652–654.

Cummings, J.L., & Benson, D.F. (1983). *Dementia: A clinical approach.* Stoneham, MA: Butterworth.

Diller, L., Ben-Yishay, Y., Gerstman, L., Goodkin, R., Gordon, W., Weinberg, J., Mandelburg, I., Schulman, P., & Shah, N. (1974). *Studies in cognition and rehabilitation in hemiplegia.* (Rehabilitation Monograph No. 50.) New York: New York University Medical Center, Institute of Rehabilitation Medicine.

Edwards, D.F., Baum, C.M., & Duel, R.K. (1991). Constructional apraxia in Alzheimer's disease: Contributions to functional loss. *Physical and Occupational Therapy in Geriatrics, 9,* 53–68.

Evans, D.A., Funkenstein, H., Albert, M.S., Scherr, P.A., Cook, N.R., Chown, M.J., Herbert, L.E., Hennekins, C.H., & Taylor, J.O. (1989). Prevalence of Alzheimer's disease in a community population of older persons. *Journal of the American Medical Association, 262,* 2551–2556.

Folstein, M.F., Folstein, S.E., & McHugh, P.R. (1975). Minimental state—A practical method for grading the cognitive state of patients for the clinician. *Journal of Psychiatric Research, 12,* 189–198.

Giles, G., & Clark-Wilson, J. (1988). The use of behavioral techniques in functional skills training after severe brain injury. *American Journal of Occupational Therapy, 42,* 658–665.

Giles, G., & Shores, M. (1989). A rapid method for teaching severely brain injured adults how to wash and dress. *Archives of Physical Medicine and Rehabilitation, 70,* 156–158.

Gilhome-Herbst, K., & Humphry, C. (1980). Hearing impairment and mental state in the elderly living at home. *British Medical Journal, 281,* 903–905.

Glickstein, J.K. (1988). *Therapeutic interventions in Alzheimer's disease: A program of functional communication skills for activities of daily living.* Gaithersburg, MD: Aspen Publishers.

Hartley, L., & Griffith, A. (1989). A functional approach to the cognitive-communication deficits of closed head injured clients. *Journal of Speech Language Pathology Association, 13*(2) 51–57.

Jacobs, H. (1988). The Los Angeles head injury survey: Procedures and initial findings. *Archives of Physical Medicine and Rehabilitation, 69,* 425–431.

Kahana, E.A. (1979). Congruence model of person-environment fit. In F. Carp (Chair), *Alternative conceptions of the person environment interaction.* Symposium conducted at the meeting of the Gerontological Society. Washington, DC.

Katzman, R. (1986). Alzheimer's disease. *The New England Journal of Medicine, 314,* 964–973.

Kay, T. (1986). *Minor head injury: An introduction for professionals.* Framingham, MA: National Head Injury Foundation, Inc.

Kovich, K., & Bermann, D. (1988). *Head injury: A guide to functional outcomes in occupational therapy.* Gaithersburg, MD: Aspen Publishers.

Kraus, J., Black, M., Hessol, N., Ley, D., Rokaw, W., Sullivan, C., Bowers, S., Knowlton, S., & Marshall, L. (1984). The incidence of acute brain injury and serious impairment in a defined population. *American Journal of Epidemiology, 119,* 186–201.

Larsson, C., & Ronnberg, J. (1987). Memory disorders as a function of traumatic brain injury. *Scandinavian Journal of Rehabilitation Medicine, 19,* 99–104.

Lawton, M.P., & Nahemow, L. (1973). Ecology and the aging process. In C. Eisdorfer & M.P. Lawton (Eds.), *The psychology of adult development and aging.* Washington, DC: American Psychological Association.

Levy, L.L. (1986). A practical guide to care of the Alzheimer's disease victim: The cognitive disability perspective. *Topics in Geriatric Rehabilitation, 2,* 16–26.

Levy, L.L. (1987). Psychosocial intervention and dementia, part II: The cognitive disability perspective. *Occupational Therapy in Mental Health, 7,* 13–36.

Levy, L.L. (1989). Activity adaptation in rehabilitation of the physically and cognitively disabled aged. *Topics in Geriatric Rehabilitation, 4,* 53–66.

Llorens, L. (1986). Activity analysis: Agreement among factors in a sensory processing model. *American Journal of Occupational Therapy, 40,* 103–110.

Liu, L., Gautier, L., & Gautier, S. (1991). Spatial disorientation with early senile dementia of the Alzheimer's type. *American Journal of Occupational Therapy, 45,* 67–74.

Malkmus, D., Booth, B., & Kodimer, C. (1980). *Rehabilitation of the head injured adult: Comprehensive cognitive management.* Downey, CA: Professional Staff Association of Rancho Los Amigos Hospital, Inc.

McKhann, G., Drachman, D., Folstein, M., Katzman, R., Price, D., & Stadlan, E.M. (1984). Clinical diagnosis of Alzheimer's disease: Report of the NINCDS-ARDRA work group under the auspices of the Department of Health and Human Services Task Force on Alzheimer's Disease. *Neurology, 34,* 939–144.

Mortimer, J.A., Schuman, L.M., & French, L.R. (1981). Epidemiology of dementing illness. In L.M. Schuman & J.A. Mortimer (Eds.), *The epidemiology of dementia* (pp. 3–23). New York: Oxford University Press.

National Institute of Neurological Disorders and Stroke. (1989). *Interagency head injury task force report.* Bethesda, MD: Author.

Nolen, N.R. (1988). Functional skill regression in late stage dementias. *American Journal of Occupational Therapy, 42,* 666–669.

Ommaya, A., & Gennarelli, T. (1974). Cerebral concussion and traumatic unconsciousness. *Brain, 97,* 633–654.

Poole, J. (1991). Application of motor learning principles in occupational therapy. *American Journal of Occupational Therapy, 45,* 531–537.

Powell, L.S., & Courtice, K. (1983). *Alzheimer's disease: A guide for families.* Reading, MA: Addison-Wesley.

Rehabilitation Research and Training Center, State University of New York at Buffalo. (1992). A formula to estimate incidence. *Community Integration, 3,* 8–9.

Reisberg, B., Ferris, S.H., de Leon, M.J., Kluger, A., Franssen, E., Borenstien, J., & Alba, R.C. (1989). The stage specific temporal course of Alzheimer's disease: Functional and behavioral concomitants based upon cross-sectional and longitudinal observation. *Progress in Clinical and Biological Research, 317,* 23–41.

Russell, W., & Nathan, P. (1946). Traumatic amnesia. *Brain, 69,* 280–330.

Select Committee on Aging. (1990). *Sharing the caring: Options for the 90's and beyond* (Publication No. 101-750). Washington, DC: Author.

Smith, S., & Wrinkler, P. (1990). Traumatic head injuries. In A. Umphred (Ed.), *Neurological Rehabilitation* (rev. ed.) (pp. 347–397). Toronto: Mosby.

Sohlberg, M., Sprunk, H., & Metzebar, K. (1988). Efficiency of an external cuing system in an individual with severe frontal lobe damage. *Cognitive Rehabilitation, 6*(4), 36–41.

Sudevan, P., & Taylor, D. (1987). The cuing and priming of cognitive operations. *Journal of Experimental Psychology: Human Perception and Performance, 13,* 89–103.

Swan, K. (1988). Management of severe head injury. In A. Ropper & S. Kennedy (Eds.), *Neurological and neurosurgical intensive care* (pp. 165–185). Gaithersburg, MD: Aspen Publishers.

Szekeres, S. F., Ylvisaker, M., & Cohen, S. (1987). A framework for cognitive rehabilitation therapy. In M. Ylvisaker (Ed.), *Head injury rehabilitation: Children and adults* (pp. 87–136). Boston: College Hill Press.

Tate, R.L. (1987a). Behavior management techniques for organic psychosocial deficit incurred by severe head injury. *Scandinavian Journal of Rehabilitation Medicine, 19*, 19–24.

Tate, R.L. (1987b). Issues in the management of behavior disturbance as a consequence of severe head injury. *Scandinavian Journal of Rehabilitation Medicine, 19*, 13–18.

Teasdale, G., & Jennett, B. (1974). Behavior management techniques for organic psychosocial deficits incurred by severe head injury. *Scandinavian Journal of Rehabilitative Medicine, 19*, 19–24.

Toglia, J.P. (1991). Generalization of treatment: A multicontext approach to cognitive perceptual impairment in adults with brain injury. *American Journal of Occupational Therapy, 45*, 505–516.

Wang, P. (1990). Assessment of cognitive competency. In D. Tupper & K. Cicerone (Eds.), *The neuropsychology of everyday life: Assessment and basic competencies* (pp. 219–228). Boston: Kluwer Academic Publishers.

Weale, R.W. (1963). *The aging eye.* New York: Harper & Row.

Wehman, P., Kreutzer, J., Sale, P., West, M., Marton, M., & Dicambra, J. (1989). Cognitive impairment and remediation: Implications for employment following traumatic brain injury. *Journal of Head Trauma Rehabilitation, 4*, 66–75.

Zahara, D., & Cuvo, A. (1984). Behavioral applications to the rehabilitation of traumatically head injured persons. *Clinical Psychology Review, 4*, 477–491.

Zencius, A., Lane, I., & Wesolowski, M. (1991). Assessing and treating non-compliance in brain-injured clients. *Brain Injury, 5*, 369–374.

13

Self-Care Strategies in Intervention for Psychosocial Conditions

Carol A. Leonardelli Haertlein

Margaret C. Blodgett

Carol A. Leonardelli Haertlein, PhD, OTR, FAOTA, is Associate Professor at and Director of the Occupational Therapy Program at the University of Wisconsin-Milwaukee, Milwaukee, WI.

Margaret C. Blodgett, MS, OTR, is Associate Lecturer at the Occupational Therapy Program at the University of Wisconsin-Milwaukee, Milwaukee, WI.

Chapter 13 Outline

Self-Care and Psychosocial Impairment

Schizophrenia

Dysfunction in Self-Care

Mood Disorders

Dysfunction in Self-Care

Personality Disorders

Dysfunction in Self-Care

Substance Abuse and Dependence

Dysfunction in Self-Care

Self-Care Assessment of Persons With Psychosocial Conditions

Self-Care Management

Psychoeducational Models

Educational Guidelines

Learning Principles

Sample Group Protocol

Criteria for Participation

Group Member Learning Objectives

Strategies Used in the Group

Reevaluation and Monitoring Procedures

Outcome Goals

Program Characteristics

References

Occupational therapy assessment and intervention for psychosocial conditions must always contend with the dilemma of defining the scope of practice (Bonder, 1993). Should therapy focus on the evaluation and development of the neuromotor, cognitive, psychological, and social abilities underlying the performance of occupation? Or should it directly address the skills necessary to complete work/educational, play/leisure, and self-maintenance tasks? Are both realms of concern—the performance components and the occupational behaviors themselves—appropriate targets for occupational therapy intervention with psychosocially disabled individuals?

Current literature in this area (Borg & Bruce, 1991; Hemphill, Peterson, & Werner, 1991) includes both realms as fitting for therapy. And inherently this makes good sense. A depressed person may not only lack the work skills to earn a living to support a family, but also need to develop the self-esteem and motivation necessary to acquire those skills. Someone with schizophrenia may lack the necessary problem-solving and interpersonal abilities needed to plan and shop for weekly meals as well as be unable to use the bus to get to the store. Both the underlying abilities for successful performance of occupations and the direct performance skills are both appropriate for occupational therapy intervention.

This chapter focuses on assessment and intervention for meeting self-care requirements for persons with psychosocial disabilities. Specific attention is devoted to schizophrenia, mood disorders, personality disorders, and substance abuse. It is our belief that self-care intervention should be primarily targeted to the level of performance skills. Psychosocial and cognitive abilities (e.g., motivation, self-concept, information processing, etc.), which affect performance of self-care tasks, can be secondarily treated while specific performance skills are addressed. They are certainly appropriate for occupational therapy intervention in their own right, through use of selected tasks and activities. But the development of self-care skills can be addressed as a viable treatment area on its own. When an individual's motivation or problem-solving abilities have improved through other therapeutic means, he or she will have the necessary knowledge and skills to perform the occupation of self-care successfully.

The following case study illustrates how the interaction of performance components and occupational behaviors is necessary to establish independence in daily living skills in an individual with a long history of mental illness.

Case Study 1.

B.T. is a 40-year-old man with a 22-year history of mental illness, specifically chronic schizophrenia and dependent personality disorder. B.T. had his first psychotic incident during exam week of his first semester in college. Following a hospitalization of several months, he returned to the university to continue his education. For about 3 years he was able to live independently and attend classes with the help of two roommates and his mother.

As the time approached to make an employment decision, and when his roommates graduated and moved away, B.T. experienced another psychotic episode, with severe depression. This hospitalization was for a longer period, extended by his setbacks any time a trial discharge or extended home pass occurred.

The intervening years, from this point until age 37, consisted of several hospitalizations, group home placements, and brief periods of living with his mother. Each of these settings seemed only to increase his dependency and his belief that he was unable to meet his most basic self-care needs.

At age 37 B.T. was admitted to a Community Support Program (CSP), and initially attended groups in a day treatment setting. These groups focused on learning the skills that would lead to independent living (i.e., personal hygiene, meal planning, grocery shopping, cooking, budgeting, and home care). Once he found an apartment, with the help of his occupational therapist/case manager, he began the process of doing those activities independently.

The occupational therapist now meets with B.T. every other week to help him with his grocery shopping. He prepares his own meal plan and shopping list prior to the trip. The therapist reports that B.T. is independent in most tasks, but needs some encouragement and support to deal with difficult situations, such as the crowds at the grocery store or confronting the landlord about repairs.

B.T. credits the one-on-one feedback and the constant encouragement from his occupational therapist/case manager and other CSP staff with his ability to live independently for the last 3 years. "I thought I took care of myself before, but I really didn't know how. I only knew how to get others to take care of me. With the help of my occupational therapist I now know that I can take care of myself and my apartment. I'm even budgeting my money so I can take a trip soon!"

As B.T. acquired the knowledge and skills necessary for independent living, his self-esteem and motivation increased to the point where he was willing to engage in the necessary occupational behaviors.

Self-Care and Psychosocial Impairment

Self-care as defined by Christiansen (1991b) refers to those activities of daily living that are required for independent living, specifically grooming and hygiene, bathing, dressing, meal-time management (eating and drinking), medication management, and functional communication.

Self-care is included in the category of self-maintenance or activities of daily living (ADL) which is one of the three areas of occupational performance commonly identified in occupational therapy literature (AOTA, 1989; Christiansen, 1991b). Occupation takes on meaning from the context in which it occurs (occupational form) and the actual doing of the activity or task (occupational performance) (Nelson, 1988).

The form of occupation consists of the physical dimensions of the environment in which its performance occurs (the materials, immediate location, other people involved, and temporal context) and the sociocultural reality (family, community, etc.) that surround it (Nelson, 1988). These are the parameters that give meaning to the occupation's performance. For the psychosocially impaired, the performance of a self-care activity, such as bathing, is only meaningful if the individual is motivated to respond to sociocultural norms of acceptable hygiene, including frequency; is able to maintain physical health through proper hygiene; can respond to feedback from others regarding the practice of or (more likely) the lack of adequate bathing routines; and has the knowledge to use the supplies and equipment necessary for successful bathing safely. The individual is unlikely to bathe if he or she is indifferent to sociocultural expectations and feedback from others, lacks sufficient self-esteem to maintain his or her own health, or lacks the knowledge to use equipment and supplies in a particular environment.

The actual doing of an occupation—the motor, cognitive, sensory, and perceptual abilities required for its execution—comprise occupational performance (Nelson, 1988).

Expanding the example of bathing, the psychosocially disabled individual needs adequate manual dexterity to manipulate faucets and shampoo bottles; strength, flexibility, and balance to enter and exit the tub; tactile sensitivity to regulate water temperature; kinesthetic awareness to wash all body parts; and information-ordering ability to organize bathing tasks.

In this framework, executing self-care activities is highly complex and includes the environment, other people, societal norms, and the person's own abilities. For the psychosocially disabled, this complexity is enhanced by dysfunction in habits, roles, values, interests, self-concept, motivation, interpersonal skills, and emotional expression. The potential manifestations of this disability are total lack of performance of self-care activities, partial or incomplete performance, performance that does not meet the socially accepted standards, or performance that is insufficient to meet the individual's needs. These same manifestations of disability may be present in the other areas of occupational performance: that is, work/education and play/leisure. But the potential impact of impaired performance of self-care activities may be somewhat different. Self-care activities include the very essence of survival on a daily basis and the foundation skills—acceptable hygiene, adequate nourishment, communication, medication management—to be successful in work and leisure occupations. Research supports this assumption.

Stein and Test (1980) identified the ability to perform necessary daily living activities as one of six factors critical to a psychosocially impaired individual's success in functioning in the community. These authors did not mention the relevance of work or leisure abilities.

An analysis of the characteristics of persons with serious mental illness in the Michigan public mental health system (Hazel, Herman, & Mowbray, 1991) found poor self-care and community living skills to be among the most common problems in the population studied (80% lived in supported environments). Lack of abilities necessary for employment (37% were unemployed and 31% were unemployable due to lack of skills) suggests that work is less relevant than self-care to this population. Leisure abilities and skills were not among the variables chosen to study. The impact of deficits in self-care abilities and skills for the psychosocially disabled mandates direct intervention at the level of performance in order to address the client's needs in a timely and efficient manner. Simultaneous intervention for performance components—cognitive, neuromotor, and so forth—would support the development of the performance skills of self-care.

Schizophrenia

Schizophrenia is a pervasive and usually chronic disorder that is diagnosed when a person shows deterioration from a previous level of function in work, self-care, or interpersonal relations. There are a wide range of characteristics in schizophrenia, not all of which are found in all persons diagnosed with the condition. Typically there are disturbances in affect and mood, behavior, and thought—both its content and form. Mood impairment in schizophrenia manifests itself as blunted, flat, and emotionless; inappropriate (e.g., laughter at sad news) or fluctuating (labile); and apathetic but alert. Behavior changes include social withdrawal and isolation, peculiar conduct, psychomotor manifestations (e.g., retardation, twitching), and impairment in function at work, school, and home. Thought disturbances are especially profound and appear as delusional ideation (e.g., mind control), hallucinations (e.g., visual, auditory), incoherence, looseness of associations, changes in speech patterns, and odd beliefs or magical thinking (Bonder, 1991; Sarason & Sarason, 1989).

Schizophrenia management has been improved over the past 30 years, so that the most debilitating symptoms (i.e., delusions, hallucinations, and behaviors) can be controlled successfully with antipsychotic drugs. However, it is worth noting that symptom relapse is not unusual, even with the effective use of medication. Some persons may have the damaging side effect of tardive dyskinesia from long-term antipsychotic drug use (injury to the nervous system causing involuntary movements). Other management techniques for schizophrenia include social skills training, behavior therapy (psychoeducational approach) for self-care skills, family support and intervention, and community support programs (Sarason & Sarason, 1989).

A typical clinical picture of schizophrenia begins with an acute episode of up to 6 months duration, occurring in late adolescence or early adulthood, with fluctuating remissions and exacerbations for the next several years. Long-term studies show that the most deterioration occurs in the first 5 years of the illness (Sarason & Sarason, 1989). Severity of symptoms is not always a good indicator of the outcome, with 20% to 25% of those stricken able to avoid severe and chronic behavior deterioration (Bonder, 1991; Sarason & Sarason, 1989). The prognosis improves with acute onset at a later age, the presence of a clear precipitating factor, no family history, a normal IQ, and good premorbid adjustment. But the majority of individuals with schizophrenic disorders are chronically disabled and function marginally in all aspects of occupational performance throughout their lives (Depoy & Kolodner, 1991).

Dysfunction in Self-Care

A change in self-care manifests itself as one of the most noticeable early symptoms of schizophrenia. The stricken individual ceases or changes personal care habits of bathing, shaving, hair care, and so forth. At times women adopt inappropriate and attention-seeking uses of makeup (e.g., excessive eye shadow and liner, unusual lipstick color and application). Changes in dress may also appear, and the person often becomes unkempt, slovenly, or dirty. Inappropriate attire is very common—for example, clothes that are too casual or dressy for the occasion, or inappropriate for the weather—especially for persons with a long history of the disease. This sometimes occurs in response to hallucinations or delusional ideation.

An interesting example of this is R.F., a 40-year-old man diagnosed with chronic paranoid schizophrenia, who always wears a long-sleeved shirt, and often a sweater or jacket too, even in very warm weather. He feels he must do this to keep the panther, tattooed on his forearm, from biting him or from coming alive and attacking someone else.

A typical secondary effect of deterioration in personal care habits is others' adverse responses. Family and friends may react with concern or denial, but strangers will almost always respond with avoidance, contributing to the individual's delusional thought processes, social withdrawal, or other symptomatic behavior. The interaction of declining self-care and interpersonal rejection becomes a self-perpetuating, downward cycle.

Eating habits of the person with schizophrenia may deteriorate, and he or she may have a total disregard for good nutrition. It has sometimes appeared to these authors that cigarettes and coffee replace food! Persons with schizophrenia may start overeating at meals, eat junk food in excess, or avoid certain foods or meals in conjunction with other bizarre behaviors. Daily medication management is very difficult for many of these individuals and usually has to be supervised by someone else. Reminders of appointments for medication checkups or reviews may also be needed. There is a noticeable change in interpersonal communication, which lacks both responsiveness and initiative. This behavior, coupled with a tendency toward social isolation and emotionless expression, interferes with functional communication, and, consequently, getting need fulfillment at several levels. For example, even though they experience hunger, people with schizophrenia may not seek information from others regarding the time of the next meal. Their lack of responsiveness may cause them to miss the call or reminder for that meal. At this point they are still hungry, and typically manage to find their way to the area vending machine where they fill up on junk food.

In early manifestations of the illness (late adolescence through early adulthood) individuals may have never developed the abilities that facilitate good self-care (i.e., organizational skills, awareness of socially accepted standards, etc.). More often, those who have had frequent or long-term hospitalizations lose skills and abilities (Bonder, 1991), lose motivation and interest in maintaining self-care routines, and stop responding to external cues in the environment (i.e., time, events, temperature, etc.). The most socially debilitating effects of schizophrenia may be the functional impairments that usually occur when symptoms are managed with antipsychotic medications (Bonder) (e.g., the foot tapping and pin rolling finger motions that may bring embarrassing attention from others). Even when self-care habits and social standards are not affected, individuals may be unable to manage the more complex self-maintenance skills of meal planning and preparation, money management, clothing care, and transportation in the community.

In summary, the self-care deficits typically seen in schizophrenia are:

1. a decline or change in personal hygiene habits (bathing, shaving, teeth care, hair care, makeup use),
2. unkempt or inappropriate clothing,
3. poor eating habits and neglect of nutrition,
4. the inability to manage medications, and
5. lack of responsiveness and initiation in interpersonal relationships, even when basic needs are not met.

Mood Disorders

Mood, or affective, disorders include a wide range of conditions, from sadness and grief to the more severe bipolar disorders and major depression. Self-care is more likely to be affected by depression than by a manic condition.

Major depression and the depressive condition of bipolar disorder are characterized by a depressed mood, feelings of worthlessness, and loss of interest or pleasure in most activities (Sarason & Sarason, 1989). For example S.T., a 35-year-old woman diagnosed with a bipolar disorder, depressed, had difficulty recognizing such simple pleasures as the feeling of a warm bath or the taste of a hot cup of coffee on a cold day. Behavior manifestations of a depressive disorder include changes in appetite and sleep patterns, and lethargy or agitation. Thought disturbances are seen in decreased ability to concentrate, delusions, and suicidal ideation.

Treating depression with psychotropic drugs is usually effective, although it is generally accepted that most depressive episodes will resolve themselves with or without treatment in about 6 months (Bonder, 1991; Sarason & Sarason, 1989). Psychotherapy is usually considered to be helpful for depression as well, and can take many forms, including cognitive therapy, self-monitoring behavioral approaches, psychoanalysis, and social-learning-based treatment. Electroconvulsive treatment is sometimes used and is considered to be effective for specific symptoms—suicidal tendencies, severe delusional thinking, and nonresponsiveness to drug therapy (Sarason & Sarason).

The course of a depressive episode varies, but most people experience depressed mood and loss of interest as well as some of the symptoms named above. Onset may be sudden or gradual over several weeks. Recurrence is seen in about half of those afflicted, with the recurring episode coming within 2 years of the first (Sarason & Sarason, 1989). According to Klemman, suicide attempts occur in about 30% of those diagnosed with depression (cited in Bonder, 1991).

Dysfunction in Self-Care

The range of self-care dysfunction in persons with depressive disorders is wide, from no self-care dysfunction to the person who is unable to get out of bed and engage in any occupational behaviors. The deficits in self-care are not from loss of skills or undeveloped abilities, as found in schizophrenia, but as secondary manifestations of the altered mood, and behavioral and thought disturbances. However, because of the habitual nature of the performance of most self-care activities, direct intervention at the performance level not only reestablishes routines, but alters self-perceptions and cognition at the same time.

A fairly common behavioral change in self-care habits seen in depression is altered appetite. This may appear as decreased eating resulting in weight loss and potentially inadequate nutrition, or increased appetite secondary to agitation with subsequent weight gain. Personal hygiene may be neglected due to the depressed mood, loss of interest, impaired concentration, and lethargy. Medication management may be impaired because of lowered concentration. Dressing and appearance of clothes may suffer due to loss of interest and depressed mood. Functional communication may be impaired as the depressed mood, loss of interest, and behavioral manifestations elicit negative reactions and avoidance responses from others. In addition to these self-care deficits, the more complex occupations of self-maintenance or the instrumental activities of daily living may be impaired.

In summary, self-care deficits that may be found in depression are:

1. changes in eating, resulting in weight loss or gain with potential nutritional compromise;

2. neglected personal hygiene, including dressing;

3. the inability to manage medication or other tasks of organization; and

4. the inability to express needs to others.

Personality Disorders

Personality disorders are often characterized as exaggerations of traits found in people without psychiatric disturbances (Depoy & Kolodner, 1991). There is typically a long-term behavioral pattern that is dysfunctional throughout life, with the affected person learning little or nothing from these experiences. It is only when the personality decompensates in the face of crisis, or the individual seeks help for another psychiatric condition, that the disorder is diagnosed.

Within the 11 classifications of personality disorders found in the *Diagnostic and Statistical Manual of Mental Disorders* (American Psychiatric Association, 1987), there is a range of disturbances found in mood and behavior. Examples of mood variations include being limited emotionally (schizoid), detached (schizotypal), labile (borderline), self-absorbed (narcissistic), fearful (dependent), and sulky (passive-aggressive). Behavioral manifestations of personality disorders are also wide ranging, and include social isolation (schizoid), manipulation and dishonesty (antisocial), seductivity (histrionic), and perfectionism (obsessive-compulsive). A commonality across the conditions is absence of a thought disorder. Although there may be some suspiciousness or indecisiveness, there is usually no evidence of delusional thinking, impaired concentration, or other symptoms of impaired thought.

Treating personality disorders is difficult at best. Interventions may include medications, skill training, behavioral interventions, hospitalization, and psychotherapy, depending on the manifestation of symptoms (Bonder, 1991). Personality patterns tend to be stable and often are not problematic if the individual learns effective stress management techniques as a way of preventing crises.

The clinical picture of the person with a personality disorder is as varied as the specific diagnoses and the affected individuals. Because the problems caused by personality disorders are often not severe, many people who might be categorized as such never seek help, and the course of their condition cannot be documented (Depoy & Kolodner, 1991).

It is important to note the increasing incidence and subsequent attention being given to multiple personality disorder (MPD). As an extreme disassociative phenomenon thought to arise from abusive childhood situations, MPD is often misdiagnosed (Braun, 1990). Psychiatric treatment aims toward reintegration of the two or more personalities controlling the person's behavior. Typically, during the reintegration process, patients with MPD can become dysfunctional, with diminished social and self-care skills (Fike, 1990a).

Dysfunction in Self-Care

Although the potential exists within classifications of personality disorder for self-care skills to be dysfunctional (as noted with MPD), typically this is not the case. Occupational function is more often problematic at the level of work and leisure behaviors, due to the interpersonal interactions often expected in those performance areas. Dysfunction in self-care, when present, is not symptomatic of skill deficits but rather is a manifestation of the disorder. For example, the person with schizoid personality disorder may exhibit unkempt dressing due to a lack of interpersonal feedback resulting from social isolation. The person with histrionic personality disorder may use excessive makeup and dress seductively as part of the attention-seeking behavior (Bonder, 1991). The impulsivity of the person with borderline personality disorder may lead to abandonment of hygiene and eating routines as value systems fluctuate, relationships waiver, and there is a steady stream of inconsistencies. There is potential for dysfunction in the more complex self-maintenance activities for many of the personality disorder classifications, particularly in money management and care of the home, clothing, and others. A common feature among all the personality disorders is impaired interpersonal relationships. All self-maintenance activities that affect interactions with others are impaired in persons with personality disorders.

In summary, deficits in self-care performance often seen in persons with personality disorders are:

1. manifestations of the exaggerated human trait that characterizes the particular disorder (e.g., unkempt appearance in the person with socially isolated schizoid personality; neglect of nutrition in the person with impulsive borderline personality; attention-getting clothes in the person with narcissistic personality); and

2. impairment in all self-care and self-maintenance activities that involve human interactions or relatedness, because relationships are impaired in all personality disorders.

Substance Abuse and Dependence

The psychiatric diagnoses of substance abuse and dependence are often seen in conjunction with other psychiatric diagnostic categories (e.g., the depressed individual who drinks to avoid feelings of hopelessness) or as situational responses to a physical condition (e.g., the individual who abuses prescription drugs to cope with pain and develops a physical and psychological dependence on them). *Abuse* is defined as the regular intake of a substance that may or may not be intoxicating but interferes with some aspect of function. *Dependence* is more severe and interferes with most aspects of function, increases tolerance for the substance, elicits withdrawal symptoms, and renders efforts to decrease the use of the substance unsuccessful (Depoy & Kolodner, 1991). Familiar substances that are abused and considered to be more psychologically than physically addictive are caffeine and cocaine. The substances that more likely create physical as well as psychological dependence are alcohol, nicotine, amphetamines, and barbiturates (Sarason & Sarason, 1989). Substance dependence is of interest to researchers because individual responses differ greatly and seem to be in accordance with each person's physiological and psychological makeup (Sarason & Sarason).

There are manifestations of changes in mood, behavior, and thought when substance abuse or dependence is present. Mood changes range from lethargy (e.g., alcohol and barbiturates) to excitability and elation (e.g., cocaine and heroin). Behavior usually becomes erratic and unpredictable in response to the chemical effects of the substances. With a physical or psychological addiction, behavior becomes focused on obtaining the substance rather than on involvement in meaningful occupational behaviors. Life-style changes evolve from these altered behaviors (e.g., loss of job, changes in leisure activities). Interpersonal relationships are almost always affected as individuals with similar life-styles and behaviors are more accepting of and acceptable to the abusing or dependent person. Impaired judgment and concentration appear as the addictive characteristics of the substance increase. The person becomes preoccupied with thoughts of seeking and using the addictive substance.

The management and course of substance abuse and dependence vary with the underlying causes (e.g., situational response to physical pain, socioeconomic forces, simultaneous psychoses). For most addictions, recognition of the problem and willingness to do something about it are important first steps (Bonder, 1991). Behavioral interventions, self-help groups, medications for physiological withdrawals, cognitive therapies, and other psychotherapeutic interventions have all met with varying success.

Dysfunction in Self-Care

The potential for dysfunction in all areas of occupational behavior is substantial, particularly as the individual progresses from substance abuse to substance dependence. Work and leisure are commonly affected, with work being neglected and leisure focusing on obtaining and using the substance. Self-care is impaired when individuals lose interest in eating, hygiene, and other personal-care habits as the need for the substance supersedes all other occupations. Central nervous system changes are most apparent during intoxication but may persist and increase if abuse continues, causing impaired judgment, altered motor activity, and forgetfulness. These changes may manifest themselves as loss of skills in self-care activities and in the more complex self-maintenance activities of money management, shopping, and so forth.

In summary, the deficits in self-care seen with substance abuse and dependence are:

1. neglect of self-care activities, as obtaining and using the substance supersedes all other occupations; and

2. loss of self-care and self-maintenance skills, as ongoing substance use causes central nervous system damage.

Self-Care Assessment of Persons With Psychosocial Conditions

Much has recently been written about the assessment of function in occupational therapy (Dickie & Robertson, 1991; Fisher, 1992; Smith, 1992). All of these authors note that discrepancies abound in the definitions of function, the purposes for which it is measured, how it should be measured, and what should be measured. At least there seems to be a recognition that self-care (or daily living skills) is a part of the domain called *function* and that it is assessed and treated at the level of occupational performance of skill, especially in psychiatry. Both Dickie and Robertson and Fisher emphasize the importance of placing an individual's function, and the assessment of it, in a social and cultural context. Fisher further emphasizes the importance of examining the interrelationship of occupational performance and the performance components. But the "concern with the prerequisite neuromotor, psychosocial, and cognitive-perceptual performance capacities is framed in their impact on occupational performance" (p. 184). In the self-care performance of persons with psychosocial conditions, the components affecting function may be cognitive (lack of knowledge, or impaired intellect or judgment) or psychosocial (decreased motivation or lowered self-esteem). These performance capacities, although within the realm of occupational therapy to treat, might be better left to other mental health professions, most notably psychology and social work, for assessment. This idea is supported by Dickie and Robertson when they make a case for *multiperspective* assessments that provide qualitative information for individual treatment decisions (the *diagnostic* purpose discussed by Smith) as compared to global measures that assume homogeneity within the population, are more quantitative, and provide information for research or quality assurance (the *outcome* purpose discussed by Smith).

The distinction between assessing at the level of occupational performance versus the level of performance components was addressed by Bonder (1993). She maintains that psychosocial variables (by definition) consist of psychological variables and social variables. She writes that "Psychological variables address internal unobservable processes that provide the person's drive toward activity" (p. 212). Social variables "...include the knowledge and ability required to relate to others" (p. 213) and "also exist at the occupational performance level, where a person's constellation of social activities (club memberships, family interactions, etc.) is at issue" (p. 213).

This distinction is important because it illustrates that self-care is not a psychosocial variable per se, but is influenced by psychosocial factors. Information on the self-care abilities of persons with psychosocial conditions may indicate the presence of occupational performance deficits, but it does not provide direct information about psychological or social status. Assessment should begin at the level of performance, then performance components should be considered as necessary.

This perspective allows the therapist to assist someone with psychosocial disabilities to focus on what is "necessary and fulfilling" (Bonder, 1993, p. 214) to perform meaningful self-care activities, not on whether he or she is depressed or isolated. It may be helpful at some level of assessment and treatment to identify the relationship between the person's social isolation and depression. But it is probably more meaningful to assist in developing a budget and money management skills so that the person can afford to eat one meal a day at the local coffee shop, and in so doing meet his or her social needs.

Other issues surrounding assessment of self-care for persons with psychosocial conditions are criterion-based versus normative-based assessment approaches (Bonder, 1993; Smith, 1992), self-report versus behavioral observation of performance (Borg & Bruce, 1991; Christiansen, 1991a; Leonardelli, 1986), and performance capability versus performance demonstrated in a natural environment (Christiansen, 1991b, 1993). Readers are referred to these sources for more discussion about these topics.

Assessment instruments that are designed for direct observation of self-care activities performance under standardized conditions are usually considered the most valid and reliable, although the most costly in time and knowledge level of the evaluator (Christiansen, 1991a). But since self-report (including questionnaires and interviews) of self-care levels has been identified as generally unreliable in psychiatric populations, especially among people with schizophrenia (Leonardelli, 1986), the trade-off of higher costs for meaningful information is worthwhile. A discussion of the self-care assessments specifically developed for psychosocially disabled populations is presented elsewhere (Leonardelli, 1986, 1987). Some use direct observation of self-care activities more than others, although not necessarily under standardized conditions. However, all incorporate direct observation to some extent.

Two other assessments found in the occupational therapy literature include activities of self-care and rely primarily on observation of skill. They are the Routine Task Inventory (RTI) (Earhardt & Allen, 1988) and the Comprehensive Occupational Therapy Evaluation (COTE) (Brayman & Kirby, 1982). The RTI is designed for persons with cognitive impairment, which can include psychosocial conditions. The COTE is designed primarily for psychiatric populations but does not break down the category of self-care into component activities (i.e., bathing, dressing, etc.). However, both are included here because of their availability and their potential contribution to self-care assessment of persons with psychosocial conditions. Figure 1 lists the specific self-care activities that can be evaluated with the assessments currently found in the occupational therapy literature. Readers are urged to evaluate the validity, reliability, assessment protocols, clinical applications, and other supporting information for each instrument prior to using it in a clinical setting.

Self-Care Management

The proliferation of occupational therapy literature in the past decade has included little about intervention for dysfunction in self-care. This has been particularly noticeable in the treatment of persons with psychosocial conditions. There have been several books and articles published on mental health assessment including self-care, descriptions of manifestations of mental illness and how they might interfere with all areas of occupational performance, detailed analysis of performance tasks with specific goals and objectives to be used in mental health settings (Hemphill et al., 1991), and group treatment in occupational therapy, but little information about the development and remediation of self-care dysfunction. The more complex self-maintenance or instrumental activities of daily living have fared better, with some models for program development appearing in recent years (Crist, 1986; Friedlob, Janis, & Deets-Aron, 1986; Hughes & Mullins, 1981; Neistadt & Cohn, 1990; Neistadt & Marques, 1984).

One of the reasons for the paucity of literature on self-care intervention may be reluctance (or confusion) when trying to distinguish the level at which treatment should occur, just as there is confusion about the level of assessment (occupational performance

Figure 1. Activities included in self-care assessments.

Assessment Name	Self-Care Activities Included	
Routine Task Inventory (Earhardt & Allen, 1988)	Grooming Dressing Bathing Feeding	Toileting Taking medication Using telephone Communicating (Listening/talking)
Comprehensive Occupational Therapy Evaluation (COTE) Scale (Brayman & Kirby, 1982)	Appearance (six factors—clean skin, clean hair, hair combed, clean clothes, clothes ironed, clothes suitable for occasion)	
Comprehensive Evaluation of Basic Living Skills (Casanova & Ferber, 1976)	Toileting Brushing teeth Bathing Hair care Dressing	Makeup Shaving Nail care Using telephone Eating
Scorable Self-Care Evaluation (Clark & Peters, 1984)	Personal care section Appearance Hygiene (frequency) Communication (emergency) First aid	
Independent Living Skills Evaluation (Johnson, Vinnicombe, & Merrill, 1980)	Personal hygiene and clothing Clothing maintenance (bathing and grooming; dressing appropriately) Medication management and health care (medical appointments, minor illnesses, first aid) Community skills (communication/conversation)	
Milwaukee Evaluation of Daily Living Skills (Leonardelli, 1988)	Basic communication Bathing Brushing teeth Denture care Dressing Eating Eyeglass care	Hair care Makeup use Managing medication Nail care Personal health care Shaving Using telephone
Kohlman Evaluation of Living Skills (Thomson, 1993)	Appearance Frequency of self-care Safety and health (telephone, emergency, danger in home, first aid, dental and medical facilities)	

or performance components). Therapists may be hesitant to describe and discuss their programs (targeted to occupational performance) at the risk of appearing too prescriptive and not individualizing methods to specific patient deficiencies (specific performance components). A discussion here about the differences between skills (as seen in occupational performance) and abilities (or performance components) may help ameliorate the confusion about levels of treatment.

Christiansen distinguishes between abilities and skills based on the work of Fleishman and colleagues in the area of human performance analysis (cited in Christiansen, 1991b). Fleishman "defines *abilities* as general traits which are a product of genetic make-up and learning, much of which occur during childhood and adolescence" Christiansen, p. 23). Examples are written comprehension, inductive reasoning, manual dexterity, and stamina—those abilities categorized as performance components in occupational therapy. *Skill* is defined as "the level of proficiency in a specific task. The assumption is that skill in complex tasks can be explained by the presence of various underlying general abilities..." (p. 23). Self-care activities might be characterized as groupings of skills involving many abilities. For example, dressing for rainy weather conditions involves deductive reasoning (decide what to wear), information ordering (arrange process of dressing), spatial orientation (locate clothing), and several motor abilities (coordination, dexterity, strength, flexibility, stamina) to don clothes. Whether or not an individual will put any of these abilities into action depends on self-concept, motivation (intrinsic and extrinsic), and knowledge (conditions of situation, sociocultural expectations). So the actual performance of skills is dependent on abilities, knowledge, and internal or external forces driving the person to act. Yet when we treat the dressing impairment of a person with schizophrenia we don't evaluate and treat deductive reasoning and spatial orientation. We function at the level of performance of the skill—assisting the person with dressing in an acceptable manner. If the person can't decide what clothing is appropriate for rainy weather, we teach a decision-making process for clothing choices with examples and cause-effect relationships. If he or she can't locate clothing, we provide visual or written reminders of where clothing is stored. The assessment and treatment occur at the level of occupational performance, with the potential for remediation of underlying abilities (performance components) occurring at the same time. For example, the decision-making process used for selecting clothing may be applied when making food choices.

If we agree that it is acceptable to treat at the level of occupational performance *and* we agree that there are common dysfunctions in self-care for persons with psychosocial conditions, then it is possible to develop guidelines or principles to direct assessment and treatment. A review of programs described in the occupational therapy literature (Crist, 1986; Fike, 1990b; Friedlob et al., 1986; Goldstein, Gershaw, & Sprafkin, 1979; Kielhofner & Brinson, 1989; Lillie & Armstrong, 1982; Neistadt & Cohn, 1990; Neistadt & Marques, 1984; Weissenberg & Giladi, 1989) and outside of occupational therapy (Bakker & Armstrong, 1976; Goldstein, 1981; Lamb, 1976; Unger, Anthony, Sciarappa, & Rogers, 1991) that address occupational performance serves as a starting point.

Most of the programs found in the occupational therapy literature use an academic or educational model to address self-maintenance deficits in persons with psychosocial conditions (referred to here as psychoeducational programs). Often the model programs are supplemented with ongoing supportive therapy once persons have completed the educational programs, and may offer support or education for families. These last two components are reinforced in the psychiatric literature with the value of aggressive community-based support programs articulated by Arana, Hastings and Herron (1991) and the necessity of services for families of persons with mental illness discussed by Pfeiffer and Mostek (1991). This then provides the three foundation principles for the treatment of self-care deficits:

    1. develop psychoeducational programs;

2. provide *intensive* follow-up via community support programs and continuous care teams, especially for persons with chronic mental illness; and

3. offer educational or supportive programs to families.

Psychoeducational Models

The concept that we can use educational approaches to change the self-care habits, routines, and skills of psychosocially disabled persons is grounded in the belief that therapy is learning. This is not a new concept in occupational therapy; references to teaching and learning in therapy have appeared in the occupational therapy literature since the 1960s. Schwartz (1991) has provided a useful description of approaches to teaching and learning and their significance to occupational performance. In this volume, Snell presents an overview of principles for behavioral and cognitive approaches and suggests guidelines useful for planning self-care intervention. Readers are urged to study these and other sources before embarking on the development of any psychoeducational program.

Educational Guidelines

Behavioral approaches (cause–effect associations, shaping, reinforcement, behavior modification, habituation, sensitization) are most effective for the following individuals:

1. those whose cognitive abilities are impaired by psychoses (e.g., acute schizophrenia, severe depression);

2. those with normal attention span and memory abilities (e.g., personality disorders); and

3. those in situations where the environment is unchanging and responses require little or no judgment in determining what to do. For example B.F., a 64-year-old man diagnosed with chronic undifferentiated schizophrenia, lives in a large residential care facility. One of the institution's rules is that the residents are not to go into the laundry area, for safety reasons. When B.F. is evaluated by an occupational therapist, he resists participating in the laundry part of the appraisal because he understands that he will be breaking the rules and does not have the ability to judge the situation as being an exception.

Cognitive approaches (teaching how learning occurs, transferring learning, role playing, rehearsal, imagery, memory enhancement techniques) are best used:

1. when the person must learn to do situational problem solving (e.g., select appropriate clothing for weather conditions);

2. when the individual has deficits in attention span, memory, or other cognitive abilities (e.g., an institutionalized schizophrenic or substance abuser with central nervous system damage); and

3. when the skills being learned need to be generalized or transferred to other situations (e.g., using acceptable eating behaviors in a restaurant).

The following case study demonstrates how behavioral and cognitive approaches were combined when assisting a client to develop socially acceptable standards of personal hygiene.

Case Study 2.

The format of an Activities of Daily Living skills group at a community day treatment setting is open-ended and addresses the needs of individuals as determined by members on a day-to-day basis. All clients admitted to the treatment program attend the ADL group. Consequently, the group's focus varies depending on whose issues are being dealt with on a given day. Group members assume a supportive peer role and give feedback to each other about how to accomplish their goals. For some clients this may be to learn how to plan and cook a nutritious meal. For others it may be to learn how to shop in a grocery store and make appropriate, cost-effective purchase decisions. Still others need feedback on a more basic level. T.R. joined the program and initially remained a quiet, background participant in most of the activities. Some of the staff and clients had difficulty approaching T.R. because of his obvious body odor and slovenly appearance. In the context of the ADL group, his peers were able to share with T.R. the effect he had on others and how that was keeping people from approaching and getting to know him. The group used role playing and rehearsal (cognitive techniques) to help T.R. improve his personal hygiene and to learn how to use the machines at the laundromat. A group shopping trip helped him to begin to overcome his anxiety about being in crowds and having a store clerk approach him. After a few weeks he was attending the group in clean clothes and had a more pleasing odor, as he used the aftershave cologne a fellow group member had given to him as a present (reinforcement—a behavioral technique)!

Learning Principles

It is clear from these guidelines that combinations of cognitive and behavioral approaches will often be indicated for the psychosocially disabled. In Johnson's (1986) summarization of a cognitive–behavioral model of treatment for depression, some basic teaching and learning principles that combine techniques from both approaches are presented. Johnson discusses three aspects of learning that must be considered in the teaching process.

1. *Subject matter:* The information to be presented must be organized meaning-fully, with a clearly stated objective. The objective should be repeated through-out the learning session, with an opportunity for learners to determine their progress. Content to be learned should have meaning for the learners.

2. *Learning activities:* Use visual cues—handouts, overheads, videos—abundantly. Vary learning activities throughout the session—use discussion, role playing, problem-solving procedures, videotaping, and so forth.

3. *Learner receptivity:* Keep the learners' anxiety to a minimum. Develop and maintain a learning environment where small successes are reinforced, learners are prepared for occasional failure or discouragement, tasks are graded from simple to complex, and peer groups can be used for support.

The following sample group protocol shows how these learning principles can be applied. It describes a Daily Living Skills group that was run within a day treatment program setting. The sessions were held for 1 hour, 5 times per week, and involved up to 10 members in the group at one time. An open-ended format allowed members to be admitted and discharged as they reached their individual treatment goals. Duration of group involvement was decided by the client and treatment team determination of progress on goals.

Sample Group Protocol

Frequently people who have suffered from mental illness have developed a dependency on others (i.e., family, institutions, caregivers) to fulfill some of their self-care needs, as a result of never having had the opportunity to learn how to perform these skills, or having become so dependent on others that they lost the ability and motivation to do them.

Criteria for Participation

1. Impaired activities of daily living skills are reflected in the patient's comprehensive treatment plan (i.e., deficits in areas such as cooking, budgeting, independent living, housekeeping, money management, social interaction, leisure involvement, etc.).

2. The living situation is currently or potentially that of a group home or an apartment/home.

3. The person has the ability to tolerate working within a group situation.

4. The person has the ability to verbalize needs and feelings.

5. The person expresses the interest and motivation to improve the level of independence.

6. The person has the ability to understand and use basic levels of instruction (i.e., basic math, reading, measurements).

Group Member Learning Objectives

1. To learn and/or develop skills and to begin to take responsibility for self in the following areas:
   a. personal hygiene,
   b. management of personal finances,
   c. cooking,
   d. nutrition (planning and preparation of meals),
   e. housekeeping and apartment or home maintenance,
   f. laundry,
   g. transportation, and
   h. leisure awareness and use of community resources.

2. To develop awareness of self, others, and the environment.

3. To improve the ability to follow and comprehend directions.

4. To enhance self-esteem.

5. To identify areas of self-competency and limitations.

6. To make use of group interaction to develop social skills.

Strategies Used in the Group

1. Discussion and practical experience activities in various areas of daily living

2. Community outings to relate learning to real-life experiences

3. Role playing

4. Educational games and learning activities

Reevaluation and Monitoring Procedures

1. Observation of the patient's participation and interactions

2. Patient's subjective comments

3. Documentation of progress toward individual and group goals on biweekly progress notes

Outcome Goals

1. The patient verbalizes and/or demonstrates improved functioning in at least two of the following areas:

    a. ability to provide for most self-care needs independently (i.e., tends to personal hygiene, cooks meals regularly, cares for own environment, handles own finances, etc.);

    b. interest in and motivation to perform the above skills on a regular basis (i.e., has arranged for or has realistic plans to live independently); or

    c. reports improved feelings of competency and adequacy.

or

2. Attainment of treatment plan goals and/or discharge from the day treatment Program

This program includes subject matter that is meaningful to the client (and can be chosen by him or her), uses a range of learning activities, and emphasizes discussion among members and the leader to maintain client receptivity to the learning experiences.

Program Characteristics

Many of these considerations have been adopted in psychoeducational models described in the literature. Bakker and Armstrong (1976) and Lillie and Armstrong (1982) identify the importance of learners setting their own goals; using verbal, written, visual, and experiential learning with rehearsal; and applying learned skills to the natural environment in their description of an Adult Development Program for day treatment patients. Other program characteristics suggested for an individual's successful involvement in a psychoeducational program are:

1. Individuals are able to learn.

2. Enrollment in the program is voluntary.

3. Participants in the program are students and instructors, not patients and staff.

4. Students set their own goals for learning.

5. Involvement in the program is time-limited (imparts a sense of urgency to acquire skills or knowledge).

6. There is some financial cost to students.

The authors emphasize that it is important to take the "mystique" out of learning. That is, it is important to tell learners that behavior patterns are learned, everyone goes through essentially the same learning process, and behavior can be acquired or changed. As Lamb (1976) states when describing a psychoeducational model for long-term mentally ill persons, it is crucial to "help patients realize that the basic skills of everyday living are learned skills" (p. 877). Lamb reiterates the guidelines proposed by Bakker and Armstrong (1976) and feels that the key principle to success is student involvement—in establishing the goals for learning, in establishing curriculum, and in taking some responsibility for its implementation. Another key factor in this perspective is conducting the program away from the site of mental health treatment, especially for long-term patients. By doing so the patient "has acquired a new identity, that of student, and feels he can participate in activities outside of mental health centers just like other people in the community. That, plus the information imparted to him in the course, helps the student move beyond the mental health system" (p. 877).

Another psychoeducational model, Structured Learning Therapy (SLT), is described in the psychology and occupational therapy literature (Goldstein, 1981; Goldstein et al., 1979), and deserves mention here. This model was developed in the 1970s as a response to the failure of most psychotherapy approaches with persons from lower socioeconomic classes, who were felt not to benefit as much as those from upper socioeconomic classes from insight-oriented, verbal psychotherapy. The SLT program consists of modeling, role playing, performance feedback (social reinforcement), and transfer training. SLT trainers came from a wide range of disciplines, including occupational therapy, and followed a training format that used the four components of the program. Standard audio modeling tapes were the primary teaching tool, followed by role-playing sessions, group feedback, and homework assignments. Although the premise on which SLT was developed would be regarded with some skepticism today, the techniques reflect some of the principles of good instruction.

The adoption of psychoeducational models into occupational therapy programs or self-maintenance for persons with psychosocial conditions has been described by Crist (1986), Friedlob et al. (1986), Kielhofner and Brinson (1989), Neistadt and Cohn (1990), Neistadt and Marques (1984), and Weissenberg and Giladi (1989). Most of these programs emphasize the more complex self-maintenance or instrumental activities of daily living. But the format and approaches they use are easily extended to self-care programs. In addition to the educational guidelines, learning principles, and program characteristics described above, there are some commonalities, as well as other considerations in developing a sound occupational therapy program for self-care management for the psychosocially disabled:

1. Remediation is based on sound assessment of deficits and strengths, *in the social and environmental context of what the patient wants to do.*

2. Newly developed knowledge and skills are integrated into *routines, habits, and roles.*

3. New knowledge and skills allow for *mastery experiences that increase self-confidence and a perceived sense of control.*

4. Individuals are able to *reengage in valued activities.* ◆

References

American Occupational Therapy Association (AOTA). (1989). Uniform terminology for occupational therapy—2nd edition. *American Journal of Occupational Therapy, 43,* 808–815.

American Psychiatric Association. (1987). *Diagnostic and statistical manual of mental disorders* (3rd ed., rev.). Washington, DC: Author.

Arana, J.D., Hastings, B., & Herron, E. (1991). Continuous care teams in intensive outpatient treatment of chronic mentally ill patients. *Hospital & Community Psychiatry, 42,* 503–507.

Bakker, C.B., & Armstrong, H.E. (1976). The adult development program: An educational approach to the delivery of mental health services. *Hospital & Community Psychiatry, 27,* 330–334.

Bonder, B. (1991). *Psychopathology and function.* Thorofare, NJ: Slack.

Bonder, B. (1993). Issues in assessment of psychosocial components of function. *American Journal of Occupational Therapy, 47,* 211–216.

Borg, B., & Bruce, M.A. (1991). Assessing psychological performance factors. In C. Christiansen & C. Baum (Eds.), *Occupational therapy: Overcoming human performance deficits* (pp. 540–586). Thorofare, NJ: Slack.

Braun, B.G. (1990). Multiple personality disorder: An overview. *American Journal of Occupational Therapy, 44,* 971–976.

Brayman, S., & Kirby, T. (1982). The comprehensive occupational therapy evaluation. In B.J. Hemphill (Ed.), *The evaluation process in psychiatric occupational therapy* (pp. 221–226). Thorofare, NJ: Slack.

Casanova, T., & Ferber, J. (1976). The comprehensive evaluation of basic living skills. *American Journal of Occupational Therapy, 30,* 143–147.

Christiansen, C. (1991a). Occupational performance assessment. In C. Christiansen & C. Baum (Eds.), *Occupational therapy: Overcoming human performance deficits* (pp. 375–421). Thorofare, NJ: Slack.

Christiansen, C. (1991b). Occupational therapy: Intervention for life performance. In C. Christiansen & C. Baum (Eds.), *Occupational therapy: Overcoming human performance deficits* (pp. 3–43), Thorofare, NJ: Slack.

Christiansen, C. (1993). Continuing challenges of functional assessment in rehabilitation: Recommended changes. *American Journal of Occupational Therapy, 47,* 258–259.

Clark, E.N., & Peters, M. (1984). *The scorable self care evaluation.* Thorofare, NJ: Slack.

Crist, P.H. (1986). Community living skills: A psychoeducational community-based program. *Occupational Therapy in Mental Health, 6*(2), 51–64.

Depoy, E., & Kolodner, E.L. (1991). Psychological performance factors. In C. Christiansen & C. Baum (Eds.), *Occupational therapy: Overcoming human performance deficits* (pp. 305–332). Thorofare, NJ: Slack.

Dickie, V.A., & Robertson, S.C. (1991). Perspectives on human functioning. *Hospital & Community Psychiatry, 42,* 575–576.

Earhardt, C.A., & Allen, C.K. (1988). *Cognitive disabilities: Expanded activity analysis.* Los Angeles: University of Southern California Medical Center.

Fike, M.L. (1990a). Clinical manifestations in persons with multiple personality disorder. *American Journal of Occupational Therapy, 44,* 984–990.

Fike, M.L. (1990b). Considerations and techniques in the treatment of multiple personality disorder. *American Journal of Occupational Therapy, 44,* 984–990.

Fisher, A.G. (1992). Functional measures, part 1: What is function, what should we measure, and how should we measure it? *American Journal of Occupational Therapy, 46,* 183–185.

Friedlob, S.A., Janis, G.A., & Deets-Aron, C. (1986). A hospital-connected halfway house program for individuals with long-term neuropsychiatric disabilities. *American Journal of Occupational Therapy, 40,* 271–277.

Goldstein, A.P. (1981). *Psychological skill training: The structured learning technique.* New York: Pergamon Press.

Goldstein, A.P., Gershaw, N.J., & Sprafkin, R.P. (1979). Structured learning therapy: Development and evaluation. *American Journal of Occupational Therapy, 33,* 635–639.

Hazel, K.L., Herman, S.E., & Mowbray, C.T. (1991). Characteristics of seriously mentally ill adults in a public mental health system. *Hospital & Community Psychiatry, 42,* 518–525.

Hemphill, B.J., Peterson, C.Q., & Werner, P.C. (1991). *Rehabilitation in mental health: Goals and objectives for independent living.* Thorofare, NJ: Slack.

Hughes, P.L., & Mullins, L. (1981). *Acute psychiatric care: An occupational therapy guide to exercises in daily living skills.* Thorofare, NJ: Slack.

Johnson, M.T. (1986). Use of cognitive-behavioral techniques with depressed adults in day treatment. In *Depression: Assessment & treatment update, proceedings of the preconference to the American Psychiatric Association's Annual Institute on Hospital and Community Psychiatry* (pp. 49–61). Rockville, MD: American Occupational Therapy Association.

Johnson, T.P., Vinnicombe, B.J., & Merrill, G. W. (1980). The independent living skills evaluation. *Occupational Therapy in Mental Health, 1*(1), 5–18.

Kielhofner, G., & Brinson, M. (1989). Development and evaluation of an aftercare program for young chronic psychiatrically disabled adults. *Occupational Therapy in Mental Health, 9*(2), 1–25.

Lamb, H.R. (1976). An educational model for teaching skills to long-term patients. *Hospital & Community Psychiatry, 27*, 875–877.

Leonardelli, C.A. (1986). The process of developing a quantifiable evaluation of daily living skills in psychiatry. *Occupational Therapy in Mental Health, 6*(4), 17–26.

Leonardelli, C.A. (1987). The Milwaukee evaluation of daily living skills (MEDLS). In B.J. Hemphill (Ed.), *Mental health assessment in occupational therapy* (pp. 151–162). Thorofare, NJ: Slack.

Leonardelli, C.A. (1988). *The Milwaukee evaluation of daily living skills: Evaluation in long-term psychiatric care*. Thorofare, NJ: Slack.

Lillie, M.D., & Armstrong, H.E. (1982). Contributions to the development of psychoeducational approaches to mental health service. *American Journal of Occupational Therapy, 36*, 438–443.

Neistadt, M.E., & Cohn, E.S. (1990). *An independent living skills model for Level I fieldwork*. Rockville, MD: American Occupational Therapy Association.

Neistadt, M.E., & Marques, K. (1984). An independent living skills training program. *American Journal of Occupational Therapy, 38*, 671–676.

Nelson, D. (1988). Occupation: Form and performance. *American Journal of Occupational Therapy, 42*, 633–641.

Pfeiffer, E.J., & Mostek, M. (1991). Services for families of people with mental illness. *Hospital & Community Psychiatry, 42*, 262–264.

Sarason, I.G., & Sarason, B.R. (1989). *Abnormal psychology* (6th ed.). Englewood Cliffs, NJ: Prentice Hall.

Schwartz, R.K. (1991). Educational training and strategies: Therapy as learning. In C. Christiansen & C. Baum (Eds.), *Occupational therapy: Overcoming human performance deficits* (665–698). Thorofare, NJ: Slack.

Smith, R.O. (1992). The science of occupational therapy assessment. *Occupational Therapy Journal of Research, 12*, 3–15.

Stein, L.I., & Test, M.A. (1980). Alternative to mental hospital treatment. *Archives of General Psychiatry, 37*, 392–399.

Thomson, L.M. (1993). *Kohlman evaluation of living skills*. Rockville, MD: American Occupational Therapy Association.

Unger, K.V., Anthony, W.A., Sciarappa, K., & Rogers, E.S. (1991). A supported education program for young adults with long-term mental illness. *Hospital & Community Psychiatry, 42*, 838–842.

Weissenberg, R., & Giladi, N. (1989). Home economics day: A program for disturbed adolescents to promote acquisition of habits and skills. *Occupational Therapy in Mental Health, 9*, 89–103.

14

Technology for Self-Care

Roger Smith
Margie Benge
Marian Hall

Roger O. Smith, PhD, OTR, FAOTA, is Associate Director of the Trace Research and Development Center at the Waisman Center, University of Wisconsin-Madison.

Margie Benge, OTR, is a part-time Faculty Member for the Occupational Therapy Assistant Program at Sinclair Community College in Dayton, OH, and has a private practice.

Marian Hall, MBA, OTR/L, is Director of Occupational Therapy at the Rehabilitation Center, Yalesville, CT.

The authors thank Betty Hasselkus, PhD, OTR, FAOTA; Alexandra Enders, OTR; Carol Gwin, OTR; and Jerilyn Johnson for their review, professional comments, and assistance in preparing this chapter.

Chapter 14 Outline

Overview of Assistive Technologies for Self-Care and Daily Living

Self-Care Devices

Home-Care Products

Seating and Mobility

Communication

Orthotics and Prosthetics

Architecture

Environmental Control

Intervention Approaches, Including Assistive Technology

History of Self-Care and Technology

Do-it-Yourself Self-Care Devices

Commercial Self-Care Devices

Product Comparison Advances

Historical Summary

Selecting Self-Care and Independent Living Assistive Technology

Assessing the Individual's Needs and Performance

Identifying Assistive Technology Options

Locating Information on Assistive Technology

Evaluating the Quality of Available Information Resources

Refining the Alternatives

Trial Use

Training

Owner's Manual

Follow-Up

Funding

Issues Surrounding the Application of Self-Care Assistive Technology

Consumer Empowerment

Independence Versus Efficiency Trade-Off

Prescription or Open Market Purchase

Compliance: An Outmoded Concept

Vendor Roles

    Occupational Therapy Vendor

    Use of Preferred Equipment Supplier

    Open Market Suppliers

Purchase, Adapt, or Fabricate?

Family, Friends, and Consumers as Experts

Special Needs of Long-Term Care

Impoverished Settings

Training Preservice Students

Teaming With Other Professionals

The Future of Assistive Technology in Self-Care

Appendix 1: Abledata Categories of Self-Care Products

Appendix 2: OT FACT Self-Care Assessment Categories

References

In 1778 Benjamin Franklin said, "Man is a tool-making animal" (cited in *The Oxford Dictionary of Quotations*, 1980, p. 218). While his gender-specific language is more than 200 years old and outdated, his observation about the unique relationship between humans and tools is timeless. This is fortunate. Today, tools used as assistive technologies enable people with disabilities to maximize their self-care independence and efficiency.

The vast number of assistive technologies available today reflects the prominent contribution they make to independent living. It is important that occupational therapy practitioners take a central role in helping to link these technologies to the people who will benefit from them. Abledata, the national database of assistive and rehabilitation technologies, includes more than 17,000 products. Of these, a large percentage is classified as self-care. Figure 1 highlights more than 7,500 products that relate to self-care. These are the assistive technologies addressed in this chapter.

This chapter, unlike many others in this text, does not focus on a disability or an impairment area. It focuses on an intervention strategy. Although it provides some information about the self-care tools themselves, it is beyond its scope to review and discuss the pros and cons of the multitude of technologies available. Thus, this chapter highlights concepts, many of which have evolved out of core philosophies of occupational therapy practice.

Legislation in the United States is increasingly recognizing assistive technology as a cost-effective intervention to assist people with disabilities. The terms *assistive technology devices* and *assistive technology services* are becoming better integrated and institutionalized in many of the federal agencies and their regulations. The federal Rehabilitation Act of 1973 as amended, especially with the 1986 additions of rehabilitation engineering services; The Education for All Handicapped Children Act of 1975 (PL 94-142) updated in 1991 as IDEA (Individuals With Disabilities Education Act, PL 101-476); the Developmental Disabilities Act; and the Older Americans Act all incorporate an assistive technology mandate. Two federal laws, however, have had specific impact across the United States and have played an important role in increasing the nation's awareness of assistive technologies and the

Figure 1. Self-care products catalogued in Abledata.

- Personal care products (3,432)*

- Home management products (911)

- Wheeled mobility products (1,373)

- Seating products (1,078)

- Communication products (128)

- Walking products (682)

- Orthotics (569)

- Prosthetics (44)

- Architectural elements (931)

- Control products (638)

* Numbers of each type of product catalogued are in parentheses

need to accommodate people with disabilities through the use of technology. The Technology Assistance Act of 1988 ("Tech Act," PL 100-407) and The Americans with Disabilities Act of 1989 (ADA, PL 101-336) have promoted a "system change." The Tech Act provides states with a systems change mandate. Stimulated by federal monies, states are required to increase assistive technology resources available to people with disabilities and partially measure their success on "consumer responsiveness." The ADA provides basic civil rights protection for individuals with disabilities and recognizes the important role assistive technology plays in equal access and overall integration into society.

Moreover, trends like the "greying" of America point toward the increased need for assistive technologies. Assistive technologies are becoming a more critical part of daily living, both for people who are developing functional limitations or disabilities through the aging process and for people with disabilities who need more functional support as they grow older. A Swedish study (Parker & Thorslund, 1991) found that technical devices are integral to the independence of people who are aging. The researchers surveyed a rural municipality with a population of about 20,000 people. They identified those aged 75 years and older who required technical aids or who had significant functional limitations. The 57 individuals randomly selected for this study had a total of 422 technical aids in their homes. The mean number of aids for each of these individuals was more than seven. Twenty-nine percent of these devices were used for mobility, 20% for personal hygiene, 20% for communication, and 16% for environmental adaptations. Five percent were ortheses or prostheses, and 11% were other functional devices. This study concluded that it is essential for occupational therapists to be familiar with assistive technologies that aid self-care independence.

The use of assistive technology is often an inexpensive and quick method for a person with a disability to compensate for the impairments and to achieve independence in self-care activities. Effective use of an assistive device, however, involves more than pulling it off a storage shelf and handing it to the client. The appropriate device must be selected based on functional need, environmental setting, and available resources. This includes decisions about whether the device is really necessary and how long it will be needed. There are many steps, considerations, and decisions that are made when providing even the simplest assistive technologies.

Incorrect decisions range from providing unnecessary or inappropriate equipment, to providing the right equipment but not teaching the client how or why to use it, to failing to recommend a device because the practitioner doesn't know it exists. Consequences range from an assistive technology never reaching the consumer, to the consumer who receives the device but puts it in a closet and never uses it. Ultimately, not only may functional ability be hampered in the short-term, but increased incidence of secondary disability can result. Ideally, good decisions made with the consumer and delivery of the assistive technology to him or her result in successful long-term use of the device. While this process of making the right decisions is often intuitive to expert therapists, in this chapter we try to provide helpful hints and ideas to help everyone use assistive technology better.

Overview of Assistive Technologies for Self-Care and Daily Living

The variety of assistive technologies in self-care and daily living is far reaching. Devices range from low technologies, to futuristic and high technologies. For example, technology may be a swivel spoon to optimize eating independence or a robot that feeds someone who is totally dependent. High and low technologies are one way to think of the range of assistive

Figure 2. Feeding evaluation kit. (Photo provided by Fred Sammons, Inc., © BISSELL Healthcare Company)

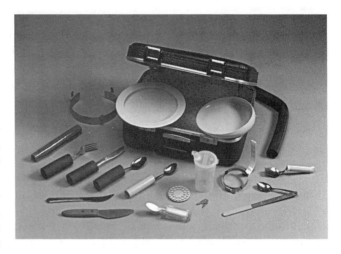

technology. There are many other ways to classify self-care technologies, too. Technology can be minimal or maximal, custom or commercial, appliances or tools (Smith, 1991). A helpful way to review the scope of these technologies is by the functions they perform.

Practitioners may see many individuals using assistive devices and help to select quite a few of them. Often, however, the range of technology encountered in a specific area of practice is narrow. To provide a broad look at assistive technology used in self-care and daily living, this section provides a cross-section of examples. The scope of technologies that occupational therapy practitioners track, just for self-care independence goals, is stunning.

Self-Care Devices

Increasing eating and drinking independence is one purpose for using assistive technologies. Special forks, knives, spoons, bibs, dishes, cups, glasses, and straws can help a person with a mild motor impairment eat independently, or make it easier. Feeding evaluation kits (see Figure 2) are available to help therapists think through the lower tech alternatives. Mealtime aids, a higher tech intervention, can help someone who has severe impairments.

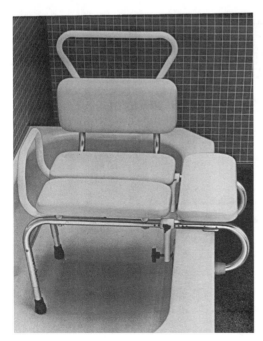

For enabling self-reliance in cleanliness, hygiene, and appearance, there are products that address dental care, eye glasses, hair care, nail care, and shaving. We take toileting and bathing for granted in our daily lives, but they require special methods and devices for many people with disabilities. Toileting technologies include catheters and accessories, ostomy supplies, and devices dealing with incontinence, commodes, toilets and urinals. For bathing, brushes and scrubbing devices, devices for seating, and equipment for helping to move in and out of tubs or showers are available (see Figure 3).

Figure 3. Tub transfer bench. (Photo provided by Fred Sammons, Inc., © BISSELL Healthcare Company)

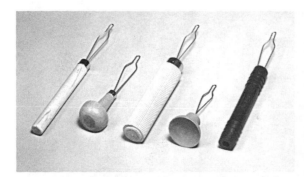

Figure 4. Button aids and amputee button hooks. (Photo provided by Fred Sammons, Inc., © BISSELL Healthcare Company)

Products for assisting in dressing and undressing independence include adaptive clothing for all ages and needs, along with shoes, helmets, dressing devices, shoe aids, stocking aids, and button aids (see Figure 4). Although smoking is clearly identified as a hazardous personal care activity, devices are available to help individuals be more independent in smoking activities. Health care professionals, such as occupational therapists, are often placed in an ethical quandary when considering helping clients become more independent in smoking. This chapter stresses that the role of an occupational therapist is to help a consumer make good decisions. This may mean facilitating the acquisition of an assistive device for smoking if that is the consumer's decision. It is important for the occupational therapist to provide consultation, professional opinions, and assistance in identifying alternatives.

A group of assistive devices for self-care addresses reaching, carrying, holding, dispensing, and transferring objects. Some of these devices are attached to wheelchairs and some to walkers as generic carrying devices like pouches and baskets. Other products hold specific objects, such as telephones or drinking glasses (see Figure 5).

Figure 5a (left). Umbrella holder for wheelchair. **Figure 5b (right).** Heavy duty attachment system for use with golf umbrella. Made by Terri Harworth, OTA student at Sinclair Community College, for individuals with C-7 quadriplegia.

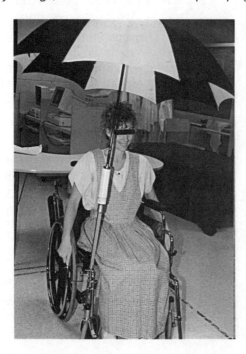
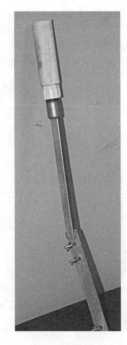

Figure 6. Medi-planner. (Photo provided by Fred Sammon, Inc., © BISSELL Healthcare Company)

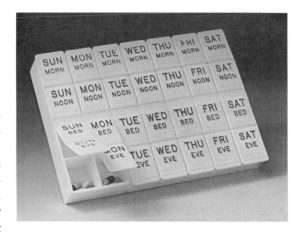

A variety of self-care assistive technologies pertain to an individual taking care of his or her own health. Arm supports and health devices, such as scales, thermometers, medication storage systems, and restraint devices fall into this category (see Figure 6). Other devices in this category have specific uses, such as special sexual devices for people with disabilities or products to assist in child care activities, such as diaper changing.

Home-Care Products

A second classification of assistive technologies includes products that allow an individual to be independent while at home (see Figure 7). These include a wide variety of kitchen appliances and cooking tools for food preparation. Housekeeping items also are a part of home management, as is specifically designed furniture, including beds, tables, chairs, and steps.

Figure 7. Lightweight extended mirror with light for high/low searching. Made by Nancy Hayes, OTA student at Sinclair Community College, for an individual with severe rheumatoid arthritis.

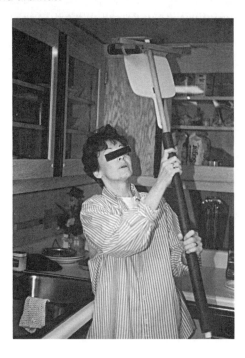
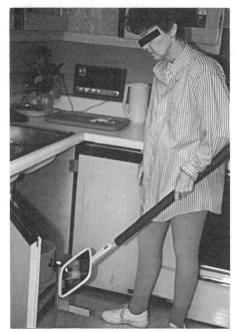

Seating and Mobility

A third major classification includes devices for mobility, and seating and positioning. Wheeled mobility devices include manual and powered wheelchairs. Wheelchair accessories, wheelchair alternatives, transporters, carts, and stretchers are related devices. For walking mobility there are canes, crutches, walkers, and standing equipment. Additionally, seating systems include support devices for parts of the body, seat cushions, car seats, and seating monitors for keeping track of pressure areas.

Communication

An important part of individual self-care is being able to communicate. Mouthwands, headwands, reading aids, book holders, writing utensils, writing guides, typing systems, telephone adaptations, and communication systems for those who are nonvocal and have speech impairments are types of assistive technology allowing an individual to communicate his or her needs (see Figure 8). A specific type of assistive device is signaling equipment. Many types of signaling products are designed for emergency situations. Advancements have been made in this area over the last several years, including monitors for people who wander. These products are triggered by emergencies and are designed to notify help. Centralized communication systems linked by radio can track the situation.

Orthotics and Prosthetics

Orthotics and prosthetics are not often considered self-care devices, but they are critical in self-care management for two reasons. First, independence or optimal efficiency may not be possible for an individual with disabilities without the assistance of some orthotic or prosthetic device. Sometimes these prostheses and orthoses are used in conjunction with other assistive technology to optimize independence and efficiency (see Figure 9). Additionally, individuals who have prosthetic or orthotic devices have special needs pertaining to the devices' maintenance and care. Orthoses and prostheses become extensions of the body and require special techniques and considerations for donning and doffing, laundering, or cleaning.

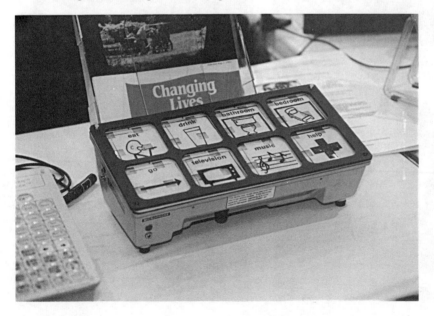

Figure 8.
Introtalker.

Figure 9. Wrist orthosis for use in self-care.

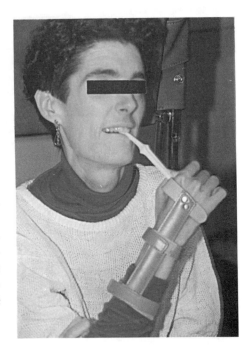

Architecture

Self-care is frequently dependent on architectural design. For example, narrow doorways can prevent self-care activities in the bathroom. It is prudent for occupational therapists to consider architectural assistive technologies in the context of independent living activities. Assistive technologies pertaining to architectural elements include door handles, door locks, hinges, special windows, floor materials, fixtures in the bathroom, public restroom accommodations, kitchen fixtures, and storage needs (see Figure 10). Lighting, safety, security devices, and vertical lifts enable personal care management and independent living.

Environmental Control

Last, controlling the environment is critical. Switching lights off and on, managing room temperature and humidity, and controlling consumer products in the home can be critical activities for independence (see Figure 11). Assistive technologies may include specific switches, remote switches, or switch interfaces that allow an individual with a disability to maintain a safe environment.

This quick overview shows the wide range of daily living assistive technologies that are available. What might not be so apparent is that if an occupational therapist fails to provide information about a product or set of products from this array of possibilities, the consumer may not reach his or her functional potential. Although consumers need to take responsibility for obtaining information about products they purchase, there is also a responsibility placed on the health care professional when dealing with medical or reha-

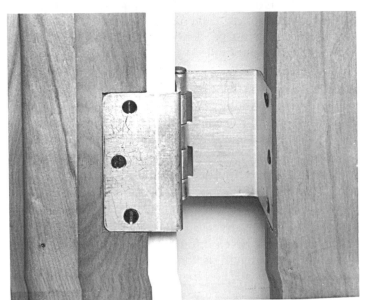

Figure 10. Offset door hinge. (Photo provided by Fred Sammon, Inc., © BISSELL Healthcare Company)

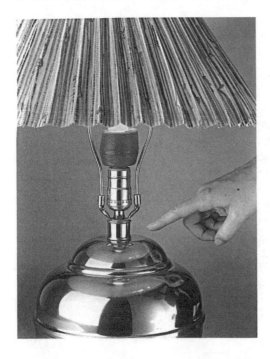

Figure 11. Touch tronic lamp converter. (Photo provided by Fred Sammon, Inc., © BISSELL Healthcare Company)

bilitative care. Occupational therapists must ensure that an individual needing assistive technology is provided with the information required to make the best decisions.

Given this responsibility, it is helpful to know that resources are available to help occupational therapy practitioners. The next section of this chapter reviews the process of choosing the most appropriate assistive technology. Charts, forms, and checklists can help occupational therapists with this task.

Intervention Approaches, Including Assistive Technology

Assistive technologies are not interventions in and of themselves. They are tools and must be integrated into the overall intervention plan to optimize the daily living independence and efficiency of an individual. Providing a piece of equipment is not an outcome. It is a part of a strategy that should be a part of a clearly identified goal. The goal should be clear to all parties involved—the client, reimbursement agency, and therapist.

Assistive technology tools are one of the five ways to help people with disabilities overcome self-care problems. At one end of the spectrum, a person with a disability can be expected to resolve the impairments causing self-care deficits. At the other end, the environment can change the expectations of the person with a disability so he or she no longer needs to perform the required self-care tasks. Examples within this spectrum of the five approaches to overcoming barriers to independence help provide a context for assistive technologies and shows how they are applied in practice.

First, what might be considered an optimal method is to reduce the impairments that result in the self-care deficits. For example, if an individual is extremely weak and is dependent for self-care, solving the weakness problem would solve the self-care deficit. No assistive technology is required with this first approach. Remediating the impairments alleviates the need for any further intervention. Total remediation, however, is not always possible.

A second type of intervention for a person with a disability is to teach compensatory techniques. For example, an individual with hemiplegia, secondary to stroke, may not be able to perform standard tasks bilaterally. Activities such as tying shoes may require new techniques, such as one-handed tying. Although remedial and compensatory techniques often work, they take time and can be costly.

In contrast, the third and fourth approaches can often be implemented more rapidly and at less cost. They require less adaptation by the person with a disability, but they too assume that the impairments are relatively static and that adaptation of other factors in the environment may be more helpful.

The third method is to use tools, or in modern terms, assistive technology. Assistive technology can make the tasks that a person with a disability cannot perform, or can perform only partially or inefficiently, easier and more efficient. A simple example is a rocker knife, which can make cutting food during meals an easier task for someone who cannot use one hand.

The fourth intervention is to change the task so the individual no longer needs to perform it. Therefore, if a person is dependent in a task and the task is removed, it becomes a moot issue. An example of this type of approach is an individual who has trouble with clothing closures and fasteners. The most effective method may be to get rid of the fasteners so they just aren't needed. Pullover shirts can be worn to avoid buttons, and pants with elastic waistbands can be worn to avoid zippers and buckles. Similarly, if someone cannot use his or her oven because of its design or location, the task can be changed by simply using a more accessible microwave oven instead.

Fifth, what a person can do alone with the assistance of technology can be supplemented with human personal assistance. Preparing table settings, providing occasional verbal cues and reminders, putting on orthoses, and placing a bath bench can each facilitate independent activities. While this approach seems least "independent" it can allow a person to make the most use of assistive technology and to maximize activities or parts of activities that can be performed independently. Figure 12 provides an example of all five of these methods through the self-care activity of tying shoelaces.

It is very important to understand that there are five methods for approaching solutions to self-care problems. Assistive technology cannot be applied in a vacuum. Technology is only one possible answer to self-care problems and interacts with all other interventions. Technology should always be considered, but only as one of the approaches that might be used.

These multiple approach concepts are not unique to occupational therapy. There is

Figure 12. Five approaches for tying shoes, including assistive technology.

For an individual who only has the use of one hand, there are five general approaches for intervention. The task of tying shoes is used in this example.

Approach 1 Reduce the impairment:	Approach 2 Build compensatory skills:	Approach 3 Use assistive technologies:	Approach 4 Change the task or task expectations:	Approach 5 Use personal assistance:
Fully rehabilitate so the individual can tie shoes using both hands.	Teach one-handed shoe-tying techniques to the individual.	Use VELCRO® closures, shoe lace button, elastic shoestrings, and so forth.	Use pull-on shoes so shoe tying is not an issue.	Spouse helps tie shoes.

a credence in the thinking that there are many different ways to solve a problem, and sometimes combinations are the best answer. Smith and Sainfort (1989) suggest a model for fitting technology into work environments, using a human factors engineering perspective. The model proposes that balancing the stress across several factors provides the best situation. These authors suggest four components that interact among themselves and with the person's skills and personal attributes: (a) the physical environment, (b) the task itself, (c) the organizational structure in which the work takes place, and (d) the technology. These comprise an overall system that determines a worker's level of stress and productivity. While not discussed in detail here, the concept of balancing approaches is a sensible one to consider in the context of self-care interventions.

History of Self-Care and Technology

Occupational therapy has been applying assistive devices to self-care activities for many decades. Hundreds of articles have been written in journals, and dozens of textbooks and monographs have been published dealing with this topic. Generally speaking, these publications have highlighted do-it-yourself approaches, described existing commercial devices, or focused on product comparisons.

Do-it-Yourself Self-Care Devices

One of the best sources of information about the do-it-yourself fabrication of assistive devices to improve self-care independence is the "New and Brief" department in the *American Journal of Occupational Therapy*. Recent titles include "An Assistive Eye-Drop Mold" (Wisher, 1991), "A Standing Belt" (King, 1989), and "A Folding Dressing Stick" (Lykouretzos & Thompson-Rangel, 1990). In the 1960s, topics included "Assistive Devices for Activities of Daily Living" (Hopkins, 1960), "Electronics for Communication" (Miller & Carpenter, 1964), and "Self-Dressing Techniques for Patients with Spinal Cord Injury" (Runge, 1967). Years before that, articles on assistive devices and self-care ranged from "Adaptations and Apparatus" (Parlin, 1948) and "Occupational Therapy for the Quadriplegic Patient" (Richert, 1950) to "Two Feeding Appliances" (Hall, 1951).

Besides journal articles, texts and monographs contain fabrication notes and construction ideas for self-care assistive devices. For example, a text titled *Assistive Devices for the Handicapped* by Charlot Rosenberg (1968), published by the American Rehabilitation Foundation, includes dozens of products with fabrication diagrams and directions. Topics include daily living, learning and communicating, working, playing, and materials methods. Other documents are more focused. The construction notes by Brown, Bottorf, DePape, and Vanderheiden (1987), for example, focus on devices that are necessary in communication activities. Ford and Duckworth (1987) wrote what is widely recognized as a comprehensive resource for people with quadriplegia.

Publications focusing on "do-it-yourself" techniques are often "fugitive literature." Many of the documents are published in small print runs and are not cited in mainstream bibliographical sources. They quickly go out of print. "Do-it-yourself" journal articles tend not to be referenced in other literature, as they often are superseded by commercially available devices.

Many books exist that describe available devices and specific applications. Comprehensive bibliographies and annotations of these resources are available in the *Assistive Technology Sourcebook* by Enders and Hall (1990).

Commercial Self-Care Devices

The computer age and electronic databases have improved our ability to stay current and go beyond hard copy books, which quickly go out of date. By using modern electronic database formats, information on an assistive technology can be updated more easily and maintained more comprehensively. Abledata is a key database developed more than a decade ago with support from the U.S. Department of Education. At that time, individuals working through a library or other program could access the national computer system using a modem. In the early 1990s, access to Abledata information was extended beyond the central database. A microcomputer desktop version of the database was developed and distributed to individuals and programs throughout the country. Currently, this database is available as "HyperAbledata" (1992) for the Macintosh and "DOS Abledata" (1992) for IBM and compatible computers. In 1992 these databases included more than 17,000 assistive devices.

Assistive devices have moved from a small set of mostly custom-fabricated devices to the thousands of devices available today in the commercial market. Abledata organizes these devices with a thesaurus of terms. The categories of devices pertaining to self-care and independent living are listed in Appendix 1. In the actual Abledata database, each category lists generic products, then the next subcategory lists individual products and brand names. For example, the "spoons" category breaks into feeding spatula, glossectomy feeding spoon, plastisol coated spoon, rubber spoon, side cutting spoon, spoon with built-up handle, spoon with extended handle, spoon with horizontal palmar handle, spoon with offset handle, spoon with vertical palmar handle, swivel spoon, and weighted spoon.

Product Comparison Advances

A third type of resource, comparison publications, evolved as the number of available products increased and the decision-making process for selecting products became more complex. Databases and other product comparison publications both list options and provide information to help compare products.

Databases such as Abledata, HyperAbledata, and DOS Abledata can help compare various product possibilities. Searching what is available and examining a variety of products helps people think through the options. This aids the consumer, because even when actual product samples are not on hand to try, at least they can be discussed. This method can also be used to locate alternative products, which can then be requested from a vendor for trial use or evaluation. In HyperAbledata, pictures of some products are included to help potential users visualize them when no literature is available. Likewise, voice samples are included for speech output devices.

An additional resource recently became available from the Rehabilitation Engineering Center at the National Rehabilitation Hospital (NRH). This Center has a federal grant to evaluate assistive devices. In the past few years, the NRH has coordinated several product evaluation projects and published reports for self-care assistive devices, including bath aids, canes, crutches, walkers, patient lifts, transfer aids, scooters, wheelchair cushions, and toilet aids (Irvine & Siegel, 1990; National Rehabilitation Hospital & ECRI, 1992). While these reports are just beginning to address the need for product comparisons in the field, they do serve somewhat as a consumer guide for these particular products. The volume titled *Independence in the Bathroom*, for example, contains 173 pages of toilet and bath aids reviews. The reviews identify product features and specifications such as type of seat (hard or padded), shape, dimensions, inclusion of lid, adjustability of support legs, type of tip on the support legs, pail capacity, type of monitoring inclusion of a splash guard, inclusion of a handle, inclusion of a cover, warranty, and so forth. This volume also discusses special considerations for choosing toilet and bath aids for people with specific disabling conditions, such as fragile skin and impaired sensation, hemiparesis, lower extremity amputation, upper extremity amputation, and confinement to bed. Other important components of this report address measuring for the appropriate device, bathroom and safety tips, care in maintenance and cleaning, related devices, common architectural modifications, choosing a contractor, funding, and a manufacturers listing.

Also, consumer magazines, such as *Consumer Reports*, are beginning to describe and rate features that are important to people with disabilities, particularly the aging population. The terminology used, however, is not medical. Nonstigmatizing language such as "ease of use," "comfort," and "safety and security" are the types of relevant descriptors.

These product evaluation and comparison volumes are significant, because they weren't available in the earlier years of self-care and independent living assistive technology. Unfortunately, so many types of technologies now exist that it is unlikely that up-to-date and exhaustive evaluative reports for all products will ever be accomplished.

Historical Summary

Several advances in self-care and independent living assistive technologies have been made over the years. Those changes have affected the role of occupational therapists. The literature highlights how there has been a slow shift from a dominating "do-it-yourself" assistive technology orientation to a commercial product orientation. While once occupational therapists needed to learn how to identify self-care problems, design assistive devices, and fabricate them, today there is a much more pressing need to know what commercial products are available and to understand how to select those most appropriate. An occupational therapist's ability to design, create, and modify devices is still an important part of his or her expertise. The need to deal effectively with the increasing numbers of commercial products, however, is an additional required skill.

The move from primarily custom-made to more widely available commercial products has also had a significant effect on occupational therapy practice. The wider availability of mass-market self-care products helps promote this consumer empowerment. Years ago, therapists and other professionals working with people with disabilities had a prescriptive role in selecting assistive devices. Consumers were usually thought of as "patients" and did not often have an active role in the process of selecting an assistive device. Today, however, the situation has changed. The overall climate has shifted from "patient" to "client" to "consumer." Consumers make their own decisions and need accurate information. Occupational therapy practitioners are in an ideal position to help people with disabilities develop consumer skills related to assistive technology.

The contributions of occupational therapy in the delivery of assistive technologies has shifted over the years as well. Many of the most helpful self-care and independent living devices for people with disabilities were developed for and are available as mass market consumer products, sold in department stores or from mail order catalogs. As consumers choose their assistive devices, occupational therapists have become a key resource: They provide information, instruction, and recommendations. Subsequent parts of this chapter further discuss this new role for occupational therapists.

Selecting Self-Care and Independent Living Assistive Technology

The process of selecting the most appropriate assistive technology with an individual is based on matching individual needs to the particular features of assistive devices. The context in which the device is to be used (both the task and the environment) is critical. The number of steps required for matching technology to individual needs varies from many (Rodgers, 1985) to a relatively simpler process. Basically, the process of selecting technology is: (a) understanding the potential of technology, (b) assessing the person within the relevant environments, (c) evaluating technology intervention alternatives, (d) selecting the most appropriate system, (e) acquiring technology, (f) training in the use, maintenance, and repair of the technology, and (g) monitoring and revising the system as appropriate (Smith, 1991). If these steps are kept in mind, decision-making errors can be minimized. The following techniques and considerations address this overall framework.

Assessing the Individual's Needs and Performance

It is critical to begin the process of selecting the most appropriate technology by comprehensively reviewing an individual's self-care and independent living skills and the environments where technologies might be added. This assessment needs to include several components (Enders, undated). First, all of the activities an individual performs need to be methodically assessed to determine the degree of independence the individual has without the assistive technology. Assistive technology is only helpful for tasks in which the person is not already independent. Second, it is essential to determine the individual's self-care priorities and how independent the individual wants to be in each of the specific self-care activities. If an individual does not share the practitioner's values about increased independence or efficiency in self-care tasks, then assistive technology is a fruitless intervention. Third, the helpfulness of assistance for each activity must be examined in terms of the type of assistance provided (e.g., assistive device, attendance, or set-up) and the amount of time it takes. Independence and time are a trade-off. Being able to do a task completely by oneself may not be worthwhile if the cost in time is too burdensome. Last, self-care activities must be viewed across all daily activities. We must not think that, for example, hygiene and appearance self-care tasks are limited only to morning. In reality, hygiene appearance activities are performed throughout the day in work or community settings. People without disabilities carry combs and brushes with them and are able to use them in various locations throughout the day. People with disabilities, therefore, should not be limited to using combs or brushes only during the morning routine. The same is true for going to the toilet or getting a drink of water. To summarize, the person's level of independence, his or her priorities, the benefits of the technology, and the frequency of its use must all be considered. Without evaluating all four, it is difficult to select self-care assistive technology.

The instrument used to assess the individual's level of independence in self-care activities must be acceptable from an occupational therapy frame of reference. In regard to assistive technology, this means it must first be able to assess an individual without the technology. Then it needs to reassess function with the assistive technology to make comparisons and to ascertain the impact of the assistive technology. Thus, the assessment instrument should be capable of measuring both the need and the outcome. It is also important that the functional assessment instrument avoid penalizing function because an individual uses assistive technology. Some assessment scoring systems inherently build assistive technology into the scale. This results in a definition that makes it impossible to be independent if one uses a device because the outcome score is less than maximum.

The assessment system OT FACT (Smith, 1992), available from the American Occupational Therapy Association, is a computerized, comprehensive, functional assessment that includes questions about self-care and independent living. Important features of OT FACT include its value as a self-care and independent living assessment, and its philosophy and recommended protocol for assessing the impact of assistive technology. OT FACT measures the impact of assistive technology on the overall level of function by using a double scoring protocol (Rust & Smith, 1992). OT FACT distinguishes among Environment-Free Scoring, Environment-Adjusted Scoring, and Environment-Assisted Scoring. Environment-Free Scoring measures how a person performs activities without any assistance or outside intervention and reflects only intrinsic abilities. This scoring is then repeated as necessary to observe the individual's abilities over time, to evaluate changes in performance. As intrinsic scores are assessed, the parallel Environment-Adjusted Scores are observed. Environment adjustments involve assistive technology and interventions, such as adapting the task. Environment-Assisted Scoring then includes assistance from an attendant, cuing from a spouse, or hand-over-hand facilitated functional movement. In this way, OT FACT helps monitor the specific needs of an individual, and not only measures the impact of occupational therapy interventions on the individual's intrinsic performance, but reflects the ability of the solutions to supplement an individual's intrinsic attributes and skills. Appendix 2 lists the OT FACT categories related to self-care. Figure 13 shows OT FACT headings scored as Environment-Free Scoring and Environmentally Adjusted Scoring for a man with a high spinal cord injury using assistive technology.

Identifying Assistive Technology Options

The second step in the selection of assistive technology is to identify the available options for the individual based on the assessed needs. This requires information on the technologies available through commercial and other sources, as well as the ability to

Figure 13. Performance with and without assistive technology as measured with OT FACT.

	No Technology	With Technology
Activities of Performance	8%	57%
A. Personal care activities	5%	43%
1. Cleanliness, hygiene, & appearance	1%	1%
2. Medical & health mgmt. activities	1%	10%
3. Nutrition activities	1%	21%
4. Sleep and rest activities	7%	100%
5. Mobility activities	1%	100%
6. Communication activities	10%	92%
B. Occupational role related activities	4%	78%
1. Home management activities	13%	64%
2. Consumer activities	8%	83%
3. Employment & volunteer prep. act.	1%	98%
4. Caregiving activities	12%	75%
5. Employer activities	1%	99%
6. Community activities	1%	89%
7. Avocational activities	1%	55%

determine the quality of the information. Decision making is facilitated if one is able to use the information to reduce the number of possible alternatives.

Locating Information on Assistive Technology

While many information searching methods are available, there is no single unassailable method. No flowcharts or formulas exist to sequence questions or to define the most appropriate answer. Several computerized expert systems that apply artificial intelligence techniques to help locate information are being studied. But state-of-the-art methods are still based on problem solving and intuitive logic and are heavily dependent on combining skill, luck, imagination, and curiosity. This is true whether one pages through catalogs, examines files, uses the library, or accesses an electronic database.

This is a complex process. The multitude of technologies on the market today and the constant changes in all the manufacturers' product lines make it virtually impossible for any one person to know about all the available technologies. In fact, as much as 30% of product information changes each year. Many occupational therapists feel that something is wrong if they cannot immediately provide all of the information needed to help someone with technology needs. It is a rare therapist, however, who can truly do this, even in a focused technology specialty. The key is to know how to use appropriate information resources in order to obtain the most up-to-date information.

To locate the most helpful information on an assistive technology topic, the search must be focused. A broad request to an information source (reference librarian, an expert in the field, or an electronic database) such as, "Please give me everything you have on X, Y, Z," usually results in a general overview of the range of information available on this broadly defined topic. Or, dangerously, an information specialist may arbitrarily define the topic and provide an entirely wrong set of information. If the information seeker is not aware of how this information was collected and provided, he or she may mistakenly assume that it is the best available. A third response to an information request that is too general is to acquire everything on the topic. Acquiring too much information may not be very helpful because combing through it could be time consuming and confusing.

With assistive technology, well-targeted questions are not always easy to formulate. Therefore, it is helpful to have a full needs assessment put together before trying to find the right assistive technology product. Figure 14 provides a framework of questions that should be answered before trying to find what assistive technologies might be appropriate.

Bias is a critical factor to remember when a vendor provides information about products. Vendors frequently make user decisions (consciously or unconsciously) on the basis of business decisions, such as what products are in stock at the time, which manufacturers have established accounts, or even which product gives the highest profit margin. Although this assertion on vendor bias is quite harsh, and the field has many ethical vendors, vendors cannot avoid the subtle bias that comes from knowing their own products the best. Even if they suspect there might be another, better, product that they don't stock, it is easiest for them to highlight their own. An occupational therapist must remain open minded to alternative vendors and products.

As obvious as it seems, it is important to remember that assistive technologies do not work the same way for every person or in different environments. For example, a grab bar may be a good solution in a clinical simulation, but in a particular home it may not work in the client's bathtub. When funding is not available to perform evaluations, site visits to the home or workplace, the consumers themselves, or a friend or family member should

Figure 14. Helpful questions to think through before selecting assistive technology.

Person and task considerations

1. What are the major tasks the user wants to accomplish?
2. What are the user's functional abilities and inabilities?
   - motor: grasp endurance, range of motion, etc.
   - sensory: visual, auditory, tactile, etc.
   - cognitive: knowledge, memory, ability to learn, etc.
   - psychosocial: willingness to try something new, gadget tolerance, frustration level, etc.
3. Will the level of disability change?
4. Is the person independent or attendant assisted?
5. Will the person need extensive training to use the equipment?
6. Is the equipment intended for long- or short-term use?
7. Are there environmental restrictions, like space or wiring?
8. Is a portable product required?
9. Will the user need accessories and other options in the future?
10. What are cleaning, maintenance, and repair requirements?
11. What resources are available for providing cleaning, maintenance, or repair for the product?
12. What are the health and safety considerations?
13. What funding is available, and are there budget limitations for purchase?
14. What funding is available, and what are the budget limitations for future repair?

Product considerations

1. What are the motor requirements (range of motion, strength) required for use of this product?
2. Is the product used independently by the consumer or with the help of an attendant?
3. What are the size dimensions and environmental requirements of the product?
4. What safety features are required for using this product?
5. What are the power requirements of the product?
6. What materials are used, and are they strong enough for the intended use?
7. What is the weight of the device?
8. Is the device portable, or does it require permanent installation?
9. How difficult is the device to clean and repair?
10. What is the process for getting the device cleaned or repaired?
11. What is the warranty?
12. Are other products needed in conjunction with this product for complete system function?
13. What is the reputation of the distributor and the manufacturer of this product?
14. Will this product soon be obsolete?
15. Are there other effective alternatives besides this product?

Figure 15. The perils of considering assistive technology outside the real environment.

An occupational therapy department always ordered a particular bath bench for everyone. In principle, it was ideal for a wide variety of people. However, in this particular department there was no real bathtub to set it up for trial use. When one of the therapists moved to another hospital where there was a real bathroom setting, the usual bath bench was only rarely used. With a bit of investigating, the therapist discovered why. It was never ordered for wheelchair users because the legs in the highest position of the seat were 4 inches below standard wheelchair seat height with a seat cushion. None of the wheelchair users who received the bench had ever complained at the old hospital—they just didn't use it. This is a real problem. Funding for a device is usually only available once in a given number of years. After being purchased, many assistive technologies cannot be returned, and there is no way to obtain a second round of funding.

be enlisted to measure the environment. Remembering to consider needs specific to each individual and particular environment can avoid unfortunate situations (see Figure 15).

Evaluating the Quality of Available Information Resources

Before an information resource is used, its content must be scrutinized. The words used to "advertise" an information book (e.g., a guide or directory) or a database usually provide a strong indication of its developers' knowledge. Phrases like "the most comprehensive," "the only up-to-date resource," "a single information resource for all of your needs," or "the complete directory available for the first time," are marketing tools and selling tactics. Information resource developers who are truly knowledgeable and ethical about the quality of their information systems rarely make these claims. They know that any information resource is just repackaged information about other programs or products. To have information available in a directory or database, the developer has to locate, abstract, enter, and edit it. This process usually takes 6 to 12 months. There is no way one source can have all of the information available on even one assistive technology specialty.

The number of entries in a specific resource also provides critical information on how complete it might be—a total listing of a few hundred products, facilities, or publications is not a comprehensive guide for assistive technologies for self-care and independent living. Some directories claiming to be comprehensive have relatively few listings.

Some information systems claim to match technology to disabilities. For these systems it is critical to know what decision-making process is used. While computerized decision aids, called "expert systems," will be one of the major advances made in the next 10 years, expert systems are now tentative and futuristic. Occupational therapy practitioners should not take for granted that any information system claiming to locate the products necessary for an individual is thorough in its evaluation and analysis of the available products. For example, every self-care activity requires a certain degree of strength, range of motion, and motivation. It is necessary to identify how these were included in the process of selecting devices. The knowledge base and credibility of the person classifying the products must be taken into consideration. It is increasingly important for occupational therapists to be able to recognize the strengths and weaknesses of "expert systems" that claim to identify appropriate self-care assistive technologies.

The assistive technology field changes rapidly. As mentioned earlier, as many as 30% of assistive technology products have information that has changed within a 12-month period (new manufacturer phone number or address, new price, new product features, obsolete products). Therefore, it is important to know how old the information is in a resource guide or database, and how often it is updated. The high frequency of information turnover also makes it prudent to know the lag time between when the information is collected and when it is received. If the lag time of a collection of data is more than 1 year, it is likely that a large percentage of the information will no longer be up-to-date. It is also helpful to know whether the update just adds more products or whether it edits the existing product entries.

Finally, it is helpful to know how the producer of the information system addresses quality control issues. Quality control usually includes technical procedures, such as standards or policies, for assigning search vocabulary or indexed keywords. Quality searches require consistency in keyword coding. Systems without careful, consistent coding may identify some key products or information, but similar items coded in a different way won't be found. At the very least, it is important to be aware that this problem can exist and to take it into consideration when strategizing an information search. If comprehensive information is being solicited, several searches using different search strategies might be required.

Refining the Alternatives

Catalogs, databases, and other information resources all help to identify assistive technology alternatives. A few specific tools are provided here to help guide the search process.

A self-care device worksheet (see Figure 16) provides students or new graduates with a way of formulating a problem-solving approach to help identify assistive device needs. Additionally, it may be helpful for an experienced practitioner to examine the parameters on this worksheet periodically to fine tune assistive device searching skills. Sometimes experienced practitioners can fall into ruts. Reconsidering that the esthetics or durability of a device might be a particularly important feature for an individual can be helpful. This worksheet is intended to stimulate thinking regarding individualized needs for clients and to provide a helpful way of taking notes to document these needs.

Figure 16. Self-care device worksheet.

ADL Problem Identified: _____

Proposed Assistive Device: _____

Consideration factors

Cost:

    Is there insurance coverage?

    Client's remaining cost?

    Client's budget?

    Other funding options?
    (church, community service clubs,
    diagnostic associations)

Psychological Factors:

    How does client feel about using device?

    Considerations they want to be aware of?

    How will device fit into client's body image?

(continued)

Figure 16. (continued)

Physical factors: Identify any special needs for using the device in the following:
 	
      Range of motion
 	
      Muscle strength
 	
      Sensation
 	
      Cognition
 	
      Perception	

Esthetics: Note any client preferences for:
 	
      Color
 	
      Materials
 	
      Style
 	
      General appearance	

Size:
 	
      Where will the item be used?
 	
      Where will the item be stored?
 	
      Will it need to be portable or transported?	

Durability:
 	
      Length of time of proposed use
 	
      Frequency of use
 	
      How hard is client on equipment?	

Maintenance:
 	
      Hygiene considerations
 	
      Replacement parts
 	
      Assistance requirements	

Availability:
 	
      When is item needed?
 	
      Is trial use recommended?	

Operation:
 	
      Will device significantly improve client's performance?
 	
      Method for retrieval, donning/doffing
 	
      Assistance available if needed?	

Miscellaneous discussion:
Does client have a personal preference for purchase source? Are family or friends able to assist with any construction?

Once a search of the assistive device alternatives has been made, it is helpful to compare one device to another. For example, five or six bath benches might be selected from a database of information and provided to a consumer to help think through the advantages and disadvantages of each. The assistive device comparison checklist (Figure 17) is a way for the practitioner and the consumer to talk through the various options to make a decision. Choosing an assistive device means working with the client and/or family in the decision-making process. This works best when an overview of the entire search and selection process is reviewed with the individual who needs to use the products, before starting the search. Once alternatives are identified, the user and the practitioner can compare the options. Ownership of the assistive technology device must transfer from the occupational therapy practitioner, who has the idea that a device might solve a functional problem, to the consumer. The consumer needs not only to own the device physically, but psychologically. If the consumer does not recognize the need and help choose the particular device, then most likely the equipment should not even be purchased.

Computers are playing more and more of a role in the product selection process. The Lifease Company announced a software program in 1992 that helps therapists identify self-care devices and adaptations for the gerontology population. The program helps

Figure 17. Assistive device comparison checklist.

	Item A	Item B	Item C	Item D	Item E
Assistive device description					
Source					
Cost					
Psychosocial factors					
Physical factors					
Esthetics					
Size					
Durability					
Maintenance					
Availability					
Operation					
Comments (pro/con)					

evaluate the needs of the individual and the environment. It then provides ideas for interventions, including devices and environmental modifications (Joe, 1992).

Trial Use

When possible, the potential device should be tried prior to its final purchase. Some devices can be designated for trial use and training within an occupational therapy department. Cooperative agreements can often be set up for therapists working independently to borrow products from other occupational therapy programs or agencies.

Equipment vendors often stock items that can be borrowed on trial if proper hygiene precautions are followed. Vendors will frequently even arrange a loan from a manufacturer's representative or from the company directly if the product isn't in stock.

Consumers can sometimes order a device directly through a vendor with an option to return it if it does not work, with the exception of bathing and toileting aids. However this may take weeks, which can delay assistive technology device decisions, and risks the cost of return shipping.

Occupational therapy practitioners can also use available resources to simulate the item being contemplated as closely as possible or can use a similar product. This might identify potential problems prior to the final decision being made. Sometimes this means trying a product similar to the one being targeted, accompanied by a discussion of how the actual targeted device differs from the particular one being examined.

Infection control measures always need to be considered prior to a client using an item involving personal hygiene contact. Items that are stocked in a department for repeated use should be cleaned and, if necessary, sterilized routinely. Some items considered expendable cannot be returned, cleaned, or reused if personal contact is made. Sometimes disposable covers can be kept on items while a client is simulating an activity. If questions arise regarding correct hygienic procedures, the infection control department of any hospital is a good resource. In today's hospitals there are special procedures for cleaning devices, especially when blood-borne pathogens are involved.

Every occupational therapy practitioner has observed low and high technology systems left unused. Home health therapists routinely find equipment stored away in closets, and clients frequently are not even aware of what they have. To avoid this problem, the consumer and his or her family must be involved in the product selection process. One way of doing this is to participate in a trial use of the item. Usually after completing a trial the client and the family are equipped to make a decision with the guidance and opinions of the therapist. An item may be rejected for multiple reasons, and it is important to identify them. Whether the therapist thinks the item is successful or not is of little consequence. If the client perceives the technology negatively in any way, it is highly probable that the equipment will not be used.

Training

Once the assistive technology decision has been made, training should be begin immediately. If the item has been ordered, it will take some time to obtain. Simulated training can sometimes be substituted. It is critical for the user to understand the device thoroughly in order to use it successfully.

Training should be directed to the user, but should not stop there. Others in the environment who will be using or dealing with the device also require training. For example, an eating utensil may be used by a particular individual, but it may be washed by others in the family. Both the consumer and the family members need specific information on relevant aspects of use and maintenance.

Training should always be done with respect to where the client will use the device. Occupational therapy does not usually occur in the individual's home environment or in the other environments where the self-care technology might be used. Some self-care tasks may be done differently in the hospital, at home, at school, or at work. Training should consider all of these settings.

The consumer of the self-care technology may need to teach others how it works. Thus, the occupational therapist may need to help the consumer feel comfortable and skillful as a trainer. The consumer is often the best conveyor of information and training to others who need to learn about a device. It can be very beneficial to have the client actually train another therapist or family member in the use of the device under the supervision of the occupational therapist. In this format, if the client has difficulties, the occupational therapist can help point out missing information or suggest other methods for explaining the features of the equipment.

To optimize therapy's efficiency, it is sometimes helpful to design assignments that the client completes at home independently. Upon return, the client and therapist can discuss how the task went. Some of the more complex assistive technologies cannot be learned through quick instruction. Augmentative communication devices and their interface technologies often require extensive training. Thus, it can be very helpful to take the assistive device into the natural environments in which it is used and report back on its success. Sometimes devices require practice, which can be done outside of therapy sessions. The client can then report on how the practice sessions have been going. Training is extremely important for many devices, but it is frequently overlooked. Self-care and independent living devices rarely come with owner's manuals.

Training is not always a one-time occurrence. Sometimes training needs to be reinforced or updated, depending on the particular needs of an individual. While this seems logical enough, if a therapist does not set up a follow-up system, it is often overlooked.

Owner's Manual

Much self-care technology is too simple to have an accompanying owner's manual from the manufacturer. It may be complex enough though, to be confusing to someone who has never seen such a device before. Assistive technologies frequently take special care and maintenance. For example, many devices are made with plastics that can only sustain low levels of heat. Microwave ovens, automatic dishwashers, hot air laundry, dryers, and car dashboards can easily exceed the plastic's heat tolerance. These kinds of details may seem obvious to an occupational therapist, but if they are not explained carefully to the consumer, the device may be inadvertently damaged.

It sometimes makes sense for a therapist to actually write an "owner's manual." Creativity and careful thinking are the keys for writing owner's manuals—they do not need to be restricted to a written format. Making a home video of the consumer using, cleaning, and storing the product is a type of owner's manual. Audiotaped messages can supplement written instructions. When written instructions are provided, illustrations or pictures are helpful.

Some of the topics that should be included in the owner's manual are proper use, maintenance, precautions, and replacement procedures. Educational research indicates that information targeted to the general public should be geared to a grade-school reading level. It is important for occupational therapy practitioners to be sensitive to this and customize the owner's manual to the particular educational, social, and cultural needs of the client. In any case, wording should be concise. The client and family should review the instructions prior to taking the device and demonstrate that they understand the manual.

Follow-Up

After an individual uses a self-care or independent living device, a follow-up procedure is almost always helpful. Follow-up is most effective when it is scheduled during the time that the individual is initially given a device. If ongoing therapy is provided, it is easy to reevaluate the use of the equipment periodically. This may not be the case if an individual lives a great distance from the occupational therapist, or if funding is not available for follow-up visits. A follow-up schedule might be set up at 6-week, 3-month, 6-month, and 1-year intervals. The success of a system can usually be evaluated and any modifications, tune-ups, or replacements can be made during those times.

If it is not possible to schedule follow-up sessions with the client, many creative options are available. These include: (a) making periodic phone calls to get feedback and to provide support to the client at home, (b) involving other health care professionals if continuing service is provided by someone else—another service provider can give feedback to the initial occupational therapist on specific issues, (c) tapping an involved case worker or ongoing advocacy person to provide feedback, and (d) instructing the client to report any problems to the occupational therapist (if the client is capable). Self-responsibility is an important characteristic, with or without a disability. Telling the client that it is his or her responsibility to stay in contact with the occupational therapist is often very successful. But therapists should not use this as an easy way out, and other follow-up mechanisms are often necessary. While follow-up is the key to maintaining a high quality of service, funding may constrain it. Occupational therapy practitioners must continually innovate and press for fundable ways to provide these important services.

Funding

Lack of adequate funding can be a major obstacle to improving functional performance through assistive technology. Funding sometimes depends on the setting in which the occupational therapist practices. Occupational therapists who charge their time directly to third party reimbursers (such as inpatient and outpatient clinics, home health) can sometimes bundle inexpensive assistive technologies into the cost of their services. Occupational therapists who do not charge their services to third party reimbursers (i.e., therapists working in school systems) may have a more difficult time acquiring devices for their clients. While it is beyond the scope of this chapter to discuss fully different funding options and methods for obtaining resources, a few comments are prudent.

Therapists should know how much assistive technologies cost. Costs should always be one of the variables that are considered when recommending a particular device. The best procedure is to make sure the client and family are aware of the various costs of the devices so they can factor this in when making their decision. Clients should never be surprised when they receive the bill for assistive technology.

Many federal laws have opened doors for paying for assistive technologies. Even funding agencies that have not yet agreed to pay for assistive technologies may someday concede that assistive technologies are a cost-effective way of improving and/or maintaining the functional abilities of individuals with disabilities.

Another important concept to consider when searching for funds for assistive technology is that any funding agency will only provide payment for specified reasons related to its mission. Medical insurance providers must believe that a particular device is necessary because of the medical needs of an individual. Educational funding providers need to believe that self-care devices are important for the education of a student within their system. Vocational funding providers need to believe that the self-care devices may affect the vocational readiness or success of an individual seeking or trying to maintain employment. Occupational therapists may need to write letters of justification to these various funding agencies and orient the wording describing the specific needs for the assistive device to reflect each agency's function.

Funding self-care and independent living assistive technologies is not a simple issue. It is intricately tied to the mechanisms of service delivery and society's perception of the importance of assistive technology (La Buda, 1988; Rein, 1988). The current funding situation is extremely complex. For many years, people assumed that health insurance would pay for all rehabilitative and assistive technology. However health insurance was initially designed to pay for health needs, not for the needed equipment to help someone become independent. In affluent times, third party payers began funding equipment in the "grey area." Today's economic situation, together with the escalation of costs associated with equipment and the amount of equipment now available to help people, threatens the easy access of funding for assistive technology. How to make insurers pay for assistive technology sometimes seems like the issue, but medical insurers never meant to pay for self-care and independent living assistive technology. There are no easy answers.

Issues Surrounding the Application of Self-Care Assistive Technology

Consumer Empowerment

The role of the consumer in selecting devices cannot be overemphasized. Occupational therapists in medical settings have historically thought of assistive technologies from an orthotic or prosthetic perspective, with the therapist and/or physician prescribing a device for the individual with a disability. This conceptual model must vanish. Over the past 20 years, it has become more and more evident from many clinical and scholarly observations that for successful assistive technology use the consumer must "buy in" to the device. The role of an occupational therapist, therefore, is not to do an assessment and select a device for an individual with a disability, but to serve as a resource for helping a consumer do a needs assessment of his or her own disabilities and functional abilities, and to provide options and suggestions for ways of overcoming barriers to optimal function. There are many ways for occupational therapists to include consumers in the process of obtaining and integrating assistive technologies into their lives (Enders, undated).

While the client's disabilities and impairments are being assessed, a technology needs assessment can be done as a joint effort between the occupational therapy practitioner and the client. Identifying the particular functional problems and impairments that contribute to the overall dependence of an individual (or, conversely, identifying what is needed to assist a person in becoming independent) can be identified by the team. Once the needs have been identified, they can be prioritized, and goals can be set. Again, a team of the occupational therapist and the client works best. When a client is not cognitively or emotionally ready to be involved in this process, other members of the client's family can act as advocates.

When goals for independence and living have been developed and prioritized, brainstorming with the client helps to identify the full range of possible solutions. Alternatives identified earlier in the chapter can be discussed with the client: (a) remedy the impairment, (b) learn skills to compensate for the impairment, (c) use assistive technologies, (d) change the task so the individual no longer needs to perform it, (e) use assistance for tasks or task components, or (f) use combinations of the above. Develop an action plan based on the alternative(s) selected. Realistically prioritize steps in the mutually agreed upon plan. If there is a question about the feasibility or availability of resources or skills, agree on a back-up plan in case the first choice doesn't work.

The client should also be involved in the training and follow-up methods needed for integrating the technology.

To highlight some of the issues and the viewpoints of a consumer during the assistive technology selection process, one of this chapter's authors interviewed a client who increasingly needed assistive technology (see Figure 18).

Figure 18. Consumer viewpoint on assistive devices.

C.H. is a 38-year-old woman who has been diagnosed with amyotrophic lateral sclerosis (ALS) for 10 years. She uses a powered wheelchair and requires maximum assistance for all self-care. She has worked with occupational therapy and used a variety of assistive devices as her status has changed over the years.

C.H.: As a patient I didn't know what was out there or what I needed, but I did know what I couldn't do. My first step was to learn what was on the market. Once I did that, trial use was the only way to really find out what would work.

OT: Would you have been comfortable purchasing an item without trying it?

C.H.: No! I have done that and it can be a waste of money.

OT: Have assistive devices been ordered that you have not used?

C.H.: Yes. Mostly things I had not tried. I didn't feel good about paying for something I didn't end up using.

OT: How do you feel about having more than one option?

C.H.: It's really important to have more than one choice. Sometimes you are not ready for something even though you really need it. Knowing what is out there and being presented choices helps with that. Pushing someone into a certain device is not a good approach to me, although I realize some people do need to be pushed. It was important for me to be believed when I said I wasn't ready for something and not be pushed. If I had ordered something I was not ready to accept, I probably wouldn't use it.

OT: What importance do you place on esthetics?

C.H.: It used to be more important to me than it is now, but I like to look as normal as I can. I like things to look as nonmedical as possible. As weak as my neck is, I don't want my head strapped unless I have to.

OT: Is cost something of a factor?

C.H.: It should always be considered. My insurance is good so it has not been a factor for me as much as some people.

OT: Has the specific company selected from which to purchase equipment been important to you?

C.H.: Not really. I wanted recommendations from therapists that knew the companies so I could use someone reputable. I wanted good follow-up if I had any problems and someone easy to contact and help with maintenance if it was needed.

(continued)

Figure 18. (continued)

> OT: What psychological factors do you think are important?
>
> C.H.: I needed mental preparation for depending on an assistive device. I found that if I was not ready in my mind, I wasn't likely to use a device. When I was ready, I'd usually think, "Why didn't I do this a long time ago?"
>
> OT: How can a therapist assist with this process?
>
> C.H.: I don't think they can, other than to provide options and be patient. It is a personal thing that needs to be dealt with in your own mind. It takes time. A good approach for me is to know what my options are. Then when I'm ready, I can pursue getting something. When I first looked at computers to assist me, it was another year before I decided I was ready to get one. When you have to depend on something, you're admitting you've lost something.
>
> OT: What do you see as an occupational therapist's role?
>
> C.H.: To work with me as a partner. No one wants to be told what to do, but we don't always know what we need. So I see the occupational therapist as a resource and someone who can help me find what will work best for me. And the only way they can do that is to work together with me.
>
> OT: How do you feel about homemade equipment versus manufactured equipment?
>
> C.H.: Homemade items are usually a lot cheaper and that can be a factor. It doesn't matter to me as long as it does the job. I have known people that can make things for me, but you lose the option of trial use before something is made.
>
> OT: If you were not cognitively able to make your decisions regarding obtaining equipment, who would you want taking this role?
>
> C.H.: Definitely my family!

Independence Versus Efficiency Trade-Off

A critical trade-off is often made when using an assistive device for self-care or independent living. Many times, assistive devices allow someone to be independent in self-care. This can be a significant cost–benefit. The cost of a device may be relatively low, and if it actually helps somebody who might otherwise require personal assistance in self-care activities, substantial savings can result. A frequent problem, however, is that even though an assistive device may make someone more independent, it may now take 10, 20, or even 50 times longer to perform the activity independently then if someone simply assisted. Early morning activities are a common example of this paradox between independence and efficiency. Although assistive technology may enable someone to be totally independent in dressing, cleanliness, hygiene, and appearance-related activities, if he or she has a severe motor disability, it might take 3 to 4 hours to perform all these functions independently. A personal assistant could help the individual achieve these tasks within 30 to 60 minutes. Fatigue is also a critical consideration. Independence may result in ineffective functioning during later parts of the day.

From a societal perspective, this is a very difficult trade-off. Society can choose to fund the assistive technology, the wages of the personal assistant, or both. This places the decision makers in an awkward position. Assuming that the assistive technology costs nothing, there is an implicit comparison between the cost of having someone provide assistance to the person with a disability and the lost time no longer available for the person if he or she performs the task independently. Personal preferences are vital. Some individuals highly value their independence, while others value their time more. Figure 19 portrays this problem as a cost–benefit formula.

Figure 19. Simple cost–benefit comparison between self-care independence and time efficiency.

- Value of being independent = **Val of Indep**

- Assistive technology device cost = **AT Cost**

- Costs of an assistant's wages = **Cost AW**

- Lost time available of the person with the disability = **LT Available**

- Resulting overall cost = **Overall Cost**

> Formula for optimizing independence:
> **Val of Indep + AT Cost + Cost AW - LT Available = Overall Cost**

If one cancels out the **AT Cost** and the **Val of Indep**, this cost–benefit problem reduces to being simply a comparison between the **Cost AW** versus the **LT Available.**

Ideally, this trade-off is not necessary. If an individual can be efficient with the use of assistive technology, then the costs reduce to only being the cost of the assistive technology. Obviously this is the optimal target.

Prescription or Open Market Purchase

The issue of consumerism reveals an important paradox. If indeed some assistive technologies and devices are available to consumers in mass market outlets, then why shouldn't they all be available on the open market? Why involve occupational therapists? A total open market system might not be any better than the prescriptive system from which we are slowly evolving. When buying laundry detergent or apples from a grocery store, consumers expect to have access to all the information they need to make good purchasing decisions. For an individual with rheumatoid arthritis who is purchasing a device, however, this may not be possible. A particular assistive device could be medically contraindicated and might actually stress joints improperly. Depending on how the catalog or department store happens to be marketing the device, a purchase might be made that aggravates the condition. Additionally, assistive technology products are not always easily understood. Assistive device consumers often do not have the information they need about options and features and the advantages and disadvantages of each. Occupational therapists play an important role as an information resource. Additionally, an individual requiring an assistive technology device for one aspect of self-care commonly has other activity difficulties that might benefit from another type of assistive technology or intervention. An occupational therapist can provide an overall perspective by asking about other needs and suggesting additional solutions. An important ingredient in this process is for occupational therapists to have the background and expertise to serve as this resource.

Compliance: An Outmoded Concept

Years ago, from the medical prescriptive model, the word *compliance* was used as a measure of successful integration of assistive technology into the lives of people with a disability. It was thought that assistive devices ended up sitting in closets because users did not comply with the direction of health care providers. This issue is important enough to be highlighted here. User selection of and satisfaction with assistive technology indicate its successful integration. Evaluating how well a client complies with the instructions of some professional is an outmoded idea for the application of assistive technology. If a user doesn't "comply" with using an assistive technology, it is likely that the consumer was not adequately involved in the selection process.

Rogers and Holm (1992) suggest that more attention be paid to the issue of successful use of assistive technology devices by people with arthritis. They report that while the literature has definitional inconsistencies with terms, and difficulties generalizing across cultures and populations, it does provide information to theorize a predictive model. Rogers and Holm propose a predictive model that includes the consumer's perspective. Because of the consumer-oriented movement, we will likely see more models that include predictive variables, such as the extent of consumer involvement in device selection and the consumer's stated need for the technology.

Vendor Roles

Occupational therapy departments have sometimes taken on the responsibility of being direct vendors of assistive technology products, particularly in the area of self-care. It made sense for occupational therapists working in inpatient or outpatient rehabilitation to be able to go to the closet and select a self-care device for use by an individual currently receiving services. Consequently a stock of inventory was developed, and occupational therapists became vendors. Obviously, there are some advantages and disadvantages to this situation, as well as advantages and disadvantages to mechanisms such as having a preferred supplier or having an open market with no supplier preference.

Occupational Therapy Vendor

An advantage of being a vendor of self-care devices is the convenience of being able to provide a device to the client on the spot. When an occupational therapy program is able to vend a product directly, third party reimbursers sometimes pay for it more readily, as it is incorporated into the occupational therapy costs. Disadvantages of this model include higher prices because of the occupational therapy department's overhead (purchasing, managing the inventory, and billing). It is also difficult to stock a wide variety of items (e.g., numerous types of wheelchair seat cushions are available, yet very few occupational therapy departments can maintain an inventory of more than a few of the options). Consumers often perceive occupational therapists who have taken this vendor role as salespeople and feel obligated to purchase the therapist's recommendation when it is handed to them for use in a therapy session. When occupational therapists are vendors themselves, they fall into the trap of vendors and tend to recommend the items that they know best, which are the ones in stock. This bias limits the consumer's options.

Use of Preferred Equipment Supplier

Another option is the use of a durable medical equipment dealer or an equipment supplier who has a business in the community. Sometimes focusing on one particular supplier is advantageous because the occupational therapist can become familiar with the inventory. Another advantage is that occupational therapists have no direct responsibility for financing the equipment. Consumers then assume some responsibility for purchasing the device from the supplier, which may lead to greater integration of the device into the person's life. A third advantage is that the consumer becomes familiar with the process of obtaining equipment from a vendor in the community and may be more confident reusing this system in the future.

Of course there are some disadvantages to this model. It is less convenient than buying from an occupational therapist, and it can be physically difficult for a consumer to get to different locations as needed. Also, there are some fraudulent businesses that only have the "bottom-line" dollar in mind, as opposed to the needs of people with disabilities, and take advantage of consumers.

Open Market Suppliers

A third vending option is for occupational therapists to stay out of product acquisition entirely and leave all of the procedures for acquiring the device up to the consumer. This sometimes can be done when a therapist provides a variety of catalogs to the consumer, who makes his or her own decisions. This can also be done in large metropolitan areas where there are many different vendors available in the community and where a therapist only needs to provide a list of them to the consumer, who can hunt around to find the device from the vendor of his or her choice.

An advantage of this model is that the consumer becomes totally responsible for self-care and decision making. This is likely to lead to a high level of product use because the consumer will have already made a substantial commitment by purchasing the device on his or her own. One disadvantage is that the consumer assumes all financial responsibility. Additionally, consumers are sometimes overwhelmed by the process and simply stop it. Thus, they fail to purchase the assistive technology device even if it may help them. And when dealing with many different companies with extremely good marketing and advertising departments, a consumer can be potentially talked into different, inappropriate items.

In this model, the consumer is responsible for evaluating the vendor. He or she may only be concerned about the purchase cost of the device and buy an item from a "fly-by-night" operation or from a vendor who provides no services whatsoever. Also, if a client needs something but depends on caregivers for its acquisition, there may be a problem if the caregivers don't understand the particular needs of the device or don't take the time to obtain it.

None of these models is perfect, but perhaps if all three were made available to the consumer, he or she could choose from the advantages and disadvantages of each.

As can be seen, there are many vending options for assistive technologies. All have their advantages and disadvantages. Perhaps the key component that allows any of these systems to work is the role the occupational therapist takes. If the occupational therapist serves as a resource for individuals with disabilities in self-care and independent living assistive devices, avoids vendor bias, and provides recommendations and options based on decisions made jointly with the consumer, any one of these models can turn out to be of major benefit.

Purchase, Adapt, or Fabricate?

If assistive technology has been decided on as a component of an individual's intervention to optimize independence and efficiency, buying a device may not be the best answer. Another approach is to take a mass market or special assistive technology device and further adapt it for the particular needs of an individual. A standard table utensil might only require a built-up handle. With the help of a technician or engineer, an occupational therapist can design and fabricate assistive technologies from scratch that exactly match the particular needs of the individual when other approaches don't work.

Cost is an obvious variable when deciding to purchase, adapt, or fabricate. Unfortunately, cost is not a simple variable. There are two types of costs involved in this discussion: the assistive technology or the parts and materials; and the time of the person who designs, adapts, or fabricates the device. These need to be examined on a case-by-case basis. In some circumstances, there are plentiful human resources available for design and fabrication, but few resources for purchasing materials or parts. Examples are a school system, veterans' administration hospital, or community agency. In these situations the professional's time is already paid for, but supplies and equipment are additional lines in the budget that are not directly reimbursed. On the other hand, some settings can pay for materials and parts, but cannot withstand personnel costs associated with the equipment's design, adaptation, and fabrication. Examples are occupational therapy departments in hospitals, home health agencies, or other medical programs where the time spent with assistive device design and fabrication would be charged to third party payers for reimbursement. When this cost is compared to the off-the-shelf price of an assistive device, it often becomes much more prudent simply to purchase the equipment.

Obviously a second major consideration in the decision to purchase, adapt, or fabricate is whether a mass market device is available, whether a device is available but needs to be adapted, or whether no device exists. Therapists must be cognizant of what assistive technologies are already available. It makes no sense to redesign the wheel when the wheel is available. Once again, this emphasizes the importance of knowing what assistive devices are available or how to find out.

Some commercially available devices are simply better made and may come with a warranty. The qualitative difference between a "do-it-yourself" versus a purchased commercial product must be considered.

Family, Friends, and Consumers as Experts

One of the most important resources available to occupational therapists is commonly missed. Many individuals begin to develop assistive technology solutions on their own before encountering an occupational therapist. It is extremely important for the occupational therapist to know what assistive technology solutions are already integrated into the person's life-style or what strategies are already being developed. In these circumstances the role of the occupational therapist can be one of encourager, facilitator, and advisor. Many consumers and their families and friends have power equipment, innovative ideas, and much untapped ingenuity that needs to be part of the assistive technology formula.

Special Needs of Long-Term Care

Clients in long-term hospitals, nursing homes, daycare programs, and community-based residential facilities are somewhat unique in their technology needs because they may not have consistent support available to them. In addition, the support personnel they encounter may have little education about assistive technologies and how they are used. Occupational therapists for assistive technology consumers in these types of settings need to help integrate the devices into the long-term-care agency. The residential team must know how to use the assistive technology appropriately so disuse does not occur by default. Even worse than disuse, it has been observed that assistive technologies that are highly valued by the consumers are sometimes withheld as punishment, or teams may unthinkingly withdraw the use of technology. Occasionally the consumers are not capable of being their own advocates due to low cognitive levels or associated behavioral problems. Therefore, it becomes important for occupational therapists to examine the environment in which the assistive technology will be used and to ensure that the support personnel understand its importance and application. If this doesn't occur, the end user loses.

Impoverished Settings

Too often we assume that health care throughout the United States and the world is like that of middle-class United States society. Unfortunately, this is not true in general or with assistive technology. Access to assistive devices is not equal for all individuals of different socioeconomic status. Dealing with disability in developing countries, impoverished inner cities, or rural areas often requires unique interventions. In many cases potential assistive technology users have limited access to medical care, even less access to rehabilitative care, and no money to purchase devices. It is extremely important for occupational therapists to understand the situation and to apply special, creative, and innovative technology solutions to individuals who do not have access to the affluent medical system for which most occupational therapists are trained.

Low-cost construction of assistive devices or second-hand strategies may be useful. For example, fabricating wheelchair-accessible work surfaces using tri-wall cardboard or surplus materials may be possible when accessible furniture cannot be purchased. Or self-fastening closures on clothing or a wash mitt may need to be sewn instead of ordering them from catalogs. The occupational therapist may need to fully utilize professional expertise and innovation in applying skills in splint making, sewing, and other fabrication technologies.

The social system's problems that prevent the appropriate application of self-care and independent living assistive technology are significant. They also may be the most difficult to remedy (Enders, 1988; Enders & Heumann, 1988). While occupational therapy practitioners should be innovative in the application of assistive technology, they must also be aware of the need to advocate system change.

Training Preservice Students

The field of assistive technology has changed dramatically over the last several decades and will continue to do so. This moving target of information is difficult to teach to new occupational therapy students. Classroom teaching and fieldwork education are constantly challenged by this. An issue that has not yet been adequately addressed by occupational therapy curricula is how self-care and independent living assistive technologies are best taught. Should there be an entire course in these assistive technologies? Should the information become part of an overall assistive technology course or should it be part of a set of technology courses? Or should it be integrated across all of the core disability-oriented courses in professional training curricula? While there are no clear best methods for teaching self-care and independent living assistive technologies, two options seem to make sense. First, self-care and independent living assistive technologies need to be taught across the preservice training curricula. Technology needs to be discussed as an intervention strategy as each type of disability area is covered. This means technology should be deliberately taught as a part of fieldwork education. Second, additional elective and independent study opportunities should be made available for the students who desire more depth in this area. The complexity of assistive technologies is increasing, and the occupational therapy profession must take great care to assure that new students receive adequate information pertaining to assistive technology.

Teaming With Other Professionals

The role of occupational therapy in self-care and independent living assistive technology seems quite evident. Occupational therapists need to assess the self-care needs of people with disabilities comprehensively and help in the matching process so consumers of technologies can make their best decisions. But occupational therapists cannot perform this function by themselves. The consumer and his or her family need to be core team members of the process. Additionally, there are other professionals who are immensely valuable members of the assistive technology team. For example, performance in self-care activities is highly dependent on mobility, and physical therapists have substantial information about the self-care technologies pertaining to walking and other mobility activities. Speech and language pathologists have extensive training and expertise in augmentative communication methods. Nurses know more than most occupational therapists about the particular self-care activities dealing with bodily functions, including bowel and bladder activities; and milieu self-care activities, such as sleeping. Additionally, technicians can help adjust, adapt, troubleshoot, and even fabricate assistive technologies for particular needs and for complex cases. Engineers are particularly qualified for design when it is necessary to invent and fabricate a piece of equipment not commercially available. This sampling of team members highlights that when applying assistive technologies, occupational therapists must function as members of a multifaceted team.

The Future of Assistive Technology in Self-Care

Higher electronic-based technologies will continue to advance and provide new opportunities for self-care management. People with severe disabilities may find more and more resources, such as using robots for their own cost-effective, self-care management. Of course, there will also be a continuing need for improvement and for better applications of the low-technology solutions. With thoughtful research, occupational therapists can apply technology more wisely and efficiently. The occupational therapist will increasingly be a key source of information. Identifying and clarifying problems, pointing out what self-care technology solutions are available, and describing how the technology may be obtained will be vital to helping consumers make good decisions (see Mann & Lane, 1991).

Occupational therapists are misleading themselves if they think they can maintain a full knowledge base of all of the assistive technologies available. This task is rapidly becoming impossible as the number of products and the different features available on them increase at a phenomenal rate. We may find larger clinics identifying assistive technology specialists, which might allow reasonable professional role expectations of occupational therapists. If every clinic had one resource person with a focused knowledge base, all staff wouldn't feel pressured to stay abreast of the latest technology developments. Funding assistive technologies in self-care will continue to be important. Although the awareness of the need for assistive technology is increasing, the implications of many societal directions are yet unknown. National health insurance may change policy decisions, which could have major effects on funding of assistive technologies for self-care.

Perhaps the most significant event that may occur in the near future pertains to decisions revolving around the five different intervention strategies defined and discussed in the first part of this chapter. The first two interventions are oriented toward education and rehabilitation. They tend to be very costly in terms of human resource personnel, but do provide optimal results if an individual can be returned to full function intrinsically. On the other hand, assistive technology or task changing strategies are frequently less costly. In the future, this may become controversial. Occupational therapy that focuses on increasing motor, sensory, and cognitive function may be poised against occupational therapy that provides assistive technology and task modification. Interest by funding agencies in functional outcome measurement may become more of a driving force to decide what societal resources can be provided to individuals with disabilities. It will be essential for occupational therapists, who comprise one of the few professions to straddle all five of these approaches and methodologies for people with disabilities, to be strong proponents for both sides and to address how integrating all five of these methods is the best strategy. Measuring the impact of what we do in occupational therapy, both in how we remediate deficits and the effect we have on environment-adjusted interventions, may be vital for occupational therapists in upcoming years (see Figure 20).

Figure 20. Independent living technology: A bridge to the future.

In October 1987, Stephen Hawking wrote in the acknowledgments of his worldwide best seller *A Brief History in Time* (1988), "This system has made the difference: In fact, I can communicate better now than before I lost my voice" (p. viii). In the introduction to *A Brief History in Time*, Carl Sagan points out that Hawking serves as the "Lucasian Professor of Mathematics at Cambridge University, a post once held by Newton and later by P.A.M. Dirac..." (p. 4). An electronic communication system enables this frontier scientist to manage his personal care.

The choice was whether to allow an operation which would remove his windpipe. It might save his life, but afterward he'd never again be able to speak or make any vocal sound. That seemed a ghastly price to pay...speech was slow and difficult to understand, but it was still speech, and his only means of communication. Without it he couldn't continue his career or even converse. What would survival be worth to him? With grave misgivings she ordered them to operate, then tried to set herself once more to give him the will to live. (Ferguson, 1991, p. 126)

Since 1980, community and private nurses had been coming for an hour or two each morning and evening to supplement care given...the cost was astronomical...The National Health Service, which in Britain is paid for by taxes, would have paid for a nursing home but could only offer a few hours of nursing care...plus help with bathing. (p. 127)

An American foundation offered fifty thousand pounds a year to pay for nurses. A computer expert...sent a computer program he'd written...which allowed the user to select words from a computer screen...a tiny movement that was still possible for him; squeezing a switch held in his hand. Should that fail him, head or eye movement could activate the switch. (p. 128)

Still too weak and ill to work on research, he practiced with his computer. Before long he could produce ten words a minute, not very fast but good enough to convince him that he could continue his career...Since then, his speed has improved. He now produces more than 15 words a minute. (p. 128)

He can send the result to a speech synthesizer, which pronounces it out loud or over the telephone, or he can save something on a disk and later print it out or rework it. (p. 128)

He can listen ahead of time to the speech synthesizer deliver a lecture, then edit and polish it. Before an audience he sends his lecture to the speech synthesizer a sentence at a time. (p. 128)

Does all of this make conversations...seem like talking to a machine—like something alien, from science fiction? At first a little, soon you forget about it. (p. 129)

...Sense of humor is contagious and likely to break out at any time. When his haggard face lights up with a smile, it's difficult to believe this man has many problems...grin is famous, and it reveals the quality of his love for his subject. (p. 130)

...He went to work again on his book. (p. 130)

Appendix 1. Abledata categories of self-care products.*

I. Personal Care Products (3,432)
  A. Eating Devices (227)
    1. feeding program (1)
    2. feeders (15)
    3. bibs (37)
    4. dishes (39)
    5. utensils (135)
      a. forks (43)
      b. knives (38)
      c. spoons (46)
      d. sporks (8)
  B. Drinking (50)
    1. cups (30)
    2. glasses (8)
    3. straws (12)
  C. Grooming and Hygiene (87)
    1. dental care (18)
      a. dental care general (7)
      b. toothbrushes (11)
    2. eyeglasses (1)
    3. hair care (36)
      a. combs (6)
      b. hair brushes (11)
      c. shampoo aids (19)
    4. mirrors (22)
    5. nail care (8)
    6. shaving (2)
  D. Toileting (680)
    1. catheters (79)
      a. catheter supplies (40)
      b. catheter hygiene (17)
      c. collection bags (22)
    2. ostomy supplies (31)
    3. incontinence (170)
      a. incontinence general (52)
      b. garments (118)
    4. commodes (201)
      a. commodes general (3)
      b. commode chairs (165)
      c. shower commodes (33)
    5. toilets (172)
      a. toilet hygiene (29)
      b. safety frames (51)
      c. toilet seats (92)
    6. urinals (27)
  E. Bathing (335)
    1. bathroom accessories (7)
    2. bathing aids (48)
      a. bath aids (14)
      b. back brushes (19)
      c. hand brushes (1)
      d. wash mitts & washcloths (5)
      e. safety treads (9)
    3. bathtub seats (92)
    4. shower chairs (118)
    5. shower stools (44)
    6. bath lifts (26)
  F. Clothing (847)
    1. clothing general (34)
    2. women's clothing (394)
      a. underwear (86)
      b. outerwear (248)
      c. nightwear (60)
    3. men's clothing (213)
      a. underwear (13)
      b. outerwear (164)
      c. nightwear (36)
    4. children's clothing (51)
    5. outdoor clothing (50)
      a. rain (8)
      b. cold (42)
    6. helmets (36)
    7. shoes (69)
  G. Dressing (116)
    1. dressing general (31)
    2. shoe aids (40)
    3. stocking aids (28)
    4. button aids (17)
  H. Smoking (12)
  I. Reaching (40)
  J. Carrying (104)
    1. carrying general (3)
    2. wheelchair (63)
    3. walker (30)
    4. crutch (8)
  K. Holding (83)
    1. holding general (19)
    2. nonslip surfaces (9)
    3. suction holders (2)
    4. drink holders (14)
    5. glass holders (9)
    6. utensil holders (23)
    7. telephone aids (7)
  L. Transfer (109)
    1. general transfer devices (41)
    2. transfer lifts (68)
  M. Dispenser Aids (4)
  N. Handle Padding (16)
  O. Arm Supports (90)
    1. body supported slings (74)
    2. mechanical arm supports (16)
  P. Health Care (605)
    1. health care general (150)
    2. heat therapy (69)
    3. cold therapy (49)
    4. thermometers (11)
    5. blood pressure instruments (10)
    6. scales (15)

*Numbers of products listed in each category are in parentheses.

7. monitors (23)
8. tracheostomy devices (18)
9. medications (98)
    a. medications general (10)
    b. pills (26)
    c. syringes (31)
    d. testing devices (31)
10. restraints (162)
    a. limb restraints (28)
    b. body restraints (126)
    c. child restraints (8)
Q. Child Care (23)
R. Sexual Aids (4)
II. Home Management (911)
  A. Food Preparation (147)
    1. food preparation (100)
      a. containers (29)
      b. kitchen tools general (29)
      c. measuring (11)
      d. mixing (5)
      e. cutting & chopping tools (26)
    2. cooking (17)
    3. appliances (30)
  B. Housekeeping (55)
    1. housekeeping general (9)
    2. cleaning (24)
    3. laundry (11)
    4. ironing (2)
    5. shopping (9)
  C. Furniture (709)
    1. furniture general (8)
    2. bedroom (417)
      a. beds (55)
      b. mattresses (72)
      c. bed aids (186)
      d. pillows (104)
    3. trays and tables (110)
    4. chairs (147)
    5. steps & stools (27)
III. Wheeled Mobility (1373)
  A. Manual Wheelchairs (315)
  B. Sport Wheelchairs (412)
  C. Powered Wheelchairs (133)
  D. Wheelchair Accessories (654)
    1. manufacturer options (13)
    2. wheelchair accessories general (53)
    3. armrests (43)
    4. batteries (28)
    5. carrying accessories (52)
    6. casters (9)
    7. exercise & sports (6)
    8. footrests (55)
    9. hand rims (16)
    10. head supports (13)
    11. lapboards (119)
    12. leg rests (31)
    13. powered wheelchair accessories (94)
    14. seats & backs (61)
    15. tires (18)

16. upholstery (16)
17. wheels (20)
18. wheel locks (7)
E. Wheelchair Alternatives (113)
F. Transporters (56)
G. Carts (51)
H. Stretchers (10)
IV. Seating (1078)
  A. Seating Systems (624)
    1. seating systems general (70)
    2. seat supports (26)
    3. back supports (100)
    4. pelvic supports (38)
    5. head & neck supports (65)
    6. trunk supports (82)
    7. leg supports (42)
    8. foot supports (30)
    9. arm supports (100)
    10. seating hardware (71)
  B. Cushions (294)
    1. cushions general (92)
    2. air (35)
    3. foam (112)
    4. gel (34)
    5. water (13)
    6. cushion covers (8)
  C. Therapeutic Seats (72)
  D. Car Seats (78)
  E. Monitors (10)
V. Communication (128)
  A. Mouthsticks (31)
  B. Headwands (22)
  C. Reading (188)
    1. reading general (73)
    2. magnifiers (87)
    3. tactile & braille (8)
    4. auditory output (8)
    5. page turners (12)
  D. Bookholders (39)
  E. Writing (198)
    1. writing general (75)
      a. writing general (19)
      b. writing tools (29)
      c. writing paper (10)
      d. writing guides (17)
    2. braille (61)
    3. braille writers (62)
  F. Typing (34)
  G. Telephones (248)
    1. telephones general (1)
    2. special dialing telephones (19)
    3. special transmission telephones (54)
    4. cordless telephones (9)
    5. telephone accessories (165)
  H. Nonvocal & Speech Impaired (354)
    1. communicators (271)
      a. communicators general (12)
      b. direct selection (83)
      c. scanning (39)

  d. encoding (9)
  e. communication boards
     & books (128)
  2. oral speech (27)
 I. Signal Systems (170)
VI. Walking (682)
  A. Canes (145)
    1. canes general (126)
    2. cane accessories (19)
  B. Crutches (117)
    1. crutches general (50)
    2. crutch accessories (67)
  C. Walkers (139)
    1. walkers general (182)
    2. specialty walkers (21)
    3. child walkers (52)
    4. walker accessories (64)
  D. Standing (101)
    1. prone standers (32)
    2. other standing equipment (69)
VII. Orthotics (569)
  A. Orthotics General (38)
  B. Upper Extremity (212)
    1. upper extremity orthoses general (32)
    2. finger orthoses (33)
    3. hand/wrist orthoses (112)
    4. elbow/shoulder orthoses (35)
  C. Lower Extremity (173)
    1. lower extremity orthoses general (34)
    2. ankle foot orthoses (56)
    3. knee orthoses (65)
    4. hip & knee orthoses (18)
  D. Head & Neck (25)
  E. Torso (121)
VIII. Prosthetics (44)
  A. Prosthetics General (1)
  B. Upper Extremity (21)
  C. Lower Extremity (22)
IX. Architectural Elements (931)
  A. Indoor (565)
    1. doors (98)
      a. doors general (14)
      b. door handles (28)
      c. door operators (40)
      d. door locks (16)
    2. windows (6)
    3. floors (8)
    4. walls (12)
    5. bathrooms (368)
      a. bathtubs (50)
      b. showers (72)
      c. toilets (12)
      d. bidets (13)
      e. sinks (10)
      f. handshowers (18)
      g. plumbing accessories (37)
      h. grab bars (156)
    6. public restrooms (26)
    7. kitchens (41)
    8. storage (6)

  D. Lighting (34)
  E. Safety & Security (95)
    1. lights (8)
    2. child proof devices (8)
    3. electric cords (6)
    4. locks (3)
    5. alarm & security systems (70)
  F. Vertical Lift (138)
    1. elevators (19)
    2. stair lifts (52)
    3. ramps (67)
X. Controls (638)
  A. Environmental Controls (117)
    1. environmental control units (48)
    2. environmental control accessories (64)
  B. Control Switches (516)
    1. electro mechanical switches (341)
      a. joysticks (30)
      b. contact switches (192)
      c. sensor switches (8)
      d. body position switches (27)
      e. pneumatic switches (31)
      f. optical switches (13)
      g. cables & switch accessories (40)
    2. remote switches (15)
    3. switch interfaces (85)
    4. assessment systems (75)
  C. Power Switches (5)

Appendix 2. OT FACT self-care assessment categories.

II. Activities of Performance
  A. Personal Care Activities
    1. Cleanliness, Hygiene, & Appearance
      a. Bathing
        1) Obtains supplies
        2) Doffs clothing
        3) Regulates water
        4) Gets in position
        5) Cleans self
        6) Shampoos hair
        7) Dries self
        8) Leaves position
      b. Toilet Hygiene
        1) Indicates need
        2) Obtains supplies
        3) Gets in position
        4) Menstrual needs
        5) Eliminates
        6) Cleans self
        7) Leaves position
        8) Flushes toilet
      c. Hand Washing
        1) Obtains supplies
        2) Regulates water
        3) Cleans hands
        4) Turns off water
        5) Dries hands
      d. Oral Hygiene
        1) Obtains supplies
        2) Brushes
        3) Stores dentures
        4) Flosses
        5) Mouthwash
      e. Grooming
        1) Shaves
        2) Cosmetics
        3) Combs/brushes hair
        4) Fingernails
        5) Toenails
      f. Dressing
        1) Selects clothing
        2) Obtains clothing
        3) Doffs clothing
        4) Dons clothing
          aa. Pullover
          bb. Front fastening
          cc. Pants/underpants
          dd. Bra
          ee. Shoes
          ff. Socks
        5) Appliances
      g. Nose Blowing
    2. Medical and Health Management Act.
      a. Health Maintenance
        and Improvement
        1) Exercise program/routine
          aa. Physical exercise
          bb. Psycho/soc. exercise
        2) Manages unhealthy
          behaviors

          aa. Smoking
          bb. Alcohol & drug use
          cc. Food consumption
          dd. Sexual practices
      b. Medication Routine
        1) Schedule
        2) Obtains medication
        3) Containers
        4) Selects/measures
        5) Administers/takes
        6) Stores medication
        7) Manages side effects
    C. Emergency Communication
        1) Accesses device
        2) Activates device
        3) Sends message
   3. Nutrition Activities
      a. Feeding/Eating
        1) Indicates need
        2) Obtains food
        3) Sets up food
        4) Utensils/tableware
          aa. Spoon
          bb. Fork
          cc. Knife
          dd. Glass
          ee. Plate
        5) Consumes soft food
          aa. Brings to mouth
          bb. Puts in mouth
          cc. Chews
          dd. Swallows
        6) Consumes solid food
          aa. Brings to mouth
          bb. Puts in mouth
          cc. Chews
          dd. Swallows
        7) Consumes liquid
          aa. Brings to mouth
          bb. Sips/tips
          cc. Swallows
        8) Uses napkin
      b. Meal Prep. & Clean-up
        1) Selects food
        2) Plans meals
        3) Prepares meal
        4) Cleans up
   4. Sleep & Rest Activities
      a. Indicates need
      b. Plans/takes sleep/breaks
      c. Relaxes/quiets self
      d. Uses appropriate locations
      e. Uses appropriate positions
      f. Regular sleep-wake cycle
      g. Sufficient sleep/rest
   5. Mobility Activities
      a. Indoor
        1) Bed mobility

        aa. Rolls over
        bb. Scoots
        cc. Bridges
        dd. Sits up
    2) Transferring
    3) Stands & sits
    4) Between rooms
    5) Between levels
  b. Outdoor/Community (private)
    1) Gets in position
    2) Uses safe procedures
    3) Manages terrains
    4) Navigates
    5) Maintains vehicle
  c. Outdoor/Community (public)
    1) Sets up transportation
    2) Gets vehicle
    3) Pays fares
    4) Enters & exits

6. Communication Activities
  a. Speaking
  b. Writing
    1) Obtains device
    2) Forms message
    3) Sends message
  c. Reading
  d. Telephone
    1) Gets to phone
    2) Uses receiver
    3) Dials
    4) Transmits message
    5) Socially proper
    6) Sets receiver
  e. Sexual Expression
    1) Recognizes behaviors
    2) Communicates sexually
    3) Performs

B. Occupational Role-Related Activities
  1. Home Management Activities
    a. Home Acquisition
    b. Menu Planning
      1) Plans meals
      2) Gets groceries
      3) Plans nutritionally
    c. Care of Clothing/Launderables
      1) Launders
      2) Dry cleaning
      3) Stores
      4) Mends
    d. Cleaning
      1) Picks up
      2) Dusts
      3) Makes bed
      4) Changes sheets
      5) Garbage
      6) Sweeps floors
      7) Scrubs/mops
      8) Plumbing fixtures
      9) Washes windows
    e. Household Repair & Maint.
    f. Household Safety

      1) Safe building/facility
      2) Safe contents
      3) Safe for people
    g. Yard Work
  2. Consumer Activities
    a. Purchasing Activities
      1) Selects products
      2) Locates items
      3) Store mobility
      4) Obtains items
      5) Transports
      6) Handles money
      7) Special returns
    b. Money Management Activities
      1) Banking
      2) Budgeting

References

Brown, B., Bottorf, C., DePape, D., & Vanderheiden, G.C. (1987). *Construction notes for laptrays, portable communication boards and adaptive pointers.* Madison, WI: Trace Research & Development Center.

DOS Abledata. (1992). [Computer program]. Madison, WI: Trace Research & Development Center.

Enders, A. (1988). Technology to assist physical function and aid independent living. In G. Drouin, (Chair), *Proceedings of ICAART 88, the 1988 RESNA Conference* (pp. 568–571). Washington, DC: RESNA.

Enders, A. (undated). *Spinal Cord Research Foundation briefing paper: Rehabilitation/technology: Daily living.* Unpublished manuscript.

Enders., A., & Hall, M. (Eds.). (1989–90). *Assistive technology sourcebook.* Washington, DC: RESNA.

Enders, A., & Heumann, J. (1988). How adults with disabilities get the everyday technology they need. *Proceedings of ICAART 88, the 1988 RESNA Conference* (pp. 580–583). Washington, DC: RESNA.

Ferguson, K. (1991). *Stephen Hawking: Quest for a theory of everything.* New York: Franklin Watts.

Ford, J., & Duckworth, B. (1987). *Physical management for the quadraplegic patient* (2nd ed.). Philadelphia: F.A. Davis.

Hall, M.E. (1951). Two feeding appliances. *American Journal of Occupational Therapy, 5,* 52–53.

Hawking, S.W. (1988). *A brief history of time from the big bang to black holes.* New York: Bantam Books.

Hopkins, H.L. (1960). Assistive devices for activities of daily living. *American Journal of Occupational Therapy, 14,* 218–220.

HyperAbledata. (1992). [Computer program]. Madison, WI: Trace Research & Development Center.

Irvine, B., & Siegel, J.D. (1990). Product comparison and evaluation: Canes, crutches, and walkers. *Request Evaluating Assistive Technology.* Washington, DC: ECRI.

Joe, B.E. (1992, June 11). Software provides independence with EASE. *OT Week,* p. 8.

King, T.I., (1989). A standing belt. *American Journal of Occupational Therapy, 43,* 471–473.

La Buda, D.R. (1988). Assistive technology for older adults: Funding resources and delivery systems. *Proceedings of ICAART 88, the 1988 RESNA Conference* (pp. 572–575). Washington, DC: RESNA.

Lykouretzos, J., & Thompson-Rangel, T. (1990). A folding dressing stick. *American Journal of Occupational Therapy, 44,* 77.

Mann, W.C., & Lane, J.P. (1991). Assistive technology for persons with disabilities: The role of occupational therapy. Rockville, MD: American Occupational Therapy Association.

Miller, J., & Carpenter, C. (1964). Electronics for communication. *American Journal of Occupational Therapy, 18,* 20–23.

National Rehabilitation Hospital & ECRI. (1992). Independence in the bathroom. *Request Evaluating assistive technology.* Washington, DC: Author.

The Oxford Dictionary of Quotations (3rd ed.). (1980). London: Oxford University Press.

Parker, M.G., & Thorslund, M. (1991). The use of technical aids among community-based elderly. *American Journal of Occupational Therapy, 45,* 712–718.

Parlin, F.W. (1948). Adaptation and apparatus. *American Journal of Occupational Therapy, 2,* 206–208.

Rein, J. (1988). Technology to assist physical function and aid independent living for children ages 0 to 21. *Proceedings of ICAART 88, the 1988 RESNA Conference* (pp. 567–579). Washington, DC: RESNA.

Richert, B.J. (1950). Occupational therapy for the quadriplegic patient. *American Journal of Occupational Therapy, 4*, 1–5.

Rodgers, B.L. (1985). *A holistic perspective: An introduction. A future perspective on the holistic use of technology for people with disabilities.* Madison, WI: Trace Research & Development Center.

Rogers, J.C., & Holm, M.B. (1992). Assistive technology device use in patients with rheumatic disease: A literature review. *American Journal of Occupational Therapy, 46*, 120–127.

Rosenberg, C. (1968). *Assistive devices for the handicapped.* Atlanta, GA: Stein.

Runge, M. (1967). Self-dressing techniques for patients with spinal cord injury. *American Journal of Occupational Therapy, 21*, 367–375.

Rust, K.L. & Smith, R.O. (1992). Use of functional outcome measure to assess covariate dimensions of function. *Confronting our future.* Chicago: AAPMR, ACRM.

Smith, R.O. (1991). Technological approaches to performance enhancement. In C. Baum & C. Christiansen (Eds.), *Occupational therapy: Overcoming human performance deficits* (pp. 747–786). Thorofare, NJ: Slack.

Smith, R.O. (1992). *OT FACT.* [Computer program]. Rockville, MD: American Occupational Therapy Association.

Smith, M.J., & Sainfort, P.C. (1989). A balance theory of job design for stress reduction. *International Journal of Industrial Ergonomics, 4*, 67–79.

Wisher, S.J. (1991). An assistive eye-drop mold. *American Journal of Occupational Therapy, 45*, 751–752.

15

The Self-Care Environment: Issues of Space and Furnishing

Pearl Sarah Bates

Pearl Sarah Bates, MA, OTR, practices in San Francisco, CA.

Karen Mae Kaeter, Jean Cole Spencer, Margaretta Newell, and June Long are thanked for their generous assistance in the preparation of this chapter. My professors in the Occupational Therapy Departments at the University of Minnesota and Texas Woman's University are thanked for teaching me the principles expressed in this chapter. My patients are thanked for teaching me about the importance of the self-care environment, and why it needs to be made accessible to all.

Chapter 15 Outline

Where is the Self-Care Environment?

Negotiability Versus Access

The Home Environment

Space and Layout in the Home

Fixtures

Bathroom Fixtures

Kitchen Fixtures

Surfaces

Furniture

Out on the Town

So-Called Public Toilets

Dining Out

Obtaining Beverages

Shopping

Health and Appearance

Taking Care of Business

Cleanliness is Next to...Impossible

Keeping the Doctor Away

On the Road

The Role of the Occupational Therapist in the Self-Care Environment

Assessment

Negotiability Rating

Recommendations

Options for Change

Factors Affecting Decisions to Change the Environment

Values Clarification: A Case Study

References

Awoman in a sports wheelchair enters the cafeteria line at a nationally known rehabilitation center. She reaches for a tray on a low shelf, and balances it carefully on her lap as she wheels to the short-order area. The ventilation fan over the grill is so loud that she cannot make herself heard. Her head is below the top of the counter. The cook cannot see her until he comes over to take the order of a standing person. When her order is ready, the cook sets it atop the 4-foot-high counter: There is a wheelchair-level counter in front of the high counter, but it is out of reach of the cook. With difficulty, the woman reaches her food and proceeds to the beverage area.

The canned sodas are in a refrigerated case on a standard 30-inch-high counter. She can reach only the lower two shelves. Her preferred selection is on the highest shelf. She looks around for assistance, but there is no one in sight, so she gives in and takes the beverage container that is within reach, even though her own brand is a mere 12 inches away.

The counters are not continuous from one area to another. To get from the beverage counter to the checkout, she has to balance her tray, unevenly weighted with plate and beverage can, on her knees while propelling her chair. She must then lift the tray from her knees to the checkout counter, pay her bill, lift the tray back onto her knees, and negotiate the ¼-inch ridge from the linoleum to the carpeted dining area without spilling. While this is not an excessive ridge from the standpoint of the law, or of a skilled wheelchair user who could easily jump a 6-inch curb, it is extremely challenging while balancing a tray on one's knees, with both hands busy pushing the wheels. Because she has complete paraplegia, the woman is unable to adjust her legs to keep the tray in balance. By a quick grab with her hand, she saves the sliding tray. She then has a choice of two types of tables: large round ones that are accessible, and small square ones that do not provide enough leg room for her wheelchair footrests. Because she is dining alone, she would prefer a small table to sitting conspicuously alone at a table for eight, but she has no choice. At last she reaches her table, and places the tray on it. Because of the slowness of the process of getting there, her meal is cold by the time she begins to eat.

The above is not a parody or a hypothetical example: It is an accurate description of part of the self-care environment, built in 1990, at a facility tailored to wheelchair users, in one of the top rehabilitation centers in the United States. The scene above was witnessed by the author.

Why do such nonfunctional environments exist? There are many reasons, obviously, but one seems to be the lack of skilled occupational therapy input. Accessibility— the ability to enter a space and move through it unobstructed—can be determined by a careful study of the relevant laws. However, it is the occupational therapist, armed with the knowledge of human function, who has the ability to determine whether an individual can operate independently in a given environment. The purpose of this chapter is to provide the therapist with a window through which to view this issue. While expertise in environmental assessment can be acquired only through experience, experience will most benefit those who attempt to look at the environment from a user's perspective. The most useful insights in this chapter are those derived from the author's experience with persons with disabilities performing, or attempting to perform, self-care activities in the existing environment.

Where is the Self-Care Environment?

Self-care is an ongoing process of maintaining one's health and well-being, and is not limited to specific activities of daily living (ADL). Self-care activities are those in which we voluntarily engage in order to preserve our organismic homeostasis. At the most basic level, they consist of the maintenance of body temperature, hydration, nutrition, elimination of wastes, and prevention of injury.

To maintain temperature, we don or doff clothing, go in or out of doors, adjust thermostats, add or remove blankets, build fires, jump in swimming pools, and vary our rate of activity. We maintain hydration by drinking beverages; and nutrition by obtaining, preparing, and consuming food. We eliminate wastes through expiration, perspiration (necessitating washing clothes and bathing), and the functions of bowel and bladder. We prevent injury to our bodies through the use of protective clothing, warning systems, and removal of environmental hazards. At any given time we are partaking of one or more of these activities, whether consciously or not.

In addition, care of the self includes related activities, such as grooming, which raise one's sense of psychosocial well-being. The "high-level" or "instrumental" activities of daily living are activities that support and make possible the basic self-care tasks. These include household management, laundry, shopping, banking and money management, telephone use, reading the newspaper, health maintenance, religious practice, and community mobility. Thus the "self-care environment" is all of the environment occupied by humans.

Negotiability Versus Access

Laws ranging from the Education for all Handicapped Children Act (1975) to The Americans with Disabilities Act (1991), along with a host of local and state regulations, mandate that public spaces be made accessible to persons with disabilities. To occupational therapists, *functional independence* is a familiar concept, and is in fact the goal of much of our patient treatment. To determine the effects of the environment on self-care, however, there is need for a third concept, joining the ideas of *access* and *independence*. Such a concept, *negotiability*, was proposed by Noris-Baker and Willems (1978). *Negotiability* refers to the ability to access a feature of the environment and use it for its intended purpose, with only one's usual adaptive equipment. The present author proposes that this be amended with the phrase "in a manner acceptable to the individual."

The need for a concept of negotiability can be made clear by examining the vignette at the beginning of this chapter. The woman in question was able to access the short-order counter. She could get as close to it as a walking person, but she could not use it independently for its intended purpose. She could not place her order with the cook unless a standing person got his attention first. The counter was accessible, but not negotiable. Conversely, she was perfectly capable of opening the beverage case and obtaining a soda can independently—but the case was too high to be accessible. It was independently usable, but not negotiable. A negotiability rating differs from most self-care or ADL assessments in that it rates the person's performance in the environment, using adaptive equipment, whereas most self-care instruments focus solely on the person's ability to perform. Instructions for carrying out a negotiability rating can be found in the assessment section of this chapter.

Negotiability involves a functional interaction among the person, environment, and equipment. Failure to consider all three aspects, and their impacts on one another, results in a less-than-optimal outcome.

Equipment issues are explored in Chapter 14, but they are also mentioned here because their impact on negotiability must be considered by the therapist when assessing a patient in his or her environment. Equipment factors bearing directly on negotiability include the size and weight of the equipment, the running noise, the type and position of controls, the type and position of signage, and the type and position of feedback systems.

Human factors bearing directly on negotiability include physical size, strength, coordination, endurance, sensation, perception, cognition, mode of mobility, the nature of the impairment, learned skills, emotional status, living arrangements, and personal values. Factors in the person that influence negotiability are dealt with in detail in the diagnosis-specific chapters of this book.

The environmental factors that affect negotiability—and, consequently, self-care performance—include structural characteristics, surface characteristics, type and location of fixtures and furnishings, lighting, temperature, acoustics, environmental press, and social press.

Structural characteristics of the environment refer to the natural and built aspects of the environment (i.e., buildings, sidewalks, hills, trees, and other relatively permanent environmental features).

Surface characteristics include traits such as friction versus slipperiness, sturdiness of wall coverings, and textural markers, such as those identifying curb cuts for the blind.

Fixtures are built-in portions of the environment that are not structural in nature, but that are added, often for the convenience of the inhabitant in the performance of self-care activities. Fixtures include such items as toilets, bath tubs, light fixtures, and built-in cabinets.

Furnishings include nonpermanent environmental features added to a structure for the physical and emotional comfort of the inhabitants.

Lighting refers to both natural and artificial sources of light. Quality, as well as amount, of light must be taken into consideration.

Acoustics refers to the behavior of sound waves in the environment, the impact of sound waves on the human ear, and, more importantly, their impact on human auditory perception.

Temperature refers simply to how warm or cold the environment is.

Press refers to the impact, both physical and emotional, of the environment on the person (Murray, 1938). Press is exerted by all factors in the environment that potentially impact a person. Thus, both people and inanimate objects exert press. Press was defined by the originator of the term, Dr. Henry A. Murray, as the "kind of effect an object or situation is exerting or could exert upon the subject...which usually appears in the guise of a threat of harm or promise of benefit to the organism" (p. 748). Thus press refers not to the way the person feels about the environment (i.e., loves it, hates it, etc.) but rather to the nature of the environmental influence itself, which, as Murray explains, is always situational. More precisely, press is the nature of the potential impact of environmental factors on the organism's ability to maintain itself (i.e., perform its self-care skills). The presence of nutritious food that can be obtained is a positive press, while the presence of food that is out of reach, as in the nonnegotiable cafeteria line, is a negative press. It should be self-evident that the press of an environment on a person who is able-bodied and cognitively and emotionally intact may be very different from the press of that same environment on an individual with impairments in any of these areas.

This is a separate issue from the individual's perceptions of the press, or what he or she believes is positive or negative in the environment, and different yet again from the apperception of the press. *Pressive apperception* refers to the expected press of an environmental factor not yet encountered. A patient may refuse to participate in community reintegration activities because of his or her apperception of the press of the community setting. For example, a new paraplegic may feel that the world outside the rehabilitation facility "is just not prepared for wheelchairs to be all over the place" (Bates, Spencer, Rintala, & Young, 1993).

Social press refers to the impact of the presence or absence of another human on the self-care performance of the subject. This includes the emotional effects of the other person's presence, as well as his or her potential to physically further or hinder the self-care process. The social press of a therapist's presence has great repercussions during bathing or toilet-transfer training. Some patients refuse training in bathroom transfers for this reason. Sensitivity to such issues is crucial for therapist-patient rapport.

The Home Environment

The most obvious setting for the performance of self-care activities is the home. We dress in our own bedrooms, bathe in our own bathrooms, and eat at our own tables. Many of the higher-level activities of self-care are also performed in the home. We balance our checkbooks at our own desks, look up numbers in our own telephone books, and cook in our own kitchens. It is only our own personal space that we can truly adapt to our own needs and wishes. Despite the great gains being made in the accessibility of public spaces with the implementation of the ADA (1991), public spaces can never be as well-tailored to the individual as private spaces are. This is not only because of discrimination, but because of the differing needs of different persons. An environment fitted solely to the needs of a wheelchair user would be inaccessible to a walking person, and a Braille signage system would be unreadable by the sighted.

Space and Layout in the Home

A well-laid-out floor plan facilitates self-care, while a poor one inhibits performance. Seven general principles need to be observed (see Figure 1).

1. *Allow enough space for ease of mobility, but no more.* Excess space forces a person to travel greater distances between tasks, and raises the cost of construction, maintenance, heating, and cooling. For example, a "strip" style kitchen, with two facing counters, can be quite negotiable. Both counters can be reached with minimal repositioning of a wheelchair, or with few steps for the person who walks with difficulty.

Figure 1. Principles for layout of the self-care environment.

1. Allow enough space for ease of mobility, but no excess.

2. Limit travel between sequential tasks.

3. Position built-in controls where most often used.

4. Limit changes in level.

5. Limit interior doors.

6. Be aware of lighting, acoustics, and temperature.

7. Build in safety features.

2. *Arrange layout so sequential tasks can be performed with little or no travel in between.* A bathroom off the bedroom requires less travel than one down the hall. A kitchen with a pass-through to the dining room eliminates many steps. Of course, for the wheelchair user the pass-through should be at a reachable level.

3. *Built-in controls (light switches, thermostats) should be placed where they are most often needed or are most convenient.* For the individual who has difficulty arising from bed, position controls where they can be reached from the bed or provide a remote-control system.

4. *Limit the number of changes in floor level.* Level change refers to any variation in the level of the floor—steps, ramps, and elevators—as well as changes in surface, such as from linoleum to raised carpeting. All level changes require extra effort on the part of persons with motor deficits, and present a risk to persons with motor, sensory, or perceptual deficits. For some wheelchair users, a small step is passable. Nonetheless, doing a "wheelie" almost guarantees that whatever the person is carrying will fall off of his or her lap. This is merely inconvenient when carrying something like laundry, but presents the risk of a severe burn in the case of a plate of hot food being spilled on the person's lap.

Steps present great risk to the person with sensory or perceptual deficits who trips or falls because the step cannot be seen. Brightly colored strips can be added to mark the edges of steps for those with residual vision. Textured strips can be used for the blind. It is safest to eliminate the step altogether.

The now-ubiquitous ramps are, of course, a boon to wheelchair users, and the author applauds their existence. Nonetheless, a ramp is less negotiable than a level floor. Traversing a ramp while using any sort of mobility aid takes effort. For the person with a prosthetic foot, a slanted surface is much harder to negotiate than a level one. Most prostheses do not allow for dorsiflexion or plantar flexion sufficient to allow walking up or down a graded surface. An individual with perceptual deficits is at greater risk on a ramp than on stairs, because he or she may not notice the grade at all, and thus may fall.

Home elevators and stair lifts may allow entry to an otherwise inaccessible top floor in an existing home. However, in designing a new space, remember that a stair lift necessitates two transfers. An elevator requires travel across the difficult-to-maneuver opening, with slots in the floor where a caster or crutch tip can get caught. Reliance on mechanical devices leaves the person vulnerable to power failure. This is especially important to remember during fire and earthquake safety planning. An alternate mode of egress must be planned for the individual who could be trapped upstairs.

5. *Limit the number of interior doors.* This recommendation is made with the recognition that some doors are unavoidable. Everything from fire codes to the need for privacy and warmth necessitate the use of doors. Within existing constraints, however, eliminate as many doors as possible. Opening and closing doors is always a challenge for the wheelchair or walker user. Many doors have sills to trip over. Doors narrow the available opening in doorways by approximately 2 inches, often enough to prevent the passage of a wheelchair. Turning door knobs is a risk for the arthritic hand. For the person with cognitive deficits, doors also present the risk of getting locked in or out.

Careful layout limits the need for privacy doors. If an individual's private bedroom has a private bath and closet, there is no need for either of these areas to have a door because no one else needs to enter the bedroom. Curtains may be used to screen either of these spaces, if desired.

6. *Plan for the sensory environment.* The impact of the environment on the human sensory system can spell the difference between dependence and independence in self-care. Lighting, acoustics, and temperature each play a part in environmental negotiability.

   Adequate light, without glare, is essential to the performance of many self-care tasks, including grooming, cooking, and money management. In addition, the ability to see out a window may have great impact on an individual's sense of well-being. Windows should be low enough for all to see out, and the controls for the windows and drapes should be within reach.

   An individual with diminished vision, relying on auditory discrimination for spatial orientation, may be rendered virtually incapable of function in a noisy environment. A person with auditory-processing deficits may be unable to discriminate what is said in an echoing room. This factor affects functional communication, including use of the telephone.

   Temperature affects muscle tone, and this increases with the cold. This has a functional impact on all persons with spasticity, including those with cerebral palsy, traumatic brain injury, stroke, and spinal cord injury. Sudden blasts of cold air, as from an air-conditioning system, can cause spasms that temporarily destroy upper extremity control. The author, as a clinical therapist, once accompanied a group of seven persons with quadriplegia to a restaurant as part of a community reintegration out-trip. All was going well until the restaurant's air conditioning system kicked in. Suddenly, one after another of the seven began having spasms and jerking their arms about, out of control. Continuing with dinner became an impossibility. Initially, some were embarrassed, but when someone commented that this was a good way to diet, everybody collapsed in a fit of the giggles. The manager was politely asked to turn down the air conditioning, and dinner proceeded without further mishap.

7. *Consider safety when laying out the floor plan.* Starting at the front door, make sure there are safety peepholes at eye-level of all inhabitants—wheelchair users and children are especially vulnerable when home alone. Built-in electronic door controls are useful for those physically unable to open or close a door.

   Safe fire egress from bedrooms must be planned. A slide makes a workable fire escape from an upstairs window. At the same time, no one wants to leave an open path for break-ins. It is difficult to balance these two concerns, and individual decisions must be made based on the relative risks in a given setting. A city home may be more liable to be broken into, while a cabin in the woods is at greater risk of fire.

Fixtures

In determining basic layout, built-in fixtures must be planned for as well. The most important and often-forgotten fact is that built-in fixtures take up space. One cannot assume that the original floor plan is negotiable until this factor is taken into consideration.

Bathroom Fixtures

A common mistake in the layout of wheelchair-accessible bathrooms is the failure to account for floor space taken up by the toilet. An adult wheelchair measures approximately 48 inches from front to back. This means that at least 48 inches of clear space must be allowed in order for the privacy door of a bathroom stall to close behind the back wheels. Many bathrooms labeled with the universal symbol of accessibility fail to meet the standards laid down in the ADA. This misleading signage is a source of much frustration for wheelchair users. To allow for transfers in a 60-inch by 60-inch space, the toilet must be in the opposite corner from the door. This layout is provided for by the ADA "standard" toilet stall (ADA, 1991, p. 35501). Any other layout makes it impossible to get into position for a transfer. The ADA's alternate stalls allow for transferring only if the person backs into the stall.

For the wheelchair user, lengthened oval pedestal sinks are helpful. Piping should be covered with insulating foam to prevent burns to insensate limbs. Cabinet-style sinks are difficult to use from a wheelchair because there is no way to face the mirror, lean over to spit toothpaste, or splash water on one's face in the morning (see Figure 2).

A roll-in shower, space permitting, is easiest for wheelchair bathing. It is important to position the spigots within reach. Towel hooks are preferred over rails because it is easier for someone with limited hand function to hang something on a hook. Also, the presence of towel rails invites their misuse as grab rails, sometimes with disastrous results. One potential problem with roll-in showers is that they are large, and tend to be chilly. A heat lamp and long shower curtain address this concern to some extent. Lacking space for a roll-in shower, the second choice is a standard shower with a tub transfer bench. The last choice is a bathtub with a tub transfer bench. This is most difficult because of the need to lift paralyzed legs over the edge of the tub in order to get into the tub bench. Sliding glass doors on bathtubs are also problematic for persons who bathe on a tub bench or tub chair. It is preferable to install a shower curtain.

Regardless of the type of shower selected, the main concern is to leave enough room to position the wheelchair for a transfer. Common problems are placement of the toilet right by the tub in order to save floor space in construction, or to save on piping by installing all fixtures close together on one "wet-wall." While these practices represent both sound plumbing and sound economics, they are not very workable for the bathroom of any individual requiring a tub bench. This includes not only wheelchairs users, but anyone too weak or unsteady to lower himself or herself into the tub (i.e., persons with strokes, Parkinson's disease, cerebral palsy, etc.). Enough space must be allowed for the individual to sit on the edge of the bench, swing the legs around without getting bruised on the toilet, and lift the legs into the tub.

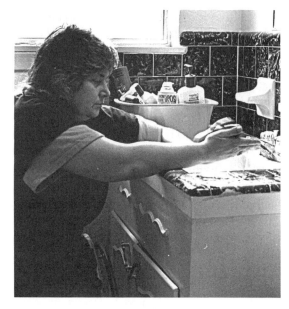

Figure 2. A cabinet-style sink is extremely awkward for the wheelchair user.

Kitchen Fixtures

The selection and positioning of kitchen features will be very strongly influenced by the type of impairments to be accommodated. Efficiency expert Lillian Gilbreth (Gilbreth, 1927; Gilbreth, Thomas, & Clymer, 1959) determined that the most efficient kitchens are organized to form a triangular path from the stove to the refrigerator to the sink. This requires much less walking than a straight-line kitchen that has all the appliances on one wall. Overall, this principle holds well; however, there are a number of ways to create the needed triangle formation, and not all work equally well for persons with various impairments. For the person who can walk but uses a walker, crutches, or two canes, the problem becomes how to carry items from one place to another. For such an individual, it is best to use a triangle with continuous countertop connecting the three "points" so heavy items can be slid over the counter on a hot pad or wheeled trivet. For the wheelchair user with good upper extremity strength, a narrow "facing" setup, with the oven and refrigerator on one wall and the sink on the other can work well, because the person would have the strength to lift a pan or bowl across the space. If the passageway were sufficiently narrow, it would not be necessary to move the wheels while doing so. For all persons, as much storage space as possible should be located between hip and shoulder level to avoid the poor body mechanics of bending or overhead reaching. If this does not provide enough total storage to meet a person's needs, very high or low cupboards can be built to house rarely used items, such as holiday serving dishes.

In addition to triangulation, height of appliances is a key factor. Standard counters are too high for the wheelchair user, but too low for a tall standing person with a back injury. Appliances requiring stooping, such as most ovens and dishwashers, are also a problem for both of these groups. If at all possible, ovens should be set up on counters between shoulder and elbow height of the user. For a wheelchair user there should be a knee hole under this counter, and a clear countertop immediately beside the oven or microwave on which to set hot food dishes. Side-opening doors, rather than swing-down doors, also enhance access. Oven racks that pull out easily and are stable in the forward position are extremely helpful.

The stovetop should be separate from the oven, and at an accessible height. The kneehole for the stovetop should be shallow, and *not* extend under the burners. Kneeholes under the burners present a risk—material may boil over and spill through the burner onto the knees of the cook. Clear counter space beside the stovetop is needed for placing hot pans.

In the case of all appliances, being able to access and operate the controls is a key factor (Steinfold et al., 1979). In most cases stove controls should be in front of the burners, not behind them. This avoids the need to reach over hot burners to turn off the stove (see Figure 3). The exception to this is the case of an individual with poor gait control or visual impairments who is at risk of bumping the stove and inadvertently turning on a burner. For such an individual, controls may be in front, but should be recessed or sit flat on the stovetop, not in a vertical layout on the front.

For a person with sensory deficits, larger dials with high-contrast letters may be of help, while for the blind person, dials with tactile feedback that "click" in at each heat level are helpful. A raised bump should mark the "off" setting for such a dial.

If it is possible to raise the dishwasher, position it so the open door is just over the lap height of the wheelchair user so he or she can get close enough to reach in. A dishwasher with a front-opening door and pull-out racks is easiest to use in this position. When in the usual under-counter position, dishwashers are virtually inaccessible (See Figure 4).

Figure 3 (top). Stove controls should be in front to minimize the risk of burns.

Figure 4 (bottom). This dishwasher is virtually inaccessible.

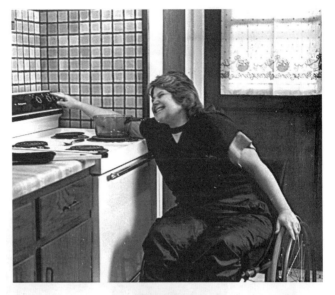

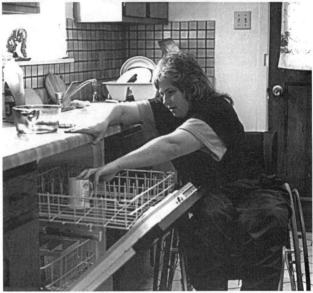

Refrigerator selection depends on individual needs. For wheelchair users, avoid the freezer-on-top style, unless the entire refrigerator is the small apartment size (see Figure 5). Side-by-side and bottom freezer models are easier to access. For the person who cannot stoop, freezer-on-top and side-by-side models are the best choices. If financially feasible, features such as exterior water or ice dispensers can be a great boon to the individual who has difficulty opening refrigerator doors.

If a separate freezer is selected, the front-opening models are much more accessible than the top-opening chests. In any case, it is necessary to allow some clear counter space next to the refrigerator or freezer, on the opening side of the door, so items can be placed there after removing them from storage.

Sinks should be at a comfortable working height for the individual, usually 2 inches to 4 inches below elbow height. A lower sink will cause back strain, while a higher one will chafe the elbow or force an uncomfortable shoulder position. Because a wheelchair sink must accommodate a 27-inch to 29-inch knee hole below, a shallow sink will fit best. Sufficient space must be left underneath for insulation to prevent hot water pipes from burning the person's knees.

It is apparent that the same sink will not provide optimal working conditions for both a wheelchair user and a standing person. In the case of a shared kitchen, a decision must be made either to build two sinks, or to let one person be the sink's primary user. Because each individual should have his or her own "work-triangle," building two sinks is far less costly than two stoves or refrigerators, so it may be a reasonable option for some families. The last factor to consider in sink selection is controls. For the person with arthritis, poor hand control, or weakness, the lever-type single control is best. For the

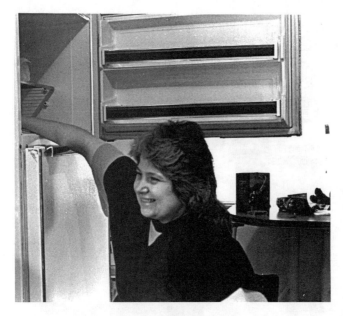

Figure 5. The refrigerator with freezer on top is a poor design for the wheelchair user.

person with incoordination, adjusting the lever-type control can be extremely difficult. Separate hot and cold faucets will allow that person to control water temperature much more easily. Dual controls are also easier for the visually impaired person to operate.

Counters for wheelchair users need to be lower than for standing persons. The height should be selected for the individual, if at all possible, as wheelchair heights and comfortable working levels vary. In general, a knee hole should allow 27 inches to 29 inches of floor-to-undersurface space. Knee holes should be deep enough to allow pulling all the way into the counter: 19 inches minimum depth and 30 inches minimum width.

Cupboard doors present access problems for the wheelchair user. The simplest solution is to have open shelves instead. In most cases, as mentioned above, the fewer doors the better. It is also true that the fewer drawers, the better. Open shelves and pull-out racks require the least reaching, bending, and maneuvering to access the contents.

Surfaces

Following layout of the space itself, the next concern is environmental surfaces. The general principle for persons with mobility impairments is that surfaces should be firm and smooth, while still providing enough traction for good control, and enough cushioning to prevent tissue breakdown. Floors present some of the greatest difficulties. For the wheelchair, walker, crutch, or cane user, a smooth, uncarpeted surface is by far the easiest to negotiate. In most cases, this means linoleum. Although wooden flooring also provides ease of mobility and is quite attractive, its cost is prohibitive for most people. In addition, the heavy maintenance requirements of a hardwood floor make it an unreasonable choice in most homes.

For southwestern style homes, ceramic tile or flagstone floors are attractive and more easily maintained than wood. Cement floors are extremely functional, but they are so cold and unattractive that they are unlikely to be selected for areas other than garages or patios. In climates too cool for tile or stone floors, carpeting is the traditional solution, providing warmth and an attractive appearance to the floor. However, the friction provided by the carpeting can be a major problem, or at the least, a real energy drain. Anyone who has attempted to propel a wheelchair through 2-inch-deep shag will appreciate this point. Whatever carpets are used should be relatively firm and flat, such as indoor-outdoor styles. They should be tightly nailed down, with no protruding nail head to puncture wheelchair tires, and their edges should be neatly covered with metal or plastic edging strips. Loose area rugs should be avoided for all persons with mobility impairments. This is true regardless of whether the impairment is of sensory, cognitive, or motoric origin.

Vertical surfaces must also be taken into consideration. For the wheelchair user, especially the novice, wall coverings should be sturdy and resistant to chipping. For the visually impaired, nonglare surfaces are preferred. Avoid decorative mirror-walls and stark-white formica. The surfaces of built-in features, such as countertops, should also be nonglare, as well as easy to clean, for those with weak hands or poor leverage for scrubbing. Wheelchair users sit too low to lean down on a counter and really scrub, so this is essential for them. Solid-color formica (not white) is probably a better choice than decorative tiles or porous wooden butcher-block countertops.

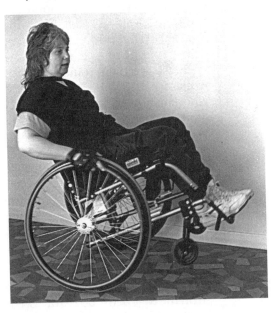

Figure 6. A tile floor is a great surface on which to tip back into a wheelie and relax awhile.

Furniture

In addition to appearance and comfort, function and quality of construction are important considerations for the consumer with a disability (see Figure 7). Some functional considerations include:

1. *Ease or difficulty of transfers onto and off of beds, chairs, and couches.* As the old saying goes, "a lot of things are easier to get into than out of!" This is especially true of waterbeds and overstuffed couches. More than one person has gotten caught in a soft couch and been unable to escape until rescued. The problem is a lack of leverage. A firm couch, level with the top of the wheelchair cushion, is the easiest for both directions of transfer.

Figure 7. Considerations in selecting furniture for persons with disabilities.

1. Ease of transfers
2. Postural support
3. Risk of skin abrasions or ulcers
4. Surface texture that aids or inhibits position or movement
5. Adjustability
6. Impact on function
7. Safety factors
8. Consumer involvement

The simple process of getting out of bed is affected by the presence or absence of bed rails, and by the height and relative firmness of the bed. Bed rails, while useful for safety and repositioning, may be designed to prevent the person in the bed from lowering them. This, obviously, makes it difficult to get out of bed unaided. (This difficult task is sometimes accomplished by persons with dementia, who do not understand that bed rails make it hard to get out of a bed!) If a bed is too high, it may be hard to get one's feet on the floor for a transfer; while if a bed is too low, it may be difficult to do an uphill transfer into a wheelchair or to rise to standing. Overall, it is best to recall the principle of limiting changes in levels. Same-level transfers are easiest in the long run. Most hospital beds are too high to allow for this, unless the wheels are removed. Many "regular" beds are either too high or too low. Bed heights are not standardized the way table heights are. If the bed is wooden, and the legs are too tall, a simple solution is to saw a few inches from the bottom of each leg. This is not particularly noticeable—few people examine the bottoms of bed posts with any degree of scrutiny. It is wise to have a professional carpenter do this so the bed does not end up lopsided. If the bed is too low, furniture leg extenders are available from rehabilitation catalogs. Chairs can be dealt with in the same manner.

2. *Quality of positioning/postural support.* Is the supporting surface firm or structured enough to provide a solid base of support for functional activities? Many people sit on the edge of the bed to dress. For such a purpose, the bed must be the correct height and sufficiently firm to lean against or to sit on in a stable manner. For the person with poor balance, it may be necessary to dress in bed. A larger bed is easier to dress on than a small one, because most people who dress in bed must roll from side to side to pull up their trousers. Bed rails may be of great use in this process, but, as mentioned above, they do often limit independent egress from the bed. An individual with a spinal cord injury of C-7 or below can push to sitting on a firm mattress, and consequently dress independently. This cannot be accomplished on a soft mattress. A C-5 or weak C-6 person with quadriplegia will likely require an electric bed to come to a sitting position in order to reach his or her feet to don slacks, socks, and shoes (Smith, 1988).

3. *Interface pressures between the person's skin and the supporting surface.* (Krouskop, 1992). Are pressures distributed to limit the risk of decubitus ulcers? Although the best pressure-control seating is probably in the wheelchair cushion, one does spend time sitting or lying on other surfaces. A medical sheepskin between the mattress and the sheet can be useful. An egg crate mattress, if used, should be placed with the flat surface up for best results. A well-baffled waterbed can provide pressure relief without making transfers inordinately difficult. Special-ized pressure-relief beds, such as those that are air-fluidized, are beyond both the needs and budgets of most people.

4. *Texture of the supporting surface.* How much shearing of the skin will occur if the person slides across the bed or couch? On the other hand, is there sufficient friction to keep the person from sliding off the chair seat, a problem that can occur with hardwood chairs? Many persons with mobility impairments select satin sheets to ease turning in bed. However, some individuals find that these do not provide enough traction for pushing to sitting.

5. *Position changes.* Is the chair/bed/couch adjustable, or does it provide only one

position? Not all persons require this feature, but for those who do, it is very important. Powered beds are helpful for individuals whose personal care is performed, completely or in part, by other people. The ability to raise the bed to an appropriate working height can prevent back strain in the caregiver.

Chairs with powered assists can help a weak individual rise to his or her feet. Care must be taken in selecting these, as too fast an assist can throw an unsteady person forward into a fall. A key safety feature is that the seat-lifter should stop lifting when the button is released. The recliner chair is useful for persons on home dialysis, who need to recline while being dialyzed. Adjustable height tables are helpful when individuals with different positioning needs use the same space at different times.

6. *Functional considerations.* Does the item of furnishing facilitate or inhibit the independent functioning of the person or people in question? Can the individual not only access the piece of furniture, but also perform whatever functional tasks are generally performed using that item? Can he or she actually write at the desk; sleep, dress, and engage in sexual activity in the bed; or watch television from the couch?

Tables and desks are simply a matter of the correct height, and, for wheelchair users, adequate knee hole. Shelves should be at a level usable by the individual—for a person with a lower extremity amputation, or anyone with a knee or back injury, low shelves are to be avoided; while for the wheelchair user, high shelves will be out of reach. In general, no shelves for anyone should be placed so high as to require neck hyperextension. Shelves are potentially messier than drawers, because they lack the front board to hold the contents in place. For this reason, fewer items can be neatly placed on a shelf than in a drawer of equivalent size. More total square feet of shelf space must be allotted than if drawers were used to store the same items. Shelves nonetheless provide more usable storage for the same floor space than drawers. A wheelchair user unable to access lower drawers because they need to be pulled out into his or her way can reach into lower shelves. He or she can also use higher shelves, while a high drawer is above visual range. In a five-drawer upright chest, only the second to the top drawer would open over the lap of a wheelchair rider, allowing him or her to see in and access the contents. A shelving unit occupying the same floor space would have usable shelves from 1 foot to 5 feet above the floor, and 3 to 5 shelves, depending on the height of each. Should the esthetics of open shelves be undesirable, the shelves can be curtained or built into the closet.

7. *Safety.* Select furnishings that limit the risk of falls or other injuries. Loose scatter rugs are accidents waiting to happen. If cushioning for the feet is desired at a sink or counter, select a thick rubber mat. Bath mats should have nonskid bottoms. They should be used only for bathing, and hung up on the side of the tub at other times to decrease the chance of slipping.

8. *Selection.* The person who will use the furniture should be present when it is chosen. No one else knows as well as the individual which pieces of furniture will work for him or her. People with disabilities have increasingly become informed consumers and active advocates on their own behalf. This movement is completely in concert with the occupational therapy principle of functional independence.

Out on the Town

The home environment can be made relatively negotiable for an individual with generally stable abilities and impairments, given adequate financial and other resources. The public self-care environment is far less user-friendly. While some improvements have been made, based on the American National Standards Institute [ANSI] regulations (1971, 1980), the Rehabilitation Act (1973), the Education for all Handicapped Children Act (1975), and, most recently, the ADA (1991), many of these are honored more in misapplication than in application.

So-Called Public Toilets

A problem with public access is, simply, the failure of either the legislators or the builders to think through functional considerations thoroughly. The two methods of wheelchair-toilet transfer illustrated in the text of the ADA (1991) are both unnecessarily difficult and risky. The easiest and safest transfer—a 45° angle approach—is not shown. Many of the bathroom layouts recommended by the law are marginally accessible at best. A quick examination of wheelchair bathrooms in local restaurants will quickly convince one that no one involved in the planning has ever spent much time in a wheelchair, ever watched anyone in a wheelchair attempt to negotiate a tight space, or even attempted to think through the process of actually trying to use the room proudly labeled with the symbol of accessibility (McClain et al., 1993). Thus, a wheelchair-accessible sink may be provided, but the paper towel dispenser is across the room and 5 feet from the floor.

Level transfers are far easier than uphill or downhill transfers. The toilets in accessible stalls should be tall, preferably 19 inches. This will also be helpful to persons who walk, but have difficulty arising.

The doors must swing toward the outside, not into the stall. There must be enough room outside the stall to maneuver into the door, as well as enough room inside to shut the door. While the standard toilet stall recommended by the ADA (1991) accommodates an average adult, 48-inch wheelchair, the alternate stall does not.

For the individual on a self-catheterization program, a toilet stall should provide a small shelf on which to place the "cath kit." One also needs 48 inches of clear space directly in front of the toilet to allow for draining the catheter into the toilet.

Beyond the problems encountered within the bathroom lies the problem of finding one in the first place. A major improvement featured by the ADA (1991) is the requirement that at least one bathroom per floor of a building be accessible. In new construction, each bathroom must have at least one accessible stall.

Dining Out

Second only to difficulties with bathrooms come difficulties with attempting to eat in public (McClain et al., 1993). Fast food restaurants are notorious for high counters (see Figures 8 and 9). Bars are filled with tall stools and tables to match. Restaurants with built-in booths may have no place to sit in a wheelchair or to transfer out of one. It is a real exercise in assertiveness to order popcorn in a crowded, noisy, cinema lobby when one's head is below the level of the counter. Carrying the popcorn through the double doors into the movie is an adventure in itself. In addition to the self-care problem inherent in the difficulty of obtaining nutrition, these situations present problems in social well-being. It is difficult and embarrassing to take a date out for dinner if one can't even use the salad bar. Salad bars are virtually unreachable from a wheelchair, due to the height and angle of the bins.

Figure 8. This snack bar is only for those who can climb.

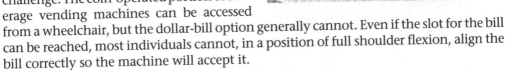

For individuals with limited ability to self-feed, the social aspects of the self-care environment may be challenging indeed. To be forced to ask someone to feed you, in public, is not easy on anybody's self-esteem. Even more difficult is the situation of someone requiring tube feeding—going out for lunch with friends moves into the realm of the impossible.

Obtaining Beverages

Even maintaining hydration can become a challenge. The coin-operated portion of beverage vending machines can be accessed from a wheelchair, but the dollar-bill option generally cannot. Even if the slot for the bill can be reached, most individuals cannot, in a position of full shoulder flexion, align the bill correctly so the machine will accept it.

Most water fountains are too high, while some wheelchair fountains are too low, or lack kneeholes. Water coolers with paper cups are a better option.

Shopping

Aside from trying to eat in public, there is the issue of obtaining food to cook and eat at home (Spencer, Krefting, & Mattingly, 1993). Some grocery stores helpfully provide power scooters with grocery baskets on the front. These are especially useful for persons who can stand briefly

to obtain items from high shelves, but lack the balance or endurance to walk all around the store. For the walker user, simply pushing a grocery cart may provide a stable alternative if one has fairly good balance and a safe place to leave one's own walker while shopping.

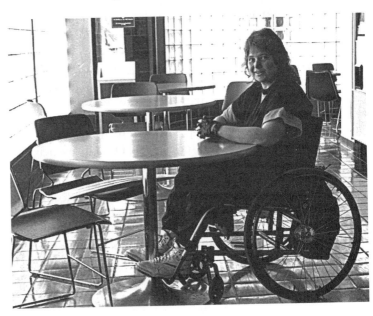

Figure 9. A pedestal table and tile floor make this snack bar easily negotiable.

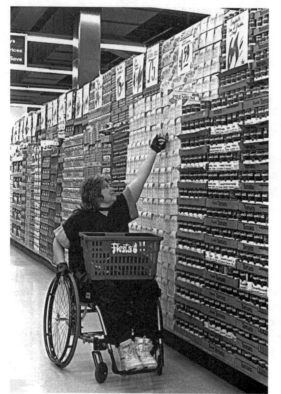

Figure 10. Most supermarket shelves have items out of reach of the wheel-chair user.

Shopping from a wheelchair presents a great challenge. The person cannot push a grocery cart, and thus is limited to what can be carried in a basket on the lap or a back pack slung behind the chair. Many items are quite simply out of reach (see Figure 10). One individual described the experience:

It seems like they are just trying to make you feel as helpless and weak and useless as possible. You're always having to ask for help when you don't want to. It's "Excuse me ma'am, would you mind doing me a favor?" all the time. I'd rather do things for myself, but I have to do my shopping somehow, and they have so much of the stuff out of reach. I just hate it.

For the individual with sensory or perceptual deficits, the overwhelming level of visual stimuli can make grocery stores very difficult environments. Glaring waxed linoleum floors further challenge the person with limited vision. For such persons, it is best always to use a single store and memorize the layout. An alternative method is to make a simple map of the store, with the locations of one's usually purchased items marked on it. Photocopy a number of the maps, and use one instead of a grocery list as a guide around the store. This system also works well for posttraumatic brain injury patients or others who easily become disoriented in the high-sensory-stimuli environment of the store.

Having purchased groceries, squeezed through the narrow aisle at the checkout, and received a brown paper bag of food, the real fun begins. How to get this bag of groceries to the car? Precariously balanced on the knees, perhaps? But what if the person is a crutch walker? Or walker user? Perhaps the sacker will help at this juncture, but the problem reappears upon arriving home. Getting the groceries out of the trunk is a real feat in leverage for the wheelchair-using shopper. It may be necessary to take the items inside in shifts, carrying a few things at a time on the lap. Or to hire a neighbor who happens to be able-bodied. A large wheelchair backpack with a relatively rigid frame can be useful. The person should be careful to avoid twisting and injuring his or her back while attempting to lift such a pack. It is better to remove items from the pack than to lift it full from the back of the chair. For the individual who walks but has limited ability to carry items, a cart can be useful.

The purchases must still be put away in the cupboards and refrigerator. And, beyond all this, the person has obtained only a small supply of groceries, due to the difficulty of transporting more than one shopping bag at a time. This entire procedure must be endured again in 2 or 3 days.

Some grocery stores will deliver for a fee, often out of reach for persons on fixed incomes, but a great advantage to those who can afford such a luxury. A chore service may also shop for individuals, or accompany them to the store. For the person who lives with another family member, it may be simplest to delegate shopping to someone else, and even it up by performing some other chore, such as paying the bills.

Health and Appearance

Some self-care activities are directed not only toward survival, but also toward health and appearance. We join health clubs to work out, buy clothes to improve our appearance, wear makeup, shave, and style our hair.

Beauty and barber shops present a real problem for wheelchair users because it is impossible for many to transfer into the barber's chair. A haircut can be given in place, but there are two negative outcomes. The wheelchair inevitably collects hair clippings, even with a drape provided; and the stylist cannot optimally position the person to cut his or her hair.

There is also the fitting room at the clothing store to contend with. As the ADA (1991) begins to affect new construction, there will be dressing rooms with benches on which to transfer to change clothes, and from which the mirror can be seen. The new regulations allow for a bench 24 inches wide and 48 inches long. This will help some individuals, but because it is not long enough for most adults to lie on, many persons will still be unable to try on clothes before buying them. Until then, trying on clothes is an option only for those who can fully dress or undress themselves in a wheelchair—and then only when the dressing room is large enough to accommodate the chair. This is a frustrating situation at best.

Another factor is maintaining personal safety while shopping. An individual attempting to transfer himself or herself, plus shopping bags, into a car is at risk for a hold-up. It is wise for him or her to carry mace or some other personal safety device. Obtaining a car phone enables the person to call for help. A cellular phone is preferable to a citizens' band radio, because with the latter anyone can answer the call. The cellular phone should have adequate range to cover at least the person's daily travels, and long distance if traveling out of town.

Working out at the gym may be impossible. Accessible equipment does exist, but is rarely available. Some YWCA or YMCA facilities are equipped for adapted swimming or provide warm water pools for people with arthritis. Free weights are an option, as are some weights on a universal gym. The real difficulties start in the locker room. The lockers may be reachable, but what about the shower? Can the person even begin to climb into the sauna or hot tub? Is there a lift to help the person into or out of the swimming pool?

Taking Care of Business

Money management is not a real access problem—but banking is. From automatic teller machines to the counter at the local bank, money-handling appears to be carried out in the standing position only. Even the table or desk provided to fill out the deposit slip is at standing height. Yet drive-through banks are too low to be reached from a van—they are designed for cars. The ADA (1991) mandates provision of automated tellers at an accessible height, which will be a major improvement over current conditions. Unfortunately, the law neglects to prescribe height requirements for drive-up tellers. This minor omission means that individuals who must drive a van—often those for whom transferring is difficult and time consuming—must transfer out in order to use the teller machine.

The post office, like the bank, is designed for quick use—everything is done in the standing position. Why is this a self-care concern? Well, it is hard to maintain one's body temperature, for example, without mailing the electric bill to keep the heating or cooling system running. And unlike banks, post offices, especially the older ones, are often built in the imposing style of federal buildings, with many stone steps running up to the front door. It has been said of such a post office that "We don't need to adapt it for wheelchair users. They never come in here anyway. . . ."

Cleanliness is Next to…Impossible

Imagine loading a basket with soiled laundry and balancing it on your lap all the way to the laundromat of your apartment complex, then attempting to negotiate the step into the laundromat, trying to fit in between the folding table and the dryers…

Whether at home or at a public laundromat, a person in a wheelchair is apt to find the top-loading washer a real frustration. The last sock will inevitably be just 2 inches out of reach. The use of a long-handled reacher is essential in this situation, so the person must carry that along, too. The folding tables are designed in most cases for the standing user— above the level of a wheelchair user's head. These factors may combine to make laundromat use impossible for the wheelchair user.

Keeping the Doctor Away

Preventive health care is a very important aspect of caring for the self. We are taught from childhood to have regular physical and dental checkups. Annual gynecological exams begin in adulthood, and mammograms at age 35. It is a rather odd paradox that the health care system can be among the least accessible of self-care settings. The ADA (1991) devotes less than a page and a half of accessibility guidelines to medical care facilities, and, in that space, physicians' offices are not even mentioned.

Consider briefly the gynecologist's table with its stirrups. Then imagine a woman with quadriplegia attempting to climb into such a device. Dentists' chairs present similar problems. A recliner wheelchair can be employed if available, but few chair-using individuals have one at their disposal, and even fewer gynecologists or dentists are so equipped.

Even rehabilitation hospitals, designed for the disabled, can be frustratingly inaccessible, as pointed out by the vignette at the beginning of this chapter. The patient rooms in such hospitals or units are generally better designed than those in other types of hospitals. There are usually closets with lowered rails, and larger bathrooms with roll-in showers. However, the rooms are often set up for nursing care, not for self-care. Thus the shower is large, and the nurse can roll the patient into it with ease, after undressing the patient and procuring the towels and soap for him or her. The nurse can then transfer the patient to the shower chair and proceed. It is a different story if the patient tries to shower independently in such a bathroom. Then its lack of user friendliness is revealed. The towels are stored in a high cabinet down the hall. There is nowhere for the person to hang his or her clothes after doffing them. There is nowhere in the shower to set the shampoo bottle and cream rinse, save on the floor. This is not a problem for the able-bodied nurse, but it is a definite problem for the wheelchair user, or, worse, the walking patient who cannot safely bend, such as someone on postsurgical or body-jacket precautions. The towel hooks are across the room on the door. A person who chills easily can become quite uncomfortable while traveling across the room wet and naked to get a towel.

Patients in rehabilitation are often taught to undress in bed, for reasons of safety. But then there is nowhere to put their doffed garments except on the floor or the bedside table—and neither is an acceptable solution. A hamper beside the bed would provide a simple solution to this self-care problem.

On the Road

Traveling is a particular challenge for the individual with special self-care needs. In an unfamiliar setting, one is constantly facing unexpected conditions, and may require forms of assistance not needed at home (Monnot, 1988) (see Figure 11). Just imagine trying to get a wheelchair into the toilet stall of an airplane. And it is not only traveling by air that may present difficulties. Cross country buses do not come under the purview of the ADA until July 1996 (Breslin, 1993). Until that date, it will remain impossible for many to climb onto the bus, let alone attempt to use the tiny toilet stall at the back.

Many individuals with mobility impairments find it easiest to travel in their own vehicles. A van or recreational vehicle is often found to be more convenient than a car. These people can, in a sense, take their own negotiable home along for the trip. There is a growing list of accessible campgrounds, found in a U.S. Forest Service booklet titled: *Design Guide for Accessible Outdoor Recreation* (1992). It is wise for the individual to call the park in advance and ask detailed questions of the park ranger, including "Has anyone with [my condition] ever stayed there, and if, so how did it work out?" A van eliminates much of the guesswork because it can be parked in virtually any campground. If the interior "conversion" is well-planned, it is possible for the person to meet many of his or her self-care needs in the vehicle. If the person is using a van lift, he or she should select one that takes up as little of the interior floor space of the van as possible. Good privacy curtains are a must. There should also be a curtain that can be drawn behind the driver's seat to obscure the view in through the windshield. It is possible to sleep and dress in the van, perform self-catheterization, or use a commode. The person may want to obtain a folding commode, if possible. For commodes, a nice touch is for the individual to obtain disposable bags with chemical inserts that solidify liquid wastes and eliminate odors. These are available from medical supply houses.

A fold-down table allows for preparing at least uncooked meals. The person can also transfer out of the van and cook and eat at a picnic table, using a lightweight backpacker's stove. If using a wheelchair inside a van, a narrow folding-frame chair is best. If the person is quite strong, it may be simplest to eliminate the chair and scoot about inside the van, having the mattress down on the floor.

Travelers soon learn to call or write to hotels in advance, specifying their needs (Molnar, 1991). Simply to ask whether a facility is accessible is insufficient—like the wheelchair symbol posted on the bathroom door, the label "accessible hotel room" is often

Figure 11. An information card may help avoid repetitive explanations.

> **Note to Flight Attendant**
>
> I have _____ (condition).
>
> Please help me with:
>
> - Taking off jacket
> - Unwrapping food
> - Fastening clothes in restroom
>
> Thank you for your assistance!
>
> Sincerely, _____

deceptive. The person must explain in detail how much negotiating room is needed between the wall and the bed—at least 32 inches to travel through, but more like 48 inches to be able to transfer into the bed. Often, the luxury suite of a hotel is larger and can be used more easily than the accessible suite. If so, it should be made available at the regular price. The closet should have both low and standard rails, and the bed should be an appropriate height and firmness. The person should be prepared, when calling, to provide the hotel manager with the dimensions of the wheelchair and to ask if it will fit into the bathroom.

The room should be safe for the user with sensory deficits. There should be a fire egress plan for the individual with mobility impairments—ideally, the room should be on the ground floor. If it is a relatively safe neighborhood, sliding glass doors directly to the courtyard provide a good exit. A member of the hotel staff should be designated to assist with fire evacuation for the person who cannot transfer extremely quickly or who has sensory deficits and may need direction in an unfamiliar setting. There should be flashing fire alarms for the hearing impaired, and braille labels for the blind on hot and cold faucets. This is especially important in geographical areas where the right/left, hot/cold convention may not be followed. A TTY phone should be available for those with a hearing impairment.

The bathroom should have a tub transfer bench (the kind that extends over the edge of the tub), not simply a shower chair. The controls should be reachable from the tub bench. Towel hooks should also be within reach. Sliding glass doors on the tub make it inaccessible to the individual who needs a tub bench. Grab rails should extend most of the length of the tub.

The sink should be a pedestal, or in a counter with a kneehole below. The toilet should be 19 inches high, and have 48 inches of clear space to one side—room to get into position for a side-side 45° angle transfer and to close the door for privacy.

Bathrooms in foreign countries often have different layouts than those in the United States. For example, in some areas of Mexico the toilet stalls are 4 inches to 6 inches above floor level, presumably to accommodate plumbing. This renders them totally inaccessible by a wheelchair user and other persons unable to negotiate a step.

The hotel restaurant and bar should be fully accessible to the mobility impaired, as well as provide Braille menus. If the restaurant is not accessible, room service should be provided at no extra charge. This should be established in advance, in writing.

Another factor affecting self-care performance while traveling has to do with sightseeing. Before going to any historical buildings or scenic locations, the person should call to find out whether accessible bathrooms and water fountains have been provided. Some historic landmarks have been exempted from the access laws. These determinations are made by the local historical societies, based on whether or not the adaptations would significantly take away from accurate historical preservation of the site.

In planning a trip, it is of inestimable value for the person to contact other individuals who have traveled to the same location, or who live in the area to which he or she is going.

The Role of the Occupational Therapist in the Self-Care Environment

Assessment

In assessing the home environment, a home visit is well worth the time involved. In some rehabilitation settings, the home visit is not performed—instead, a family member is given a list of measurements to take, such as doorway widths. This list is returned to the therapist for recommendations. While better than nothing, such a list has limited value because it enables one to check only accessibility, not negotiability. Relying on the memory of one's patient or family members to describe the home is not of much help, either. People often find it hard to describe a place that they see every day simply because it is so familiar and taken for granted that they don't pay attention to it any more. This may be a reason why many accidents occur in the home. We don't notice the hazards in our daily environment because it has always been that way. A throw rug that was put down years ago and presented no hazard to an unimpaired person, may not be mentioned in the description of the home. That same rug, now a hazard to an individual with impaired balance, could have easily been removed, if noticed.

Negotiability Rating

A thorough home visit should include a negotiability assessment. The therapist first makes a careful inventory of all features of the home environment, starting with the approach to the door. The therapist then retraces this path with the client. The client is asked to try to use each environmental feature for its intended purpose, with only his or her usual adaptive equipment—open and pass through the door, obtain water from the sink, transfer onto and off of the toilet. The client is asked to try each feature, regardless of whether or not he or she usually does so. Any environmental feature that cannot be used by the client should be noted, with a description or measurement of whatever it was that limited the function; for example, "Cupboard not negotiable—client cannot reach in—6 inches above top of comfortable reach, 3 inches above maximal reach." Once a list is completed, the negotiability rating may be obtained by computing the proportion of features negotiable by the user. This simple percentage calculation (see Figure 12) is useful for documenting measurable changes as a result of occupational therapy intervention. For example, if the therapist provides adaptive equipment making two more features negotiable, and recommends environmental adaptations making four more features negotiable, the rating increases (see Figure 13).

Figure 12. Sample negotiability calculation.

Number of environmental features: 76
Number negotiable: 42
[Calculation (42/76) x 100]
Negotiable environment = 55.26%

Figure 13. Changes in negotiability as the result of occupational therapy intervention.

Environmental features:	76
Original number negotiable:	42
Number added by OT intervention:	6
Number currently negotiable:	48
New rating: (48/76) x 100 =	63.42%
Original rating =	55.26%
Improvement =	8.24%

It must be emphasized that negotiability represents the interplay of the person, the environment, and the adaptive equipment. It cannot be assessed in general terms, only for the individual person in his or her own environment. Its strength as a concept is that it is sensitive to changes in all three arenas.

A negotiability rating is not a self-care scale in the ordinary sense. It does not rate the person's ability to perform in general. It rates only the person's ability to perform in a given environment with given equipment. The other key point is that it is not an activity-analyzed rating system. In other words, the units being rated are not units of performance, they are units of the environment. An environmental feature is negotiable—or not—for a given person, with given equipment. For an item to be negotiable, the person must be able to perform all logically related tasks or task components. That is, to negotiate a door, one unlocks a lock, turns a door knob, opens the door, passes through a door frame, and closes and locks the door.

In rating negotiability, environmental features are left in their usual positions. They may be moved later as part of the intervention. In other words, if the individual could possibly sit on a chair, but the chair is in an inaccessible corner, then the chair is not negotiable unless the individual can reposition it unaided.

It is important to make an inventory of the individual's environment to obtain an accurate rating. The list of features suggested in Figure 14 is provided merely to draw the reader's attention to areas of the self-care environment that may be neglected.

Recommendations

For each environmental feature found not to be negotiable, determine whether or not the client wishes to be able to negotiate it. Question carefully in this regard. People will sometimes deny interest in an activity because they believe it is not an option, so "why want what you can't have?" In other cases, the person genuinely has no interest in performing a given activity. Someone who has not cooked in 70 years is unlikely to start

Figure 14. Environmental features and associated functions.

Environmental Feature	Associated Function
Floor surface (each type)	Traverse floor
Light switches	Turn on and off
Doorways	Open door, traverse, close door
Chairs (each style)	Transfer onto, sit on, perform relevant functional tasks while sitting, and transfer or arise from chair
Tables/desks/counters/workbenches	Approach surface and perform appropriate tasks (e.g., eat at table, work at desk or counter)
Storage (shelves, etc.)	Place and retrieve items
Windows	Approach, open, close, operate blinds/drapes, look out each window
Appliances	Approach appliance and perform all aspects of operating it
Outdoors/yard	Work in garden, operate grill, eat at picnic table

at that juncture. If the individual does wish to be able to negotiate a given environmental feature, attempt to discern what is limiting its negotiability—is it the environmental feature? The need for adaptive equipment? The individual's status? Consider what would be involved in making changes to each area. After eliminating the medically, physically, or financially impossible, proceed to implement whatever is left. Select the area or areas of intervention that seem likely to yield the best results for the least outlay of resources. That is, if one could either purchase a stove with the controls in front, or a self-standing powered wheelchair to allow the person to reach the existing controls, the price differential makes it an easy choice. The new stove costs several hundred dollars, while the self-standing wheelchair had a 1992 sticker price of $30,000.

Options for Change

What follows are suggestions for creating self-care environments—not an exhaustive compendium. Creative problem solving is a therapist's best asset, for no existing solution may meet the needs of your present client. The local Center for Independent Living is an excellent resource for those wishing to move into or build a negotiable home. The following are familiar concepts that have worked well in the past, arranged roughly from least costly to most costly.

1. Rearrange existing furniture.
   - Eliminate unnecessary items.
   - If the person rarely transfers from the wheelchair, eliminate at least one chair from the living room and dining room.
   - Get rid of throw rugs.
   - Rearrange items on kitchen shelves to reach items most commonly used.
   - Switch rooms—if necessary, a large living room can replace an unreachable bedroom.
2. Adapt existing furniture/fixtures.
   - Add leg extenders to low chairs/beds.
   - Cut legs from high chairs/beds.
   - Put plywood under the mattress or couch cushions to add firmness.
   - Add a raiser to the toilet seat.
   - Purchase grab rails and install them in the bathroom—make sure they are mounted into the stud, and never use a towel rack for a grab rail. Towel racks are held in place only by short screws into the plaster, and pull out easily.
   - Add a lumbar cushion to chairs.
   - Add a foam wedge to the bed for positioning.
   - Remove interior doors (this adds approximately 2 inches of available space to a doorway).
   - Remove cabinet doors to create open shelves.
   - Remove doors from below cabinet-style sinks to allow knee room.
   - Remove sliding glass shower doors; replace with a curtain.
   - Lower closet rails.

3. Purchase new furniture/fixtures.
   - Purchase a commode for over-toilet or bedside use.
   - Replace the toilet with a higher style.
   - Obtain a tub transfer bench or shower chair, depending on the person's transfer skills.
   - Obtain a refrigerator with side-by-side doors or a bottom freezer for a wheelchair user, or a top freezer for a person unable to bend.
   - Obtain an environmental control system or have one installed.
   - Purchase or rent an electric bed.

4. Move to an accessible environment.

   When contemplating the cost and inconvenience of making architectural changes to one's home, especially if it is rented, it may be best simply to move to a setting that is already adapted to one's needs. This, of course, depends on the availability of such housing—in the author's home town, there is a 2-year waiting list as of this writing. As with the purchase of furniture, the individual with specialized self-care needs should carefully check out the apartment in person before moving in. A building designed for the elderly may not meet the needs of a young person with a disability, and vice-versa. Never assume that the "accessible" label means it will work for a given person. He or she should rate the apartment for negotiability, as outlined above, before moving in.

5. Make architectural changes.
   - Widen doorways.
   - Add ramps, stair-lifts, or elevators.
   - Replace carpets with tile, wood, flagstones, or linoleum.
   - Install lower counters with kneeholes in the kitchen.
   - Obtain a side-opening standard and/or a microwave oven and place it on a lowered counter.
   - Have a shallow sink positioned in a lowered counter.
   - Replace drawers with built-in shelves for the wheelchair user.

6. Build your own.

   Considering the cost and inconvenience involved in architectural changes, even to an owned home, it may be worth building a new home to the person's own specifications. If doing so, the person needs to take into account the recommendations at the beginning of this chapter regarding layout and environmental surfaces. It would also be wise for the person to work with both an occupational therapist and an architect in designing an accessible home.

Factors Affecting Decisions to Change the Environment

Although it is not possible to know what is best in each case, it is possible to state which factors probably need to be considered when deciding which of the above routes to follow in the attempt to improve the negotiability of a person's self-care environment. The following list may help.

1. Which factor is easiest to change? The environment, the equipment, the abilities of the person—or some combination?

2. What will the available funding sources pay for? This is not necessarily the least expensive option in an ultimate sense, but the determining factor in the decision may be what the sources will pay for and what they won't. Contact the insurer or government agency to find this out in advance. So-called retrofitters (professionals who adapt existing structures) may charge as much as the funding source allots, rather than what the same job would cost if done by a regular carpenter. However, some funding sources may mandate use of a retrofitter rather than a general contractor. It is also worthwhile to check out community resources. Victims of violent crimes are sometimes eligible for grants. Some religious and charitable organizations provide funds. A rehabilitation social worker can provide information about local sources of funding.

3. Is the expected result worth the effort and cost? Is it worth purchasing a $30,000 wheelchair in order to be able to stand up and slice carrots? Would the purchase of a low table be a more realistic solution?

4. What is the impact of this environmental adaptation on the other people who share the same environment? Some adaptations, such as changing bed heights, have little impact on others, while some radically affect the accessibility for other people. Kitchens work especially well for either wheelchair-level or standing cooks, but not both. Unless the person has the space and money for two sinks and two stove tops, someone's access will be limited. It is important to decide who plans on doing the majority of the cooking and dishwashing in any given kitchen.

5. Does the adaptation meet legal requirements and building codes? These vary considerably from place to place, so suffice it to state that prior to beginning a construction project of any kind it is necessary to consult the local authorities and obtain any needed permits.

Values Clarification: A Case Study

A therapist once explained to a patient that the patient's bathroom could indeed be made accessible—it was only necessary to replace the in-cabinet sink with a pedestal or wall-mounted sink, and add a sliding door in one wall. The patient made no comment. Over the course of a week, it became apparent that the patient was not motivated for therapy, but, when questioned, she denied feeling that way. Eventually the patient's daughter made a private stop at the clinic and explained the situation to the therapist.

"You see, mom has never felt comfortable with you since you told her to put in a different sink. She just got that bathroom redecorated after years of waiting, and she was really offended that you just told her to get rid of her new sink."

"But she can't get into the bathroom the way it is," protested the therapist. "She may never get into it again."

"I know," replied the daughter. "But she doesn't care about that."

"You mean, she'll take bed baths the rest of her life, and use a bedside commode, just to avoid changing her bathroom?"

"Yes," replied the patient's daughter. "That's exactly what I mean."

"So what I really need to do is help her order a bedside commode, and tell her she doesn't have to redo the bathroom after all," the therapist commented.

"Now you understand," replied the daughter.

The moral of this story is: Do not assume that your patients have the same values and beliefs that you do. The fact that to an occupational therapist functional independence is the highest goal for a patient does not mean that the patient necessarily agrees. For some individuals, the appearance of the home may be far more valuable than the ability to use it functionally. And it is their absolute right to hold such beliefs. In assessing and adapting the self-care environment, as in all occupational therapy interventions, our role is not to remake our clients according to our standards: It is to help them live according to their own. ◆

References

American National Standards Institute, Inc. (1971). *American National Standards specifications for making buildings and facilities accessible to, and usable by, the physically handicapped.* New York: Author.

American National Standards Institute, Inc. (1980). *American National Standards specifications for making buildings and facilities accessible to, and usable by, the physically handicapped.* New York: Author.

Americans With Disabilities Act (ADA). (1991). Appendix to part 1191: Accessibility guidelines for buildings and families. *Federal Register, 56*(154), 35455–35542.

Bates, P.S., Spencer, J.C., Rintala, D.H., & Young, M.E. (1993). Assistive technology and the newly disabled adult: Adaptation to wheelchair use. *American Journal of Occupational Therapy, 47,* 1014–1021.

Breslin, M.L. (1993). On the road—almost. *Mainstream, 17*(7), 12–15.

Education for all Handicapped Children Act of 1975, 20 U.S.C. § 1501, 1505, 1506, 1511 et seq., 1553 (1975).

Gilbreth, L.E.M. (1927). *The home-maker and her job.* New York: D. Appleton.

Gilbreth, L.E.M., Thomas, O.M., & Clymer, E. (1959). *Management in the home: Happier living through saving time and energy* (Rev. & Enlarged). New York: Dodd, Mead.

Krouskop, T.A. (1992). *Selecting a support surface.* Unpublished manuscript, Baylor College of Medicine, Houston, TX.

McClain, L., Beringer, D., Kuhnert, H., Priest, J., Wilkes, E., Wilkinson, S., & Wyrick, L. (1993). Restaurant wheelchair accessibility. *American Journal of Occupational Therapy, 47,* 619–623.

Molnar, M. (1991). Questions to ask before hitting the vacation trail. *Mainstream, 15*(6), 11–13.

Monnot, M. (1988). *From rage to courage: The road to dignity walk.* Northfield, MN: St. Denis Press.

Murray, H.A. (1938). *Explorations in personality.* New York: Oxford University Press.

Noris-Baker, C., & Willems, E.P. (1978). Environmental negotiability as a direct measurement of behavior-environment relationships: some implications for theory and practice. In A. D. Seidel & S. Danford (Eds.), *Proceedings of the Tenth Annual Conference of the Environmental Design Research Association* (pp. 209–214). Houston, TX.

Rehabilitation Act of 1973, 29 U.S.C. § 701 et seq., (1973).

Smith, R. (1988). Quality assurance in equipment ordering for the spinal–cord injured patient. *American Journal of Occupational Therapy, 42,* 36–39.

Spencer, J., Krefting, L., & Mattingly, C. (1993). Incorporation of ethnographic methods in occupational therapy assessment. *American Journal of Occupational Therapy, 47,* 303–309.

Steinfold, E., Schroeder, S., Duncan, J., Faste, R., Chollet, D., Bishop, M., Wirth, P., & Cardell, P. (1979). *Access to the built environment: A review of the literature.* Washington, DC: U.S. Government Printing Office.

U.S. Forest Service. (1992). *Design guide for accessible outdoor recreation.* Washington, DC: U.S. Government Printing Office.

16

Caregiver Assistance: Using Family Members and Attendants

Carolyn Baum

Patricia LaVesser

Carolyn Baum, PhD, OTR/L, FAOTA, is Elias Michael Director and Assistant Professor, Program in Occupational Therapy, and Assistant Professor of Neurology at Washington University in St. Louis, MO.

Patricia LeVesser, MA, OTR/L is an Instructor in the Program in Occupational Therapy and a doctoral student in Social Work at Washington University in St. Louis, MO.

Chapter 16 Outline

Who Are the Caregivers, and Why do They Provide Care?

Assisting the Family in Providing Care

Minimizing Burden

Applying a Family Systems Perspective

Informal Versus Formal Support

Types of Formal Support

Occupational Therapy Frameworks for Facilitating Caregiving in the Home

Attendant Selection, Supervision, and Training

Strategies to Maximize Performance of the Person With the Impairment, and the Family

Avoiding Excess Disability and Neglect

Future Policy Considerations: Options to Allow Caregivers Access to OT Services

Implications for Policy

Appendix

References

Increased survival rates following serious trauma, an aging population, the AIDS epidemic, and government policies favoring noninstitutional care are among the factors that have created a heightened interest in care provided in the home. Although family members most often provide care when it occurs in the home setting, services are also provided by personal care attendants and home health aides, particularly when a permanent disability or chronic or progressive illness is involved, reimbursement is available, and the person needing care is unable to perform basic self-care tasks without assistance. During discharge planning involving patients who require self-care assistance, the occupational therapist must view the needs of the individual and the family's ability to provide or arrange for home care as important considerations. This chapter presents an overview of current issues and provides basic information to assist the occupational therapist in providing informed discharge planning and caregiver assistance.

Under the current health care system in the United States, the family is expected to care for individuals with various types of functional impairment. Prior to the mid-1970s, individuals with cognitive deficits often were institutionalized, though not by choice. Legislation enacted over the past 15 to 20 years has supported deinstitutionalization for persons with mental illness, persons with physical disabilities, and even those with acute illness. Legislation limiting reimbursement for acute hospital stays has forced early discharges and often necessitated recovery and convalescence in the home setting.

Some programs and services exist to help the family manage the person with impairment or disability. The passage of PL 94-142, the Education for All Handicapped Children Act of 1975, assisted parents by mandating services necessary to enable participation in appropriate free public education for disabled children. This legislation was amended in 1986 with the passage of PL 99-457, which identified the family as a central focus in early intervention programs.

Public Law 98-21, enacted in 1983, initiated the Prospective Payment System, which stimulated the development of medical rehabilitation for elderly persons in the United States. All of these policy initiatives expanded the scope of occupational therapy, but placed more responsibility for the care of the impaired person on the family. Appropriately, and necessarily, the occupational therapist has become a family educator, whereby knowledge and skills necessary for effective disability management are provided to families in preparation for their roles as caregivers.

Case Study 1. Occupational therapy consultation for the home setting.

In 1975, a special education teacher and his wife were rearing two children with Down's syndrome. That year they placed their oldest son in a state institution for the mentally retarded because the mother was having difficulty providing the care the child needed, and there were no services available through the school. Soon after, the wife was diagnosed with Alzheimer's disease, and her condition deteriorated very rapidly. The husband could not manage his wife at home, and she was institutionalized. The younger child, a daughter, was of school age and her school had just begun to implement services to comply with PL 94-142 (the Education for All Handicapped Children Act of 1975).

The occupational therapist helped the teacher learn how to engage the child in classroom activities and provided consultation for solving problems related to life tasks at home. With the support of the school-based program and the help of the occupational therapist, the father was able to maintain the child at home throughout her school years and into young adulthood. She is now in her early 30s, lives in a group home, and works in a sheltered workshop. Her father believes that the assistance provided through the legislation enabled him, a single parent, to raise his daughter at home while maintaining his full-time employment.

Individuals in the immediate and extended family who share caregiving duties for an impaired family member are often referred to as a family system. Brody (1990) has estimated that 85% of the care needed by a person with a disability is given by the family system. "The household provides the context for a great deal of caregiving, and shared housing influences both the caregiving process and the stress experienced by family members" (Pruchno, 1990, p. 175).

The occupational therapist must consider a number of factors when a family member assumes the responsibility for care, particularly if the family member has to learn new skills, acquire new roles, devote considerable time to the process, or transport the person to outpatient care. Even if modified assistance is all the impaired person needs, the set up for activities is a new responsibility that requires the caregiver to learn how to analyze tasks. Many patients need supervision or minimal to moderate assistance after they leave an institution.

Families choosing to care for the impaired person may not understand what the therapist means by "set up," "physical assist," "verbal assist," or "verbal cue." This is not because providing assistance or delivering a cue is difficult; rather, unlike clinicians, families may not recognize when and how to offer help. Considering this, occupational therapists should appreciate how difficult it is to learn concepts such as agnosia, apraxia, procedural memory, or postural stability, which convey information that is quite important to the safe and effective management of a person with a functional deficit. Therapists must help the family recognize and understand the impaired person's deficits, and teach them how to recognize and manage resulting problems. Only when the necessary skills are mastered will the family feel competent in their caregiving roles.

Who Are the Caregivers, and Why Do They Provide Care?

Caregiving may be informal, as when family members, friends, or relatives provide care, or formal, involving paid attendants or helpers. Informal caregivers are primarily female family members, of whom the majority work and more than 30% are single. Caregivers with families and jobs may have difficulty providing care for a disabled person. Some level of assistance is necessary for those who choose to manage the disabled person in the community, so their other roles do not suffer.

Even if a spouse has the day-to-day responsibility of caring for an older impaired person, usually one other person in the family network also becomes a principal support. While a daughter generally becomes this predominant provider of care (Brody, 1981; Cantor, 1983; Horowitz, 1985), a son may also play a substantial role in decision making and providing financial assistance (Horowitz; Treas, 1979). When a son accepts the role of primary caregiver in the absence of a female sibling, he often provides less support and less time, and frequently the care is not in the area of concrete assistance (Horowitz). While studies have shown that female caregivers are more likely to carry out personal care and household tasks, they are also more likely to report greater burden. However, meta analysis of studies has not demonstrated significant gender differences in caregiver involvement in care (Miller & Cafasso, 1992).

Brody (1990) cites three major reasons why caregivers take on the role of managing older adults: geographic proximity (23.5 %); feelings of responsibility (16.3 %); and gender or birth order (14.3 %). Horowitz (1985) suggests that three factors explain why daughters dominate as primary caregivers: Daughters have traditionally assumed nurturing tasks; they show stronger emotional ties to the family; and if they are homemakers, they may have more flexible schedules than sons.

When a child is born with a disability, some parents automatically assume the role of caregiver, while other parents, for various reasons, cannot fulfill that role and give the child to the state for management, either formally or by abandonment. Social trends that influence the family structure make it necessary to reevaluate the notion that the family will always take responsibility for the care of the impaired family member. Marital disruption affects care. Persons who are separated or divorced provide less care to elderly parents than those with intact marriages (Cicirelli, 1983). Financial difficulties (Troll, Miller, & Atchley, 1979), practical problems with duties of everyday living (Stevens-Long, 1979), and problems in interpersonal relationships (Spanier & Hanson, 1982) are stated as reasons for providing less help by persons who are separated or divorced. In contemporary Western society, the lower birthrate, longer life expectancy, changing roles of women, and remarriage rate are additional issues that influence caregiving practices. Occupational therapists must consider these factors when planning ongoing caregiving with the family. They can help identify resources as well as help families adjust their expectations and activities.

Assisting the Family in Providing Care

When family members take on the role of caregiver, they rarely have the knowledge and skills to manage the performance deficits that accompany the impairment or disability. The occupational therapist can fulfill a major function in helping the family, and specifically the primary caregiver, to acquire the necessary skills to manage and support the independence of a person who has an impairment.

Clark and Rakowski (1983) have emphasized the importance of helping the caregiver develop the skills, attitudes, and confidence to support the disabled individual in the community. They have identified the following caregiver skills as essential:

Clinical Observation: The caregiver needs sufficient understanding of the characteristics of the disease to assess and report changes in the individual's condition accurately. The caregiver also needs the skills to report the individual's reactions to interventions to the physician, other professionals, and the family.

Direct Care Skills: The caregiver needs to learn to recognize and understand the needs of the family member and to learn the techniques necessary to help family members give appropriate assistance to facilitate the impaired person's independence.

Management: The caregiver should be familiar with services that could be helpful in managing the impaired person. Additionally, the caregiver must learn how to access and coordinate these services to benefit both the impaired person and family members. The caregiver also needs to know how to seek additional help as problems arise.

Brody (1990) notes the complexity of caregiving and the importance of viewing it with a wide-angle lens, writing that:

> Looking at different family members separately with tunnel-vision does not illuminate the complex manner in which various sets of relationships are layered and

intricately interwoven. The family situation interacts with the socioeconomic context and the service environment in which caregiving occurs, a context that plays a major role in determining how care is provided and the mental health effects on family members. (p. 31)

This suggests that by helping family members integrate their caregiving functions into existing roles and responsibilities, the occupational therapist may help them avoid unnecessary burden. *Burden* is a term that refers to the demands and resulting stress that rendering care imposes on family members and others assuming caregiving responsibilities.

Minimizing Burden

Occupational therapists must consider the effect caregiving has on caregivers. Maximizing the independence of the functionally impaired person and minimizing the burden of care on the family are major intervention goals. A brief history of burden highlights the factors the occupational therapist must consider when planning care with families.

Caregiver burden was first reported by Grad and Sainsbury in 1963 when they documented the burden of caring for the mentally impaired. In 1966, Hoenig and Hamilton identified two components of burden: subjective (related to feelings) and objective (the demands of care). McCubbin and Patterson (1983) described a model of family stress that considers the build up of stresses, family's resources, and family's interpretation of the problem. This model defines the crisis and how families adjust and adapt to it.

In an attempt to identify and quantify specific components of caregiver burden, Kosberg and Cairl (1986) developed a scale called the "cost of care index," which permits professionals to screen informal (nonpaid) care providers to estimate the impact that caregiving will have on them. Their short (20-item) measure considers five dimensions or costs that help account for the burden of care. These include restrictions on personal and social life, the impact of caregiving on physical and emotional health, the caregiver's perceptions of the value of providing care, the patient's capacity for provoking mistreatment, and the direct economic costs of caregiving. Subsequent research with this index (Kosberg & Cairl, 1990) suggests that the cost of care index can help professionals predict problems, anticipate adverse consequences, and engage in preventive interventions. Their research has also shown that competence does not predict the level of caregiver burden (Kosberg & Cairl, 1991), suggesting that interventions provided by professionals must be uniquely tailored to each caregiver's individual personality and circumstances.

In 1989, two major studies indicated that some people take pleasure from caregiving, especially when they are successful and when the impaired person responds. Kinney and Stephens (1989) report that caregivers get uplifts when they see the impaired person calm, responsive, and affectionate, and when they receive help from the family and support from their friends. One explanation for the uplifts was that even though many of the tasks were irritating, they also were predictable and controllable. The caregivers tried to find satisfaction in their helping efforts.

Lawton, Brody, and Saperstein (1989) reported that caregiver satisfaction is an achievable goal. Some caregivers report enjoyment in recognizing the impaired person's needs, being with the impaired person, knowing that the impaired person appreciates the help of the caregiver, and seeing the impaired person's pleasure. The satisfaction of feeling close and caring raised the caregivers' self-esteem. The developmental disabilities literature also reports the positive aspects of parenting children with disabilities. Wikler, Wasow, and Hatfield (1983) report that parents often benefit from the challenges of caring for their child.

Collectively, these findings suggest the importance of skill training to facilitate successful experiences in providing care. Moreover, the amount of formal and informal support caregivers use may relate to the level of burden caregivers perceive they experience (Clipp & George, 1990).

In summary, burden is a multidimensional concept that includes objective components (such as tasks of caring, demand, time in caring, use of resources) and subjective components (such as the caregiver's relationship with the person for whom care is provided, tolerance of the caregiver, and time available for meeting the personal and social needs of the caregiver). Research has shown that social support and resources may be important in mediating the burden. While the caregiving process has some satisfying aspects, the burden of care may also lead to neglect or abuse of the person needing care. Yet the relationship of burden to neglect or abuse is just beginning to be addressed.

Occupational therapists can make a major contribution to the caregiving process by helping families minimize burden. Education and training enable caregivers to feel more confident in their ability to provide care, recognize their own health and social needs, and carry out skills that lead to successful outcomes and positive relationships with the person with impairments.

Applying A Family Systems Perspective

A family is a system. In order to address the issues associated with caregiving, the therapist must consider the issues families face across the life cycle. The family life cycle is a sequence of changes that occur at different stages and time periods (Barber, Turnbull, Behr, & Kerns, 1989). As many as 24 stages have been documented. However, for the sake of simplicity, six basic stages are presented: (a) birth and early childhood, (b) elementary school years, (c) adolescence, (d) young adulthood, (e) empty nest, and (f) elderly years. Figure 1 describes the typical issues caregivers may face when the person is in the different life cycles. These should be carefully considered when planning care.

Changes in family life cycle patterns have affected the caregiving process. It is estimated that the average woman will spend 17 years raising her children and 18 years caring for her parents (Select Committee on Aging, 1987). More than 60% of women are in the work force. This frequently forces women caring for disabled children or adults into a conflict in activities and schedules (Bloom, 1986). An increasing number of couples are divorced and/or remarried. This factor causes role stress in many caregiving situations. For example, remarried couples may be contending with the demands of parenting new children at the same time that their parents need assistance.

The most profound implication of the change in family cycle patterns is the decrease in the actual number of persons, particularly family members, who are available to provide informal support. More than 5 million older Americans, or 20% of the population over 65, are childless. Without children, the elderly have less access to informal help (Johnson & Catalano, 1981; Treas, 1979).

Informal Versus Formal Support

As previously mentioned, 85% of the care the impaired person receives is provided by the family. Branch and Jette (1983) report that the extent of the impairment is the strongest predictor of the use of formal support services. Data from the 1982 National Long Term Care Survey indicate that fewer than 10 % of informal caregivers reported the use of paid helpers (Stone, Cafferata, & Sange, 1987).

Figure 1. Issues that may influence caregiving at various stages of the life cycle.

Stage 1: Birth and early childhood Ages 0–5	• severity of the diagnosis • expectations • timing of the diagnosis • uninsured financial costs • level of caregiving demands • family size, form, and support • needs of other family members • perception of stigma that may be attached to the exceptionality • income and education level • service availability
Stage 2: School age Ages 6–12	• school-based program options • establishment of new routines • adjustment to educational implications • movement away from family-centered to school-based • locating community resources • access to or availability of services • expectations
Stage 3: Adolescence Ages 13–21	• emotional adjustment to possible chronicity of exceptionality • emerging sexuality • career/vocational planning • leisure activities • expectations
Stage 4: Young adulthood	• possible need for guardianship • appropriate adult residence • transition to work force • emotional adjustment to dependency as adult • expectations
Stage 5: Middle adulthood	• time demand of care • financial demand of care • competing priorities • cognitive/physical status of care recipient • relationship with parent and/or child • marital disruption • expectations
Stage 6: Older adult	• cognitive/physical status of care recipient • age of care recipient • physical status of caregiver • time demand of care • financial demand of care • competing priorities • expectations of retirement • availability of caregiver (spouse, children) • marital disruption among adult children • interpersonal relationships with patients and adult children

Some people do not reach out for formal assistance. Birkel and Jones (1989) suggest that caregivers choose not to use assistance for cognitively impaired older adults for three reasons: the behavioral and mood disturbances of the impaired person discourage assistance, it is difficult to locate helpers trained to manage a person with cognitive loss (and perhaps severe disabilities), and bringing others in for assistance may have a negative impact on the impaired person.

Many organizations provide assistance to families. Voluntary organizations usually do not charge for their services. The appendix to this chapter lists major organizations that clinicians and families can access to get information, support, and, in some situations, loaner equipment, to facilitate the caregiving process.

Types of Formal Support

Studies of burden indicate the importance of educational programs for caregivers (Cohen, Kennedy, & Eisforder, 1984; Haley, 1983; Quayhagen & Quayhagen, 1988; Rabins, Mace, & Lucas, 1982). Although most educational programs address the disease process, general communication skills, behavioral management, basic strategies regarding activities of daily living (ADL), and information about resources (Chiverton & Caine, 1989; Goldstein & Tye, 1987; Haley, Levine, Brown, Berry, & Hughes, 1987; Kahan, Kemp, Staples, & Brummel-Smith, 1985), studies suggest that caregivers prefer to improve their effectiveness rather than decrease their stress (Chiverton & Caine; Haley et al.). Educational programs are designed primarily to impart information. Researchers have hypothesized that by having more knowledge of and skills to deal with the disease, the caregiver's burden will be reduced. Unfortunately, the effectiveness of educational programs in reducing burden has not yet been empirically established. Caregivers seek information to help them become more effective in their roles. None of the studies reviewed used an individualized assessment of both the impaired person and the caregiver to determine the specific needs to manage the problems they were facing. If more information were available about the deficits exhibited by the impaired person, caregivers could receive training in specific skills to manage the person with specific deficits. Occupational therapists can play a valuable role in this training.

Social support buffers against stress. Caregivers coping with functional dependencies, behavioral problems, new tasks, losses of relationships, shared activities, and increased financial strains of managing a household with less income, require social support interventions. Social support is a mechanism by which interpersonal relationships presumably protect people from the effects of stress. A number of authors (Brown, 1979; Caplan 1974; Cassel, 1974; Cohen & Wills, 1985; Dean & Lin, 1977; Kessler & McLeod, 1985), suggest that it reduces the adverse psychological impact of stressful life events and serves various functions, such as compensating for loss, maintaining psychological well-being, reassuring self-worth, and guidance. Bandura (1977, 1982) proposed that social resources promote adaptive coping efforts and discourage avoidance strategies.

Three categories of social support sustain the individual facing a stressful situation. According to Thoits (1986), people need information, emotional support, and assistance so they can maintain their roles while managing stressful situation. Self-efficacy increases when fears are alleviated and the skills to manage new situations are developed (Bandura, 1982). Schaefer, Coyne, and Lazarus (1981) suggest that the major support functions should be defined and assessed separately to determine their effectiveness and interrelatedness. *Emotional support* is defined as including intimacy and attachment, reassurance, and relying on and/or confiding in others. *Tangible support* involves direct aid or services (i.e., gifts of money or goods, taking care of needy persons, or doing chores for them). *Informational support* includes problem solving, information, advice, and feedback on the person's progress.

Decreasing caregiver burden through social support has not been empirically documented, although several investigations have yielded preliminary information. Kahan et al. (1985) found that a caregiver's relatively short but intensive discussion with professionals can have a positive effect on reducing some of the burden and depression; however, the authors did not follow up their study to determine its lasting effects. Clipp and George (1990) conducted a survey to determine if they could predict patterns of support based on selected caregiver characteristics, (i.e., financial resources, physical and mental health, social and recreational activities, and aspects of the caregiving situation). A major finding of the study was that caregivers' needs do not necessarily elicit support from others, and that caregivers with the lowest needs received the most assistance. No relationships among the severity of symptoms, the duration of care, and the use of support were noted. These findings suggest the importance of determining the caregivers' perceived needs before developing intervention strategies.

Respite has gained attention as one of many social support strategies designed to prolong community residence as it gives the caregiver time away from the demands of caring (Lawton, Kleban, Moss, Rovine, & Glicksman, 1989). Respite takes many forms: (a) skilled care residential facilities (such as nursing homes) for short stays, (b) daycare programs, (c) support groups, and (d) help with chores or management of the impaired person. Although the need for these services exists, utilization has been surprisingly low due to a lack of availability of, or access to, such services (Rabins et al., 1982; Caserta, Lund, Wright, & Redburn, 1987).

Lawton, Brody, and Saperstein (1989) hypothesized that respite services would result in a higher sense of well-being in the caregiver. They found no relationship between the psychological state of the caregiver and the use of respite services. Although respite did not affect the caregiver's perceived level of burden or mental health, his or her satisfaction with the services and information received was very high. Families that used respite care maintained their impaired relative significantly longer in the community (22 days). This finding, though significant, weakened the support for federally funded respite services for cognitively impaired older adults, because the small increase in the number of days in the community did not justify the cost of the provision of the service. Perhaps other studies can be conducted by occupational therapists who look not only at the use of respite, but also at the effect of teaching the caregiver to train others who are willing act as caregivers. In this way, the resistance to using others because of their lack of skills when interacting with the impaired person may be lessened or eliminated.

In addition to these supportive strategies, other interventions can be employed. The Occupational Therapy Department at the Veterans Administration Hospital in Minneapolis conducts a daycare program where cognitively impaired older adults participate in activities that include folding laundry, binding ace bandages, wrapping food, collating and stapling brochures, labeling and sealing envelopes, and engraving name tags. The activities tap and preserve existing skills. Additionally, these tasks provide exercise and stimulation. The patients are able to engage in work tasks for 74% of their time in the program. Although carry-over in the home is not reported, caregivers do report fewer destructive behaviors and affected persons who sleep through the night (Burns & Buell, 1990).

Seltzer, Irvy, & Litchfield (1987) reported a program where family members were trained as case managers to build partnerships between the formal and informal support networks. They found that family members were able to perform a number of case management tasks for their elderly relatives. Additionally, they found that the duration of service was significantly shorter than when a social worker functioned as the case manager. Their findings suggest that families are willing to assume case management responsibilities when trained and supported by professional staff.

The goal of intervention is to maximize the performance of the impaired person while minimizing the burden on the caregiver. In order to achieve this goal, comprehensive programs need to be developed that are aimed at determining the best strategy for each caregiving unit to address the family's unique problems.

Occupational Therapy Frameworks for Facilitating Caregiving in the Home

Because the issues related to managing the impaired person are complicated and need to be individualized, helping the caregiver develop skills is the most appropriate strategy. The person must function in the home; therefore, it is in the home that training and skill development should occur.

Occupational therapists who are interested in family-centered training programs should: (a) undertake training in the instruments to assess the family and the impaired person in the community; (b) adopt a training, rather than a treatment, philosophy; (c) recognize and employ the contributions of other health care professionals to the restorative and preventive model of care; and (d) learn of available community resources. Treatment should help the caregiver and the family provide support to the impaired person. The goal should be to establish an ongoing consultation role for when new problems arise.

Schaaf and Mulrooney (1989) propose an early intervention, family-centered approach. Although originally constructed for children, the model could be applied to the caregiving process at any age. The Family-Centered Framework for Early Intervention is a synthesis of concepts from the Model of Human Occupation (Kielhofner & Burke, 1980). This ecological framework emphasizes viewing the person and his or her family within the context of their life environments. The values, interests, habits, routines, and skills of the person receiving care must be given primary consideration in the evaluation and intervention processes.

Hasselkus (1989) conceptualizes the caregiver as a lay practitioner who is involved in the clinical reasoning and ethical dilemmas integral to the provision of health care for the care receiver. The caregiver's judgments regarding the priority, ordering, and attainment of goals determines the caregiving activities. The goal of the clinical encounter must be to devise a plan that preserves the caregiver's values and represents a mutual understanding between the therapist and the caregiver. She reminds us that services must be tailored to fit the family caretaking system "however unstructured and cumbersome. . . . Both the therapist and the family caregiver (1) bring knowledge and experience to the situation, (2) produce data to identify options, and (3) bring their own code of ethics to the course of action. If the therapist and caregiver can collaborate on the process, then tension can be minimized and a shared responsibility and shared ethical decision making can result" (Hasselkus, p. 653).

In order to implement a preventive strategy for the caregiver, it is necessary to suggest approaches for him or her to achieve a balance of activities that are personally important. Caregivers must understand that respite assistance enables them to spend time on activities that are pleasant to them and that contribute to their sense of life satisfaction (Hasselkus, 1989). The occupational therapist can create a situation in which the caregiver and clinician share expertise, values, and interests. This will support the caregiver in his or her role.

The family's resources should be determined; in addition the expectations, attitudes toward providing care, and motivation for taking on the caregiver role should be assessed. Figure 2 identifies some instruments that can help the occupational therapist get a perspective on the family. Informal interviews can also provide invaluable information.

Figure 2. Selected instruments for assessing family needs and resources.

Carolina Parent Support Scale Bristol, M.M. (1983) University of North Carolina.	Assesses availability and perceived adequacy of supports to parents, taking into account both informal and formal support systems.
Daily Routine Recording Form Vincent, L., Davis, J., Brown, P., Teicher, J., & Weynand, P. (1983). Madison: University of Wisconsin.	Provides parent record of what the child and parent do during each 30-minute time period of the day. Specific activities, frequency of activity, and assistance required by child during activity are noted.
Early Coping Inventory Zeitlin, S., Williamson, G.G., & Szczepanski, M. (1988). Bensenville, IL: Scholastic Testing Service.	Assesses children aged 4 to 36 months (chronologically and/or developmentally) in three categories: Sensorimotor Organization, Reactive Behavior, and Self-Initiated Behavior.
Family Inventory of Life Events and Changes (FILE) McCubbin, H.I., Patterson, J.M., & Wilson, L.R. (1992). St. Paul: University of Minnesota, Family Social Science.	Identifies the stresses a family has experienced and assesses their "cumulative risk" (effect) through a 72-item inventory. Subheadings include Intra-Family Strains, Marital Status, Pregnancy and Childbearing Strains, Finance and Business Strains, Work-Family Illness and Family "Care" Strains, Losses, and Transitions.
Family Needs Scale Dunst, C.J., Cooper, C.J., Weeldreyer, J.C., Snyder, K.D., & Chase J.H. (1988). In C.J. Dunst, C.M. Trivette, & A.G. Deal (Eds.), *Enabling and empowering families: Principles and guidelines for practice* (p. 115). Cambridge, MA: Brookline.	Identifies the extent of a family's needs for various resources and supports. Nine categories are considered, including food and shelter, finances, child care, and transportation. Scores include the total number of areas of need and the perceived importance of each.
Family Planning Questionnaire Stevens-Dominiguez, M. (1988). Albuquerque: University of New Mexico, Developmental Disabilities Division.	Serves as a planning tool for families to identify needed information and services. Families are asked to specify when and where they would like to meet with program staff.
Family Resource Scale Leet, H.E., & Dunst, C.J. (1988). In C.J. Dunst, C.M. Trivette, & A.G. Deal (Eds.), *Enabling and empowering families: Principles and guidelines for practice* (p. 141). Cambridge, MA: Brookline.	Identifies whether a family has adequate resources to meet its needs.
Family Support Scale Dunst, C.J., Jenkins, V., & Trivette, C.M. (1988). In C.J. Dunst, C.M. Trivette, & A.G. Deal (Eds.), *Enabling and empowering families: Principles and guidelines for practice* (p. 157). Cambridge, MA: Brookline.	Identifies the availability and helpfulness of 18 sources of formal and informal support. Indicates the total number of supports and parental perceptions of the helpfulness of these supports.

(continued)

Figure 2 (continued).

Functional Behavior Profile (FBP)
Baum, C.M., Edwards, D.F., & Morrow-Howell, N. (1993). Identification and measurement of productive behaviors in senile dementia of the Alzheimer's type. *The Gerontologist, 33*(3), 403–408.

Measures the presence and frequency of productive behaviors associated with patients with SDAT. Can serve as a guide for developing individualized caregiving strategies by helping the caregiver focus on the presence of behaviors useful in managing the impaired person.

Home Screening Questionnaire
Coons, C.E., Gay, E.C., Fandal, A.W., Ker, C., & Frankenburg, W.K. (1981). Denver, CO: Denver Developmental Materials.

Provides a short form of the Home Observation for Measurement of the Environment (Bradley & Caldwell, 1984) and is designed to assess children's home environments, including availability of toys.

Home Skills Performance Scale
Rodel, D.M. (1978). Minneapolis, MN: Minneapolis Public Schools.

Assesses how consistently a child performs various daily tasks in the home. Three areas are identified: Self-Help/Adaptive, Personal/Social, and Motor Performance.

Infant Behavior Questionnaire
Rothbart, M.K. (1987). Eugene: University of Oregon, Department of Psychology.

Assesses an infant's temperament in a variety of areas. Parents answer questions related to feeding, sleeping, bathing and dressing, play, daily activities, and soothing techniques.

Inventory of Social Support
Trivette, C.M., & Dunst, C.J. (1988). In C.J. Dunst, C.M. Trivette, & A.G. Deal (Eds.), *Enabling and empowering families: Principles and Guidelines for practice* (pp. 161–163). Cambridge, MA: Brookline.

Lists the various types of assistance provided by individuals, groups, or agencies, and identifies the frequency and results of family members' contacts with these sources. Information helps to identify type, utilization, and access to supports.

Life Experience Survey
Sarason, I.G., Johnson, J.H., & Siegal, J.M. (1978). *Journal of Consulting and Clinical Psychology, 46,* 932–946.

Lists various incidents, such as personal events, financial changes, and changes in the family that may adversely affect a family's functioning, and assesses their impact on family members.

Mothers' Perceptions of Their Needs and Supports
Vincent, L., & Laten, S. (1985). Madison: University of Wisconsin.

Parents choose five needs from a list of 38 about which they feel most concerned. Parents also identify two resources that would help meet each of the five needs. Subcategories include Working With the Schools and Other Professionals; My Child's Development and Needs at Home; Personal and Emotional Needs of Parents; Family Needs; and Dealing With Family, Friends, and Relatives.

Parent Needs Survey
Seligman, M., & Daring, R. (Eds.). (1989). In *Ordinary Families*. New York: Guilford.

Used in conjunction with a parent interview to identify needs for services. Parents rate a variety of items on how much help they need.

Personal Network Matrix, Version I
Trivette, C.M., & Dunst, C.J. (1988). In C.J. Dunst, C.M. Trivette, & A.G. Deal (Eds.). *Enabling and empowering families: Principles and Guidelines for Practice* (pp. 161–163). Cambridge, MA: Brookline.

Family member indicates frequency of contact with specified individuals. Respondent also lists 10 needs or projects and indicates which members of his or her support network could provide assistance with each. Information on frequency of contact (quantitative) and dependability is useful in defining a family's network.

Survey of Family Needs
Bailey, D., & Simeonsson, R. (1985). Chapel Hill: University of North Carolina.

Checklist for families regarding their needs in the areas of financial and social supports, community-based services, overall family functioning, and methods of conflict resolution.

Adapted from *Family Centered Care: An Early Intervention Resource Manual* (pp. 3-53–3-55) by B. Hanft (Ed.), 1989, Rockville, MD: American Occupational Therapy Association. Copyright © 1989 by AOTA.

Attendant Selection, Supervision, and Training

The use of paid attendants or home health aides constitutes a more formal approach to providing care in the home setting. Although the idea of hiring assistance for home care seems straightforward enough, successful arrangements are not easily attained. Considerable care must be taken in the selection, training, and supervision of paid attendants to achieve success. When persons needing care and their families are prepared for these functions, the results can help obtain a significantly higher quality of life for all concerned.

The following excerpt from Ruby Heine, who has a spinal cord injury, illustrates the importance of attendant care in the lives of persons with disabilities:

> Only through other people have I been able to survive out of a hospital. You can learn to have enough confidence in yourself and how to take care of yourself so that you can take a stranger off the street at a moment's notice and calmly, intelligently explain to that person how to take care of you in the rocking bed and pneumobelt, how to fold the wheel chair, and how to get you in and out of bed. You will feel like you're taking care of yourself through other people's hands. (Laurie, 1977, p. 98)

Attendant care and the use of personal care attendants are services associated with the independent living movement, which began in the early 1970s. The concept of independent living focuses on allowing people with disabilities to live as they choose in their communities rather than confining them to institutions (DeJong & Wenker, 1983).

A personal care attendant is "a paid employee who provides in-home assistance with essential activities of daily living to a severely disabled person who is unable to perform the activities alone" (Hutchins, Thornock, Lindgre, & Parks, 1978). The attendant care model assumes that individuals who are functionally dependent and require the scope of assistance provided by a paid attendant are cognizant of their own health care needs and have the necessary ability and skills to direct and monitor their own personal care (Crewe & Zola, 1983). This model is usually applied to working age or older adults, and because of reimbursement issues, criteria to qualify for an attendant vary from state to state. For example, to be eligible for attendant care services in Massachusetts, a person must be at least 18 years old, limited in upper extremity use, psychologically and medically stable, and eligible for Medicaid (Crewe & Zola).

Crewe and Zola (1983) have compared the models of attendant care and home health care services. The attendant care model views the person with a disability as a consumer. In the home health model, the person is a patient. Both models are needed. The home health model provides acute restorative care during a period of illness or recuperation following hospitalization. The attendant care model provides ongoing routine care and is an alternative to long-term institutionalization. Figure 3 summarizes the differences between these two models described in the literature (Crewe & Zola; Ulicny & Jones, 1985).

The Independent Living Movement describes the relationship between people with disabilities and attendants as an employer to employee relationship (Ulicny & Jones, 1985). The lack of management skills on the part of these new "employers" (those with disabilities) is the most common problem. Procedures to enable people with disabilities to train and manage their attendants more effectively have been developed by the Research and Training Center on Independent Living at the University of Kansas. These materials help the occupational therapist prepare the disabled person with the new life skill of "attendant manager."

Attendants must be trained. The specific characteristics of the disabled person must

Figure 3. A comparison of models for home caregiving.

Home Health Services Medical Model	Attendant Care Services Independent Living Model
Physician as decision maker	Consumer as decision maker
Recipient of care treated as patient	Recipient of care treated as consumer
Home health aide recruited and supervised by home health agency	Attendant recruited and supervised by consumer
Condition requiring care tends to be acute	Condition requiring care tends to be permanent or chronic
Nature of care is restorative/episodic	Care is of a maintenance or continuing nature
Service viewed as a "health care" benefit	Service viewed as a "social service" benefit

be reflected in how the attendant performs the activities. In a sense, the attendant provides technological support, which is exactly the kind of support that everyone gets when they ask someone else to do a task for which they lack either the necessary strength and/or skills. It takes a person with special skills to be an attendant, because the support he or she gives must not overshadow the person who receives the assistance.

Getting to the point where the attendant supports the needs and idiosyncrasies of the disabled person requires specific training and management on the part of the disabled person. Finding, training, and retaining an attendant is one of the most difficult challenges confronting the disabled person who needs such assistance to live in the community.

Selection and recruitment can be facilitated through the use of carefully defined sets of tasks. Ulicny and Jones (1985) propose the use of performance checklists to outline certain job tasks for the attendant. Specific work routines, such as housekeeping or environmental maintenance, are outlined to identify the frequency of the task, the materials needed to support the task, and the set up. Checklists provide specific instructions and help the employer monitor, evaluate, and provide feedback on the attendant's performance. Once training is completed, checklists can be used for continued supervision.

The process for developing a checklist is straightforward. First, the person with the disability identifies those personal care tasks that require assistance. Then the identified tasks are analyzed and procedures are developed to support the tasks. The resulting task and procedure lists become the checklist.

Checklists should be used in the interview process so that the prospective employee knows what will be expected of him or her. After the attendant is hired, the checklist can

Case Study 2. John's caregiver.

John sustained an injury while he was in college. His spinal cord was severed at level C-4 to C-5. He had a supportive environment and the resources to continue in school, and he made a commitment to do so. I first met John when I served on a committee that he chaired. In order to manage his papers, have access to water, eat, and perform basic ADL, he required an attendant. His attendant is a very kind, lovely man who is quite enjoyable to talk with; however, when he is at work as John's attendant, his efforts must be directed toward supporting the physical needs of his employer, who is running a meeting, reading reports, and demonstrating his superb leadership abilities.

serve as part of the job responsibility contract and a record of the attendant's performance. Once the attendant is hired, he or she must be trained. Figure 4 describes the training process that supports a successful relationship between the disabled person and the attendant.

Employing this model of attendant care will help the disabled person develop management skills and provide clear expectations to both the attendant and the disabled person. An effective system of attendant care should demonstrate cost effectiveness by allowing the disabled person to become what he or she wants. Assistance from an attendant provides support in home, work, and leisure activities.

The model described above embraces the idea that it is much less expensive and more effective to train one person systematically in a specific routine (that person being the one requiring the attendant; the specific routine being the ability to hire, train, and manage an attendant) than to train the dozen or more different attendants that person will require in his or her lifetime.

Occupational therapists play a very important role in helping a disabled person understand how an attendant can help him or her accomplish personal objectives and goals. This process should begin during the rehabilitation program (Opie & Miller, 1989). Early in the rehabilitation process the occupational therapist should help the patient clarify his or her needs and expectations regarding relationships, work, and family. It is important to encourage the person to become assertive and to discuss personal care needs (Opie & Miller). The therapist should help the disabled person understand the choices necessary to achieve independence. What is important to the disabled person? Should he or she struggle for more than an hour getting dressed alone? If so, how much energy will be left for the rest of the day? Some will find it very important to be independent. Others may find that the challenge of work and the pleasures of the family are enhanced when they receive assistance from a person whom they have chosen and trained to help with self-care and other daily requirements. Therapists should avoid making assumptions about the care recipient's needs and recognize that the ability to manage assistants represents a choice for interdependence. For many people, the acceptance of this strategy and the acquisition of attendant management skills each represent important milestones in the rehabilitation process.

The ability to manage a personal care attendant effectively requires the acquisition of new skills for most people. These necessary management skills include the ability to communicate expectations in terms of standards of performance, provide appropriate and timely feedback, and terminate employment when necessary. Possessing the competence and self-confidence to oversee one's personal care often requires special

Figure 4. Process for establishing a training program.

1. Training should help the attendant understand and develop skills in each aspect of the task that will support the needs and wishes of the person with the disability.

2. The person with the disability should review the tasks that are to be performed and provide feedback until a satisfactory level of performance is achieved.

3. The person with the disability should provide ongoing feedback, both when the performance is satisfactory and when improvement is needed, until routines are well-established.

4. The person with the disability should remember that the attendant is an employee who requires recognition as well as respect for his or her ideas.

consultation and training. The occupational therapist can be a valuable resource in the skill building process to enhance the person's ability to manage his or her personal affairs (Crewe & Zola, 1983).

How a person with a disability arranges his or her attendant care depends on the individual's situation, personality, goals, and resources. The occupational therapist must explore attendant care as an option and lay the groundwork for successful experiences that will facilitate independence. The occupational therapist could begin the process of making checklists and have the disabled person practice training and supervisory procedures as part of the rehabilitation process. The skills that will be developed in this effort will certainly prepare the person for independence after the formal rehabilitation process is complete. The occupational therapist may also serve as a consultant to the disabled person and attendant as they explore and solve complex issues after the person is discharged from the rehabilitation facility.

Strategies to Maximize Performance of the Person With the Impairment, and the Family

The previous section stressed the importance of the disabled person taking control by selecting and training an attendant to provide assistance to support self-reliance. The same principles of task analysis and training should be applied to the family. Some persons cannot afford an attendant because they are not skilled for employment or

Case Study 3. Mr. Smith: A little knowledge can be a dangerous thing.

Mr. Smith attended a training session that the author of this chapter and a colleague presented at a local community center. The topic was "Strategies to Support Cognitively Impaired Elderly." During the presentation, we discussed the importance of breaking tasks down into simple steps and verbally supporting the person as he or she performed the activity. After the session, Mr. Smith told us this was "exactly the information I need." He said he would begin using it the following morning. We gave him our business cards and told him to call us to let us know how things were going.

Two weeks after the session Mr. Smith appeared at my office exclaiming, "If I had paid for that session, I'd ask for my money back." I asked him to explain his disparaging remark. He told me that he and his wife went to the store. When they returned home, he remembered that he had forgotten to stop at the post office. He said that, deciding to try his new technique, "I gave her a one-step command, just like you said." When Mr. Smith was asked to describe what he had said, he replied: "I told her 'put away the groceries.'" Hoping that this was not what he interpreted as a one-step command, I asked, "Did you say anything else?" Mr. Smith replied, "I bought some pork chops, and there were four small ones in one package and two small ones and one big one in the other package. I told her to put the small ones in the freezer, two to a package, and put the large one in a package by itself. When I came home she was sitting in the middle of the kitchen floor crying, groceries all over the place, and the ice cream had melted. Your advice wasn't worth a damn."

Obviously, the information Mr. Smith received set up an expectation that he would be able to communicate more effectively with his wife. But Mr. Smith needed much more than the information provided during the presentation he attended. He needed training, reinforcement, and a series of successful experiences. Often, such training can be provided by the occupational therapist while the person to be cared for is receiving treatment. The most appropriate place for this training is in the home, where the caregiver and person with the impairment can interact in real situations.

cannot find a job. However, the Americans with Disability Act should make it possible for more disabled persons to find work. The fundamental difference between hiring, training, and supervising an attendant and being cared for by a family should be quite obvious. Anything the occupational therapist can do to assist the family in developing the attitudes and skills to support the self-reliance of the disabled person should enhance independence and motivate the person to pursue his or her own goals.

Some people, particularly those with severe cognitive deficits, need a caregiver to provide essential assistance to ensure safety. If a person cannot initiate, sequence, or organize a task, or if he or she cannot attend or be safe in the performance of a task, then a caregiver is necessary. A caregiver providing such assistance needs skills that can be taught by the occupational therapist as part of the rehabilitation process. Caregivers need to know how to modify environments, perform basic self-care tasks, and engage the impaired person in activities and social interactions. They also need to learn how to break down tasks and deliver both gestural and verbal cues. Imparting the necessary knowledge and skill for these attendant responsibilities cannot be achieved without systematic training. The caregiver, like the attendant, must be trained, and the training must be performed and monitored for a significant period of time. Caregivers do not have the same observational skills that trained occupational therapists possess.

Case Study 4. Mr. A.

Mr. A. was a plumber. When he could no longer work, he continued to follow his routine of rising, taking his plumbing tool belt to the kitchen, eating breakfast, and putting on his belt. He then spent the day fixing pipes around the house. His wife did not mind the occasional water on the floor because his "work" allowed her to do her "work."

This had been the routine for nearly 18 months when one day Mrs. A. came home to find that Mr. A. had unhooked the kitchen stove. She immediately took his tools away from him, which resulted in an instant change in his behavior. He was hostile, began wandering, became argumentative, and was sleeping during the day and staying awake most of the night.

Mrs. A. was very upset by this. Not only did she see her husband in distress, but her life had been totally altered. Mrs. A. told her occupational therapist of her worries and it was suggested that she have her sons and neighbors build a plumbing work station for Mr. A. in the back of the garage. They did. This enabled Mr. and Mrs. A. to reestablish their "work" routine, which has continued on a satisfactory basis ever since.

Avoiding Excess Disability and Neglect

Many people with a disability do not require acute medical intervention and, therefore, neither they nor their families have access to rehabilitative services that could help them learn to manage the problems associated with their impairment. As a result, the person with disabilities is a prime target for a condition called excess disability.

Excess disability, as defined by Kahn (1965), exists when a person's dysfunction is greater than it should be considering the degree of his or her impairment. Brody, Morton, Lawton, and Moss (1974) first reported that subjects who received individualized care improved in their ability to participate in activities. This improvement was facilitated by designing an enriched environment (both in terms of facilities and staff interaction) for persons in a long-term-care institution. The goal of an intervention designed to minimize excess disabilities would be the same as a goal to avoid unnecessary disabling conditions.

Occupational therapists provide services and must train families to care for persons with chronic disabling conditions. If the caregiver is not trained in the skills necessary to identify and manage a person with a disability, the impaired person will not function at his or her potential. Though improvement in the disease is not possible, a higher level of function may allow the caregiver to manage the person without experiencing unnecessary burden.

To implement a model where the caregiver is included in designing the care, it is necessary to understand the caregiver's commitment to the role of caregiving. Hasselkus (1989) identified three goals of the caregiving activity: getting things done, achieving a sense of health and well-being for the care receiver, and achieving a sense of health and well-being for the caregiver.

Clinicians should fit into the family's caretaking system even if it is cumbersome. "Both the clinician and the family caregiver (a) bring knowledge and experience to the situation, (b) produce data to identify options, and (c) bring their own code of ethics to the course of action. If the therapist and caregiver can collaborate on the process tension can be minimized and shared responsibility and shared ethical decision making can result" (Hasselkus, 1989, p. 653).

For a caregiver to maintain health, he or she must balance the caregiver duties with other activities. Persuading people to balance their daily activities is difficult; however, by discovering a caregiver's understanding of a balance and helping him or her to accept assistance, there may be more time for the person to pursue personally satisfying activities. With this approach, a partnership may evolve between the caregiver and the clinician where expertise, values, and interests are shared.

Traditionally, medically based professionals provide treatment. Most health insurance plans stress a treatment goal and deny payment for patient and caregiver education. When clinicians incorporate educational goals into treatment, it has often been necessary to deemphasize education and training in order to obtain reimbursement. Vitaliano, Russo, Breen, Vitiello, & Prinz (1986) suggest that providing information about the patient's function could "do much to modify the stress that arises from the uncertainties [of a condition] and allow family members to better anticipate problems before they fully develop" (p. 45).

Future Policy Considerations: Options to Allow Caregivers Access to OT Services

Davies (1987) suggests that it is important to target the services, screen for eligibility, assess the user's circumstances, plan the care to take advantage of the resources available within the patient's environment, and monitor the services. To establish such a system, the government will need to address this problem in a coordinated manner and provide payment options for families who require assistance to manage the impaired person in the community.

The following alternatives suggest how services to support families could be financed. Some of these recommendations require policy considerations by the government and/or the employer.

1. Some families could purchase the services from their own resources.

2. Employers, in an effort to attract and retain qualified employees, could offer a range of services and educational programs. This benefit, coupled with payment for daycare and respite service, should attract and retain qualified employees. By offering these services, companies could expand their daycare benefits across groups of employees to include adults managing their parents, in addition to

working parents with children. Some major corporations are currently exploring such programs. Travelers Insurance, Con Edison, Mobil, and Ciba-Geigy have implemented educational programs and are developing strategies for sharing the costs of respite care and work-sponsored adult daycare (Select Committee on Aging, 1987). Flexible-time could also offer an important alternative for families who would like to provide the care themselves. This is an impressive start, but to help those in need of assistance, more will need to be done to ensure that employees have access to information and services, and employers have productive workers.

3. Medicare could expand its coverage to allow 6 to 8 weeks of in-home support and training of caregivers and families of older adults as a preventive health measure. By financing an in-home training program under specifically defined criteria, the family would benefit from having the skills to manage the problem. This approach could be coupled with family leave policies so working caregivers could receive the benefit. Now that the Family Leave Act has been enacted, many families would be able to take time away from work to learn new skills to provide care. This option would require changing the Medicare law.

4. Medicaid could be expanded to cover a program for the poor as an alternative to institutional placement, for families who want to maintain the impaired person in the community. This approach would take advantage of a less expensive model of care, as well as tap the resources of the family in providing informal care. Studies would need to be conducted, perhaps under a waiver program, to demonstrate the cost–benefit ratio of such an approach. This would require changes in the current regulations.

5. An additional method of support for the working caregiver is the Dependent Care Assistance Plan. This employee benefit plan is allowed under the Internal Revenue Service. It excludes the value of employer-provided dependent care from an employee's gross income. The cost of the care is a deductible business expense for the employer. In 1986 an estimated 1,000 employers offered such a plan for child care, but none reported using it for elder care. The major reason it was not used for the elderly was that for tax purposes the elder must be a dependent of the employee and qualify by having very limited income. This plan could offer assistance to some; however, the regulations must be modified to address the issue of dependence before it will benefit most people who need it (Select Committee on Aging, 1987).

Implications for Policy

In the United States, the family, the marketplace, and, to some extent, the church, have traditionally been responsible for meeting the needs of the individual. Society has resisted expanding the scope of programs beyond minimal efforts (Wilensky & Lebeaux, 1965). The United States has continued to build an institutionally based medical care system that leaves the elder and the family vulnerable to the consequences of chronic conditions in old age (Select Committee on Aging, 1987).

Amenta and Skocpol (1989) point out that the U.S. has an incomplete system of social insurance because it takes too narrow a view of public policy. They suggest that public policies are characterized by (a) an emphasis on spending programs with divisible, rather than collective, benefits; and short-lived benefits rather than permanent ones; (b) a system of taxation that is overburdened with distributive and economic goals; (c) the reliance on nationalistic macroeconomic policies, avoiding both classical market liberalism and selective economic interventions; (d) extensive, but ambiguous, public employment; and (e) selective social spending policy, with certain groups, such as veterans, the aged, and widows considered deserving, and those considered undeserving subject to surveillance. This approach has made it very difficult to apply public solutions to social problems. However, the scope of the problems associated with managing disabled persons may bring many of these policies into focus.

Caring for a family member with a disability strikes at all of our domestic policies: housing, taxation, employment, health, and social welfare. A fragmented selective policy approach will not build a system that will support families. Industry, normally indifferent to the family issues of its workers, may be forced to address these issues. Because of tight labor markets in the years ahead, employers will need to build incentives to support working caregivers. Seventy-five percent of new jobs will be in service-product industries. These jobs are traditionally held by women, and flexibility and resources will be required to help the employees manage aging parents (Bloom, 1986) in order to attract and retain them in the work force. Innovative personnel practices will relieve financial and complex logistic burdens on children who are caregivers to their elderly parents.

Caring for disabled persons affects both the family and the productivity of workers who must be absent from their jobs to manage the problems associated with providing the care. These issues need to be addressed because family caregiving is no longer solely a woman's issue. Men also provide informal services to parents, and are now suffering the consequences of the restrictions on their time and increased family responsibilities.

Somers (1982) suggests that our problems result from trying to fit the new needs of our elderly into outmoded policy. She states:

> What is needed is a new policy that takes changes in both health needs and family structure into account, acknowledges that the quality of life is at least as important as the quantity, and recognizes that costs can be contained only through appropriate controls applied consistently and fairly to both long-term and acute care. (p. 223)

Somers indicates that a reorientation cannot be achieved quickly, but that there is a growing consensus that there should be a shift to (a) focus on functional independence, (b) emphasize prevention, (c) build mechanisms to help families cope, (d) focus on community and home care rather than on acute care, and (e) include persons other than physicians in the delivery of care. Since 1983 we have begun to see these changes.

Advocacy for the development of a needed system for personal assistance is growing. Delegates to the World Congress on Disability, held in Oakland, California, in 1991, drafted a resolution (see Figure 5) on personal assistance services, which includes a statement of principles. This document provides insight into the need for services and standards for personal assistance.

Polices are needed so persons with disabilities and their families can be assured of access to the services that will provide them with the skills to enable a more independent and self-reliant life-style. In the meantime, it is important for occupational therapists to view families as integral parts of intervention.

Figure 5. Resolution on personal assistance services.

Passed by participants of the International Personal Assistance Services Symposium, sponsored by the World Institute on Disability, Convened September 29 to October 1, 1991, in Oakland, California.

RESOLUTION

WE, THE PEOPLE WITH DISABILITIES AND OUR ALLIES, have come together from across the United States and around the world from September 29–October 1, 1991, in Oakland, California at the symposium entitled EMPOWERMENT STRATEGIES FOR THE DEVELOPMENT OF A PERSONAL ASSISTANCE SERVICES SYSTEM.

This conference has focused on personal assistance services as an essential factor in independent living, which itself encompasses the whole area of human activities, including but not limited to housing, transportation, community access, education, employment, economic security, family life and interpersonal relationships of choice, leisure, and political influence.

Recognizing our unique expertise derived from our experience, we're taking the initiative in the development of policies that directly affect all people with disabilities.

People with disabilities are entitled to be enabled to achieve the highest possible level of personal functioning and independence through appropriate education, health care, social services and assistive technology, including, as necessary, the assistance of other people.

We firmly uphold our basic human and civil rights to full and equal participation in society as called for in the Americans With Disabilities Act and the United Nations Universal Declaration of Human Rights. We consider independent living and the availability of support services to be critical to the exercise of our full human and civil rights, responsibilities and privileges.

To this end, we condemn forced segregation and institutionalization as direct violations of our human rights. Government policies and funding should not perpetuate the forced segregation, isolation, or institutionalization of people with disabilities of any age. The Americans With Disabilities Act was passed into law to promote the equalization of opportunity. The passage of comprehensive federal personal assistance legislation is essential to realizing the historic promise of the Act.

The recommendations of the United Nations World Programme of Action (s 115) specifically state that "Member states should encourage the provision of support services to enable disabled people to live as independently as possible in the community and in so doing should ensure that persons with a disability have the opportunity to develop and manage these services for themselves."

In support of the international movement of disabled people and in Disabled Peoples' International, which has a special commitment to setting up a network of initiatives for personal assistance services as part of the implementation of the equalization of opportunities, we call on governments and policy makers to assure greater and more equitable access to personal assistance services based on the following principles:

PRINCIPLES:

1. Personal assistance services are a human and civil right. These services shall serve people of all ages, from infancy throughout a person's lifetime, when the person's functional limitation(s) shall necessitate the services. This right is irrespective of disability, personal health, income, marital and family status, and without discrimination on the basis of race, national origin, cultural background, religion, gender, sexual preference, or geography.

2. All people with disabilities (and their self-designated or legal representative if applicable) shall be informed about their rights and options related to personal assistance services in

---

(continued)

Figure 5. (continued)

accessible formats and appropriate languages. All levels of personal assistance services should respect the privacy and confidentiality of the user.

3. Personal assistance users shall be able to choose from a variety of personal assistance services models which together offer the choice of various degrees of user control. User control, in our view, can be exercised by all people regardless of their ability to give legally informed consent or their need for support in decision making or communication.

4. Services shall enable the users to exercise their rights and to participate in every aspect of sociocultural life including, but not limited to, home, school, work, cultural and spiritual activities, leisure, travel, and political life. These services shall enable disabled people, without penalty, if they so choose, to establish a personal, family and community life and fulfill all the responsibilities associated with those aspects of life.

5. No individual shall be forced into or kept in an institutionalized setting because of lack of resources, high costs, sub-standard or non-existent services or the refusal and/or denial of any or all services.

6. These services must be available for up to seven days a week for as many hours as needed during the 24-hour period of the day, on long-term, short-term and emergency bases. These services shall include, but are not limited to, assistance with personal body functions, communicative, household, mobility, work, emotional, cognitive, personal, and financial affairs, community participation, parenting, leisure, and other related needs. The user's point of view must be paramount in the design and delivery of services. Users must be able to choose or refuse services.

7. Government funding shall be an individual entitlement independent of marital status and shall not be a disincentive to employment.

8. Government funding must include competitive wages (based on consumer cost experience within the private sector) and employment benefits for assistants and related administrative and management expenses.

9. Payments to the user shall not be treated as disposable, taxable income and shall not make the user ineligible for other statutory benefits or services.

10. Sufficient governmental funding shall be made available to ensure adequate support, outreach, recruitment, counseling, and training for the user and the assistant. Government efforts shall ensure that a pool of qualified, competent assistance shall be available for users to access through a variety of personal assistance services models, including, but not limited to, individual providers and full services agencies.

11. The user should be free to select and/or hire as personal assistants whomever s/he chooses, including family members.

12. Children needing personal assistance services shall be offered such services as part of their right to inclusive education as well. Such education and personal assistance services shall include age appropriate opportunities to learn to use and control personal assistance services effectively.

13. There shall be a uniform appeals procedure which is independent of funders, providers, and assessors that is effected in an expeditious manner and allows the applicant/user to receive advocacy services and legal counsel at the expense of the statutory authority.

14. In furtherance of all the above, users must be formally and decisively involved and represented at all levels of policy making through ongoing communication and outreach in planning, implementation, design, and development of personal assistance services.

Appendix. Resources.

AIDS

American Red Cross
18th and E Streets, N.W.
Washington, DC 20006

Gay Men's Health Crisis
Box 274, 132 West 24th Street
New York, NY 10011
212-807-7035

Alcoholism

Alcoholics Anonymous
P.O. Box 459, Grand Central Station
New York, NY 10163
212-686-1100

Al-Anon Family Group Headquarters, Inc.
P.O. Box 182, Madison Square Station
New York, NY 10159-0182
212-683-1771

National Clearinghouse for Alcohol Information
P.O. Box 2345
Rockville, MD 20852
301-468-2600

Alzheimer's Disease

Alzheimer's Disease and Related Disorders
  Association, Inc.
70 East Lake Street
Chicago, IL 60601
312-853-3060

Amputation

National Amputation Foundation, Inc.
12-45 150th Street
Whitestone, NY 11357-1790
212-767-0596

Amyotrophic Lateral Sclerosis

The ALS Association
15300 Ventura Boulevard
Sherman Oaks, CA 91403
213-990-2151

Arthritis

Arthritis Foundation
1314 Spring Street, N.W.
Atlanta, GA 30309
404-872-7100

Autism

National Society for Children and Adults With
  Autism
1234 Massachusetts Avenue, N.W.
Washington, DC 20005
202-783-0125

Birth Defects

March of Dimes Birth Defects Foundation
1275 Mamaroneck Avenue
White Plains, NY 10605
914-428-7100

Blindness

American Foundation for the Blind
15 West 16th Street
New York NY 10011
212-620-2000

National Federation for the Blind
1800 Johnson Street
Baltimore, MD 21230
301-659-9314

Helen Keller National Center for the Deaf-Blind
  Youth and Adults
111 Middle Neck Road
Sands Point, NY 11050
516-944-8900

Burn Injuries

Phoenix Society, Inc.
National Organization for Burn Victims
  and Their Families
11 Rust Hill Road
Levittown, PA 19056
215-946-4788

Cancer

American Cancer Society
90 Park Avenue
New York, NY 10016
212-599-8200

Cerebral Palsy

United Cerebral Palsy Association, Inc.
66 East 34th Street
New York, NY 10016
212-481-6300

National Easter Seal Society
2023 West Ogden Avenue
Chicago, IL 60612
312-243-8400
TDD: 312-243-8000

Deafness

National Information Center on Deafness
Gallaudet College
900 Florida Avenue, N.E.
Washington, DC 20002
202-651-5109
TDD: 202-651-5976

Diabetes

National Diabetes Information Clearinghouse
Box NDIC
Bethesda, MD 20892
301-468-2162

Epilepsy

Epilepsy Foundation of America
4351 Garden City Drive
Landover, MD 20785
301-459-3700

Guillain-Barré Syndrome

Guillain-Barré Syndrome National Foundation
1538 Acacia Road
Akron, OH 44313
216-666-3053

Head Injury

National Head Injury Foundation
P.O. Box 567
Framingham, MA 01701

Heart Disease

American Heart Association
7320 Greenville Avenue
Dallas, TX 75231
214-750-5300

Huntington's Disease

National Huntington's Disease Association, Inc.
1182 Broadway
New York, NY 10001
211-684-2781

Learning Disabilities

Foundation for Children With Learning
 Disabilities
99 Park Avenue
New York, NY 10016

Mental Illness

National Alliance for the Mentally Ill
1901 North Fort Meyer Drive
Arlington, VA 22209-1604
703-524-7600

Mental Retardation

Association for Retarded Citizens of the United
 States
P.O. Box 6109
2501 Avenue J
Arlington, TX 76006
817-640-0204

Special Olympics
1350 New York Avenue, N.W.
Washington, DC 20005
202-628-3630

Multiple Sclerosis

National Multiple Sclerosis Society
205 East 42nd Street
New York, NY 10017
212-986-3240

Muscular Dystrophy

Muscular Dystropy Association
810 7th Avenue
New York, NY 10019
212-586-0808

Parkinson's Disease

American Parkinson Disease Foundation
116 John Street
New York, NY 10038
212-732-9550

Spinal Cord Injury

National Spinal Cord Injury Association
149 California Street
Newton, MA 02158
617-964-0521

Paralyzed Veterans of America
801 18th Street, N.W.
Washington, DC 20006
202-872-1300

Stroke

National Stroke Association
1420 Odgen Street
Denver, CO 80219
303-839-1992

Stroke Clubs International
805 12th Street
Galveston, TX 77550
409-762-1022

North American Riding for the Handicapped
  Association, Inc.
P.O. Box 100, R.I.B. 218
Ashburn, VA 22011
703-471-1621

From *Occupational Therapy: Overcoming Human Performance Deficits* (pp. 837–842) by C. Christiansen & C. Baum (Eds.), 1991, Thorofare, NJ: Slack. Copyright © 1992 by Slack. Reprinted by permission.

**Organizations Providing Resource
  Information**

Clearinghouse on the Handicapped
U.S. Department of Education
Switzer Building, Room 3132
Washington, DC 20202-2319
202-732-1241

HEALTH Resource Center (Higher Education
  and the Handicapped)
One DuPont Circle
Washington, DC 20036

National Handicapped Sports and Recreation
  Association
P.O. Box 33141, Farragut Station
Washington, DC 20033
202-783-1441

National Library Service for the Blind and
  Physically Handicapped
The Library of Congress
Washington, DC 20542
202-287-5100

National Organization on Disability
2100 Pennsylvania Avenue, N.W.
Washington, DC 20037
202-293-5960

National Rehabilitation Information Center
Catholic University of America
4407 Eighth Street, N.E.
Washington, DC 20017
202-635-5826 (telephone or TDD)
800-346-2742

References

Amenta, E., & Skocpol, T. (1989). Taking exception: Explaining the distinctiveness of American public policies in the last century. In F.G. Castles (Ed.), *The comparative history of public policy* (pp. 292–333). New York: Oxford University Press.

Bandura, A. (1977). Self-efficacy: Toward a unifying theory of behavioral change. *Psychological Review, 84*, 191–215.

Bandura, A. (1982). Self-efficacy mechanism in human agency. *American Psychologist, 37*, 122–147.

Barber, P.A., Turnbull, A.P., Behr, S.K., & Kerns, G.M. (1989). A family systems perspective on early childhood special education. In S.L. Odom & M.B. Karnes (Eds.), *Early intervention for infants and children with handicaps: An empirical base* (pp. 179-197). Baltimore: Paul H. Brookes.

Birkel, R.C., & Jones, C.J. (1989). A comparison of the caregiving networks of dependent elderly individuals who are lucid and those who are demented. *Gerontologist, 29*, 114–119.

Bloom, D.E. (1986). Women and work. *American Demographics, 8*, 25–30.

Bradley, B.M., & Caldwell, R.H. (1984). *Home observation for measurement of the environment.* Seattle: University of Washington, School of Nursing.

Branch, L.G., & Jette, A.M. (1983). Elders' use of informal long-term care assistance. *Gerontologist, 23*, 51–56.

Brody, E.M. (1981). Women in the middle and family help to older people. *Gerontologist, 21*, 471–480.

Brody, E.M. (1990). The family at risk. In E. Light & B.D. Lebowitz (Eds.), *Alzheimer's disease treatment and family stress: Directions for research* (pp. 2–49). New York: Hemisphere.

Brody, E.M., Morton, H.K., Lawton, M.P., & Moss, M. (1974). A longitudinal look at excess disabilities in the mentally impaired aged. *Journal of Gerontology, 29*(1), 79–84.

Brown, G.W. (1979). A three-factor causal model of depression. In J.E. Barrett (Ed.), *Stress and mental disorder* (pp. 111–129). New York: Raven Press.

Burns, T., & Buell, J. (1990). The effectiveness of work programming with an Alzheimer population. *Occupational Therapy Practice, 1*(2), 64–73.

Cantor, M.H. (1983). Strain among caregivers: A study of experience in the United States. *Gerontologist, 23*, 597–604.

Caplan, G. (1974). *Support systems.* New York: Basic Books.

Caserta, M.S., Lund, D.A. , Wright, S.D., & Redburn, D.E. (1987). Caregivers to dementia patients: The utilization of community services. *Gerontologist, 27*, 209–214.

Cassel, J. (1974). Psychosocial processes and stress: Theoretical formulations. *International Journal of Health Service, 4*, 471–482.

Chiverton, P., & Caine, E.D. (1989). Education to assist spouses in coping with Alzheimer's disease: A controlled trial. *Journal of the American Geriatrics Society, 37*, 593–598.

Cicirelli, V.G. (1983). A comparison of helping behavior to elderly parents of adult children with intact and disrupted marriages. *Gerontologist, 23*, 619–625.

Clark, N.M., & Rakowski, W. (1983). Family caregivers of older adults: Improving helping skills. *Gerontologist, 23*, 627–642.

Clipp, E.C., & George, L.K. (1990). Caregiver needs and patterns of social support. *Journal of Gerontology, 45*(3), 102–111.

Cohen, D., Kennedy, G., & Eisforder, C. (1984). Phase of change in the patient with Alzheimer's dementia: A conceptual dimension for defining health care management. *Journal of the American Geriatrics Society, 32*, 11–15.

Cohen, S., & Wills, T.A. (1985). Stress, social support and the buffering hypothesis. *Psychological Bulletin, 98*, 310–357.

Crewe, N.M., & Zola, I.K. (1983). *Independent living for physically disabled people.* San Francisco: Jossey-Bass.

Davies, B. (1987). Equity and efficiency in community care: Supply and financing in an age of fiscal austerity. *Aging and Society, 7*, 161–174.

Dean, A., & Lin, N. (1977). The stress-buffering role of social support. *Journal of Nervous and Mental Disorders, 165*, 403–413.

DeJong, G., & Wenker, T. (1983). Attendant care. In N.M Crewe & I.K. Zola (Eds.), *Independent living for physically disabled people* (pp. 157–170). San Francisco: Jossey-Bass.

Goldstein, R., & Tye, S. (1987). Social work management of the Alzheimer's patient: Who needs the support? *The Mount Sinai Journal of Medicine, 51*(1), 86–92.

Grad, J., & Sainsbury, P. (1963). Mental illness and the family. *Lancet, 1*, 544–557.

Haley, W.E. (1983). A family-behavioral approach to the treatment of the cognitively impaired elderly. *Gerontologist, 23*, 18–20.

Haley, W.E., Levine, E.G., Brown, S.L., Berry, J.M., & Hughes, G.H. (1987). Psychological, social and health consequences of caring for a relative with senile dementia. *Journal of the American Geriatrics Society, 35*, 405–411.

Hasselkus, B.R. (1989). The meaning of daily activity in family caregiving for the elderly. *American Journal of Occupational Therapy, 43*, 649–656.

Hoenig, J., & Hamilton, M.W. (1966). Elderly psychiatric patients and the burden on the household. *Psychiatric Neurology, 154*, 281–293.

Horowitz, A. (1985). Sons and daughters as caregivers to older parents: Differences in role performance and consequences. *Gerontologist, 25*, 612–617.

Hutchins, T.K., Thornock, M., Lindgre, B., & Parks, J. (1978). Profile in in-home attendant care workers. *American Rehabilitation, 4*(2), 18–22.

Johnson, C.L., & Catalano, D.J. (1981). Childless elderly and their family supports. *Gerontologist, 21*, 610–618.

Kahan, J., Kemp, B., Staples, F.R., & Brummel-Smith, K. (1985). Decreasing the burden in families caring for a relative with a dementing illness. A controlled study. *Journal of the American Geriatrics Society, 33*, 664–670.

Kahn, R.L. (1965). The mental health system and the future aged. *Gerontologist, 15*, 24–31.

Kessler, R.C., & McLeod, J. (1985). Social support and psychological distress in community surveys. In S. Cohen & L. Syme (Eds.), *Social support and health* (pp. 219–240). New York: Academic Press.

Kielhofner, G., & Burke, J., (1980). A model of human occupation, part 1: Conceptual framework and content. *American Journal of Occupational Therapy, 34*, 572–581.

Kinney, J.M., & Stephens, M.A. (1989). Hassles and uplifts of giving care to a family member with dementia. *Psychology of Aging, 4*, 402–408.

Kosberg, J.I., & Cairl, R.E. (1986). The cost of care index: A case management tool for screening informal caregivers. *Gerontologist, 26*, 273–278.

Kosberg, J.I., & Cairl, R.E. (1990). Components of burden: Interventive implications. *Gerontologist, 30*, 236–242.

Kosberg, J.I., & Cairl, R.E. (1991). Burden and competence in caregivers of Alzheimer's disease patients: Research and practice implications. *Journal of Gerontological Social Work, 18*(1–2), 85–96.

Laurie, G. (1977). *Housing and home services for the disabled.* New York: Harper & Row.

Lawton, M.P., Brody, E.M., & Saperstein, A.R. (1989). A controlled study of respite service for caregivers of Alzheimer's patients. *Gerontologist, 29*, 8–16.

Lawton, M.P., Kleban, M.H., Moss, M., Rovine, M., & Glicksman, A. (1989). Measuring caregiving appraisal. *Journal of Gerontology, 44*(3), 61–71.

McCubbin, H., & Patterson, J.M. (1983). The family stress process: The double ABCX Model of adjustment and adaptation. *Marriage and Family Review, 6*, 7–37.

Miller, B., & Cafasso, L. (1992). Gender differences in caregiving. Fact or artifact? *Gerontologist, 32*, 498–507.

Opie, N.D., & Miller, E.L. (1989). Personal care attendants and severely disabled adults: Attributions for relationship outcomes. *Archives of Psychiatric Nursing, 3*, 205–210.

Pruchno, R.A. (1990). Alzheimer's disease and families: Methodological advances. In E. Light & B.D. Lebowitz (Eds.), *Alzheimer's disease treatment and family stress: Directions for research* (pp. 174–197). New York: Hemisphere.

Quayhagen, M.P., & Quayhagen, M. (1988). Alzheimer's stress: Coping with the caregiving role. *Gerontologist, 28*, 391–396.

Rabins, P., Mace, H.L., & Lucas, M.J. (1982). The impact of dementia on the family. *Journal of the American Medical Association, 248*, 333–335.

Schaaf, R.C., & Mulrooney, L.L. (1989). Occupational therapy in early intervention: A family centered approach. *American Journal of Occupational Therapy, 43*, 745–754.

Schaefer, C., Coyne, J.C., & Lazarus, R.S. (1981). *Journal of Behavioral Medicine, 4*, 381–426.

Select Committee on Aging (House of Representatives). (1987). *Exploding the myths: Caregiving in America* (Committee Publication No. 96-611). Washington, DC: U.S. Government Printing Office.

Seltzer, M.M., Irvy, J., & Litchfield, L.C. (1987). Family members as case managers: Partnership between the formal and informal support networks. *Gerontologist, 27*, 722–728.

Somers, A. (1982). Long-term care for the elderly: A new health priority. *New England Journal of Medicine, 307*, 221–225.

Spainer, G.B., & Hanson, S. (1982). The role of extended kin in the adjustment to marital separation. *Journal of Divorce, 5*, 33–48.

Stevens-Long, J. (1979). *Adult life: Developmental process.* Palo Alto, CA: Mayfield.

Stone, R., Cafferata, G.L., & Sange, J. (1987). Caregivers of the frail elderly: A national profile. *Gerontologist, 27*, 616–626.

Thoits, P.A. (1986). Social support as coping assistance. *Journal of Consulting and Clinical Psychology, 54*, 416–423.

Treas, J. (1979). Intergenerational families and social change. In P. Ragan (Ed.), *Aging parents* (pp. 58–65). Los Angeles: The University of Southern California Press.

Troll, L.E., Miller, S.J., & Atchley, R.C. (1979). *Families in late life.* Bellmont, CA: Wadsworth.

Ulicny, G., & Jones, M.L. (1985). Enhancing the attendant management skills of persons with disabilities. *American Rehabilitation, 2*(2), 18–20.

Vitaliano, P.P., Russo, J., Breen, A.R., Vitiello, M.V., & Prinz, P.N. (1986). Functional decline in the early stages of Alzheimer's disease. *Psychology of Aging, 1*(1), 41–46.

Wikler, L., Wasow, M., & Hatfield, E. (1983). Seeking strengths in families of developmentally disabled children. *Social Work, 28,* 313–315.

Wilensky, H., & Lebeaux, C. (1965). *Industrial society and social welfare.* New York: Free Press.

Index

A

Abledata, 383
  categories of self-care products, 416–418
Above elbow amputation
  bilateral, 296–299
  unilateral, 287–291
Access, 426
Activities of daily living, 4
  AOTA recommended terminology, 5
  burn, 319–320
  domains, 4
  scales, 67–69
  self-care, 4–6
Adaptation, symptom, 31
Adaptive device. *See also* Assistive device
  self-care, 17–19
    consumer rating factors, 19, 20
Adaptive equipment
  motor disorder, 260–273
  self-feeding, 124–125
Adaptive system, self-care, 17–19
  consumer rating factors, 19, 20
Aging, stroke, 232
Ankylosing spondylitis, 166
Architectural barrier, 33–34
Architecture, 389
Arthritis
  American College of Rheumatology Functional Classification, 170
  defined, 161
  disease variability, 170

endurance, 169–170
equipment, 170–174
fatigue, 169–170
joint protection techniques, 170
medication, 168–169
self-care, 161–185
self-care assessment, 168
Assisted mobility, 145–152
  children requiring, 145
Assistive device
  bathing, 180–181, 182
  communication, 388
  dressing, 179–180, 181
  eating, 184
  elbow, 174, 177
  grooming, 180, 182
  hand, 174, 175–176
  hip, 178–179, 180
  housekeeping, 181, 183
  knee, 176–178, 179
  meal preparation, 183, 184, 185
  neck, 174–176, 178
  rheumatic disease, 170–184
  shoulder, 174, 177
  spinal cord injury, 221–223
  toileting, 181, 183
Assistive technology
  adaption, 411–412
  assessment, 395–396
  comparison checklist, 402

compliance, 409–410

consumer empowerment, 406–408

equipment supplier, 410–411

evaluating information, 399–400

experts, 412

fabrication, 411–412

finding information, 397–399

follow-up, 405

funding, 405–406

future trends, 414–415

independence vs. efficiency, 408–409

long-term care, 412–413

occupational therapy vendor, 410

open market purchase, 409

open market suppliers, 411

option identification, 396–397

overview, 384–390

owner's manual, 404–405

poverty, 413

prescription, 409

preservice student training, 413

purchase, 411–412

selection, 394–406

teaming with other professionals, 413–414

training, 403–404

trial use, 403

vendor roles, 410–411

Ataxia, defined, 258

Athetosis, defined, 258

Attendant, 20–21, 453–475

factors, 460

formal support, 459–463

types, 461–463

future policy, 471–473

occupational therapy framework, 463

reasons for providing care, 456–457

selection, 466–469

strategies, 469–471

supervision, 466–469

training, 466–469

who provides care, 456–457

Augmentative communication, 138–145

classroom, 144–145

direct selection, 140–141

encoding, 141–142

home, 144–145

indications for, 138–139

mounting, 142

positioning, 142–143

scanning mode, 141

selection, 139–142

skills enhancement, 143–144

B

Banking, 441

Barthel Index, 63

Bathing, 134–138, 200–201, 210, 211, 219

assistive device, 180–181, 182

defined, 5

issues, 134–135

motor delay, 135–137

infant, 135–137

skill development, 134, 135

tactile defensiveness, 136

Bathroom fixture, 430–431

Beauty

cultural stereotypes, 43–45

grooming, 43–45

Behavior problem, feeding, 121–122

Below elbow amputation, 284–287, 294–296

Bipolar disorder, self-care, 364

Bladder care, 204–205, 217, 220

Body function
    class, 29–31
    culture, 29–31
    ethnicity, 29–31
Bowel care, 204–205, 217, 220
Bradykinesia, defined, 258
Brain injury, definition, 344
Burn
    activities of daily living, 319–320
    acute care phase, 314–316
    acute care phase assessment, 312–313
    acute rehabilitation, 326–327
    case examples, 325–330
    depth, 308–309
    facial scar, 324
    home program content, 320
    injury severity, 310
    inpatient phase assessment, 313–314
    inpatient rehabilitation, 326–327
    mechanism of injury, 309
    morbidity, 307
    occupational therapy, 311–312
    outpatient phase, 320–324
    outpatient phase assessment, 313–314
    outpatient rehabilitation, 327–328, 329–330
    percent total body surface area involved, 309–310
    positioning, 315
    reconstruction, 324–325
    recovery phases, 308
    rehabilitation phase, 316–320, 326–327
    scar formation, 310–311
    self-care, 305–330
    survival, 307
    wound care, 310
    wound characteristics, 309
Button aid, 386

C

Caregiver, 453–475. *See also* Attendant
    factors, 460
    formal support, 459–463
        types, 461–463
    future policy, 471–473
    occupational therapy framework, 463
    reasons for providing care, 456–457
    strategies, 469–471
    who provides care, 456–457
Cerebrovascular accident. *See* Stroke
Cervical spinal cord, functional levels, 194–195
Child
    developmental deficit, 101–153
        family variables, 106–108
        parent-child interaction, 108
        variables, 106
    self-care, 101–153
        development, 105–106
Chorea, defined, 258
Chronicity, symptom, 31
Class
    body function, 29–31
    body part, 29–31
    symptom, 29–31
Client-centered assessment, 54–59
Cognition, factors affecting, 337
Cognitive deficit, self-care, 333–353
Cognitive functioning scale, 347
Communication, 203–204, 215–217, 220
    assistive device, 388
    movement disorder, 267–269, 270–271
Community transportation, 213
Compensatory training, 16
Compliance, assistive technology, 409–410
Connective tissue disease, self-care, 161–185

Consumer empowerment, assistive technology, 406–408

Cuing program, traumatic brain injury, 348–349

Culture

body function, 29–31

body part, 29–31

symptom, 29–31

D

Decision making, self-care, 10–15, 18

Degenerative joint disease, 161–162, 163

Dementia, 336–343

Dental care, 199, 208

Dependence, self-care, 14–15

Depression, self-care, 364

Developmental deficit

child, 101–153

family variables, 106–108

parent-child interaction, 108

variables, 106

dressing, 125–134

functional mobility, 145–152

self-care, 101–153

Developmental disability, feeding, 110

Deviance disavowal, dressing, 41–43

Dining out, 438–439

Disability

self-identity, 8–9

stigma, 9–10

Discharge planning, stroke, 250–253

Dressing, 41, 202–203, 214–215, 219–220, 441

assistive device, 179–180, 181

defined, 5

developmental deficit, 125–134

developmental sequence, 125, 126

deviance disavowal, 41–43

dyspraxia, 133–134

interventions, 127–134

motor impairment, 127–130

self-expression, 43–45

stigma, 41–43

tactile defensiveness, 130, 133

Driving assessment, stroke, 238–239

Dysfunction, hierarchy, 12–13

Dysphagia, assessment, 238

Dyspraxia, dressing, 133–134

Dystonia, defined, 258

E

Eating, 197–198, 205–206, 218–219

assistive device, 184

defined, 5

public, 438–439

Ecological inventory, 80

Elbow, assistive device, 174, 177

Emergency response, defined, 5

Endurance, arthritis, 169–170

Environmental assessment, 80

Environmental control, 389–390

Environmental control unit, 262

Environmental modification, self-care, 19–20

Equipment supplier, assistive technology, 410–411

Ethnicity

body function, 29–31

body part, 29–31

symptom, 29–31

F

Facial scar, burn, 324

Family, 453–475

assisting in providing care, 457–459

child with developmental deficit, 106–107

division of labor, 34–36

factors, 460

formal support, 459–463

    types, 461–463

future policy, 471–473

instruments for assessing, 464–465

occupational therapy framework, 463

reasons for providing care, 456–457

self-care, 20–21

strategies, 469–471

who provides care, 456–457

Family life cycle, 108–109

Family systems perspective, 459

Fatigue, arthritis, 169–170

Feeding, 37–41, 109–125. *See also* Specific type

    behavior problem, 121–122

    defined, 5

    developmental disability, 110

    family mealtime, 112–113

    food texture progression, 119

    functional problems, 111

    motor delay, 113–116

        facilitation, 114

        handling techniques, 114

        inhibition, 114

        jaw and tongue support, 114, 115

        positioning, 113–114

        sensory aspects of food, 115–116

    nutritional considerations, 110

    parent-child interaction, 112

    as social event, 112

    tactile defensiveness, 116–118

Feeding evaluation kit, 385

Food choice, 38–39

Function, hierarchy, 12–13

Functional Assessment Inventory, 63–66

Functional communication, 138–145

    defined, 5

Functional independence, 426

Functional Independence Measure, 66–67

Functional mobility

    defined, 5

    developmental deficit, 145–152

Functional Status Index, 67

Funding, assistive technology, 405–406

Furnishing, 423–450

G

Graduated guidance, self-care skill teaching, 93

Grooming, 41, 199, 208, 211, 219, 441

    assistive device, 180, 182

    beauty, 43–45

    defined, 5

    deviance disavowal, 41–43

    stigma, 41–43

H

Habilitation, 16

Hand, assistive device, 174, 175–176

Hand amputation

    bilateral partial, 292–294

    unilateral partial, 282–284

Health, defined, 3

Health care, 442

Hip, assistive device, 178–179, 180

Home-care product, 387

Home environment, 428–437

    bathroom fixture, 430–431

    fixtures, 430–437

    furniture, 435–437

    kitchen fixture, 432–434

layout, 428–430

space, 428–430

surfaces, 434–435

Homemaking, movement disorder, 271

Hook, 280–281

Hospital, 36–37

Housekeeping, assistive device, 181, 183

Human agency, self–identity, 8

Hygiene, 199, 208, 211, 441

Hyperkinesia, defined, 258

Hypokinesia, defined, 258

I

Illness, defined, 3

Illness narrative, symptom, 29–32

Independence, self-care, 14–15

Institutional care, 36–37

Instrumental Activities of Daily Living Scale, 69

Instrumental reasoning, 11

Introtalker, 388

J

Juvenile rheumatoid arthritis, 167

K

Katz Index of ADL, 67–68

Kenny Self-Care Evaluation, 68

Kitchen fixture, 432–434

Klein-Bell ADL Scale, 68–69

Knee, assistive device, 176–178, 179

L

Laundry, 442

Learning, 82–83

stages, 82

Least prompts, 92–93

Lumbar spinal cord, functional levels, 196

M

Makeup application, 210, 211

Manual wheelchair, 212–213

Meal, 39–41

Meal preparation, 199, 207, 218–219

assistive device, 183, 184, 185

movement disorder, 264–265, 271–272

Medi-planner, 387

Medication, 198–199, 206–207

arthritis, 168–169

Medication routine, defined, 5

Milwaukee Evaluation of Daily Living Skills, 69

Mobility, 201–202, 211–213, 219, 388

development, 146

movement disorder, 265–267

Mood disorder, 363–364

self-care, 364

Morning stiffness, 169

Motor delay

bathing, 135–137

infant, 135–137

feeding, 113–116

facilitation, 114

handling techniques, 114

inhibition, 114

jaw and tongue support, 114, 115

positioning, 113–114

sensory aspects of food, 115–116

self-bathing, 137–138

adapted equipment, 137

intervention approaches, 137–138

Motor impairment

adaptive equipment, 260–273

dressing, 127–130

self-dressing, 131–133

activities, 131–132

adapted equipment, 133

adapted techniques, 132
appropriate clothing, 132–133
motor analysis, 131, 132
Motorized wheelchair, 213
Movement disorder
adaptive strategies using routines, 269–273
facilitation, 272–273
adaptive strategy choice, 260–273
communication, 267–269, 270–271
homemaking, 271
manifestations, 259
meal preparation, 264–265, 271–272
mobility, 265–267
occupational therapy, 259–260
presenting problems, 259
self-care, 255–273
framework for identifying problems, 257–259
social supports, 269–273
facilitation, 272–273
terminology, 258
Multi-infarct dementia, 336
Myoelectric hand, 280–281

N

Narrative reasoning, 11–12
Neck, assistive device, 174–176, 178
Negotiability, 426
Negotiability rating, 445–446
Non-oral feeding, 118–121
oral feeding transition, 120–121
recommending, 118

O

Observation, self-care assessment, 57–59
Occupational performance, 360
domains, 4

play or leisure occupations, 4
self-maintenance occupations, 4
work and productive occupations, 4
Occupational therapist, self-care environment, 444–450
assessment, 444–445
change decision factors, 448–449
change options, 447–448
negotiability rating, 445–446
recommendations, 446–447
Occupational therapy
consultation for home setting, 455–465
diagnosis, 15
diagnosis formulation, 12–13
family roles, 107
movement disorder, 259–260
process model, 13
Occupational therapy vendor, assistive technology, 410
Older Americans Resource Service (OARS) Multidimensional Functional Assessment Questionnaire, 69
Oral feeding, 109–118
development, 109–110
transition from non-oral, 120–121
Oral hygiene, defined, 5
Orthotics, 388
Osteoarthritis, 161–162, 163
OT FACT assessment system, 395–396
OT FACT self-care assessment, categories, 419–420
Owner's manual, assistive technology, 404–405

P

Paraplegia
T-1 through T-6, 218–220
bathing, 219
bladder care, 220

bowel care, 220
communication, 220
dressing, 219–220
eating, 218–219
grooming, 219
meal preparation, 218–219
mobility, 219
sink hygiene, 219
T-7 through S-5, 220–221
Personal assistive services resolution, 474–475
Personal device care, defined, 5
Personality disorder, 364–365
self-care, 365
Physical Self-Maintenance Scale, 69
Post office, 441–442
Powered wheelchair, 148–149
Preprosthetic therapy program, upper extremity amputation, 279–280
Prompting, self-care skill teaching, 82
Prosthetics, 388
Psoriatic arthritis, 165–166
Psychosocial condition
psychoeducational models, 371–375
self-care assessment, 367–368, 369
self-care management, 368–375
Public toilet, 438
PULSES Profile, 70

Q

Quadriplegia
C-1 through C-4, 197–205
bathing, 200–201
bladder care, 204–205
bowel care, 204–205
case study, 197
communication, 203–204
dental care, 199

dressing, 202–203
eating, 197–198
grooming, 199
hygiene, 199
meal preparation, 199
medication, 198–199
mobility, 201–202
transfer, 201
transportation, 202
wheelchair, 201–202
C-5 through C-6
bathing, 210
dental care, 208
grooming, 208
hair combing, 209
hygiene, 208
makeup application, 210
shaving, 209, 210
washing face and hands, 210
C-5 through C-8, 205–217
bladder care, 217
bowel care, 217
communication, 215–217
community transportation, 213
dressing, 214–215
eating, 205–206
manual wheelchair, 212–213
meal preparation, 207
medication, 206–207
mobility, 211–213
motorized wheelchair, 213
telephone, 215–216
transfer, 211–212
writing, 215
C-7 through C-8
bathing, 211
grooming, 211

hair combing, 211

hair washing, 211

hygiene, 211

makeup application, 211

shaving, 211

washing face and hands, 211

R

Rheumatic disease, 161

   assistive device, 170–184

Rheumatoid arthritis, 162–165

Rigidity, defined, 258

Routine Task Inventory, 70

S

Sacral spinal cord, functional levels, 196

Satisfaction With Performance Scaled Questionnaire, 70

Scaffolding, self-care skill teaching, 82

Schizophrenia, 361–363

   self-care, 362–363

Scooter, 149–150

Scorable Self-Care Evaluation, 71

Seating, 388

Self-bathing, motor delay, 137–138

   adapted equipment, 137

   intervention approaches, 137–138

Self-care

   adaptive device, 17–19

      consumer rating factors, 19, 20

   adaptive system, 17–19

      consumer rating factors, 19, 20

   arthritis, 161–185

   bipolar disorder, 364

   burn, 305–330

   child, 101–153

      development, 105–106

   cognitive deficit, 333–353

connective tissue disease, 161–185

daily living skills, 4–6

decision making, 10–15, 18

dependence, 14–15

depression, 364

developmental deficit, 101–153

environmental modification, 19–20

experiences, 32–46

family, 20–21

goals, 14–15

importance of self, 32–46

independence, 14–15

intervention strategy factors, 10–12

mood disorder, 364

movement disorder, 255–273

   framework for identifying problems, 257–259

personal care attendant, 20–21

personal meaning, 29–46

personality disorder, 365

planning, 15–21

psychosocial conditions, 357–375

public policy, 34–35

schizophrenia, 362–363

social world significance, 6–7

socioanalytic perspective, 7

spinal cord injury, 189–223

stigma, 9–10

strategies, 17–21

   social considerations, 17

stroke, 227–253

   precautions, 231–232

substance abuse, 366–367

training, 17

upper extremity amputation, 277–303

Self-care assessment, 53–72

   client capability, 58

   client centered, 54–59

client priorities, 59

communication, 59–60

data sources, 58

instrument, 60–71

   characteristics, 60–71

   evaluation process, 60

   reliability, 61

   selection, 59

   validity, 61, 62

observation, 57–59

performance components, 55–57

purpose, 53–54

self-report, 57–59

strategy, 59–60

terminology, 53

validation, 59–60

Self-care device, 385–387

commercial, 393

do-it-yourself, 392

worksheet, 400–401

Self-care environment, 423–450. *See also* Specific type

acoustics, 427

fixtures, 427

furnishings, 427

lighting, 427

negotiability vs. access, 426–428

occupational therapist, 444–450

   assessment, 444–445

   change decision factors, 448–449

   change options, 447–448

   negotiability rating, 445–446

   recommendations, 446–447

press, 427

public, 438–441

structural characteristics, 427

surface characteristics, 427

temperature, 427

Self-care skill teaching, 17, 79–99

age appropriateness, 79–80

antecedent

   instructional cues, 90–91

   prompts, 91

artificial prompt, 90

assessment data, 84

chained behavior, 84–85

consequences, 94

   following correct or approximate responses, 94–95

   following errors, 95–96

direct assessment of skills, 83–89

discrete behavior, 84–85

ecological inventory, 80

feedback, 90

function appropriateness, 79–80

graduated guidance, 93

learning evaluation, 96–98

   baseline data, 96

   data usage, 97–98

   probe data, 96

   training data, 96–97

learning stage, 82–83

natural prompt, 90

observational data, 84

planning, 79–83

principles, 79–81

prompting, 82

scaffolding, 82

strategies, 89–96

system of least prompts, 92–93

task analysis, 81, 85–89

task types, 84–89

teaching evaluation, 96–98

   baseline data, 96

   data usage, 97–98

   probe data, 96

training data, 96–97

test data, 84

time delay, 93–94

training data, 84

Self-care technology, 379–415

comparison publications, 393–394

history, 392–394

Self-dressing

intervention approaches, 130–133

motor impairment, 131–133

activities, 131–132

adapted equipment, 133

adapted techniques, 132

appropriate clothing, 132–133

motor analysis, 131, 132

Self-expression

dressing, 43–45

overcoming barriers, 45–46

Self-feeding, 122–125

adaptive equipment, 124–125

development, 122–123

handling techniques, 123–124

intervention approaches, 123–125

positioning, 123, 124

Self-identity, 7–10

disability, 8–9

human agency, 8

role of narrative, 8

Self-maintenance tasks, AOTA recommended terminology, 5

Self-propelled wheelchair, 148

Self-report, self-care assessment, 57–59

Senile dementia of the Alzheimer's type, 336–343

Sexual expression, defined, 5

Shaving, 209, 210, 211

Shopping, 439–441

Shoulder, assistive device, 174, 177

Shoulder disarticulation amputation

bilateral, 299

unilateral, 291–292

Showering, defined, 5

Sick role, 9

Sink hygiene, 219

Social skills

assessment, 21–23

intervention, 21–23

social impression management, 21–23

training, 21

Socialization, defined, 5

Space, 423–450

Spasticity, defined, 258

Special equipment, 33–34

Spinal cord injury

assistive device, 221–223

Frankel grading system, 196

prevalence, 193–194

self-care, 189–223

Stigma

defined, 42

disability, 9–10

dressing, 41–43

grooming, 41–43

self-care, 9–10

Stroke

aging, 232

case descriptions, 233–234

compensation techniques, 239–241

contextual training, 239–241

cultural factors, 236–237

discharge planning, 250–253

driving assessment, 238–239

functional problems associated, 229–230

medical problems associated, 229–230

prognosis, 230–231

psychosocial factors, 236–237

remediation techniques, 247–250

self-care, 227–253

    precautions, 231–232

self-care skills assessment, 234–239

specialized evaluations, 237–239

successful outcome predictors, 232–233

treatment, 239–250

    case descriptions, 241–247

work assessment, 239

Substance abuse, 366–367

    self-care, 366–367

Symptom

    adaptation, 31

    chronicity, 31

    class, 29–31

    culture, 29–31

    defining in occupational terms, 31–32

    ethnicity, 29–31

    illness narrative, 29–32

    meaning, 29–32

Systemic lupus erythematosus, 166–167

Systemic sclerosis, 167

T

Tactile defensiveness

    bathing, 136

    dressing, 130, 133

    feeding, 116–118

Task analysis, self-care skill teaching, 85–89

Telephone, 215–216

Time delay, self-care skill teaching, 93–94

Toileting, 33

    assistive device, 181, 183

    defined, 5

Training, social skills, 21

Transfer, 201, 211–212

Transport chair, 146–148

Transportation, 202, 443–444

Traumatic amputation, 282

Traumatic brain injury, 344–352

    case study, 349–352

    cuing program, 348–349

    definition, 344

    factors affecting cognition, 345

    frames of reference, 345–346

    medical management, 344

    self-care management strategies, 346–352

    severity, 344–345

Traveling, 443–444

Tremor, defined, 258

Tub transfer bench, 385

U

Unified ADL Form, 71

Upper extremity amputation

    below elbow amputation, 284–287, 294–296

    bilateral above elbow amputation, 296–299

    bilateral amputation, 282

    bilateral partial hand amputation, 292–294

    bilateral shoulder disarticulation amputation, 299–302

    bilateral wrist disarticulation, 294–296

    functional issues, 280–303

    hook, 280–281

    myoelectric hand, 280–281

    preprosthetic therapy program, 279–280

    self-care, 277–303

    traumatic amputation, 282

    unilateral above elbow amputation, 287–291

    unilateral amputation, 281–282

unilateral partial hand amputation, 282–284

unilateral shoulder disarticulation amputation, 291–292

unilateral wrist disarticulation, 284–287

V

Values clarification, 449–450

W

Washing face and hands, 210, 211

Wheelchair, 145–152, 201–202, 212–213. *See also* Specific type

    components, 146

    fitting, 151–152

    functional use, 152

    positioning, 151–152

    powered, 148–149

    selection, 146

    self-propelled, 148

    standard powered, 150–151

    variations, 149

Work assessment, stroke, 239

Wrist disarticulation

    bilateral, 294–296

    unilateral, 284–287

Writing, 215